SECOND EDITION

Essentials of Patient
Education

Susan B. Bastable, EdD, RN
Professor Emerita and Founding Chair
Department of Nursing
Le Moyne College

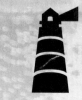

JONES & BARTLETT
LEARNING

World Headquarters
Jones & Bartlett Learning
5 Wall Street
Burlington, MA 01803
978-443-5000
info@jblearning.com
www.jblearning.com

Jones & Bartlett Learning books and products are available through most bookstores and online booksellers. To contact Jones & Bartlett Learning directly, call 800-832-0034, fax 978-443-8000, or visit our website, www.jblearning.com.

Substantial discounts on bulk quantities of Jones & Bartlett Learning publications are available to corporations, professional associations, and other qualified organizations. For details and specific discount information, contact the special sales department at Jones & Bartlett Learning via the above contact information or send an email to specialsales@jblearning.com.

13121-5

Production Credits

VP, Executive Publisher: David D. Cella
Executive Editor: Amanda Martin
Editorial Assistant: Lauren Vaughn
Associate Production Editor: Juna Abrams
Senior Marketing Manager: Jennifer Scherzay
Product Fulfillment Manager: Wendy Kilborn
Composition: S4Carlisle Publishing Services

Cover Design: Kristin E. Parker
Associate Director of Rights & Media: Joanna Lundeen
Rights & Media Specialist: Wes DeShano
Media Development Editor: Troy Liston
Cover Image: © wanchai/Shutterstock
Printing and Binding: Edwards Brothers Malloy
Cover Printing: Edwards Brothers Malloy

Library of Congress Cataloging-in-Publication Data
Names: Bastable, Susan Bacorn, editor.
Title: Essentials of patient education / edited by Susan B. Bastable.
Description: Second edition. | Burlington, Massachusetts : Jones & Bartlett Learning, [2017] | Includes bibliographical references and index.
Identifiers: LCCN 2016002966 | ISBN 9781284104448 (paperback)
Subjects: | MESH: Education, Nursing—methods | Learning | Patient Education as Topic—methods | Teaching
Classification: LCC RT90 | NLM WY 18 | DDC 615.5/071—dc23
LC record available at http://lccn.loc.gov/2016002966

6048

Printed in the United States of America
20 19 18 17 16   10 9 8 7 6 5 4 3 2 1

Dedication

*To nursing students and professional colleagues
who over the years have shared their patient teaching
experiences as well as their knowledge, skills, ideas,
and reflections on the principles of teaching and
learning.*

Contents

PART I   Perspectives on Teaching and Learning   1

1   Overview of Education in Health Care   3

Susan B. Bastable and Kattiria M. Gonzalez

2   Ethical, Legal, and Economic Foundations of the Educational Process   23

M. Janice Nelson and Kattiria M. Gonzalez

7   Literacy in the Adult Patient Population   187
Susan B. Bastable and Gina M. Myers

8   Gender, Socioeconomic, and Cultural Attributes of the Learner   239
Susan B. Bastable and Deborah L. Sopczyk

9   Educating Learners with Disabilities   295
Deborah L. Sopczyk

PART III   Techniques and Strategies for Teaching and Learning   345

10   Behavioral Objectives and Teaching Plans   347
Susan B. Bastable and Eleanor Price McLees

11   Teaching Methods and Settings   379
Kathleen Fitzgerald and Kara Keyes

Preface

This text has been written primarily as a resource for staff nurses in practice, as well as for undergraduate nursing students learning to become the professional nurses of tomorrow, for whom the role of teacher is a significant component of their daily caregiving activities. The content of this text focuses on patients and their family members as the audience of learners and provides nurses with enough depth of information necessary to carry out the essentials of patient teaching.

Teaching patients and their families or significant others has been the responsibility of nurses since the profession began during the era of Florence Nightingale. Since then, the scope of nursing practice has evolved and grown. For many years professional nurses functioning at all levels of education have had the legal, ethical, and moral obligation to teach clients, as mandated by the nurse practice acts in all states and territories, as expected by the national and regional standards of nursing organizations and accrediting bodies, and as required by the policies and procedures of local healthcare institutions and agencies.

This text is a timely resource to address the pressing issues of the growing demand for nurses to deliver the highest quality of care possible, the significant problem of consumer health literacy, the healthcare reform movement with the recent Affordable Care Act legislation, the technological advances making health care even more complex, the changing demographics of the population, the increasing emphasis on health promotion and disease prevention, and the rise in chronic illnesses, to name a few important trends. Not only is it recognized that patient education by nurses can significantly improve client health outcomes, but also today's consumers are expected to independently manage more of their own care.

Nevertheless, most nurses acknowledge that they have not had the formal preparation to successfully and securely carry out their role as patient educators. Every nurse must have the knowledge and skills to competently and confidently teach clients with various needs in a variety of settings. Also, they must be able to do so with efficiency and effectiveness based on a solid mastery of the principles of teaching and learning.

However, nurses are not born with the innate ability to teach or to understand the ways in which people learn. The act of teaching takes special expertise about how to best communicate information and about how that information is most successfully acquired by the learner. Patient teaching is critical to the delivery of quality nursing care, and nurses must capture this domain as an important and unique aspect of the profession's holistic approach to practice.

The content of this text reflects a balance between theories and models associated with teaching and learning and their application to the real world of patient education. This latest edition fully acknowledges the changing role of the professional nurse as well as the consumer of health care with respect to accountability and responsibility for teaching and learning. No longer should the nurse be the giver of information only, but must function as the guide by the side and the facilitator in partnership with the consumer, who must assume a much greater role in learning. This interdependence between the teacher and learner in the process of patient education is emphasized throughout the chapters.

All chapters include updated references, but classic works relevant to the field of education have been retained. Many chapters have been reformatted to enhance and simplify the content, current statistics reflect changes in population trends, and new tables and figures have been added to visually summarize the information presented. In addition, websites are provided throughout the text as sources of further information on particular topics. And, by popular demand, case study scenarios have been added to the end of each chapter for application of teaching and learning principles to nursing practice.

Thus, the focus of this text is on the nurse's role in teaching patients, well or ill, to maintain optimal health and to prevent disease and disability by assisting them to become as independent as possible in self-care activities. It is comprehensive in scope, taking into consideration the basic foundations of the education process, the needs and characteristics of learners, the appropriate techniques and strategies for instruction, and the methods to evaluate the achievement of educational outcomes. In essence, this text addresses answers to questions that pertain to the teaching process—who, what, where, when, how, and why.

Best wishes to all readers who are striving to become adept at delivering patient education based on the principles of how the nurse can best teach and how the consumer can best learn. As nurses, we must never forget our solemn duty to make a positive difference in the lives of those we serve, and patient teaching is a major factor that influences the health and well-being of our clients.

Contributors

Susan B. Bastable, EdD, RN
Professor Emerita and Founding Chair
Department of Nursing
Purcell School of Professional Studies
Le Moyne College
Syracuse, New York

Margaret M. Braungart, PhD
Professor Emerita of Psychology
Center for Bioethics and Humanities
State University of New York
Upstate Medical University
Syracuse, New York

Richard G. Braungart, PhD
Professor Emeritus of Sociology and
International Relations
Maxwell School of Citizenship and
Public Affairs
Syracuse University
Syracuse, New York

Kathleen Fitzgerald, MS, RN, CDE
Patient Educator (retired)
St. Joseph's Hospital Health Center
Syracuse, New York

Kattiria M. Gonzalez, MS, RN
Clinical Coordinator—Instructor
Department of Nursing
Purcell School of Professional Studies
Le Moyne College
Syracuse, New York

Pamela R. Gramet, PhD, PT
Associate Professor and Chair
(retired)
Department of Physical Therapy
State University of New York
Upstate Medical University
Syracuse, New York

Diane Hainsworth, MS, RN-C, ANP
Clinical Case Manager—Oncology
(retired)
University Hospital
State University of New York
Upstate Medical University
Syracuse, New York

Kara Keyes, MS, RN-BC, doctoral candidate
Professor of Practice
Department of Nursing
Purcell School of Professional Studies
Le Moyne College
Syracuse, New York

Sharon Kitchie, PhD, RN
Adjunct Instructor
Keuka College
Keuka Park, New York
Director of Patient Education and
Interpreter Services (retired)
University Hospital
SUNY Upstate Medical University
Syracuse, New York

Eleanor Price McLees, MS, RN, CNM
Administrator/Part-Time Faculty
Department of Nursing
Purcell School of Professional Studies
Le Moyne College
Syracuse, New York

Gina M. Myers, PhD, RN, CDRN
Adjunct Faculty
Department of Nursing
Purcell School of Professional Studies
Le Moyne College
Syracuse, New York

M. Janice Nelson, EdD, RN
Professor and Dean Emerita
College of Nursing
State University of New York
Upstate Medical University
Syracuse, New York

Eleanor Richards, PhD, RN
Associate Professor and Chair
(in memoriam)
Department of Nursing
State University of New York at New Paltz
New Paltz, New York

Deborah L. Sopczyk, PhD, RN
Dean of the Health Sciences
Excelsior College
Albany, New York

Priscilla Sandford Worral, PhD, RN
Coordinator of Nursing Research
University Hospital
State University of New York
Upstate Medical University
Syracuse, New York

Acknowledgments

A special appreciation is extended to the original authors of the chapters to the first *Essentials* text whose valuable work provided the foundation for revising information and adding new material to this most recent edition. In memoriam, I wish to honor Dr. Eleanor Richards, a dear friend and colleague whose brilliant mind was able to initially organize and make sense of concepts and theories on compliance and motivation presented in Chapter 6. For this second edition, I am grateful for both the loyalty of the original contributors who agreed to edit their own work for this text and for a group of new colleagues who joined the team to contribute their professional knowledge, practice expertise, and fresh perspectives in revising the content of the remaining chapters. Every one of them dedicated their efforts to updating information and simplifying material contained in all 14 chapters for the benefit of the intended audience of readers.

Also, I extend my sincerest thanks to the entire publishing staff of the nursing division of Jones & Bartlett Learning for making this new edition possible. In particular, I would like to acknowledge Amanda Martin, executive editor; Rebecca Myrick, associate acquisitions editor; Lauren Vaughn, editorial assistant; Juna Abrams, associate production editor; Wesley DeShano, rights and media specialist; and Jennifer Scherzay, senior marketing manager, for their technical advice and guidance, organizational skills, and constant support, understanding, and encouragement throughout the process of launching this publication. Also, I'd like to acknowledge the incredible copyediting skills of Janet Kiefer. All of them together are a very talented team of professionals!

Also instrumental in the preparation of this manuscript was Cathleen Scott, science librarian at Le Moyne College. She worked diligently behind the scenes in locating relevant and current references used to update the content of many chapters.

And lastly, but certainly not least, my husband, Jeffrey, deserves the deepest gratitude from me for his steadfast support during the countless hours and endless months that I devoted to research, writing, and editing, which was key to making this second edition a reality.

About the Author

Susan Bacorn Bastable earned her MEd in community health nursing and her EdD in curriculum and instruction in nursing at Teachers College, Columbia University, in 1976 and 1979, respectively. She received her diploma in nursing from Hahnemann Hospital School of Nursing (now known as Drexel University of the Health Sciences) in Philadelphia in 1969 and her bachelor's degree in nursing from Syracuse University in 1972.

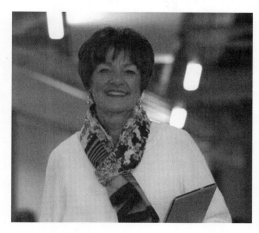

    Dr. Bastable was professor and founding chair of the Department of Nursing at Le Moyne College in Syracuse, New York for 11 years. She retired in May 2015 and was honored with the title of professor emerita. She began her academic career in 1979 as assistant professor at Hunter College, Bellevue School of Nursing in New York City, where she remained on the faculty for 2 years. From 1987 to 1989, she was assistant professor in the College of Nursing at the University of Rhode Island. In 1990, she joined the faculty of the College of Nursing at the State University of New York (SUNY) at Upstate Medical University in Syracuse, where she was associate professor and chair of the undergraduate program for 14 years. In 2004, she assumed her leadership position at Le Moyne College and successfully established an RN-BS completion program; an innovative 4-year undergraduate dual-degree partnership in nursing (DDPN) supported by a Robert Wood Johnson Foundation grant in conjunction with the associate's degree program at St. Joseph's College of Nursing in Syracuse; a BS-MS bridge program; a post-baccalaureate RN-MS certificate program; a master of science program and three post-MS certificate programs with tracks in nursing education, nursing administration, and informatics; and most recently a family nurse practitioner program with a post-MS FNP option.

    Dr. Bastable has taught undergraduate courses in nursing research, community health, and the role of the nurse as educator, and courses at the master's and post-master's level in the academic faculty role, curriculum and program development, and educational assessment and evaluation. For 31 years she served as consultant and external faculty member for Excelsior College (formerly known as Regents College of the University of the State of New York). Her clinical practice includes experiences in community health, oncology, rehabilitation and neurology, occupational health, and medical/surgical nursing.

Dr. Bastable received the President's Award for Excellence in Teaching at Upstate Medical University and the SUNY Chancellor's Award for Excellence in Teaching. Also, she was recognized for the Women in Leadership award from the Greater Syracuse Chamber of Commerce and was honored with the Distinguished Achievement Award in Nursing Education from Teacher's College, Columbia University. In addition to authoring four editions of *Nurse as Educator*, she is the main editor of the textbook *Health Professional as Educator*.

PART I

Perspectives on Teaching and Learning

© wanchai/Shutterstock

Overview of Education in Health Care

Susan B. Bastable | Kattiria M. Gonzalez

Chapter Highlights

- Historical Foundations for Patient Education in Health Care
- The Evolution of the Teaching Role of Nurses
- Social, Economic, and Political Trends Affecting Health Care
- Purposes, Goals, and Benefits of Patient Education
- The Education Process Defined
- The Contemporary Teaching Role of the Nurse
- Barriers to Teaching and Obstacles to Learning
  - *Factors Affecting the Ability to Teach*
  - *Factors Affecting the Ability to Learn*
- Questions to Be Asked About Teaching and Learning

Key Terms

barriers to teaching
education process
learning
obstacles to learning
patient education
teaching/instruction

Objectives

After completing this chapter, the reader will be able to

1. Discuss the evolution of patient education in health care and the teaching role of nurses.
2. Recognize trends affecting the healthcare system in general and nursing practice in particular.
3. Identify the purposes, goals, and benefits of patient education.
4. Compare the education process to the nursing process.
5. Define the terms *education process, teaching, learning,* and *patient education.*
6. Identify reasons why patient education is an important duty for nurses.
7. Discuss the barriers to teaching and the obstacles to learning.
8. Formulate questions that nurses in the role of patient teachers should ask about the teaching–learning process.

Patient education in health care today is a topic of utmost interest to nurses in every setting in which they practice. Teaching is an important aspect of the nurse's professional role (Friberg, Granum, & Bergh, 2012). The current trends in health care are making it essential that clients be prepared to assume responsibility for self-care management. These trends make it imperative that nurses in the workplace be accountable for the delivery of high-quality care. The focus of modern health care is on outcomes that demonstrate the extent to which patients and their significant others have learned essential knowledge and skills for independent care.

According to Friberg and colleagues (2012), patient education is an issue in nursing practice and will continue to be a significant focus in the healthcare environment. The term **patient education** is defined as "any set of planned educational activities, using a combination of methods (teaching, counseling, and behavior modification), that is designed to improve patients' knowledge and health behaviors" (Friedman, Cosby, Boyko, Hatton-Bauer, & Turnbull, 2011). Because so many changes are occurring in the healthcare system, nurses are increasingly finding themselves in challenging, constantly changing, and highly complex positions (Gillespie & McFetridge, 2006). Nurses in the role of patient teachers must understand the forces, both historical and present day, that have influenced and continue to influence their responsibilities in practice.

One purpose of this chapter is to shed light on the historical evolution of patient education in health care. Another purpose is to offer a perspective on the current trends in health care that make the teaching of clients a highly visible and required function of nursing care delivery. In addition, this chapter clarifies the broad purposes, goals, and benefits of the teaching–learning process; presents the philosophy of the nurse–patient partnership in teaching and learning; compares the education process to the nursing process; and identifies barriers to teaching and obstacles to learning. The focus is on the overall role of the nurse in teaching and learning, with the patient as the audience. Nurses must have a basic understanding of the principles and processes of teaching and learning to carry out their professional practice responsibilities with efficiency and effectiveness.

Historical Foundations for Patient Education in Health Care

"Patient education has been a part of health care since the first healer gave the first patient advice about treating his (or her) ailments" (May, 1999, p. 3). Although the term *patient education* was not specifically used, considerable efforts by the earliest healers to inform, encourage, and caution patients to follow appropriate hygienic and therapeutic measures occurred even in prehistoric times (Bartlett, 1986). Because these early healers—physicians, herbalists, midwives, and shamans—did not have a lot of effective diagnostic and treatment interventions, it is likely that education was, in fact, one of the most common interventions (Bartlett, 1986).

From the mid-1800s through the turn of the 20th century, described as the formative period by Bartlett (1986), several key factors influenced the growth of patient education.

The emergence of nursing and other health professions, technological developments, the emphasis on the patient–caregiver relationship, the spread of tuberculosis and other communicable diseases, and the growing interest in the welfare of mothers and children all had an impact on patient education (Bartlett, 1986). In nursing, Florence Nightingale emerged as a resolute advocate of the educational responsibilities of district public health nurses and authored *Health Teaching in Towns and Villages*, which advocated for school teaching of health rules as well as health teaching in the home (Monterio, 1985).

In the first few decades of the 20th century, patient teaching continued to be delivered by nurses as part of their clinical practice, but this responsibility was overshadowed by the increasing technology that was being introduced into health care (Bartlett, 1986). Then in the early 1950s, the first references in the literature to patient education began to appear (Falvo, 2004). In 1953, Veterans Administration (VA) hospitals issued a technical bulletin titled *Patient Education and the Hospital Program*. This bulletin identified the nature and scope of patient education and provided guidance to all hospital services involved in patient education (Veterans Administration, 1953).

In the 1960s and 1970s, patient education began to be seen as a specific task where emphasis was placed on educating individual patients rather than providing general public health education. Developments during this time, such as the civil rights movement, the women's movement, and the consumer and self-help movement, all affected patient education (Bartlett, 1986; Nyswander, 1980; Rosen, 1977). In 1971, two significant events occurred: (1) A publication from the Department of Health, Education, and Welfare, titled *The Need for Patient Education,* emphasized a concept of patient education that provided information about disease and treatment as well as teaching patients how to stay healthy, and (2) President Richard Nixon issued a message to Congress using the term *health education* (Falvo, 2004). Nixon later appointed the President's Committee on Health Education, which recommended that hospitals offer health education to families of patients (Bartlett, 1986; Weingarten, 1974). Although the terms *health education* and *patient education* were used interchangeably, this recommendation had a great impact on the future of patient education because a health education focal point was established in what was then the Department of Education and Welfare (Falvo, 2004).

As a result of this committee's recommendations, the American Hospital Association (AHA) appointed a special committee on health education (Falvo, 2004). The AHA committee suggested that it was a responsibility of hospitals as well as other healthcare institutions to provide educational programs for patients and that all health professionals were to be included in patient education (AHA, 1976). Also, the healthcare system began to pay more attention to patient rights and protections involving informed consent (Roter, Stashefsky-Margalit, & Rudd, 2001). Also in the early 1970s, patient education was a significant part of the AHA's *Statement on a Patient's Bill of Rights* (1973). This document outlines patients' rights to receive current information about their diagnosis, treatment, and prognosis in understandable terms as well as information that enables them to make informed decisions about their health care.

In the 1980s, national health education programs once again became popular as healthcare trends focused on disease prevention and health promotion. The U.S. Department of

Health and Human Services' *Healthy People 2000: National Health Promotion and Disease Prevention Objectives* (USDHHS, 1990), followed by *Healthy People 2010* (USDHHS, 2000) and *Healthy People 2020* (USDHHS, 2010), established specific and important goals and objectives for the public health of the nation. Patient education is a fundamental component of these far-reaching national initiatives.

Also, in recognition of the importance of patient education by nurses, The Joint Commission (TJC), formerly the Joint Commission on Accreditation of Healthcare Organizations (JCAHO), established nursing standards for patient education as early as 1993 (JCAHO, 2001). These standards required nurses to achieve positive outcomes of patient care through teaching activities that must be patient centered and family oriented. More recently, TJC expanded its expectations to include an interdisciplinary team approach in providing patient education as well as evidence that patients and their significant others participate in care and decision making and understand what they have been taught. This requirement means that all healthcare providers must consider the literacy level, educational background, language skills, and culture of every client during the education process (Cipriano, 2007; Davidhizar & Brownson, 1999; JCAHO, 2001).

The Evolution of the Teaching Role of Nurses

Nursing is unique among the health professions in that patient education has long been considered a major component of standard care given by nurses. Since the mid-1800s, when nursing was first acknowledged as a unique discipline, the responsibility for teaching has been recognized as an important role of nurses as caregivers. The focus of nurses' teaching efforts is on the care of the sick and promotion of the health of the well public.

Florence Nightingale, the founder of modern nursing, was the ultimate educator. Not only did she develop the first school of nursing, but she also devoted a large portion of her career to teaching nurses, physicians, and health officials about the importance of proper conditions in hospitals and homes to improve the health of people. Nightingale also emphasized the importance of teaching patients the need for adequate nutrition, fresh air, exercise, and personal hygiene to improve their well-being. By the early 1900s, public health nurses in the United States clearly understood the significance of the role of the nurse as teacher in preventing disease and in maintaining the health of society (Chachkes & Christ, 1996). It is from these roots that nurses have expanded their practice to include the broader concepts of health and illness (Glanville, 2000).

As early as 1918, the National League of Nursing Education (NLNE) in the United States (now the National League for Nursing [NLN]) observed the importance of health teaching as a function within the scope of nursing practice. Two decades later, this organization recognized nurses as agents for the promotion of health and the prevention of illness in all settings in which they practiced (NLNE, 1937). In similar fashion, the American Nurses Association (ANA, 2015) has for years issued statements on the functions, standards, and qualifications for nursing practice, of which patient teaching is a key element. In addition, the International Council of Nurses (ICN, 2012) has long endorsed the nurse's role as patient educator to be an essential component of nursing care delivery.

Today, all state nurse practice acts (NPAs) include teaching within the scope of nursing practice responsibilities. Nurses, by legal mandate of their NPAs, are expected to provide instruction to consumers to assist them to maintain optimal levels of wellness and manage illness. Nursing career ladders often incorporate teaching effectiveness as a measure of excellence in practice (Rifas, Morris, & Grady, 1994). By teaching patients and families, nurses can achieve the professional goal of providing cost-effective, safe, and high-quality care.

A variety of other health professions also identify their commitment to patient education in their professional documents (Falvo, 2004). Standards of practice, practice frameworks, accreditation standards, guides to practice, and practice acts of many health professions delineate the educational responsibilities of their members. In addition, professional workshops and continuing education programs routinely address the skills needed for quality patient and staff education. Although specific roles vary according to profession, directives related to contemporary patient education clearly echo Bartlett's (1986) assertion that it "must be viewed as a fundamentally multidisciplinary enterprise" (p. 146).

Since the 1980s, the role of the nurse as educator has undergone a paradigm shift, evolving from what once was a disease-oriented approach to a more prevention-oriented approach. In other words, the focus is on teaching for the promotion and maintenance of health (Roter et al., 2001). Education, which was once done as part of discharge planning at the end of hospitalization, has expanded to become part of a comprehensive plan of care that occurs across the continuum of the healthcare delivery process (Davidhizar & Brownson, 1999).

As described by Grueninger (1995), this transition toward wellness entails a progression "from disease-oriented patient education (DOPE) to prevention-oriented patient education (POPE) to ultimately become health-oriented patient education (HOPE)" (p. 53). Instead of the traditional aim of simply imparting information, the emphasis is now on empowering patients to use their potential, abilities, and resources to the fullest (Glanville, 2000). Along with supporting patient empowerment, nurses must be mindful to continue to ensure the protection of "patient voice" and the therapeutic relationship in patient education against the backdrop of ever-increasing productivity expectations and time constraints (Roter et al., 2001).

Social, Economic, and Political Trends Affecting Health Care

In addition to the professional and legal standards various organizations and agencies have put forth, many social, economic, and political trends nationwide that affect the public's health have focused attention on the role of the nurse as teacher and the importance of patient education. The following are some of the significant forces influencing nursing practice in particular and healthcare practice in general (Ainsley & Brown, 2009;

Berwick, 2006; Birchenall, 2000; Bodenheimer, Lorig, Holman, & Grumbach, 2002; Cipriano, 2007; Glanville, 2000; IOM, 2011; Lea, Skirton, Read, & Williams, 2011; Osborne, 2005; USDHHS, 2010; Zikmund-Fisher, Sarr, Fagerlin, & Ubel, 2006):

- The federal government, as discussed earlier, published *Healthy People 2020,* a document that set forth national health goals and objectives for the next decade. Achieving these national priorities would dramatically cut the costs of health care, prevent the premature onset of disease and disability, and help all Americans lead healthier and more productive lives. Among the major causes of morbidity and mortality are those diseases now recognized as being lifestyle related and preventable through educational intervention. Nurses, as the largest group of health professionals, play an important role in making a real difference by teaching patients to attain and maintain healthy lifestyles.
- The Institute of Medicine (IOM, 2011) established recommendations designed to enhance the role of nurses in the delivery of health care. This includes nurses functioning to the fullest extent of their education and scope of practice. Patient and family education is a key component of the nurse's role.
- The U.S. Congress passed into law in 2010 the Affordable Care Act (ACA), a comprehensive healthcare reform legislation. The ACA is designed to provide cost-effective, accessible, equitable, quality health care to all Americans with the intent of improving their health outcomes. Universal accessibility to health care has the potential to transform the healthcare system, and nurses will play a major role in meeting the demands and complexities of this increasing population of patients.
- The growth of managed care has resulted in shifts in reimbursement for healthcare services. Greater emphasis is placed on outcome measures, many of which can be achieved primarily through the health education of patients.
- Health providers are recognizing the economic and social values of reaching out to communities, schools, and workplaces, all settings where nurses practice, to provide public education for disease prevention and health promotion.
- Consumers are demanding increased knowledge and skills about how to care for themselves and how to prevent disease. As people are becoming more aware of their needs and desire a greater understanding of treatments and goals, the demand for health information is expected to grow. The quest for consumer rights and responsibilities, which began in the 1990s, continues into the 21st century.
- An increasing number of self-help groups exist to support clients in meeting their physical and psychosocial needs. The success of these support groups and behavioral change programs depends on the nurse's role as teacher and advocate.
- Demographic trends, particularly the aging of the population, require nurses to emphasize self-reliance and maintenance of a healthy status over an extended life span. As the percentage of the U.S. population older than age 65 years climbs dramatically in the next 20 to 30 years, the healthcare needs of the baby-boom generation of the post–World War II era will increase as this vast group of people deals with degenerative illnesses and other effects of the aging process.

- The increased prevalence of chronic and incurable conditions requires that individuals and families become informed participants to manage their own illnesses. Patient teaching can facilitate an individual's adaptive responses to illness and disability.
- Advanced technology increases the complexity of care and treatment in home and community-based settings. More rapid hospital discharge and more procedures done on an outpatient basis force patients to be more self-reliant in managing their own health. Patient education assists them in following through with self-management activities independently.
- Healthcare providers increasingly recognize patient health literacy as an essential skill to improve health outcomes nationwide. Nurses must attend to the education needs of their patients to be sure that they adequately understand the information to promote, maintain, and restore their health. Better understanding by patients and their families of the recommended treatment plans can lead to increased cooperation, decision making, satisfaction, and independence with therapeutic regimens.

Nurses recognize the need to develop their expertise in teaching to keep pace with the demands for patient education. As they continue to define their role, body of knowledge, scope of practice, and professional expertise, they are realizing, more than ever before, the significance of their role as teachers. Nurses have many opportunities to carry out health education. They are the healthcare providers who have the most continuous contact with patients and their families, are usually the most accessible source of information for the consumer, and are the most highly trusted of all health professionals. In Gallup polls conducted since 1999, nurses continue to be ranked number 1 in honesty and ethics among 45 occupations (McCafferty, 2002; Riffkin, 2014; Saad, 2008).

Purposes, Goals, and Benefits of Patient Education

The purpose of patient education is to increase the competence and confidence of clients for self-management. The ultimate goal is to increase the responsibility and independence of patients and their families for self-care. This can be achieved by supporting them through the transition from being dependent on others to being self-sustaining in managing their own care and from being passive listeners to active learners. An interactive, partnership education approach provides them with opportunities to explore and expand their self-care abilities (Cipriano, 2007).

The single most important action of nurses as teachers is to prepare patients for self-care. If patients cannot independently maintain or improve their health status when on their own, nurses have failed to help them reach their potential (Glanville, 2000). The benefits of patient education are many. For example, effective teaching by the nurse can do the following:

- Increase consumer satisfaction
- Improve quality of life
- Ensure continuity of care
- Decrease patient anxiety

- Effectively reduce the complications of illness and the incidence of disease
- Promote adherence to treatment plans
- Maximize independence in the performance of activities of daily living
- Energize and empower consumers to become actively involved in the planning of their care

Because patients and their families must handle many health needs and problems at home, people must be educated on how to care for themselves—that is, both to get well and to stay well. Illness is a natural life process, but so is humankind's ability to learn. Along with the ability to learn comes a natural curiosity that allows people to view new and difficult situations as challenges rather than as defeats. As Orr (1990) observes, "Illness can become an educational opportunity . . . a 'teachable moment' when ill health suddenly encourages [patients] to take a more active role in their care" (p. 47). This observation remains relevant today.

Numerous studies have documented the fact that informed patients are more likely to comply with medical treatment plans, more likely to find innovative ways to cope with illness, and less likely to experience complications. Overall, they are more satisfied with care when they receive adequate information about how to manage for themselves. One of the most frequently cited complaints by patients in litigation cases is that they were not adequately informed (Reising, 2007).

The Education Process Defined

The **education process** is a systematic, sequential, logical, scientifically based, planned course of action consisting of two major interdependent operations: teaching and learning. This process forms a continuous cycle that also involves two interdependent players: the teacher and the learner. Together, they jointly perform teaching and learning activities, the outcome of which leads to mutually desired behavior changes. These changes foster growth in the learner and, it should be acknowledged, growth in the teacher as well. Thus the education process is a framework for a participatory, shared approach to teaching and learning (Carpenter & Bell, 2002). This process is similar across the practice of many of the health professions.

The education process can be compared to the nursing process because the steps of each process run parallel to the steps of the other (Figure 1–1). Like the nursing process, it consists of the basic elements of assessment, planning, implementation, and evaluation. The two are different in that the nursing process focuses on the planning and implementation of care based on the assessment and diagnosis of the physical and psychosocial needs of the patient. The education process, in contrast, focuses on the planning and implementation of teaching based on an assessment and prioritization of the client's learning needs, readiness to learn, and learning styles (Carpenter & Bell, 2002).

The outcomes of the nursing process are achieved when the physical and psychosocial needs of the client are met. The outcomes of the education process are achieved when changes in knowledge, attitudes, and skills occur. Both processes are ongoing,

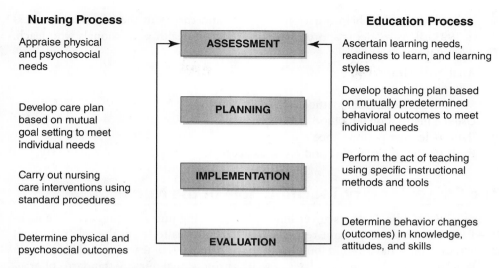

Nursing Process		Education Process
Appraise physical and psychosocial needs	**ASSESSMENT**	Ascertain learning needs, readiness to learn, and learning styles
Develop care plan based on mutual goal setting to meet individual needs	**PLANNING**	Develop teaching plan based on mutually predetermined behavioral outcomes to meet individual needs
Carry out nursing care interventions using standard procedures	**IMPLEMENTATION**	Perform the act of teaching using specific instructional methods and tools
Determine physical and psychosocial outcomes	**EVALUATION**	Determine behavior changes (outcomes) in knowledge, attitudes, and skills

Figure 1–1 Education process parallels nursing process

with assessment and evaluation perpetually redirecting the planning and implementation phases. If mutually agreed-on outcomes in either process are not achieved, as determined by evaluation, the process can and should begin again through reassessment, replanning, and reimplementation.

Note that the actual act of **teaching** or **instruction** is merely one component of the education process. Teaching and instruction—terms that are often used interchangeably—are deliberate interventions that involve sharing information and experiences to meet intended learner outcomes in the cognitive, affective, and psychomotor domains according to an education plan. Teaching and instruction are often thought of as formal, structured, organized activities, but they also can be informal, spur-of-the-moment education sessions that occur during conversations and incidental encounters with the learner. The cues that someone has a need to learn can be communicated in the form of a verbal request, a question, a puzzled or confused look, a blank stare, or a gesture of defeat or frustration. In the broadest sense, then, teaching is a highly versatile strategy that can be applied in preventing, promoting, maintaining, or modifying a wide variety of behaviors in a learner who is receptive and motivated (Duffy, 1998).

Learning is defined as a change in behavior (knowledge, attitudes, and/or skills) that can be observed or measured and that occurs at any time or in any place as a result of exposure to environmental stimuli. Learning is an action by which knowledge, skills, and attitudes are consciously or unconsciously acquired such that behavior is altered in some way. The success of the nurse's endeavors in teaching is measured not by how much content is shared, but rather by how much the person learns (Musinski, 1999).

Specifically, patient education is a process of assisting people to learn health-related behaviors that they can incorporate into everyday life with the goal of achieving optimal health and independence in self-care. The ASSURE model is a useful paradigm originally developed to help nurses to organize and carry out the education process (Rega, 1993). This model is appropriate for use by all health professionals who teach. The acronym stands for

Analyze the learner
State the objectives
Select the instructional methods and materials
Use the instructional methods and materials
Require learner performance
Evaluate the teaching plan and revise as necessary

The Contemporary Teaching Role of the Nurse

Over the years, organizations governing and influencing nurses in practice have identified teaching as an important responsibility. For nurses to fulfill the role of patient teacher, they must have a solid foundation in the principles of teaching and learning.

Legal and accreditation mandates as well as professional nursing standards of practice have made the teaching role of the nurse an essential part of high-quality care to be delivered by all registered nurses, regardless of their level of nursing school preparation. Given this fact, it is imperative to examine the present teaching role expectations of nurses (Gleasman-DeSimone, 2012). The role of the nurse as teacher of patients and families should stem from a partnership philosophy. A learner cannot be made to learn, but an effective approach in educating others is to create the teachable moment, rather than just waiting for it to happen, and to actively involve learners in the education process (Bodenheimer et al., 2002; Lawson & Flocke, 2009; Tobiano, Bucknell, Marshall, Guinane, & Chaboyer, 2015; Wagner & Ash, 1998).

Although all nurses are expected to teach as part of their licensing criteria, many lack formal preparation in the principles of teaching and learning (Donner, Levonian, & Slutsky, 2005). Obviously, a nurse needs a great deal of knowledge and skill to carry out the teaching role with efficiency and effectiveness. Although all nurses are able to function as givers of information, they need to acquire the skills of being a facilitator of the learning process (Musinski, 1999).

A growing body of evidence suggests that effective education and learner participation go hand in hand. The nurse should act as a facilitator, creating an environment conducive to learning that motivates individuals to want to learn and makes it possible for them to learn (Musinski, 1999). Both the educator and the learner should participate in the assessment of learning needs, the design of a teaching plan, the implementation of instructional methods and materials, and the evaluation of teaching and learning. Thus the emphasis should be on the facilitation of learning from a nondirective rather than a didactic teaching approach (Donner et al., 2005; Knowles, Holton, & Swanson, 1998; Mangena & Chabeli, 2005; Musinski, 1999).

No longer should teachers see themselves as simply transmitters of content. Indeed, their role has shifted from the traditional position of being the giver of information to that of a process designer and coordinator. This role alteration from the traditional teacher-centered perspective to a learner-centered approach is a paradigm shift that requires nurses to possess skill in needs assessment as well as the ability to involve learners in planning, link learners to learning resources, and encourage learner initiative (Knowles et al., 1998; Mangena & Chabeli, 2005).

Instead of the teacher teaching, the new educational paradigm focuses on the learner learning. That is, the teacher becomes the guide on the side, assisting the learner in his or her effort to determine objectives and goals for learning, with both parties being active partners in decision making throughout the learning process. To increase comprehension, recall, and application of information, clients must be actively involved in the learning experience (Kessels, 2003; London, 1995). Glanville (2000) describes this move toward assisting learners to use their own abilities and resources as "a pivotal transfer of power" (p. 58).

Certainly, patient education requires a collaborative effort among healthcare team members, all of whom play more or less important roles in teaching. However, physicians are first and foremost prepared "to treat, not to teach" (Gilroth, 1990, p. 30). Nurses, by comparison, are prepared to provide a holistic approach to care delivery. The teaching role is a unique part of nursing's professional domain. Because consumers have always respected and trusted nurses to be their advocates, nurses are in an ideal position to clarify confusing information and make sense out of nonsense. Amidst a fragmented healthcare delivery system involving many providers, the nurse serves as coordinator of care. By ensuring consistency of information, nurses can support patients and their families in efforts to achieve the goal of optimal health (Donovan & Ward, 2001).

Barriers to Teaching and Obstacles to Learning

It has been said by many educators that adult learning takes place not by the teacher initiating and motivating the learning process, but rather by the teacher removing or reducing obstacles to learning and enhancing the process after it has begun. The nurse as teacher should not limit learning to the information that is intended, but rather should clearly make possible the potential for informal, unintended learning that can occur each and every day with each and every teacher–learner encounter (Carpenter & Bell, 2002). The evidence supports that interactions between learner and teacher are central to the development of teachable moments, regardless of the obstacles or barriers that may be encountered (Lawson & Flocke, 2009).

Unfortunately, nurses must confront many barriers in carrying out their responsibilities for educating others. Also, learners face a variety of potential obstacles that can interfere with their learning. For the purposes of this text, **barriers to teaching** are defined as those factors that impede the nurse's ability to deliver educational services. **Obstacles to learning** are defined as those factors that negatively affect the ability of the learner to pay attention to and process information.

Factors Affecting the Ability to Teach

The following barriers (Figure 1–2) may interfere with the ability of nurses to carry out their roles as educators (Carpenter & Bell, 2002; Casey, 1995; Chachkes & Christ, 1996;

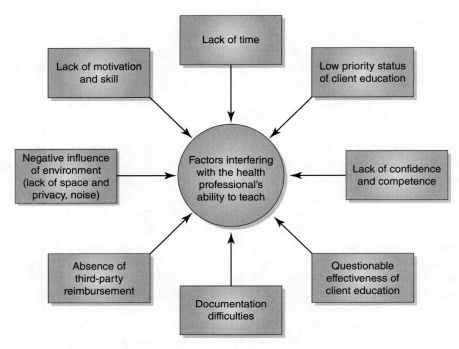

Figure 1–2 Barriers to teaching

Donovan & Ward, 2001; Duffy, 1998; Friberg et al., 2012; Glanville, 2000; Honan, Krsnak, Petersen, & Torkelson, 1988; Tobiano et al., 2015):

1. Lack of time to teach is cited by nurses as the greatest barrier to being able to carry out their role effectively. Early discharge from inpatient and outpatient settings often results in nurses and patients having fleeting contact with each other. In addition, the schedules and responsibilities of nurses are very demanding. Finding time to allocate to teaching is very challenging in light of other work demands and expectations. In one survey by TJC, 28% of nurses claimed that they were not able to provide patients and their families with the necessary instruction because of lack of time during their shifts at work (Stolberg, 2002). Nurses must know how to adopt an abbreviated, efficient, and effective approach to patient education, first by adequately assessing the learner and then by using appropriate teaching methods and instructional tools at their disposal. Discharge planning is playing an ever more important role in ensuring continuity of care across settings.

2. Many nurses and other healthcare personnel admit that they do not feel competent or confident with their teaching skills. As stated previously, although nurses are expected to teach, few have ever taken a specific course on the principles of teaching and learning. The concepts of patient education are often integrated throughout nursing curricula rather than being offered as a specific course of

study. As early as the 1960s, Pohl (1965) found that one third of 1500 nurses, when questioned, reported that they had no preparation for the teaching they were doing, while only one fifth felt they had adequate preparation. Almost 30 years later, Kruger (1991) surveyed 1230 nurses in staff, administrative, and education positions regarding their perceptions of the extent of nurses' responsibility for and level of achievement of patient education. Although all three groups strongly believed that patient education is a primary responsibility of nurses, the vast majority of respondents rated their ability to perform educator role activities as unsatisfactory. Many of the other health professions share similar views. Only a few additional studies have been forthcoming on nurses' perceptions of their teaching role (Friberg et al., 2012; Kelo, Martikainen, & Eriksson, 2013; Lahl, Modic, & Siedlecki, 2013; Trocino, Byers, & Peach, 1997). Today, preparation for the role of the nurse as educator still needs to be strengthened in undergraduate nursing education.

3. Personal characteristics of the nurse play an important role in determining the outcome of a teaching–learning interaction. Motivation to teach and skill in teaching are prime factors in determining the success of any educational endeavor.

4. Until recently, administration and supervisory personnel assigned a low priority to patient teaching. With the strong emphasis of TJC mandates, the level of attention paid to the education needs of consumers has changed significantly. However, budget allocations for educational programs remain tight and can interfere with the adoption of innovative and time-saving teaching strategies and techniques.

5. The environment in the various settings where nurses are expected to teach is not always conducive to carrying out the teaching–learning process. Lack of space, lack of privacy, noise, and frequent interferences caused by patient treatment schedules and staff work demands are just some of the factors that may negatively affect the nurse's ability to concentrate and effectively interact with learners.

6. An absence of third-party reimbursement to support patient education relegates teaching and learning to less than high-priority status. Nursing services within healthcare facilities are subsumed under hospital room costs and, therefore, are not often specifically reimbursed by insurance payers. In fact, patient education in some settings, such as home care, often cannot be incorporated as a legitimate aspect of routine nursing care delivery unless specifically ordered by a physician. Because there are no separate billing codes for patient education, it is difficult to make this process an area of focus; instead, it must be integrated into a therapeutic intervention for many health professionals (Hack, 1999).

7. Some nurses and physicians question whether patient education is effective as a means to improve health outcomes. They view patients as impediments to teaching when patients do not display an interest in changing behavior, when they demonstrate an unwillingness to learn, or when their ability to learn is in

question. Concerns about coercion and violation of free choice, based on the belief that patients have a right to choose and that they cannot be forced to comply, explain why some professionals feel frustrated in their efforts to teach. It is essential that all healthcare members buy into the utility of patient education (that is, they believe it can lead to significant behavioral changes and increased compliance with therapeutic regimens).

8. The type of documentation system used by healthcare agencies has an effect on the quality and quantity of patient teaching. Both formal and informal teaching are often done (Carpenter & Bell, 2002) but not written down because of insufficient time, inattention to detail, and inadequate forms on which to record the extent of teaching activities. Many of the hard-copy forms or computer software used for documentation of teaching are designed to simply check off the areas addressed rather than allowing for elaboration of what was actually accomplished. In addition, most nurses do not recognize the scope and depth of teaching that they perform on a daily basis. Communication among healthcare providers regarding what has been taught needs to be coordinated and appropriately delegated so that teaching can proceed in a timely, smooth, organized, and thorough fashion.

Factors Affecting the Ability to Learn

The following obstacles (Figure 1–3) may interfere with a learner's ability to attend to and process information (Beagley, 2011; Billings & Kowalski, 2004; Glanville, 2000; Kessels, 2003; Weiss, 2003):

1. Lack of time to learn resulting from rapid patient discharge from care and the amount of information a client is expected to learn can discourage and frustrate the learner, impeding his or her ability and willingness to learn.

2. The stress of acute and chronic illness, anxiety, and sensory deficits in patients are just a few problems that can diminish learner motivation and interfere with the process of learning. However, illness alone seldom acts as an impediment to learning. Rather, illness is often the impetus for patients to attend to learning, make contact with the healthcare professional, and take positive action to improve their health status.

3. Low literacy and functional health illiteracy have been found to be significant factors in the ability of patients to make use of the written and verbal instructions given to them by providers. Almost half of the American population reads and comprehends at or below the eighth-grade level, and an even higher percentage suffers from health illiteracy.

4. The negative influence of the hospital environment itself, which results in loss of control, lack of privacy, and social isolation, can interfere with a patient's active role in health decision making and involvement in the teaching–learning process.

5. Personal characteristics of the learner have major effects on the degree to which behavioral outcomes are achieved. Readiness to learn, motivation and

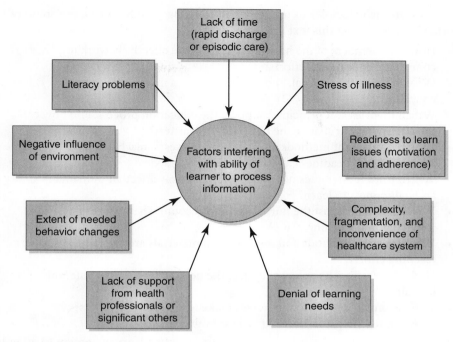

Figure 1–3 Obstacles to learning

compliance, developmental-stage characteristics, and learning styles are some of the prime factors influencing the success of education efforts.

6. The extent of behavioral changes needed, both in number and in complexity, can overwhelm learners and discourage them from attending to and accomplishing learning objectives and goals.

7. Lack of support and lack of ongoing positive reinforcement from the nurse and significant others serve to block the potential for learning.

8. Denial of learning needs, resentment of authority, and lack of willingness to take responsibility (locus of control) are some psychological obstacles to accomplishing behavioral change.

9. The inconvenience, complexity, inaccessibility, fragmentation, and dehumanization of the healthcare system often result in frustration and abandonment of efforts by the learner to participate in and comply with the goals and objectives for learning.

Questions to Be Asked About Teaching and Learning

To maximize the effectiveness of patient education, the nurse must examine the elements of the education process and the role of the nurse as teacher. Many questions arise related to the principles of teaching and learning. The following are some of the important questions that this text addresses:

- How can members of the healthcare team more effectively work together to coordinate educational efforts?
- What are the ethical, legal, and economic issues involved in patient education?
- Which theories and principles support the education process, and how can they be applied to change the behaviors of learners?
- Which assessment methods and tools can nurses as teachers use to determine learning needs, readiness to learn, and learning styles?
- Which learner attributes negatively and positively affect an individual's ability and willingness to learn?
- Which elements must the nurse take into account when developing and implementing teaching plans?
- What teaching methods and instructional materials are available to support teaching efforts?
- How can teaching be tailored to meet the needs of specific populations of learners?
- Which common mistakes do nurses make when teaching others?
- How can teaching and learning be best evaluated?

Summary

Nurses can be considered information brokers—teachers who can make a significant difference in how patients and families cope with their illnesses and disabilities as well as how the public benefits from education directed at prevention of disease and promotion of health. As the United States moves forward in the 21st century, many challenges and opportunities lie ahead for nurses in the role of teachers in the delivery of health care.

The teaching role is becoming even more important and more visible as nurses respond to the social, economic, and political trends affecting health care today. The foremost challenge for nurses is to be able to demonstrate, through research and action, that definite links exist between education and positive behavioral outcomes of the learner. In this era of cost containment, government regulations, and healthcare reform, the benefits of patient education must be made clear to the public, to healthcare employers, to healthcare providers, and to payers of healthcare benefits. To be effective and efficient, nurses must be willing and able to work collaboratively with one another to provide consistently high-quality education to patients and their families.

Nurses can demonstrate responsibility and accountability for the delivery of care to the consumer in part through education based on solid principles of teaching and learning. The key to effective education of the varied audiences of learners is the nurse's understanding of and ongoing commitment to his or her role in patient education.

Review Questions

1. Which key factors influenced the growth of patient education during its formative years?
2. How far back in history has teaching been a part of the nurse's role?
3. Which nursing organization was the first to recognize health teaching as an important function within the scope of nursing practice?
4. Which legal mandate universally includes teaching as a responsibility of nurses?
5. How have the ANA, NLN, ICN, AHA, and TJC influenced the role and responsibilities of the nurse for patient education?
6. What is the current focus and orientation of patient education?
7. Which social, economic, and political trends today make it imperative that patients be adequately educated?
8. What are the similarities and differences between the education process and the nursing process?
9. What are three major barriers to teaching and three major obstacles to learning?
10. Which factor serves as both a barrier to education and an obstacle to learning?

Case Study

As part of Lackney General Hospital's continuous quality improvement plan, and in preparation for the next Joint Commission accreditation visit, all departments in the hospital are in the process of assessing the quality and effectiveness of their patient education efforts. When the professional nursing staff on your unit are asked about their opinions on this topic, you are surprised at the frustration they express. Liz states, "Although I am incredibly frustrated by the lack of administrative support for patient education, I do believe that patient education makes a difference." Jeremiah jumps in and says, "I am sick of continuously being interrupted when trying to educate my patients." Finally, Johaun comments, "I have no idea how I am supposed to fit education in with all the other tasks I need to complete, especially when the patient is clearly not willing to learn." Because the nursing staff obviously have some strong feelings about the department's education efforts, your manager feels that a SWOT (strengths, weaknesses, opportunities, threats) analysis is a good place to begin to gather information about the issues and problems.

1. Use the section titled "Barriers to Teaching and Obstacles to Learning" as a beginning framework for the weaknesses and threats section of the SWOT analysis, and then describe five potential barriers to teaching on your unit that the nurses might identify.
2. Use the section titled "Barriers to Teaching and Obstacles to Learning" as another framework for the weaknesses and threats section of the SWOT analysis, and then describe five potential obstacles to learning on your unit that the nurses might identify.
3. Provide possible solutions to the barriers and obstacles identified that would serve to enhance patient education.

References

Ainsley, B., & Brown, A. (2009). The impact of informatics on nursing education: A review of the literature. *Journal of Continuing Education, 40*(5), 228–232.

American Hospital Association (AHA). (1973). Statement on a patient's bill of rights. *Hospitals, 47*(4), 41.

American Hospital Association (AHA). (1976). Statement on the role and responsibilities of hospitals and other health care institutions in personal and community health education. *Health Education, 7*(4), 23.

American Nurses Association (ANA). (2015). *Scope and standards of practice* (3rd ed.). Silver Spring, MD: Nursebooks.org.

Bartlett, E. E. (1986). Historical glimpses of patient education in the United States. *Patient Education and Counseling, 8,* 135–149.

Beagley, L. (2011). Educating patients: Understanding barriers, teaching styles, and learning techniques. *Journal of PeriAnesthesia Nursing, 26*(5), 331–337.

Berwick, D. (2006, December 12). *IHI launches national campaign to reduce medical harm in U.S. hospitals: Building on its landmark 100,000 lives campaign.* Retrieved from http://www.ihi.org

Billings, D., & Kowalski, K. (2004). Teaching learners from varied generations. *Journal of Continuing Education in Nursing, 35*(3), 104–105.

Birchenall, P. (2000). Nurse education in the year 2000: Reflection, speculation and challenge. *Nurse Education Today, 20,* 1–2.

Bodenheimer, T., Lorig, K., Holman, H., & Grumbach, K. (2002). Patient self-management of chronic disease in primary care. *Journal of the American Medical Association, 288*(19), 2469–2475.

Carpenter, J. A., & Bell, S. K. (2002). What do nurses know about teaching patients? *Journal for Nurses in Staff Development, 18*(3), 157–161.

Casey, F. S. (1995). Documenting patient education: A literature review. *Journal of Continuing Education in Nursing, 26*(6), 257–260.

Chachkes, E., & Christ, G. (1996). Cross cultural issues in patient education. *Patient Education and Counseling, 27,* 13–21.

Cipriano, P. F. (2007). Stop, look, and listen to your patients and their families. *American Nurse Today, 2*(6), 10.

Davidhizar, R. E., & Brownson, K. (1999). Literacy, cultural diversity, and client education. *Health Care Manager, 18*(1), 39–47.

Donner, C. L., Levonian, C., & Slutsky, P. (2005). Move to the head of the class: Developing staff nurses as teachers. *Journal for Nurses in Staff Development, 21*(6), 277–283.

Donovan, H. S., & Ward, S. (2001, third quarter). A representational approach to patient education. *Journal of Nursing Scholarship,* 211–216.

Duffy, B. (1998). Get ready—Get set—Go teach. *Home Healthcare Nurse, 16*(9), 596–602.

Falvo, D. F. (2004). *Effective patient education: A guide to increased compliance* (3rd ed.). Sudbury, MA: Jones and Bartlett.

Friberg, F., Granum, V., & Bergh, A. L. (2012). Nurses' patient-education work: Conditional factors: An integrative review. *Journal of Nursing Management, 20*(2), 170–186.

Friedman, A. J., Cosby, R., Boyko, S., Hatton-Bauer, J., & Turnbull, G. (2011). Effective teaching strategies and methods of delivery for patient education: A systematic review and practice guideline recommendations. *Journal of Cancer Education, 26,* 12–21.

Gillespie, M., & McFetridge, B. (2006). Nursing education: The role of the nurse teacher. *Journal of Clinical Nursing, 15,* 639–644.

Gilroth, B. E. (1990). Promoting patient involvement: Educational, organizational, and environmental strategies. *Patient Education and Counseling, 15,* 29–38.

Glanville, I. K. (2000). Moving towards health oriented patient education (HOPE). *Holistic Nursing Practice, 14*(2), 57–66.

Gleasman-DeSimone, S. (2012). *How nurse practitioners educate their adult patients about healthy behaviors: A mixed method study* (Unpublished dissertation in partial fulfillment of requirements for the degree of Doctor of Philosophy). Capella University, Minneapolis, MN.

Grueninger, U. J. (1995). Arterial hypertension: Lessons from patient education. *Patient Education and Counseling, 26,* 37–55.

Hack, L. M. (1999). Health policy implications for patient education in physical therapy. *Journal of Physical Therapy Education, 13*(3), 57–61.

Honan, S., Krsnak, G., Petersen, D., & Torkelson, R. (1988). The nurse as patient educator: Perceived responsibilities and factors enhancing role development. *Journal of Continuing Education in Nursing, 19*(1), 33–37.

Institute of Medicine (IOM). (2011). *The future of nursing: Leading change, advancing health.* Washington, DC: National Academies Press.

International Council of Nurses (ICN). (2012). *International Council of Nurses fact sheet.* Retrieved from http://www.icn.ch/about-icn/about-icn/

Joint Commission on Accreditation of Healthcare Organizations. (2001). *Patient and family education: The compliance guide to the JCAHO standards* (2nd ed.). Retrieved from http://catalog.hathitrust.org/Record/003169433

Kelo, M., Martikainen, M., & Eriksson, E. (2013). Patient education of children and their families: Nurses' experiences. *Pediatric Nursing, 39*(2), 71–79.

Kessels, R. P. C. (2003). Patients' memory for medical information. *Journal of the Royal Society of Medicine, 96,* 219–222.

Knowles, M. S., Holton, E. F., & Swanson, R. A. (1998). *The adult learner: The definitive classic in adult education and human resource development* (5th ed., pp. 198–201). Houston, TX: Gulf Publishing.

Kruger, S. (1991). The patient educator role in nursing. *Applied Nursing Research, 4*(1), 19–24.

Lahl, M., Modic, M. B., & Siedlecki, S. (2013, July–August). Perceived knowledge and self-confidence of pediatric nurses as patient educators. *Clinical Nurse Specialist Journal,* 188–193.

Lawson, P. J., & Flocke, S. A. (2009). Teachable moments for health behavior change: A concept analysis. *Patient Education and Counseling, 76,* 25–39.

Lea, D. H., Skirton, H., Read, C. Y., & Williams, J. K. (2011). Implications for educating the next generation of nurses on genetics and genomics in the 21st century. *Journal of Nursing Scholarship, 43*(1), 3–12.

London, F. (1995). Teach your patients faster and better. *Nursing, 95*(68), 70.

Mangena, A., & Chabeli, M. M. (2005). Strategies to overcome obstacles in the facilitation of critical thinking in nursing education. *Nurse Education Today, 25,* 291–298.

May, B. J. (1999). Patient education: Past and present. *Journal of Physical Therapy Education, 13*(3), 3–7.

McCafferty, L. A. E. (2002, January 7). Year of the nurse: More than four out of five Americans trust nurses. *Advance for Nurses,* 5.

Monterio, L. A. (1985). Florence Nightingale on public health nursing. *American Journal of Public Health, 75,* 181–186.

Musinski, B. (1999). The educator as facilitator: A new kind of leadership. *Nursing Forum, 34*(1), 23–29.

National League of Nursing Education (NLNE). (1937). *A curriculum guide for schools of nursing.* New York, NY: Author.

Nyswander, D. V. (1980). Public health education: Sources, growth and educational philosophy. *International Quarterly of Community Health Education, 1*, 5–18.

Orr, R. (1990). Illness as an educational opportunity. *Patient Education and Counseling, 15*, 47–48.

Osborne, H. (2005). *Health literacy A to Z: Practical ways to communicate your health message.* Sudbury, MA: Jones and Bartlett.

Pohl, M. L. (1965). Teaching activities of the nursing practitioner. *Nursing Research, 14*(1), 4–11.

Rega, M. D. (1993). A model approach for patient education. *MEDSURG Nursing, 2*(6), 477–479, 495.

Reising, D. L. (2007, February). Protecting yourself from malpractice claims. *American Nurse Today, 39*, 44.

Rifas, E., Morris, R., & Grady, R. (1994). Innovative approach to patient education. *Nursing Outlook, 42*(5), 214–216.

Riffkin, R. (2014, December 18). Americans rate nurses highest on honesty, ethical standards. Retrieved from http://gallup.com/p011/180260/americans-rate-nurses-highest-honesty-ethical-standards.aspx

Rosen, G. (1977). *Preventive medicine in the United States, 1900–1995.* New York, NY: Prodist.

Roter, D. L., Stashefsky-Margalit, R., & Rudd, R. (2001). Current perspectives on patient education in the U.S. *Patient Education and Counseling, 44*, 79–86.

Saad, L. (2008, November 24). *Nurses shine, bankers slump in ethics ratings. Gallup Poll.* Retrieved from http://www.gallup.com

Stolberg, S. G. (2002, August 8). Patient deaths tied to lack of nurses. *New York Times.* Retrieved from http://www.nytimes.com/2002/08/08/health/08NURS.html?pagewanted=1

Tobiano, G., Bucknell, T., Marshall, A., Guinane, J., & Chaboyer, W. (2015, June 21). Nurses' view of patient participation in nursing care. *Journal of Advanced Nursing,* 1–12.

Trocino, L., Byers, J. F., & Peach, A. G. (1997). Nurses' attitudes toward patient and family education: Implications for clinical nurse specialists. *Clinical Nurse Specialist: The Journal for Advanced Nursing Practice, 11*(2), 77–84.

U.S. Department of Health and Human Services (USDHHS), Office of Disease Prevention and Health Promotion. (1990). *Healthy People 2000.* Retrieved from http://www.cdc.gov/nchs/healthy_people/hp2000.htm

U.S. Department of Health and Human Services (USDHHS), Office of Disease Prevention and Health Promotion. (2000). *Healthy People 2010.* Retrieved from http://www.cdc.gov/nchs/healthy_people/hp2010.htm

U.S. Department of Health and Human Services (USDHHS), Office of Disease Prevention and Health Promotion. (2010). *Healthy People 2020.* Retrieved from http://www.cdc.gov/nchs/healthy_people/hp2020.htm

Veterans Administration. (1953). *Patient education and the hospital program* (TB 10–88). Washington, DC: Author.

Wagner, S. P., & Ash, K. L. (1998). Creating the teachable moment. *Journal of Nursing Education, 37*(6), 278–280.

Weingarten, V. (1974). Report of the findings and recommendations of the President's Committee on Health Education. *Health Education Monographs, 1*, 11–19.

Weiss, B. D. (2003). *Health literacy: A manual for clinicians.* Chicago, IL: American Medical Association & American Medical Association Foundation.

Zikmund-Fisher, B. J., Sarr, B., Fagerlin, S., & Ubel, P. A. (2006). A matter of perspective: Choosing for others differs from choosing for yourself in making treatment decisions. *Journal of General Internal Medicine, 21*, 618–622.

Ethical, Legal, and Economic Foundations of the Educational Process

M. Janice Nelson | Kattiria M. Gonzalez

Chapter Highlights

- A View of Ethics, Morality, and the Law
- Evolution of Ethical and Legal Principles in Health Care
- Application of Ethical Principles to Patient Education
  - *Autonomy*
  - *Veracity*
  - *Confidentiality*
  - *Nonmaleficence*
  - *Beneficence*
  - *Justice*
- Ethics of the Patient–Provider Relationship in Practice Settings
- The Patient's Right to Education and Information
- Legal and Financial Implications to Documentation
- Economic Factors in Healthcare Education
- Financial Terminology
  - *Direct Costs*
  - *Indirect Costs*
  - *Cost Savings*
  - *Cost Benefit*
  - *Cost Recovery*
- Program Planning and Implementation

Key Terms

autonomy
beneficence
confidentiality
cost benefit
cost recovery
cost savings
direct costs
ethical
ethical dilemmas
ethics
fixed costs
hidden costs
indirect costs
justice
legal rights and duties
malpractice
moral values
negligence
nonmaleficence
practice acts
revenue generation
variable costs
veracity

Objectives

After completing this chapter, the reader will be able to

1. Identify major ethical principles related to education in health care.
2. Distinguish between ethical and legal dimensions of the healthcare delivery system with respect to patient education.

3. Describe the importance of nurse practice acts and the code of ethics for the nursing profession.
4. Recognize the potential ethical consequences of power imbalances between the nurse and the patient in practice settings.
5. Describe the legal and financial implications of documentation.
6. Delineate the ethical, legal, and economic importance of federal, state, and accrediting body regulations and standards in the delivery of healthcare services.
7. Differentiate among financial terms associated with the development, implementation, and evaluation of patient education programs.

Approximately 45 years ago, the field of modern Western bioethics arose in response to the increasing complexity of medical care and decision making. New and unique challenges in health care continually stem from such influences as technological advances, changes in laws, and public awareness of scientific research findings. The field of bioethics provides thoughtful approaches, based on theory and practice experiences, for handling such complex issues and the dilemmas. As a result, programs of study for health professionals, including nurses, now provide formal and sometimes mandated ethics education. Healthcare providers who commit ethical violations while in training or practice may be referred for ethics remedial instruction by their programs or specialty licensing boards, or they may risk disapproval or punishment by their professional bodies.

In the popular media, bioethical issues arise frequently, such as stem cell research, organ transplantation, genetic testing, and other sensational innovations. But every day, far from the spotlight, nurses confront commonplace and troubling ethical dilemmas. Consider a patient who refuses a routine but lifesaving blood transfusion. Should he or she be allowed to refuse this treatment, or should the nursing staff persuade the patient otherwise? Suppose a nurse witnesses a confused patient signing a consent form for a procedure. Should he or she ask whether the patient has the ability to make the decision to agree to have the procedure done? Or suppose a surgeon misleads a family by indicating that a surgical error was really a complication. Should the nurse who observed the error inform her or his supervisor?

These scenarios describe not only practice issues but also moral problems. They happen so frequently that convening an ethics committee to address every one of them is impractical. Increasingly, staff nurses are being called upon to reason through both medical and ethical issues. However, knowledge of basic ethical principles and concepts does not always suffice. As the healthcare field has developed, so has a critical awareness of individual rights stemming from both natural and constitutional law. Healthcare organizations have many laws and regulations ensuring clients' rights to high-quality standards of care, to informed consent, and subsequently to self-determination. Further, in the interest of justice, it is worthwhile to acknowledge the relationship between costs to the healthcare facility and providing health services. Consequently, it is important that nurses inform patients of their rights, and it is equally important that nursing staff be continually educated about the ethics of care delivery.

Although the physician is primarily held legally accountable for prescribing medical treatment, it is a known fact that patient education generally falls to the nurse. Indeed, given the close relationship of the nurse to patients and their families, the role of the nurse in patient education is absolutely essential and is mandated in the scope of nursing practice through each state nurse practice act.

Today's enlightened consumers are aware of and demand recognition of their individual constitutional rights regarding freedom of choice and self-determination. In fact, it may seem strange to some that federal and state governments, accrediting bodies, and professional organizations find it necessary to legislate, regulate, or provide standards and guidelines to ensure the protection of human rights in matters of health care. The answer, of course, is that the federal government, which once had a historical hands-off policy toward the activities of physicians and other health professionals, has now become heavily involved in the oversight of provider practices. This is due to shocking abuses of human rights in the name of biomedical research that were first discovered in the mid-20th century and, unfortunately, continue to this day.

These issues of human rights are fundamental to the delivery of high-quality healthcare services. They are equally fundamental to the patient education process, in that the intent of the nurse should be to empower patients and their families to identify and articulate their values and preferences, to acknowledge their role in the teaching-learning process, and to make well-informed choices by being aware of the alternatives and consequences of those choices. Thus, the role of the nurse as teacher must include the ethical and legal foundations of the patient education process.

The purpose of this chapter is to provide the ethical, legal, and economic foundations that are essential to carrying out patient education initiatives, on the one hand, and the rights and responsibilities of the healthcare provider, on the other hand. This chapter describes the differences between ethical, moral, and legal concepts. It explores the foundations of human rights based on ethics and the law, and it reviews the ethical and legal dimensions of health care. Furthermore, this chapter examines the importance of documentation of patient teaching while highlighting the economic factors that must be considered in the delivery of patient education programs in healthcare settings.

A View of Ethics, Morality, and the Law

Although ethics as a branch of philosophy has been studied throughout the centuries, by and large these studies were left to the domains of philosophical and religious thinkers. More recently, because of the complexities of modern-day living and the heightened awareness of an educated public, ethical issues related to health care have surfaced as a major concern of both consumers and healthcare providers. It is now a widely held belief that the patient has the right to know his or her medical diagnosis, the treatments available, and the expected outcomes. This information is necessary so that patients can make informed choices about their health and their care options with advice offered by health professionals.

Ethical principles related to human rights are based on natural laws, which guide human society. Inherent in these natural laws are, for example, the principles of respect for others, truth telling, honesty, and regard for life. Ethics as a discipline interprets these basic principles of behavior in broad terms that direct moral decision making in all aspects of human activity (Tong, 2007).

Likewise, the legal system and its laws are based on ethical and moral principles that, through experience and over time, society has accepted as behavioral norms (Hall, 1996; Lesnick & Anderson, 1962). In fact, the terms *ethical*, *moral*, and *legal* are often used interchangeably. It should be made clear, however, that although these terms are certainly interrelated, they are not the same.

Ethics refers to the guiding principles of behavior, and **ethical** refers to norms or standards of behavior accepted by the society to which a person belongs. Although the terms *moral* and *morality* are generally used together with the terms *ethics* and *ethical*, nurses can differentiate between the notion of moral rights and duties from the notion of ethical rights and duties. **Moral values** refer to an internal belief system (what one believes to be right). This value system, defined as morality, is expressed externally through a person's behaviors. **Ethical dilemmas** are a "specific type of moral conflict in which two or more ethical principles apply but support mutually inconsistent courses of action" (Dwarswaard & van de Bovenkamp, 2015, pp. 1131–1132). An example that these authors provide is that the nurse must respect patient autonomy and individual patient responsibility when encouraging and supporting self-management behaviors, but the ethical principle of the patient's right to self-determination may clash with professional values that promote health and help achieve medical outcomes. **Legal rights and duties**, in contrast, refer to rules governing behavior or conduct that are enforceable by law under threat of punishment or penalty, such as a fine, imprisonment, or both.

The intricate relationship between ethics and the law explains why ethics terminology, such as *informed consent, confidentiality*, and *justice*, can be found within the language of the legal system. In keeping with this practice, nurses may cite professional commitment or moral obligation to justify the education of patients as one dimension of their role. In reality, this role is legally mandated by the nurse practice act that exists in the particular state where the nurse resides, is licensed, and is employed.

Practice acts are documents that define a profession, describe that profession's scope of practice, and provide guidelines for state professional boards to grant entry into a profession via licensure and to take disciplinary actions against a professional when necessary. Practice acts were developed to protect the public from unqualified practitioners and to protect the professional title, such as registered nurse (RN), occupational therapist (OT), and physical therapist (PT). A model practice act (American Nurses Association, 1978) serves as a template for individual states to follow, with the ultimate goal of minimizing variability of professional practice from state to state. From the model, a state or other jurisdiction can develop its own practice act that addresses the basic information regarding scope of practice, licensure requirements, and so forth (Flook, 2003). In essence, a professional practice act is not only legally binding but also protected by the police authority of the state in the interest of protecting the public (Brent, 2001; Mikos, 2004).

Evolution of Ethical and Legal Principles in Health Care

In the past, ethics was, as stated before, almost exclusively a concern of philosophers and religious orders. Likewise, from a historical perspective, medicine and nursing were considered humanitarian and charitable occupations. Often these services were provided by members of religious communities and others considered to be caring in nature, courageous, dedicated, and self-sacrificing. Public respect for doctors and nurses was so strong that for many years, healthcare organizations in which they worked were considered to be charitable institutions and, thus, were largely immune from legal action (Lesnik & Anderson, 1962). In the same way, these healthcare practitioners of the past were usually regarded as Good Samaritans who acted in good faith and who also were exempt from lawsuits.

Although numerous court records of lawsuits involving hospitals, physicians, and nurses can be found dating back to the early 1900s, their numbers were very few in comparison with the volumes being generated on a daily basis in today's world (Reising & Allen, 2007). Further, despite the horror stories that have been handed down through the years regarding inhumane and often torturous treatment of prisoners, the mentally ill, the disabled, and the poor, in the past there was only limited focus on ethical aspects of that care. In turn, little thought was given to legal protection of the rights of such mentally, physically, or socioeconomically challenged people.

Clearly, this situation has changed dramatically. For example, informed consent—a basic principle of the ethical practice of health care—was established in the courts as early as 1914 by Justice Benjamin Cardozo. Cardozo determined that every adult of sound mind has a right to protect his or her own body and to determine how it shall be treated (Hall, 1992; *Schloendorff v. Society of New York Hospitals*, 1914). Although the Cardozo decision had considerable impact, governmental interest in the bioethics of human rights in the delivery of healthcare services did not really surface until after World War II.

Before that time, federal and state governments did not get involved in issues of biomedical research or physician–patient relationships. However, the human atrocities committed by the Nazis in the name of biomedical research during World War II shocked the world into critical awareness of gross violations of human rights. Unfortunately, such abuses were not just happening in wartime Europe. On U.S. soil, for example, the lack of treatment of African Americans with syphilis in Tuskegee, Alabama; the injection of live cancer cells into uninformed, nonconsenting older adults at the Brooklyn Chronic Disease Hospital; and the use of institutionalized mentally retarded children to study hepatitis at the Willowbrook State School on Staten Island, New York, startled the nation and raised public awareness of disturbing breaches in the physician–patient relationship (Brent, 2001; Centers for Disease Control and Prevention, 2005; Rivera, 1972; Thomas & Quinn, 1991; Weisbard & Arras, 1984).

Stirred to action by these disturbing examples, in 1974, Congress created the National Commission for the Protection of Human Subjects of Biomedical and Behavioral Research (U.S. Department of Health and Human Services [USDHHS], 1983). As an outcome, institutional review boards (IRBs) for the protection of human subjects were mandated to be established at the local level in hospitals, academic medical centers, agencies, or organizations conducting research on human subjects. To this day, the primary function of these IRBs is to safeguard all human study subjects by insisting that research procedures include voluntary participation and withdrawal, confidentiality, truth telling, and informed consent, and that they address additional specific concerns for vulnerable populations such as infants, children, prisoners, and persons with mental illnesses.

In addition, in 1975, the American Hospital Association (AHA) distributed a document titled *A Patient's Bill of Rights*, which was revised in 1992 (Association of American Physicians and Surgeons, 1995). A copy of these patient rights is framed and posted in a public place in every healthcare facility across the United States. In addition, federal standards developed by the Centers for Medicare & Medicaid Services (CMS) require that each patient be provided with a personal copy of these rights, either at the time of admission to the hospital or long-term care facility or prior to the initiation of care or treatment when admitted to a surgery center, health maintenance organization (HMO), home care, or hospice. In fact, many states have adopted the statement of patient rights as part of their state health code law, which makes them legally enforceable by threat of penalty.

As early as 1950, the American Nurses Association (ANA) developed and adopted an ethical code for professional practice, titled the *Code of Ethics for Nurses with Interpretative Statements,* that has since been revised and updated in 1976, 1985, 2001, and most recently in 2015. This code sets forth nine provisions for professional values and moral obligations in relation to the nurse-patient relationship and in support of the profession and its mission. Lachman (2009a, 2009b) outlines and clarifies the nursing role in this document. The nursing profession's code has been recognized as exemplary and has been used as a template by other health disciplines in crafting their own ethics documents. In the end, however, it is up to the individual healthcare provider to take his or her professional ethics code to heart.

Application of Ethical Principles to Patient Education

In considering the ethical and legal responsibilities inherent in the process of patient education, nurses can turn to a framework of six major ethical principles—including the so-called big four principles initially proposed by Beauchamp and Childress (1977)—that are specified in the ANA's *Code of Ethics* (2015) and in the AHA's *A Patient's Bill of Rights* (1992). These principles are as follows:

Autonomy

The term **autonomy** is derived from the Greek words *auto* ("self") and *nomos* ("law") and refers to the right of self-determination (Tong, 2007). Laws have been passed to protect the patient's right to make choices independently. Informed consent, a government mandate, must be evident in every application for federal funding to support biomedical research. The local IRBs assume the role of judge and jury to determine that this regulation is enforced (Dickey, 2006).

The Patient Self-Determination Act, which was passed by Congress in 1991 (Ulrich, 1999), is a clear example of the principle of autonomy enacted into law. Any healthcare facility, including acute- and long-term care institutions, surgery centers, HMOs, hospices, or home care organizations, that receives Medicare and/or Medicaid funds must comply with the Patient Self-Determination Act. This law requires that, either at the time of hospital admission or prior to the initiation of care or treatment in a community health setting,

> every individual receiving health care be informed in writing of the right under state law to make decisions about his or her health care, including the right to refuse medical and surgical care and the right to initiate advance directives. (Mezey, Evans, Golob, Murphy, & White, 1994, p. 30)

Although ultimate responsibility for discussing treatment options and a plan of care as well as obtaining informed consent rests with the physician, Mezey and colleagues point out that it is the nurse's responsibility to ensure informed decision making by patients. This includes, but is certainly not limited to, advance directives (e.g., living wills, durable power of attorney for health care, and designation of a healthcare agent). Evidence of such instruction must appear in the patient's record, which is the legal document validating that informed consent took place (Hall, Prochazka, & Fink, 2012).

Veracity

Veracity, or truth telling, is closely linked to informed decision making and informed consent. The landmark decision by Justice Cardozo, as mentioned previously, identified an individual's fundamental right to make decisions about his or her own body. This ruling provides a basis in law for patient education or instruction regarding invasive medical procedures. Nurses are often confronted with issues of truth telling, as was exemplified in the *Tuma vs. Board of Nursing* case (Rankin & Stallings, 1990). In the interest of full disclosure of information, the nurse (Tuma) had advised a patient with cancer of alternative treatments without consulting the client's physician. Tuma was sued by the physician for interfering with the medical regimen that he had prescribed for care of this particular patient. Although Tuma was eventually freed from professional misconduct charges, the case emphasizes a significant point of law to be found in the New York State Nurse Practice Act (New York State Nurses Association, 1972), which states that nursing actions must be consistent with current medical therapies prescribed by physicians. However, others insist that failure to instruct the patient properly relative to invasive procedures is equivalent to battery (Creighton, 1986; Hall et al., 2012). Therefore, in some instances, the nurse may find himself or herself in a double bind. If in such a dilemma, the nurse has a variety of actions available. One possibility would be to inform the physician of the professional double bind and engage with him or her in achieving a course of action that best meets the patient's medical needs while respecting the patient's autonomy. The second possibility is to seek out the institutional ethics committee or an ethics consultant for assistance in negotiating interactions with both the physician and the patient (Cisar & Bell, 1995).

Confidentiality

Confidentiality refers to personal information that is protected as privileged information by a healthcare standard or code or legal contract. When this information is acquired from a patient, healthcare providers may not disclose it without consent of that patient. If sensitive information were not to be protected, patients would lose trust in their providers and would be reluctant to openly share problems with them or even seek medical care at all.

A distinction must be made between the terms *anonymous* and *confidential*. Information is anonymous, for example, when a patient's identity cannot be linked to the medical record of that person. Information is confidential when identifying materials that appear on patients' records can be accessed only by the healthcare providers (Tong, 2007). Only under special circumstances may secrecy be ethically broken, such as when a patient has been the victim or subject of a crime to which the nurse or doctor is a witness (Lesnick & Anderson, 1962). Other exceptions to confidentiality occur when nurses or other health professionals suspect or are aware of child or elder abuse, narcotic use, legally reportable communicable diseases, gunshot or knife wounds, or the threat of violence toward someone. To protect others from bodily harm, health professionals are legally permitted to breach confidentiality.

The 2003 updated Health Insurance Portability and Accountability Act (HIPAA) ensures nearly absolute confidentiality related to distributing patient information, unless the patient himself or herself authorizes release of such information (Kohlenberg, 2006). One goal of the HIPAA policy, first enacted by Congress in 1996, is to limit disclosure of patient healthcare information to third parties, such as insurance companies or employers. This law, which requires patients' prior written consent for release of their health information, was never meant to interfere with consultation between professionals but is intended to prevent, for example, "elevator conversations" about private matters of individuals entrusted to the care of health professionals. In a technologically advanced society such as exists in the United States today, this law is a must to ensure confidentiality (Tong, 2007). Currently, in some states and under certain conditions, such as death or impending death, a spouse or members of the immediate family can be apprised of the patient's condition if this information was previously unknown to them. Despite federal and state legislation protecting the confidentiality rights of individuals, the issue of the ethical/moral obligation of the patient with HIV/AIDS or genetic disease, for example, to voluntarily share his or her condition with others who may be at risk remains largely unresolved (Legal Action Center, 2001).

Nonmaleficence

Nonmaleficence is defined as "do no harm" and refers to the ethics of legal determinations that have to do with negligence and/or malpractice. According to Brent (2001), **negligence** is defined as "conduct which falls below the standard established by law for the protection of others against unreasonable risk of harm" (p. 54). She further asserts that the concept of professional negligence "involves the conduct of professionals (e.g., nurses, physicians, dentists, and lawyers) that falls below a professional standard of due care" (p. 55). As clarified by Tong (2007), due care is "the kind of care healthcare professionals give patients when they treat them attentively and vigilantly so as to avoid mistakes" (p. 25). For negligence to exist, there must be a duty between the injured party and the person whose actions (or nonactions) caused the injury. A breach of that duty must have occurred, it must have been the immediate cause of the injury, and the injured party must have experienced damages from the injury (Brent, 2001).

The term **malpractice**, by comparison, "refers to a limited class of negligent activities committed within the scope of performance by those pursuing a particular profession involving highly skilled and technical services" (Lesnick & Anderson, 1962, p. 234). More recently, malpractice has been specifically defined as "negligence, misconduct, or breach of duty by a professional person that results in injury or damage to a patient" (Reising & Allen, 2007). Thus malpractice is limited in scope to those whose life work requires special education and training as dictated by specific educational standards. In contrast, negligence refers to all improper and wrongful conduct by anyone arising out of any activity.

Reising and Allen (2007) describe the most common causes for malpractice claims specifically against nurses, but these causes are also relevant to the conduct of other health professionals within the scope of their practice responsibilities:

1. Failure to follow standards of care
2. Failure to use equipment in a responsible manner
3. Failure to communicate
4. Failure to document
5. Failure to assess and monitor
6. Failure to act as patient advocate
7. Failure to delegate tasks properly

The concept of *duty* is closely tied to the concepts of negligence and malpractice. Nurses' duties are spelled out in job descriptions at their places of employment. Policy and procedure manuals of a particular facility are certainly intended to protect the patient and ensure good quality care, but they also exist to protect both the employee—in this instance, the nurse—and the employer against litigation. Policies are more than guidelines. Policies and procedures determine standards of behavior (duties) expected of employees of a particular institution and can be used in a court of law in the determination of negligence (Weld & Bibb, 2009; Yoder-Wise, 2015).

Beneficence

Beneficence is defined as "doing good" for the benefit of others. It is a concept that is legalized through properly carrying out critical tasks and duties contained in job descriptions; in policies, procedures, and protocols set forth by the healthcare facility; and in standards and codes of ethical behaviors established by professional nursing organizations. Adhering to these various professional performance criteria and principles, including adequate and current patient education, speaks to the nurse's commitment to act in the best interest of the patient. Such behavior emphasizes patient welfare, but not necessarily to the harm of the healthcare provider.

The effort to save lives and relieve human suffering is a duty to do what is right only within reasonable limits. For example, when AIDS first appeared, the cause of and means to control this fatal disease were unknown. Some health professionals protested that the duty of beneficence did not include caring for patients who put them at risk for this deadly, infectious, and untreatable disease. Others maintained that part of the decision to become a health professional involves the acceptance of certain personal risks: It is part of the job. Nevertheless, once it became clear that HIV transmission through occupational exposure was quite small, the majority of healthcare practitioners agreed with the opinion of the AMA that ethically they must treat seropositive patients as long as the providers are competent to do so (Tong, 2007).

Justice

Justice speaks to fairness and the equitable distribution of goods and services. The law is the justice system. The focus of the law is the protection of society; the focus of health law is the protection of the consumer. It is unjust to treat one person better or worse than another person in a similar condition or circumstance, unless a difference in treatment can be justified with good reason. In today's healthcare climate, professionals must be as objective as possible in allocating scarce medical resources in a just manner. Decision making for the fair distribution of resources includes the following criteria as defined by Tong (2007):

1. To each, an equal share
2. To each, according to need
3. To each, according to effort
4. To each, according to contribution
5. To each, according to merit
6. To each, according to the ability to pay (p. 30)

According to Tong (2007), professional nurses may have second thoughts about the application of these criteria in particular circumstances because one or more of the criteria could be at odds with the concept of justice. "To allocate scarce resources to patients on the basis of their social worth, moral goodness, or economic condition rather than on the basis of their medical condition is more often than not wrong" (p. 30).

As noted earlier, the requirement to adhere to *A Patient's Bill of Rights* is legally enforced in most states. In turn, the nurse, or any other health professional, can be subjected to penalty or to litigation for discrimination in denying care. Regardless of his or her age, gender, physical disability, sexual orientation, or race, for example, the client has a right to proper instruction regarding risks and benefits of invasive medical procedures. She or he also has a right to proper instruction regarding self-care activities, such as home dialysis, for example, that are beyond normal activities of daily living for most people.

Furthermore, when a nurse is employed by a particular healthcare facility, she or he enters into a contract to provide nursing services in accordance with the policies of the facility. Failure to provide nursing care (including educational services) based on patient diagnosis or providing substandard care based on client age, diagnosis, culture, national origin, sexual preference, and the like can result in liability for breach of contract with the employing institution (Emanuel, 2000).

Ethics of the Patient–Provider Relationship in Practice Settings

With respect to the patient–provider relationship, nurses and the patients they care for have their own worldviews that come together in the practice setting. These perspectives must be negotiated and understood by each party for the process of patient education to occur with a sense of trust.

It is important to recognize the balance of power that exists between a nurse and a patient. The nurse possesses medical expertise: keys to the patient's health, well-being, and ability to work, play, go to school, or engage in social relationships. For those reasons, the ethics of being a patient typically includes respecting nurses and trusting them to have the patient's best interests at heart. Patients have a moral claim on the nurse's competence and on the use of that competence for the patient's welfare (Pellegrino, 1993).

The blurring of professional–personal boundaries also is an area of ethical importance common to nurses' relationships with their patients. The potential for blurred boundaries between professionals and patients is particularly evident because of the intimacies of the practice setting. Patient education can take place when patients are wearing little clothing, are lying down in a bed, are sharing personal information with the nurse, or are in the context of medically related physical contact. Nurses can use the following specific criteria to distinguish between interactions that are appropriate in the context of the patient educational process and those that are less appropriate or even frankly inappropriate (Martinez, 2000):

- Risk of harm to the patient or to the patient–teacher relationship
- Presence of coercion or exploitation
- Potential benefit to the patient or to the patient–teacher relationship
- Balance of the patient's interests and the teacher's interests
- Presence of professional ideals

These five criteria can assist the teacher in being fully honest with himself or herself regarding the appropriateness of counseling the patient and can serve as an extremely useful guide in uncertain situations.

Nurses are obligated to remain mindful of the power imbalance between themselves and their patients, to put the patient's welfare before their own concerns, and to reflect honestly on the consequences of blurred boundaries to the patient and to their relationship with the patient in the practice setting.

Out of a respect for patient autonomy, a model of medical decision making shared between health professionals and patients has become a priority in the practice setting (deBocanegra & Gany, 2004; Donetto, 2010; Freedman, 2003; Visser, 1998). This model supports imparting health-related information selected by the health professional to the patient for the purposes of the patient making his or her choices and preferences known. Although health professionals engaging in this process may mean well, the unidirectional nature of this model of patient education succeeds in reinforcing the power that health professionals have over patients by virtue of their technical knowledge. Therefore, ethical decision making is necessary in ensuring patients' safety and well-being.

New evidence indicates that concerns may arise regarding healthcare professionals' ethical competency. Park (2012) developed an integrated model consisting of six steps designed to better guide ethical decision making:

1. The identification of an ethical problem
2. The collection of information to verify the problem and develop solutions
3. The development of alternatives for analysis and comparison
4. The selection of the best alternatives and justification
5. The development of diverse, practical ways to implement ethical decisions and actions
6. The evaluation of effects and development of strategies to prevent a similar occurrence

Park (2012) acknowledges that the use of this model does not guarantee ethically right or good decisions, but it does support an improved process of making ethical decisions.

Patients are autonomous agents. They may choose to follow the recommended course of treatment because they trust their health professional and believe that what has been recommended will improve their condition. They may also follow recommendations because they understand the rationale for the treatment, they consider the treatment to be acceptable or at least tolerable, the treatment fits into their lifestyle and values, they can afford it financially, and for many other reasons.

Furthermore, some patients believe that they should behave like good patients by taking all medications or doing all exercises as prescribed, adhering to a recommended diet, not complaining, and so forth, so that their health professional will like them, consider them worthy of their time, and want to continue to take care of them (Buckwalter, 2007; Freedman, 2003). This desire to be a good patient underscores how dependent and vulnerable patients can feel. Even when presenting for a screening mammogram or follow-up urine culture, patients are not at their best. At every medical encounter, there exists the potential for discovering something that merits concern.

In the practice setting, it is plausible that a nurse providing discharge instructions to a patient might not necessarily give the patient a fair share of his or her time or be open to all the patient's questions if the nurse knows he or she will never see that patient again. Admittedly, the better the patient education, the longer the patient will likely remain out of the hospital. However, if the nurse is extremely busy with other competing priorities or is tired from having worked two shifts in a row, he or she may not reflect on how fatigue or work demands lead to a failure to focus primarily on this particular patient's welfare. It may be easier for the nurse to assume a let-someone-else-deal-with-it attitude. Short-term relationships can result in a lack of focus on the welfare, time, and interests of each patient.

All professional nurses will face a conflict of values, ethically and professionally, at some point in their career. Nurses need to demonstrate at all times ethical behaviors. Nurses can take the lead in anticipating ethical challenges and focusing on appropriate professional values. Key to ethical nurse leadership is a willingness to collaborate with colleagues, apply evidence-based practice to remain competent, and invite feedback from others for ethical decision making (Gallagher & Tschudin, 2010).

The Patient's Right to Education and Information

The patient's right to adequate information regarding his or her physical condition, medications, risks, and access to information regarding alternative treatments is specifically spelled out in *A Patient's Bill of Rights* (AHA, 1992; ANA, 2015; Association of American Physicians and Surgeons, 1995; President's Advisory Commission, 1998). As noted earlier, many states have adopted these rights as part of their health code, thus making them legal and enforceable by law. Patients' rights to education and information also are regulated through standards put forth by accrediting bodies such as The Joint Commission (TJC, 2015). Although these standards are not enforceable in the same manner as law, lack of conformity can lead to loss of accreditation, which in turn can hurt the facility's eligibility for third-party payment, such as private and Medicare and Medicaid reimbursement, and also can lead to loss of public confidence in the institution.

All these laws and professional standards serve to ensure the fundamental rights of every person as a consumer of healthcare services. **Table 2–1** outlines the relationship of ethical principles to the laws and professional standards applicable to each principle.

In general, physicians are responsible and accountable for proper patient education. In reality, however, nurses are expected to carry out patient education, which "is central to the culture of nursing as well as to its legal practice" (Redman, 2008, p. 817) according to respective state nurse practice acts. The issue regarding patient education is not necessarily one of failure to teach on anyone's part, but rather lack of proper documentation that teaching has, in fact, been done.

Legal and Financial Implications to Documentation

When the U.S. Congress passed a public law in 1965 creating the entitlements of Medicare and Medicaid, this guaranteed health care for older adults and people who are socioeconomically deprived. The act stressed the importance of disease prevention and rehabilitation in health care. Thus, to qualify for Medicare and Medicaid reimbursement, "a hospital has to show evidence that patient education has been a part of patient care" (Boyd, Gleit, Graham, & Whitman, 1998, p. 26). Proper documentation provides written testimony that patient education has indeed occurred.

Casey (1995) pointed out many years ago that of all lapses in documentation, patient teaching was identified as "probably the most undocumented skilled service because nurses do not recognize the scope and depth of the teaching they do" (p. 257). Lack of documentation continues to reflect negligence in adhering to the mandates of nurse practice acts. This is unfortunate because patient records can be required for court evidence. Appropriate documentation can be the determining factor in the outcome of legal rulings. Pure and simple, if the instruction isn't documented, it didn't occur!

Table 2–1 Linkages Between Ethical Principles, the Law, and Practice Standards

Ethical Principles	Legal Actions/Decisions and Standards of Practice
Autonomy (self-determination)	Cardozo decision regarding informed consent Institutional review boards Patient Self-Determination Act *A Patient's Bill of Rights* Joint Commission/CMS standards
Veracity (truth telling)	Cardozo decision regarding informed consent *A Patient's Bill of Rights* *Tuma* decision Joint Commission/CMS standards
Confidentiality (privileged information)	Privileged information *A Patient's Bill of Rights* Joint Commission/CMS standards HIPAA
Nonmaleficence (do no harm)	Malpractice/negligence rights and duties Nurse practice acts *A Patient's Bill of Rights* *Darling vs. Charleston Memorial Hospital* State health codes Joint Commission/CMS standards
Beneficence (doing good)	*A Patient's Bill of Rights* State health codes Job descriptions Standards of practice Policy and procedure manuals Joint Commission/CMS standards
Justice (equal distribution of benefits and burdens)	*A Patient's Bill of Rights* Antidiscrimination/affirmative action laws Americans with Disabilities Act Joint Commission/CMS standards

Furthermore, documentation is a vehicle of communication that provides critical information to other health professionals involved with the patient's care. Failure to document not only makes other staff potentially liable but also renders the facility liable and in jeopardy of losing its accreditation as well as losing its appropriations for Medicare and Medicaid reimbursement.

Economic Factors in Healthcare Education

In addition to the legal mandates for patient education and the importance of documentation, another ethical principle speaks to both quality of care and justice, which refer to the equitable distribution of goods and services. In the interest of patient care, the patient as a human being has a right to good-quality care regardless of his or her economic status, national origin, race, and the like. Furthermore, health professionals have a duty to ensure that such services are provided, and the healthcare organization has the right to expect that it will receive its fair share of reimbursable revenues for services provided.

Thus, as an employee of a healthcare institution or agency, the nurse has a duty to carry out organizational policies and mandates by acting in an accountable and responsible manner. In an environment characterized by shrinking healthcare dollars, continuous shortages of staff, and dramatically shortened lengths of stay yielding rapid patient turnover, organizations are challenged to be sure their professional staff are competent to provide educational services while at the same time doing so in the most efficient and cost-effective manner possible. This is an interesting dilemma considering that patient education is identified as a legal responsibility of nurses in their state practice acts.

The principle of justice is a critical consideration in patient education. The rapid changes and trends in contemporary health care are, for the most part, economically driven. Described as chaotic by some, the U.S. healthcare system in many ways is challenged to maintain its humanistic and charitable origins that have characterized healthcare services in this country across the decades. Indeed, organizations that provide health care are caught between the need to allocate scarce resources and the necessity to provide just, yet economically feasible, services.

On the one hand, the managed care approach results in shrinking revenues. This trend, in turn, dictates shorter patient stays in hospitals and doing more with less. Despite continued shortages of healthcare personnel in most geographic areas of the United States, health facilities are continuing to expand their clinical offerings into satellite types of ambulatory and home care services in a bid to increase their revenues. On the other hand, these same organizations are held to the exact standards of care written in *A Patient's Bill of Rights* (AHA, 1992). In addition, hospital accreditation is required to be considered eligible for third-party reimbursement in both the public and private sectors. Thus the regulated right of clients to health education carries a corresponding duty of healthcare organizations to provide that service.

Financial Terminology

Given the fact that the role of the nurse as teacher is an essential aspect of care delivery, this section provides an overview of financial terms that directly relate to the delivery of patient education. Such educational services are not provided without having to cover the cost of human and material resources. Thus, it is important to know that expenses are essentially classified into two categories: direct costs and indirect costs (Gift, 1994). The sources of revenue (profit) that an institution or agency can accumulate as a result of patient education efforts are known as cost savings, cost benefit, and cost recovery (Abruzzese, 1992; Ghebrehiwet, 2005; Mitton & Donaldson, 2004; Wasson & Anderson, 1993).

Direct Costs

Direct costs are usually easily identified and predictable expenses, which include personnel salaries, employment benefits, and equipment. This share of an organization's budget is almost always the largest percentage of the total costs to operate any healthcare facility. Because of the labor-intensive function of nursing care delivery, the costs of nurses' salaries and benefits usually account for at least 50% of the total facility budget. Of course, the higher the educational level of nursing staff, the higher the salaries and benefits, and, therefore, the higher the institution's total direct costs.

Time, however, is also considered a direct cost, but it is often difficult to predict how long it will take nurses to plan, implement, and evaluate the individual patient teaching encounters and the educational programs being offered. Although the purpose of salary is to buy an employee's time and particular expertise, planning and carrying out patient education may exceed the time allocated for care, and the nurse educator draws overtime pay. That extra cost may not have been anticipated in the budget planning process. If the time it takes to prepare and offer patient education programs is greater than the financial gain to the institution, the facility may seek other ways of providing this service, such as computerized programmed instruction or a patient television channel.

Also, equipment is classified as a direct cost. No organization can function without proper materials and tools, which also means there is the need to replace them when necessary. Teaching requires written materials, audiovisual tools, and equipment for the delivery of instruction, such as handouts and brochures, models, closed-circuit televisions, computers, and copy machines. Although renting or leasing equipment may sometimes be less expensive than purchasing it, rental and leasing costs are still categorized as direct costs.

Direct costs are divided into two types: fixed and variable. **Fixed costs** are those expenses that are predictable, remain the same over time, and can be controlled. Salaries, for example, are fixed costs because they remain relatively stable and can also be manipulated. The facility usually makes annual decisions to give employee raises, to freeze salaries, or to cut positions, thereby influencing the budgeted amount for direct cost expenditures. In addition, mortgages, loan repayments, and the like are included as fixed costs.

Variable costs are those costs that, in the case of healthcare organizations, depend on volume. The number of meals prepared, for example, depends on the patient census. From an educational perspective, the demand for patient teaching depends on the number and diagnostic types of patients. For example, if the volume of total hip replacement patients is low, educational costs may be high resulting from the fact that intensive one-to-one instruction must be offered to each patient admitted. On the other hand, if the volume of total hip replacement surgeries is high, it is relatively less expensive to provide standardized programs of instruction via group teaching sessions. Supply-related costs—another direct, variable cost—can change depending on the amount and type needed.

Indirect Costs

Indirect costs are those costs not directly related to the actual delivery of an educational program. They include, but are not limited to, institutional overhead such as heating and air conditioning, lighting, space, and support services of maintenance, housekeeping, and security. Such services are necessary and ongoing whether or not a teaching session is in progress.

Hidden costs—a type of indirect cost—cannot be anticipated or accounted for until after the fact. Low employee productivity can produce hidden costs, for example. Organizational budgets are prepared on the basis of what is known and predictable, with projections for variations in patient census included. Personnel budgets are based on levels of staff needed (e.g., number of registered nurses, licensed practical nurses, and nursing assistants) to accommodate the expected patient volume. This is determined by an annual projection of patient days and the number of patients for whom an employee can effectively care on a daily basis. Low productivity of one or two personnel on a nursing unit, for example, can have a significant impact on the workload of others, which in turn leads to low morale and employee turnover. Turnover increases recruitment and new employee orientation costs. In this respect, the costs are appropriately identified as hidden.

Cost Savings

Hospitals incur **cost savings** when patient lengths of stay are shortened or fall within the allotted diagnosis-related group time frames. Patients who have fewer complications and use less expensive services will yield a cost savings for the institution. In an ambulatory care setting, cost savings may occur when patient education keeps people healthy and independent for a longer period of time, thereby preventing overuse of expensive diagnostic testing or inpatient services. Perhaps most important, patient education becomes even more essential when a pattern of early discharge results in frequent readmissions to a facility. In such a scenario, the facility comes under scrutiny by the government for Medicare and Medicaid reimbursements and may be penalized when services are not paid for—in which case any cost savings may be offset by the amount of revenue lost.

Cost Benefit

Cost benefit occurs when there is increased patient satisfaction with the services an institution provides, including educational programs such as childbirth classes, weight and stress reduction sessions, and cardiac fitness and rehabilitation programs. Patient satisfaction is critical to the individual's return for future healthcare services. Such programs may represent an opportunity for an institution to capture a patient population for lifetime coverage.

Cost Recovery

Cost recovery results when either the patient or the insurer pays a fee for educational services that are provided. Cost recovery may be captured by offering health education programs for a fee. Also, under Medicare and Medicaid guidelines, reimbursement may be made for programs and services if they are deemed reasonable, appropriate, and necessary to treat a person's illness or injury (Kaiser Family Foundation, 2005). The key to success in obtaining third-party reimbursement is the ability to demonstrate that as a result of education, patients can manage self-care at home and consequently experience fewer hospitalizations.

To take advantage of cost recovery, hospitals and other healthcare agencies develop and market a number of health education programs that are open to all members of a community. If well attended, these fee-for-service programs can result in revenues for the institution. The critical element, of course, is not just the recovery of costs but also the generation of revenue. **Revenue generation** (i.e., profit) refers to income earned that is over and above the costs of the programs offered.

To offset the dilemma of striving for cost containment in an environment of shrinking fiscal resources, healthcare organizations have developed alternative strategies for patient education to realize cost savings, cost benefit, cost recovery, or revenue generation. For example, Wasson & Anderson (1993) explained that a preoperative teaching program for surgical patients given prior to admission to the hospital was found to lower patient anxiety, increase patient satisfaction, decrease nursing hours devoted to patient education during hospitalization, and lessen the length of the hospital stay.

Program Planning and Implementation

The key elements to consider when planning a patient education offering intended to make revenue include an accurate assessment of direct costs such as paper supplies, printing of program brochures, publicity, rental space, and professional time (based on an hourly rate) required of nurses to prepare and offer the service. If an hourly rate is unknown, a simple rule of thumb is to divide the annual base salary by 2080, which is the standard number of hours for which people working full-time are paid in the course of 1 year.

If the program is to be offered at the facility, there may be no need to plan for a rental fee for space. However, indirect costs such as housekeeping and security should be factored in as an expense. Such a practice not only is good fiscal management but also provides an accounting of the contributions of other departments to the educational efforts of the facility.

Fees for a program should be set at a level high enough to cover the total costs of program preparation and delivery. If an education program is intended to result in cost savings for the facility, such as education classes for patients with diabetes to reduce the number of costly hospital admissions, then the aim may be to break even on costs. In such a case, the price is set by dividing the calculated cost of the program by the number of anticipated attendees. If the goal is for the institution to improve cost benefits, then success can be measured by increased patient satisfaction (as determined by questionnaires or evaluation forms) or by increased use of the facility's services (as determined by record keeping). If the intent is to offer a series of classes for smoking cessation or childbirth preparation to improve the wellness of the community and to generate income for the facility, then the fee is set higher than cost so as to make a profit (cost recovery). An annual report to administration of the time and money spent on education efforts in outpatient and inpatient care units may be required to determine if the institution made a profit in terms of cost savings, cost benefit, or cost recovery (Demeerec, Stouthuysena, & Roodhooft, 2009).

Summary

Ethical and legal dimensions of human rights provide the justification for patient education, particularly as it relates to issues of self-determination and informed consent. These rights are enforced through federal and state regulations and through performance standards of accrediting bodies and professional organizations for implementation at the local level. The nurse's role as teacher is addressed in the individual nurse practice act in the state where nurses are licensed and employed, and by codes of ethics governing professional conduct in various employment settings.

Patient education is a nursing duty that is grounded in justice; that is, the nurse has a legal responsibility to provide education to all patients, regardless of their age, gender, culture, race, ethnicity, literacy level, religious affiliation, or other defining attributes. All patients have a right to receive health education relevant to their physical and psychosocial needs. Justice also dictates that education programs be designed to meet the needs of patients to be informed, self-directed, and in control of their own health, and ultimately of their own destiny.

Review Questions

1. What are the definitions of the terms *ethical*, *moral*, and *legal*, and how do they differ from one another?
2. Which government and professional organizations legislate, regulate, and provide standards to ensure the protection of human rights in matters of health care?
3. How are the six ethical principles applied to the delivery of patient education?
4. What are four examples of direct costs and five examples of indirect costs in the provision of patient education?
5. What are the definitions of the following terms: *fixed direct costs*, *variable direct costs*, *indirect costs*, *cost savings*, *cost benefit*, and *cost recovery*?

Case Study

Laura is a nursing staff member on a medical–surgical unit. She notices that there has been focused attention on one particular patient who is now receiving comfort care measures. The patient does not appear in any distress or pain. The family members, however, have been difficult to manage and have made constant demands for the patient to receive increased doses of medication to be sure their loved one does not suffer. Laura witnesses a staff nurse, who is assigned to the comfort care of the patient, tell another nurse that she is going to give a "nurse's dose" of morphine because she is "tired of the family's criticism" of the care she is giving.

1. What actions should Laura take at this point?
2. Which legal and ethical reasons could Laura rely on to justify the actions she takes?
3. Which of Laura's actions seem the most justified from a moral and ethical standpoint?

References

Abruzzese, R. S. (1992). *Nursing staff development: Strategies for success*. St. Louis, MO: Mosby.

American Hospital Association (AHA). (1975). *A patient's bill of rights*. Chicago, IL: Author.

American Hospital Association (AHA). (1992). *A patient's bill of rights*. Retrieved from http://www .patienttalk.info/AHA-Patient_Bill_of_Rights.htm

American Nurses Association (ANA). (1978). *Model nurse practice act*. Washington, DC: Author.

American Nurses Association (ANA). (2015). *Code of ethics for nurses with interpretive statements*. Washington, DC: Author. Retrieved from http://www.ANACodeofEthicsforNurses.aspx

Association of American Physicians and Surgeons. (1995). *Patients' bill of rights*. Retrieved from http:// www.aapsonline.org/patients/billrts.htm

Beauchamp, T., & Childress, J. (1977). *Principles of biomedical ethics*. New York, NY: Oxford University Press.

Boyd, M. D., Gleit, C. J., Graham, B. A., & Whitman, N. I. (1998). *Health teaching in nursing practice: A professional model* (3rd ed.). Stamford, CT: Appleton & Lange.

Brent, N. J. (2001). *Nurses and the law* (2nd ed.). Philadelphia, PA: Saunders.

Buckwalter, J. G. (2007). The good patient. *New England Journal of Medicine, 357*(25), 2534–2535.

Casey, F. S. (1995). Documenting patient education: A literature review. *Journal of Continuing Education in Nursing, 26*(6), 257–260.

Centers for Disease Control and Prevention. (2005). *Tuskegee timeline*. Retrieved from http://www.cdc .gov/nchstp/od/tuskegee/time.htm

Cisar, N. S., & Bell, S. K. (1995). Informed consent: An ethical dilemma. *Nursing Forum, 30*(3), 20–28.

Creighton, H. (1986). Informed consent. *Nursing Management, 17*(10), 11–13.

Darling v. Charleston Memorial Hospital, 211 N.E.2d 253 (Ill 1965).

deBocanegra, H. T., & Gany, F. (2004). Good provider, good patient: Changing behaviors to eliminate disparities in healthcare. *American Journal of Managed Care, 10*, SP20–SP28.

Demeerec, N., Stouthuysena, K., & Roodhooft, F. (2009). Time-driven activity-based costing in an outpatient clinic environment: Development, relevance and managerial impact. *Health Policy, 92*(2–3), 296–304.

Dickey, S. B. (2006). Informed consent: Ethical issues. In V. D. Lachman (Ed.), *Applied ethics in nursing* (pp. 25–38). New York, NY: Springer.

Donetto, S. (2010). Medical students' views of power in doctor–patient interactions: The value of teacher–learner relationships. *Medical Education, 44*, 187–196.

Dwarswaard, J., & van de Bovenkamp, H. (2015). Self-management support: A qualitative study of ethical dilemmas experienced by nurses. *Patient Education and Counseling, 98*, 1131–1136.

Emanuel, E. J. (2000). Justice and managed care: Four principles for the just allocation of health care resources. *Hastings Center Report, 30*(3), 8–16.

Flook, D. M. (2003). The professional nurse and regulation. *Journal of PeriAnesthesia Nursing, 18*(3), 160–167.

Freedman, T. G. (2003). Prescriptions for health providers: From cancer patients. *Cancer Nursing, 26*(4), 323–330.

Gallagher, A., & Tschudin, V. (2010). Educating for ethical leadership. *Nurse Education Today, 30,* 224–227.

Ghebrehiwet, T. (2005). The ICN code of ethics for nurses: Helping nurses make ethical decisions. *Reflections on Nursing Leadership, 31*(3), 26–28. Retrieved from http://www.nursingsociety.org/RNL/3Q_2005/features/features6.html

Gift, A. G. (1994). Understanding costs. *Clinical Nurse Specialist, 8*(2), 90.

Hall, D. E., Prochazka, A. V., & Fink, A. S. (2012). Informed consent for clinical treatment. *Canadian Medical Association, 184*(5), 533–540.

Hall, J. K. (1996). *Nursing ethics and the law*. Philadelphia, PA: Saunders.

Hall, K. L. (1992). *The Oxford Companion to the Supreme Court of the United States*. New York, NY: Oxford University Press.

The Joint Commission. (2015). *Accreditation, health care, and certification*. Retrieved from http://www.jointcommission.org

Kaiser Family Foundation. (2005). *Navigating Medicare and Medicaid, 2005*. Retrieved from http://kff.org/medicare/7240.cfm

Kohlenberg, E. M. (2006). Patients' rights and ethical issues. In V. D. Lachman (Ed.), *Applied ethics in nursing* (pp. 39–46). New York, NY: Springer.

Lachman, V. D. (2009a). Practical use of the nursing code of ethics: Part I. *MEDSURG Nursing, 18*(1), 55–57.

Lachman, V. D. (2009b). Practical use of the nursing code of ethics: Part II. *MEDSURG Nursing, 18*(3), 191–194.

Legal Action Center. (2001). *HIV/AIDS: Testing, confidentiality, and discrimination*. New York, NY: Legal Action Center of the City of New York.

Lesnick, M. J., & Anderson, B. E. (1962). *Nursing practice and the law*. Philadelphia, PA: Lippincott.

Martinez, R. (2000). A model for boundary dilemmas: Ethical decision-making in the patient–professional relationship. *Ethical Human Sciences and Services, 2*(1), 43–61.

Mezey, M., Evans, L. K., Golob, Z. D., Murphy, E., & White, G. B. (1994). The patient self-determination act: Sources of concern for nurses. *Nursing Outlook, 42*(1), 30–38.

Mikos, C. A. (2004). Inside the nurse practice act. *Nursing Management, 35*(9), 20, 22, 91.

Mitton, C., & Donaldson, C. (2004). Health care priority setting: Principles, practice and challenges. *Cost Effectiveness and Resource Allocation, 2*(3). Retrieved from http://www.resource-allocation.com/content/2/1/3

New York State Nurses Association. (1972). *New York state nurse practice act*. Retrieved from http://www.op.nysed.gov/prof/nurse/nurse-omrdd-mou-regents.htm

Park, E. (2012). An integrated ethical decision-making model for nurses. *Nursing Ethics, 19*(1), 139–159.

Pellegrino, E. (1993). The metamorphosis of medical ethics: A thirty-year retrospective. *Journal of the American Medical Association, 269,* 1158–1162.

President's Advisory Commission on Consumer Protection and Quality in the Healthcare Industry. (1998). *Consumer bill of rights and responsibilities*. Retrieved from http://www.hcquality commission.gov/final/append_a.html

Rankin, S. H., & Stallings, K. D. (1990). *Patient education: Principles and practices.* Philadelphia, PA: Lippincott.

Redman, B. K. (2008). When is patient education unethical? *Nursing Ethics, 15*(6), 813–820.

Reising, D. L., & Allen, P. N. (2007). Protecting yourself from malpractice claims. *American Nurse Today, 2*(2), 39–44.

Rivera, G. (1972). *Willowbrook: A report on how it is and why it doesn't have to be that way.* New York, NY: Vintage Books.

Schloendorff v. Society of New York Hospitals, 211 NY 125, 128, 105 N.E. 92,93 (1914).

Thomas, S. B., & Quinn, S. C. (1991). The Tuskegee Syphilis Study, 1932 to 1972: Implications for HIV education and AIDS risk education programs in the black community. *American Journal of Public Health, 81*(11), 1498–1505. Retrieved from http://ajph.aphapublications.org/cgi/content/abstract/81/11/1498

Tong, R. (2007). *New perspectives in health care ethics.* Upper Saddle River, NJ: Pearson Prentice Hall.

Ulrich, L. P. (1999). *The Patient Self-Determination Act: Meeting the challenges in patient care.* Washington, DC: Georgetown University Press.

U.S. Department of Health and Human Services (USDHHS). (1983). Protection of human subjects: Reports of the President's Commission for the Study of Ethical Problems in Medicine and Biomedical and Behavioral Research. *Federal Register, 481*(146), 34408–34412.

Visser, A. (1998). Ethical issues in patient education and counseling. *Patient Education and Counseling, 35*, 1–3.

Wasson, D., & Anderson, M. (1993). Hospital–patient education: Current status and future trends. *Journal of Nursing Staff Development, 10*(3), 147–151.

Weisbard, A. J., & Arras, J. D. (1984). Commissioning morality: An introduction to the symposium. *Cardozo Law Review, 6*(4), 223–241.

Weld, K. K., & Bibb, S. C. G. (2009). Concept analysis: Malpractice and modern-day nursing practice. *Nursing Forum, 44*(1), 1–10.

Yoder Wise, P. S. (2015). *Leading and managing in nursing* (6th ed.). St. Louis, MO: Mosby.

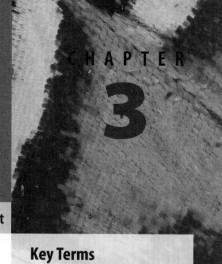

Applying Learning Theories to Healthcare Practice

Margaret M. Braungart | Richard G. Braungart | Pamela R. Gramet

Chapter Highlights

Key Terms

behaviorist learning
cognitive development
cognitive learning
defense mechanisms
feedback
gestalt perspective
hierarchy of needs
humanistic learning
information processing
learning
learning theory
mental practice
motor learning
motor performance
operant conditioning
practice
psychodynamic learning
respondent conditioning
role modeling
social cognition
social learning
spontaneous recovery
stages of motor learning
systematic desensitization
vicarious reinforcement

Objectives

After completing this chapter, the reader will be able to

1. Analyze the major differences in how teaching and learning are approached in the five learning theories.
2. Describe the role of the teacher according to each theory.
3. Discuss at least three ways to motivate learners based on the learning theories.
4. Outline how to teach patients new information using different learning theories.
5. Explain specific teaching strategies to use for each stage of Fitts and Posner's three stages of motor learning.
6. Give examples of how different types of practice and feedback variables in motor learning can be applied to patient teaching.

Learning is defined in this chapter as a relatively permanent change in thinking, emotional functioning, skill, and/or behavior as a result of experience. It is the process by which individuals gain new knowledge or skills and change their thoughts, feelings, attitudes, and actions. Although people in every culture have beliefs about how teaching and learning should occur, there are several major theories of learning that have been tested with research. Each theory describes or explains how learning occurs and has its own vocabulary, perspectives on learning, and generalizations about teaching and learning. The major learning theories are widely applicable and form the foundation for the field of education, health education, psychological and psychiatric counseling, workplace organization and human resources management, and marketing and advertising.

Learning allows individuals to adapt to demands and changing circumstances and is crucial in health care—whether for patients and families struggling with ways to improve their health and adjust to their medical conditions, for students gaining the information and skills necessary to become a nurse, or for staff nurses developing more effective approaches to educating and treating patients. Despite the significance of learning to each individual's development, functioning, health, and well-being, debate continues about how learning occurs, which kinds of experiences assist or slow the learning process, and what ensures that learning becomes relatively permanent.

A **learning theory** is a logical framework describing, explaining, or predicting how people learn. Whether used singly or in combination, learning theories have much to offer the practice of health care. Increasingly, health professionals—including nurses—must demonstrate that they regularly use sound methods and a clear rationale in their education efforts, patient and client interactions, staff management and training, and continuing education and health promotion programs (Ferguson & Day, 2005).

Given the current structure of health care in the United States, nurses, in particular, are often responsible for designing and implementing plans and procedures for improving health education and encouraging wellness. Beyond one's profession, however, knowledge of the learning process relates to nearly every aspect of daily life. Nurses can apply learning theories at the individual, group, and community levels to understand and teach new material and tasks, solve problems, change unhealthy habits, build constructive relationships, manage emotions, and develop effective behavior.

This chapter reviews the psychological and motor learning theories that are useful to health education and clinical practice. Behaviorist, cognitive, and social learning theories are most often applied to patient education as an aspect of professional nursing practice. This chapter also treats psychodynamic and humanistic perspectives as learning theories because they encourage a patient-centered approach to care and add much to our understanding of human motivation and emotions in the learning process. Emotions and feelings, it is argued, are critical to understanding learning (Goleman, 1995), especially in a healthcare setting (Halpern, 2001). Why? Emotional reactions are often learned as a result of experience, they play a significant role in the learning process, and they are a vital consideration when dealing with health, disease, prevention, wellness, medical treatment, recovery, healing, and relapse prevention. In addition, motor learning is included as a theory because it offers a framework for nurses teaching motor skills to patients.

The goals of this chapter are to provide a framework for understanding subsequent chapters in this text and to offer a toolbox of approaches that nurses can use to enhance learning and change in patients, oneself, and others. After completing the chapter, readers should be able to describe the basic principles of learning, discuss various ways in which teaching and learning can be approached, and develop alternative strategies to change attitudes, behaviors, and skills of learners in different settings.

Psychological Learning Theories

This section summarizes some of the basic principles of the behaviorist, cognitive, social learning, psychodynamic, and humanistic learning theories. While reviewing each theory, readers are asked to consider the following questions:

1. What is the basic focus of each theory in explaining how learning and motivation occur?
2. What motivates individuals to learn?
3. What is the role of the nurse as teacher in the learning process?

Behaviorist Learning Theory

According to the **behaviorist learning** theory, learning is the result of connections made between the stimulus conditions in the environment (S) and the individual's responses (R) that follow—sometimes termed the S–R model of learning. Whether dealing with animals or people, the learning process is relatively simple. Generally ignoring what goes on inside the individual, behaviorists closely observe a person's responses to the environment and then manipulate stimuli in the environment to bring about the intended learning and behavioral change. Currently in educational and clinical psychology, behaviorist theories are more likely to be used in combination with other learning theories, especially cognitive theory (Bush, 2006; Dai & Sternberg, 2004). Behaviorist theory continues to be considered useful in nursing practice for the delivery of health care.

To encourage people to learn new information or to change their attitudes and responses, behaviorists recommend altering conditions in the environment and reinforcing positive behaviors after they occur. Motivation is explained as the desire to reduce some drive (drive reduction), such as the desire for food, security, recognition, or money. This is why individuals who are satisfied or who have what they want may have little motivation to learn new behaviors or change old behaviors. Getting behavior to transfer from the initial learning situation to other settings is largely a matter of practice (strengthening habits). Transfer of learning occurs when there is a similarity in the stimuli and responses in the initial learning situation to future situations where behavior is expected to occur. Essentially there are two ways to change behavior and encourage learning using the behaviorist principles of respondent conditioning and operant conditioning.

First identified and demonstrated by Russian physiologist, Ivan Pavlov, **respondent conditioning** (also termed *classical* or *Pavlovian conditioning*) emphasizes the importance of stimulus conditions in the environment and the associations formed in the learning process (Ormrod, 2016). Although it may seem complicated at first, the explanation for learning or conditioning is really quite simple. A neutral stimulus (NS)—a stimulus that has no particular value or meaning to the learner—is paired with a naturally occurring unconditioned or unlearned stimulus (UCS) and unconditioned response (UCR) (**Figure 3–1**). After a few such pairings, the neutral stimulus alone (i.e., without the unconditioned stimulus) elicits the same response. Often without thought or awareness, learning occurs when the newly conditioned stimulus (CS) becomes associated with the conditioned response (CR).

Consider an example from health care. Someone without much experience with hospitals (NS) may visit a relative who is ill. While in the relative's room, the visitor may smell offensive odors (UCS) and feel queasy and light-headed (UCR). After this initial visit and later repeated visits, hospitals (now the CS) may become associated with feeling anxious and nauseated (CR), especially if the visitor smells odors similar to those encountered during the first experience (see Figure 3–1).

Respondent conditioning highlights the importance of what is going on in the environment in health care. Often without thinking or reflection, patients and visitors make associations as a result of their hospital experiences, providing the basis for long-lasting

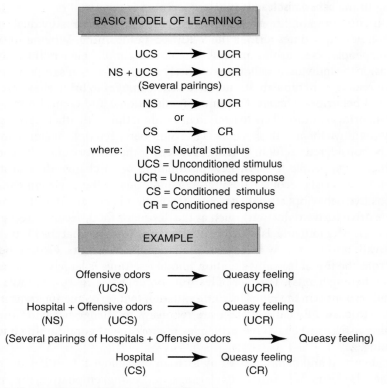

Figure 3–1 Respondent conditioning model of learning

attitudes toward medicine, healthcare facilities, and health professionals. Principles of respondent conditioning may be used to get rid of or eliminate a previously learned response, which is especially useful in teaching people to reduce their anxiety or break bad habits. In this case, old responses or habits can be weakened if the presentation of the conditioned stimulus is not accompanied by the unconditioned stimulus over time. Thus, if the visitor who became dizzy after smelling offensive odors in one hospital goes to other hospitals to see relatives or friends without smelling offensive odors, then her discomfort and anxiety about hospitals may lessen after several such experiences and she has learned—or been conditioned to—a new response to hospitals (CR).

Systematic desensitization is a technique based on respondent conditioning that is used by psychologists to reduce fear and anxiety in their clients (Wolpe, 1982). The assumption is that fear of a particular stimulus or situation is learned; thus it can also be unlearned or extinguished. With this approach, fearful individuals are first taught relaxation techniques. While they are in a state of relaxation, the fear-producing stimulus is gradually introduced at a nonthreatening level so that anxiety and emotions are not aroused. After repeated pairings of the stimulus under relaxed, nonfrightening conditions, the individual learns that no harm will come to him from the once fear-inducing stimulus. Finally, the client is able to confront the stimulus without being anxious and afraid.

In healthcare research, respondent conditioning has been used to extinguish chemotherapy patients' anticipatory nausea and vomiting (Lotfi-Jam et al., 2008; Stockhurst, Steingrueber, Enck, & Klosterhalfen, 2006), while systematic desensitization has been used to treat drug addiction (Piane, 2000), phobias (McCullough & Andrews, 2001), dental anxiety (Armfield & Heaton, 2013; Heaton, Leroux, Ruff, & Coldwell, 2013), and body image disturbance in women with eating disorders (Bhatnagar, Wisniewski, Solomon, & Heinberg, 2013). Also, it has been used to teach children with attention-deficit/hyperactivity disorder (ADHD) or autism to swallow pills (Beck, Cataldo, Slifer, Pulbrook, & Guhman, 2005). Prescription drug advertisers regularly use conditioning principles to encourage consumers to associate a brand-name medication with happy and improved lifestyles; once conditioned, consumers will likely favor the advertised drug over competitors' medications and the much less expensive generic form. As another example, taking the time to help patients relax and reduce their stress when applying some medical intervention—even a painful procedure—lessens the likelihood that patients will build up negative and anxious associations about medicine and health care.

It is worth noting that although a response may appear to be extinguished, it may recover and reappear at any time (even years later), especially when stimulus conditions are similar to those in the initial learning experience. This is called **spontaneous recovery**, which helps us understand why it is so difficult to completely eliminate unhealthy habits and addictive behaviors such as smoking, alcoholism, and drug abuse.

Operant conditioning is another behaviorist approach to learning, which was developed primarily by B. F. Skinner (1974, 1989). **Operant conditioning** focuses on the behavior of the organism and the reinforcement that occurs after the response. A reinforcer is a stimulus or event applied after a response that strengthens the probability that the response will be performed again. Praise, hugs, money, and prizes are examples of positive reinforcers. When specific responses are reinforced on the proper schedule, behaviors can be either increased or decreased.

The best way to increase the probability that a response will occur again is to apply positive reinforcement or rewards after the behavior occurs. As an illustration, although a patient moans and groans as she attempts to get up and walk for the first time after an operation, praise and encouragement (reward) for her efforts at walking (response) will improve the chances that she will continue struggling toward independence.

Decreasing a response, such as breaking a bad habit, is accomplished by using either nonreinforcement or punishment. Skinner (1974) maintained that the simplest way to get rid of a response is not to provide any kind of reinforcement for some unwanted action. For example, unpleasant jokes in the workplace may be handled by showing no reaction. After several such experiences, the joke teller, who more than likely wants attention, may stop his use of offensive humor. Keep in mind, too, that desirable behavior that is ignored may lessen as well if its reinforcement is withheld.

If nonreinforcement does not work, then punishment may be used as a way to decrease responses. For example, if the obnoxious joke teller does not respond to reinforcement, then someone might announce that the joke is offensive to the group, which might serve as punishment—unless, of course, the joke teller most wants attention, and to some people negative attention is preferable to no attention. However, there are risks to using punishment, especially because the learner may become so emotional (sad or angry) that he does not even remember why he is being punished. The purpose of punishment is not to do harm or to serve as a release for anger. The goal is to get someone's attention to decrease a specific behavior and to instill self-discipline. If punishment is used as a last resort, it should be immediate, reasonable, and focused clearly on the behavior, not the person.

For operant conditioning to be effective, it is necessary to assess which kinds of reinforcement are likely to increase or decrease behaviors for each individual. Not every client, for example, finds health practitioners' terms of endearment rewarding. Comments such as, "Very nice job, dear," may be offensive to some clients. A second issue involves the timing of reinforcement. The success of operant conditioning procedures partially depends on when the reinforcement is applied. According to this theory, in the early stages, learning needs to be reinforced every time it occurs. Once a response is well established, however, behavior needs to be reinforced only every so often, because the goal is for the learner to internalize the response and build good habits without being supervised.

Operant conditioning techniques provide relatively quick and effective ways to change behavior. Carefully planned programs using behavior modification procedures can readily be applied to health care. For example, computerized instruction and tutorials for patients and staff rely heavily on operant conditioning principles in structuring learning programs. Operant conditioning has even been used as a simple method of helping staff reduce noise levels in a resource-constrained neonatal intensive care unit (Ramesh et al., 2012). In the clinical setting, the families of patients with chronic back pain have been taught to minimize their attention to the patients whenever they complain and behave in dependent, helpless ways, but to pay a lot of attention when the patients attempt to function independently, express a positive attitude, and try to live as normal a life as possible. Some patients respond so well to operant conditioning that they report experiencing less pain as they become more active and involved. For example, recent studies have shown that operant conditioning by a physiotherapist has proved to be more effective than a placebo as an intervention in reducing short-term pain in patients with subacute low back pain (Bunzli, Gillham, & Esterman, 2011) and as a promising strategy for the prevention of chronic low back pain (Brunner, De Herdt, Minguet, Baldew, & Probst, 2013).

The behaviorist theory is simple and easy to use. It does, however, require careful analysis of what is happening in the environment that affects people's behavior and what factors influence a person's responses. Nevertheless, some criticisms and cautions must be considered. For one thing, learners are assumed to be relatively passive and easily manipulated, which raises the ethical question: Who is to decide what the desirable behavior should be? Too often the desired response is conformity and cooperation to make someone's job easier or more profitable.

In addition, the theory's emphasis on rewards and incentives reinforces and promotes materialistic values and doing things only for some personal gain. Another concern is that research evidence supporting behaviorist theory is often based on animal studies, the results of which may not be applicable to human behavior. A final shortcoming of behaviorist techniques is that changed behavior in patients may weaken over time, especially once they are back in the environment that may have caused their problems in the first place. The basic principles of behaviorist learning are:

- Focus on the learner's drives, the external factors in the environment that influence a learner's associations, and on reinforcements that increase or decrease responses.
- The teacher's task is first to assess conditions in the environment that lead to specific responses, the learner's past habits and history of S–R connections, and what is reinforcing the learner. Then teachers must effectively manipulate conditions to build new associations, provide appropriate reinforcement, and allow for practice to strengthen connections between stimuli in the environment and a person's responses or behavior.

The next section moves from focusing on responses and behavior to considering the role of mental processes in learning.

Cognitive Learning Theory

In contrast to behaviorist theory, **cognitive learning** theory focuses on what goes on inside the mind of the learner. Cognitive theory is assumed to be made up of a number of subtheories and is widely used in education and counseling. According to this perspective, for individuals to learn, they must change their perceptions and thoughts and form new understandings and insights. The individual largely directs the learning process by organizing information based on what is already known, and then reorganizing the information into a new understanding.

Unlike behaviorists, cognitive psychologists maintain that rewarding people for their behavior is not necessary for learning. More important are learners' goals and expectations, which create tensions that motivate them to act. Teachers and those trying to influence the learning process must recognize that any learning situation is influenced by learners' past experiences, perceptions, and ways of incorporating and thinking about information in relation to their goals, expectations, and the social influences on the situation. To promote remembering, the learner must think about or act on the information. Similar patterns in the initial learning situation and subsequent situations aid memory and the ability to transfer learning from one situation to the next.

Cognitive learning theory includes several well-known perspectives, such as gestalt, information processing, cognitive development, and social cognition theory. More recently, attempts have been made to incorporate considerations related to emotions within cognitive theory. Each of these perspectives emphasizes a particular feature of cognition; collectively, when pieced together, they indicate much about what goes on inside the learner.

One of the oldest psychological theories is the **gestalt perspective**, which emphasizes the importance of perception in learning and laid the groundwork for the various other cognitive perspectives that followed (Kohler, 1947, 1969; Murray, 1995). Rather than focusing on individual stimuli, gestalt refers to the configuration or patterned organization of cognitive elements, reflecting the maxim that "the whole is greater than the sum of its parts." A principal assumption is that each person perceives, interprets, and responds to any situation in his or her own way. While many gestalt principles worth knowing have been identified (Hilgard & Bower, 1966), the discussion here focuses on those that relate to health care.

A basic gestalt principle is that people strive toward simplicity, equilibrium, and regularity. For example, study the bewildered faces of some patients listening to a complex, detailed explanation about their disease; what they actually desire most is a simple, clear explanation that settles their uncertainty and relates directly to them and their familiar experiences. Another central gestalt principle is that perception is selective, which has several implications. First, because no one can attend to all possible surrounding stimuli at any given time, individuals pay attention to certain features of an experience while screening out or ignoring other features. Patients who are in severe pain or who are worried about their hospital bills, for example, may not attend to patient education information, no matter how well presented. Second, what individuals select to pay attention to and what they ignore are influenced by a host of factors such as past experiences, needs, motives and attitudes, and the particular structure of the information and the situation (Sherif & Sherif, 1969). Because individuals vary widely with regard to these and other characteristics, they will perceive, interpret, and respond to the same event in different ways, perhaps distorting information to fit their goals, expectations, and what they want to hear. This tendency helps explain why an approach that is effective with one client may not work with another client. People with chronic illnesses—even different people with the same illness—are not alike, and helping any patient with disease or disability includes recognizing each person's unique perceptions and subjective experiences (Imes, Clance, Gailis, & Atkeson, 2002).

Information processing is a second cognitive perspective that emphasizes thinking, reasoning, the way information is encountered and stored, and memory functioning

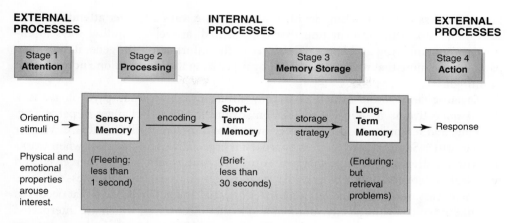

Figure 3–2 Information-processing model of memory

(Gagné, 1985; Sternberg & Sternberg, 2012). How information is incorporated and retrieved is useful for nurses to know, especially in relation to older people's learning (Hooyman & Kiyak, 2011; Kessels, 2003). **Figure 3–2** illustrates an information-processing model of memory functioning.

The stages are:

- *Attention.* Certain information is focused on while other information in the environment is ignored. Attention is viewed as the key to learning. Thus, if a patient is not concentrating on what the nurse is saying, perhaps because the patient is weary or distracted, it would be wise to try the explanation at another time when the patient is more receptive and attentive.

- *Processing.* Information is processed using one or more of the senses. Here it becomes important to consider the client's preferred mode of sensory processing (visual, hearing, or by using touch or motor skills). It is also important to determine whether there are any sensory deficits, such as hearing loss or poor eyesight.

- *Memory storage.* Information is transformed and incorporated (encoded) briefly into short-term memory, after which it suffers one of two fates: The information is disregarded and forgotten, or it is stored in long-term memory. Information is stored in long-term memory by using a strategy, such as forming a mental picture (visual imagery), associating the information with what is already known, repeating or rehearsing the information, or breaking the information into smaller units or chunks. Although long-term memories are enduring, a central problem is retrieving the stored information at a later time.

- *Action.* The action or response that the individual makes is based on how the information was processed and stored. Responses must be observed carefully in case corrections need to be made, although there is always a question as to whether any performance is a true indicator of someone's learning and competence. People may not really know the answer but guess correctly, or they may know the answer but not perform correctly for some reason.

From this perspective, teaching involves assessing the ways a learner attends to, processes, and stores the information that is presented, as well as finding ways to encourage remembering and being able to recall the information. In general, cognitive psychologists note that memory is helped by organizing the information and making it meaningful.

Cognitive development, which is heavily influenced by gestalt psychology, is a third perspective on learning. It focuses on advancements and changes in perceiving, thinking, and reasoning as individuals grow and mature (Crandell, Crandell, & Vander Zanden, 2012; Santrock, 2013). This approach is especially useful to know when working with children and teenagers. How information and experiences are perceived and represented depends on an individual's stage of development and readiness to learn. A principal assumption is that learning is a sequential and active process that occurs as the child interacts with the environment and makes discoveries, which are interpreted in keeping with what she knows (schema) and is capable of understanding.

Jean Piaget is the best known of the cognitive developmental theorists. His observations of children's perceptions and thought processes at different ages have contributed much to our recognition of the special ways that young people reason, the changes in their abilities to reason, and the limitations in their ability to understand, communicate, and perform (Piaget & Inhelder, 1969). By watching, asking questions, and listening to children, Piaget identified and described four successive stages of cognitive development (sensorimotor, preoperational, concrete operations, and formal operations) that unfold sequentially over the course of infancy, early childhood, middle childhood, and adolescence. (See Chapter 5 for more on developmental stages.)

According to this theory, children take in information as they interact with people and the environment. They either make their experiences fit with what they already know (assimilation) or change their perceptions and interpretations in keeping with the new information (accommodation). Nurses and family members need to determine what children are perceiving and thinking in a given situation. As an illustration, young children usually do not comprehend fully that death is final. They respond to the death of a loved one in their own way, perhaps asking God to give back the dead person or believing that if they act like a good person, the deceased loved one will return to them (Gardner, 1978).

Advocates of the cognitive development perspective have some differences in their views that are worth considering by nurses. For example, while Piaget stresses the importance of perception in learning and views children as little scientists exploring, interacting, and discovering the world in a relative solitary manner, Russian psychologist Lev Vygotsky (1986) emphasizes the significance of language, social interaction, and adult guidance in the learning process. When teaching children, Vygotsky says the job of adults is to interpret, respond, and give meaning to children's actions. Rather than the discovery method favored by Piaget, Vygotsky encourages clear, well-designed instruction that is carefully structured to advance each person's thinking and learning.

In practice, some children may learn more effectively by discovering and putting pieces together on their own, whereas other children benefit from a more social and directive approach. It is the nurse's responsibility to identify the child's or teenager's stage of thinking, to provide experiences at an appropriate level for the child to actively discover and participate in the learning process, and to determine whether a child learns best through language and social interaction or through perceiving and experimenting in his or her own way.

What do cognitive developmental theorists say about adult learning? First, some adults never reach the formal operations stage. These adults may learn better from simple, concrete approaches to health education. In addition, while some older adults may demonstrate an advanced level of reasoning gained from their wisdom and life experiences, others may reflect lower stages of thinking resulting from lack of education, disease, depression, stress, or the effects of medications (Hooyman & Kiyak, 2011). Research indicates that adults generally do better when offered opportunities for self-directed learning (emphasizing learner control, independence, and initiative), a clear rationale for learning, a problem-oriented rather than subject-oriented approach, and opportunities to use their experiences and skills to help others (Tennant, 2006). Also, teachers must keep in mind that anxiety, the demands of adult life, and childhood experiences may interfere with learning in adulthood.

The **social cognition** approach is a fourth perspective in cognitive psychology, which emphasizes the effects of social factors on perception, thought, and motivation. According to this view, the players in any healthcare setting would be expected to have differing perceptions, interpretations, and responses to a situation that are strongly colored by their social and cultural experiences. For example, patients with certain religious views or a particular type of parental upbringing may believe that their disease is a punishment for their sins, whereas other patients may blame their disease on the actions of others. From this perspective, patients' explanations for their diseases may or may not promote wellness and well-being. The route to changing health behaviors is to change distorted beliefs and explanations. With America's rapidly changing age and ethnic composition, the social cognition approach will become especially useful in the healthcare setting.

Cognitive theory has been criticized for neglecting emotions, and recent efforts have been made to incorporate considerations related to emotions within a cognitive framework (Eccles & Wigfield, 2002; Goleman, 1995; Greene, Sommerville, Nystrom, Darley, & Cohen, 2001; Hoffman, 2000). When working with patients, family, and staff, nurses need to exhibit and encourage empathy and emotional intelligence, which refers to managing one's emotions, motivating oneself, reading the emotions of others, and working effectively in interpersonal relationships (Goleman, 1995). Emotional intelligence can play a moderating role in the experience of job stress for nurses (Gorgens-Ekermans & Brand, 2012; Karimi, Leggat, Donohue, Farrell, & Couper, 2014), and high emotional intelligence may increase well-being in female nursing and allied health students by reducing the experience of stress (Ruiz-Aranda, Extremera, & Pineda-Galan, 2014).

H. O'Sullivan and McKimm (2014) stress the importance of emotions in the everyday practice of medical care. Research indicates that the development of cognitive emotional perspectives in self and patients is associated with a greater likelihood of healthy behavior, psychological well-being, optimism, and meaningful social interactions (Brackett, Lopes, Ivcevic, Mayer, & Salovey, 2004). When applied to health care, cognitive learning theory encourages an appreciation of the individuality and rich diversity in how people learn and process experiences. Cognitive theory has proved useful in formulating exercise programs for breast cancer patients (Rogers et al., 2004), understanding individual differences in bereavement (Stroebe, Folkman, Hansson, & Schut, 2006), and dealing with adolescent depression in girls (Papadakis, Prince, Jones, & Strauman, 2006). The challenge in teaching is to identify a learner's level of cognitive development, his or her goals and expectations, ways of perceiving and processing information, and the social influences that affect learning. Once identified, teachers can find novel ways to encourage new insights and to solve problems. To summarize, the basic principles of cognitive learning theory are:

- Focus on internal factors within learners, such as their developmental stage of reasoning; perceptions; thoughts; ways of processing and storing information in memory; and the influence of social factors on attitudes, thoughts, and actions. Realize that learning is motivated by the learner's goals and expectations, as well as by a feeling of imbalance, tension, and a desire to restore equilibrium.
- The role of the teacher is first to assess each learner's developmental stage, goals and expectations, preferred style of learning, and ways of processing, storing, and retrieving information. The next steps are to foster curiosity (imbalance); organize learning experiences and make them meaningful; encourage understanding, insight, problem solving, and creativity in learners; and keep learning simple and at an appropriate level.

The next learning theory combines principles from both the behaviorist and cognitive theories.

Social Learning Theory

Most learning theories assume the individual must have direct experiences in order to learn. According to the **social learning** theory, much of learning occurs by observation—watching other people and determining what happens to them. Learning is often a social process, and other individuals, especially significant others, provide compelling examples as role models for how to think, feel, and act.

Social learning theory is largely based on the work of Albert Bandura (1977, 2001), who mapped out a perspective on learning that includes consideration of the personal characteristics of the learner, behavior patterns, and the environment. In early discussions of this theory, Bandura emphasized behaviorist features and the imitation of role models; later, the focus shifted to cognitive considerations, and more recently, Bandura's attention has turned to the impact of social factors and the social context within which learning and behavior occur. **Figure 3–3** illustrates the dynamics of social learning based on Bandura's work.

Role modeling is a central concept of the social learning theory. As an example, a more experienced nurse who demonstrates desirable professional attitudes and behaviors sometimes serves as a mentor for a less experienced nurse, while medical students, interns, and residents are mentored by attending physicians. **Vicarious reinforcement** is another concept from social learning theory and involves viewing other people's

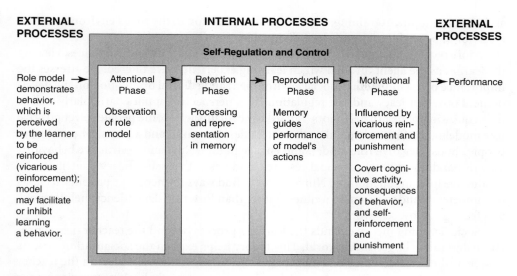

Figure 3–3 Social learning theory

emotions and determining whether role models are perceived as rewarded or punished for their behavior. Reward is not always necessary, however, and a learner may imitate the behavior of a role model even when no reward is available to either the role model or the learner. Nevertheless, in many cases, whether the model is viewed by the observer as rewarded or punished may have a direct influence on learning. This relationship may be one reason why it is difficult to attract health professionals to geriatric care. Although some highly impressive role models work in this field, geriatric health care is often accorded lower status with less pay in comparison to other specialty areas.

Although social learning theory is based partially on behaviorist principles, the self-regulation and control that the individual exerts in the learning process is critical and reflects cognitive principles. Bandura (1977) outlines a four-step, largely internal process that directs social learning. As seen in Figure 3–3, the first step in Bandura's model is the attentional phase, a necessary condition for any learning to occur. Research indicates that role models with high status and competence are more likely to be observed, although the learner's own characteristics (needs, self-esteem, competence) may be the more significant determiner of attention. Second is the retention phase, which involves the storage and retrieval of what was observed. Third is the reproduction phase, when the learner copies the observed behavior. Mental rehearsal, immediate enactment, and corrective feedback strengthen the reproduction of behavior. Fourth is the motivational phase, which indicates the learner's level of motivation to perform a certain type of behavior.

Reinforcement or punishment of a role model's behavior, the learning situation, and the appropriateness of subsequent situations where the behavior is to be displayed all combine to affect a learner's performance (Bandura, 1977; Gage & Berliner, 1998). This organized approach to learning, which is well suited to conducting patient education and staff development training, requires paying attention to the social environment, the behavior to be performed, and the individual learner (Bahn, 2001).

More recently, Bandura (2001) shifted his focus to sociocultural influences, viewing the learner as the agent through which learning experiences are filtered. He stresses the importance of the individual's social environment and cultural orientation on the development of self-efficacy and self-regulation. This perspective applies particularly well to the acquisition of health behaviors. It partially explains why some people select positive role models and effectively regulate their attitudes, emotions, and actions, whereas other people choose negative role models and engage in unhealthy and destructive behaviors. One of Bandura's (2001) principal research findings is that self-efficacy contributes to productive human functioning. Nurses need to find ways to encourage patients' feelings of competency and to promote wellness rather than fostering dependency, helplessness, and feelings of low self-worth.

Social learning theory extends the learning process beyond the teacher–learner relationship to the larger social world. This theory helps explain the socialization process as well as the breakdown of behavior in society. Responsibility is placed on the teacher or leader to act as a positive role model and to choose socially healthy experiences for individuals to observe and repeat (requiring the careful evaluation of learning materials for stereotypes, mixed or hidden messages, and negative effects). Yet simple exposure to role models correctly performing a behavior that is rewarded (or performing some undesirable behavior that is punished) does not guarantee learning. Attention to the learner's self-system and the dynamics of self-regulation may help sort out the varying effects of the social learning experience.

In health care, nurses and other health professionals have applied social learning principles to working with teenage mothers (Stiles, 2005), developing a sexual counseling intervention for post-myocardial infarction patients (Steinke, Mosack, Hertzog, & Wright, 2012), facilitating simulation learning (Bethards, 2014; Burke & Mancuso, 2012), exploring the risk of obesity (Christakis & Fowler, 2007), and the dynamics of smoking cessation (Christakis & Fowler, 2008).

The basic principles of social learning theory are:

- Focus on role models, the reinforcement that a model has received, the social environment, and the self-regulating processes within the learner.
- The role of the teacher is to act as a stellar role model, to use effective role models in teaching that are rewarded for their behavior, to assess the internal regulation of the learner, and to provide feedback for the learner's performance.

The final two theories reviewed in this chapter focus on the importance of emotions and feelings in the learning process.

Psychodynamic Learning Theory

Although not usually treated as a learning theory, some of the concepts from **psychodynamic learning** theory (based on the work of Sigmund Freud and his followers) have significant implications for learning and changing behavior (Hilgard & Bower, 1966; Slipp, 2000). Largely a theory of motivation, the emphasis in psychodynamic theory is on emotions rather than on responses to the environment or on perceptions and thoughts. A central principle of this theory is the notion that behavior may be conscious or unconscious—in other words, people may or may not be aware of their motivations and why they feel, think, and act as they do.

According to the psychodynamic view of personality development, the most primitive source of motivation comes from the id, which involves our most basic instincts, impulses, and desires. The id includes two components: *eros* (the desire for pleasure and sex, sometimes called the "life force") and *thanatos* (aggressive and destructive impulses, or "death wish"). Patients who survive or die despite all predictions to the contrary provide illustrations of such primitive motivations. The id, according to Freud, operates on the basis of the pleasure principle—to seek pleasure and avoid pain. For example, patient education provided by nurses who go through the motions of presenting content without much enthusiasm or emotion inspire few patients to listen to the information or follow the advice being given. This does not mean, however, that only pleasurable patient education encounters are acceptable (Hilgard & Bower, 1966).

The id, with its primitive drives, is held in check by the superego, which involves the societal values and standards children are taught. The superego forms the basis for a conscience. According to Freud, if a conscience is not formed by adolescence, it is unlikely to develop later in life. Because the id and superego are in such conflict, they need to be mediated by the ego, which operates on the basis of the reality principle. Thus, rather than insisting on immediate gratification, people learn to take the long road to pleasure and to weigh the choices in the conflict between the id and the superego (Hilgard & Bower, 1966).

Healthy ego (self) development is an important consideration in healthcare fields. For example, patients with ego strength can cope with painful medical treatments because they recognize the long-term value of enduring discomfort and pain to achieve a positive outcome. Patients with weak ego development, in contrast, may miss their appointments and treatments or engage in short-term pleasurable activities that work against their healing and recovery. Helping patients develop ego strength and adjust realistically to a changed body image or lifestyle brought about by disease and medical interventions is a significant aspect of the learning and healing process.

Nurses and other health professionals also require personal ego strength to cope with the numerous predicaments in the everyday practice of delivering care as they face conflicting values, ethical responsibilities, and medical demands. Professional burnout, for example, is rooted in an overly idealized concept of the healthcare role and unrealistic expectations for the self in performing the role. Malach-Pines (2000) notes that burnout may stem from nurses' childhood experiences with lack of control.

A particularly useful psychodynamic concept for health professionals to know involves the use of ego **defense mechanisms**. When the ego is threatened, as can easily occur in a stressful healthcare setting, defense mechanisms may be employed to protect the self. The short-term use of defense mechanisms is a way of coming to grips with reality. The danger arises from the overuse of or long-term reliance on defense mechanisms, which allows individuals to avoid reality and may act as a barrier to learning and transfer.

Table 3–1 Ego Defense Mechanisms: Ways of Protecting the Self From a Perceived Threat

Denial: Ignoring or refusing to acknowledge the reality of a threat
Rationalization: Excusing or explaining away a threat
Displacement: Taking out hostility and aggression on other individuals rather than directing anger at the source of the threat
Depression: Keeping unacceptable thoughts, feelings, or actions from conscious awareness
Regression: Returning to an earlier (less mature, more primitive) stage of behavior as a way of coping with a threat
Intellectualization: Minimizing anxiety by responding to a threat in a detached, abstract manner without feeling or emotion
Projection: Seeing one's own unacceptable characteristics or desires in other people
Reaction formation: Expressing or behaving the opposite of what is really felt
Sublimation: Converting repressed feelings into socially acceptable action
Compensation: Making up for weaknesses by excelling in other areas

Table 3–1 describes some of the more commonly used defense mechanisms. Because of the stresses involved in health care, knowledge of defense mechanisms is useful, whether for nursing students who are struggling with the challenges of nursing education; staff nurses who are dealing with the challenges of working in hospitals, community agencies, and long-term care facilities; or patients and their families who are learning to cope with illness.

As an example of defense mechanisms in health care, Kübler-Ross (1969) points out that many terminally ill patients' initial reaction to being told they have a serious threat to their health and well-being is to employ the defense mechanism of denial. Patients typically find it too overwhelming to process the information that they are likely to die. Although most patients gradually accept the reality of their illness, the dangers are that if they remain in a state of denial, they may not seek treatment and care, and if their illness is contagious, they may not protect others against infection.

In turn, a common defense mechanism employed by healthcare staff is to intellectualize the significance of disease and death rather than to deal with these issues realistically at an emotional level. This defense mechanism may contribute to the reported tendency of oncologists to often ignore, rather than address, the emotions that patients express during communication (Friedrichsen & Strang, 2003; Friedrichsen, Strang, & Carlsson, 2000; Pollak et al., 2007). One study found that oncologists, in responding to patients expressing fear, more often addressed the topic causing the fear rather than addressing the emotion itself (Kennifer et al., 2009). Telford, Kralik, and Koch (2006) report that nurses may strive to buttonhole terminally ill patients within a denial–acceptance framework too quickly and, as a result, may not listen to patients as they attempt to tell their stories and interpret their illness experiences. Protecting the self (ego) by dehumanizing patients and treating them as diseases and body parts rather than as whole individuals (with spiritual, emotional, and physical needs) is an occupational hazard for nurses and other health professionals.

Another central assumption of psychodynamic theory is that personality development occurs in stages, with much of adult behavior derived from earlier childhood experiences and conflicts. For example, people's behavior when they are sick may reflect their emotional feelings and conflicts from childhood. One of the most widely used models of personality development is Erikson's (1968) eight stages of life, a model organized around a psychosocial crisis to be resolved at each stage. For example, during infancy, the psychosocial crisis to be resolved is trust versus mistrust. The early childhood years involve issues of autonomy versus doubt, followed by initiative versus guilt. The school-aged child comes to terms with industry versus inferiority. Adolescence involves the crisis of intimacy versus isolation. Middle-aged adults focus on generativity versus stagnation. Older adults struggle with integrity versus despair. Erickson noted that the two most significant periods of personality growth occur during adolescence and older adulthood—an important observation for health professionals to consider when working with members of these two age groups. (See Chapter 5 for more on developmental stages.)

Treatment regimens, communication, and health education need to include considerations of the patient's stage of personality development. For example, in working with 4- and 5-year-old patients, where the crisis defined by Erikson is initiative versus guilt, nurses should encourage the children to offer their ideas and to make and do things themselves. Staff also must be careful not to make these children feel guilty for their illness or misfortune. As a second example, the adolescent's psychosocial developmental needs to have friends and to find an identity require special attention in health care. Adolescent patients may need help and support in adjusting to a changed body image and in addressing their fears of weakness, lack of activity, and social isolation. One danger is that young people may treat their illness or impairment as a significant dimension of their identity and self-concept.

The psychodynamic approach reminds nurses to pay attention to emotions, unconscious motivations, and the psychological growth and development of all those involved in health care and learning. The teacher's role is to listen and ask questions. Teachers need to recognize how conscious and unconscious motivations affect learning and to work with id–superego conflicts. The goal is to promote ego strength in learners. Forgetting information may be due to a desire not to remember it or as a result of emotional barriers to learning. Psychodynamic theory is well suited to understanding patient and family noncompliance (Menahern & Halasz, 2000), trauma and loss (Duberstein & Masling, 2000), palliative care and the deeply emotional issues of terminal illness (Chochinov & Breitbart, 2000), the anxieties of working with long-term psychiatric residents (Goodwin & Gore, 2000), and the stress of working with people who have learning disabilities and complex needs (Storey, Collis, & Clegg, 2011). It can even be useful in helping nursing students reflect on the emotional issues arising in their clinical placements (Allan, 2011) and in understanding why some nurse managers use bullying techniques and fail to formally report incidents of violence and aggression (Ferns, 2006).

One problem with the psychodynamic approach is that much of the analysis of learners is open to different interpretations. Health professionals' biases, emotional conflicts, and motivations may distort their evaluation of other persons and situations. Psychodynamic theory also can be used inappropriately; it is not the job of nurses with little clinical psychology or psychiatric training to probe into the private lives and feelings of patients so as to uncover deep, unconscious conflicts. Another danger is that nurses and other health professionals may depend on the many psychodynamic principles as reasons to explain away, rather than deal with, people as individuals who need emotional care. When applied to learning, the basic principles of psychodynamic theory are:

- Focus on the learner's personality development, significant childhood experiences, conscious and unconscious motivations, id–ego–superego conflicts, and defensive behaviors.
- The teacher's role is to listen, ask probing questions about motivations and wishes, assess emotional barriers to learning, and make learning pleasurable while working to promote ego strength in learners.

Humanistic Learning Theory

Underlying the **humanistic learning** theory is the assumption that each individual is unique and that all individuals have a desire to grow in a positive way. Unfortunately, say the humanists, positive psychological growth may be damaged by some of society's values and expectations (e.g., males are less emotional than females, some ethnic groups are inferior to others, making money is more important than caring for people) and by adults' mistreatment of their children and one another (e.g., inconsistent or harsh discipline, humiliation and belittling, abuse and neglect). Spontaneity, the importance of emotions and feelings, the right of individuals to make their own choices, and human creativity are the cornerstones of a humanistic approach to learning (Rogers, 1994; Snowman & McCown, 2015). Humanistic theory is especially compatible with nursing's focus on caring and patient centeredness—an orientation that is increasingly being challenged by the emphasis in medicine and health care on science, technology, cost efficiency, for-profit medicine, bureaucratic organization, and time pressures.

Like the psychodynamic theory, the humanistic theory is largely a motivational theory. From a humanistic perspective, the motivation to act stems largely from each person's needs, feelings about the self, and the desire to grow in positive ways. Remembering information and transferring learning to other situations are helped by encouraging curiosity and a positive self-concept, as well as having open situations where people respect individuality and freedom of choice. Under such conditions, flexibility in problem solving and creativity is enhanced.

One of the best known humanistic theorists is Abraham Maslow (1954, 1987), who identified a **hierarchy of needs** (**Figure 3–4**) to explain human motivation. At the bottom of Maslow's hierarchy are physiological needs (food, water, warmth, sleep); next come safety needs; then the need for belonging and love; followed by self-esteem. At the top of the hierarchy is the need for self-actualization (maximizing one's potential). Within this model, it is assumed that basic-level needs must be met before individuals can be concerned with learning and self-actualizing. Thus clients who are hungry, tired,

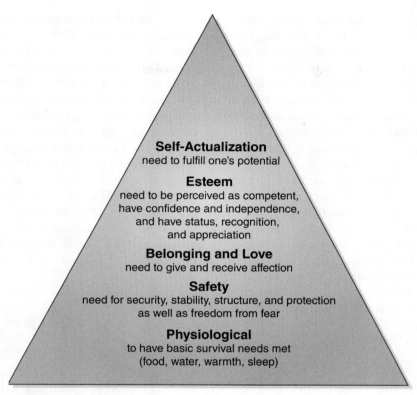

Figure 3–4 Maslow's hierarchy of needs

Modified from Maslow, A. (1987). *Motivation and personality* (3rd ed.). New York, NY: Harper & Row.

and in pain are motivated to get these biological needs met before they will be open to learning about their illness, rules for self-care, and health education. Although this model is intuitively appealing, research has not been able to support Maslow's hierarchy of needs with much consistency. For example, although some people's basic needs may not be met, they may nonetheless engage in creative activities, extend themselves to other people, and enjoy learning (Pfeffer, 1985).

Besides personal needs, humanists believe that self-concept and self-esteem are necessary considerations in any learning situation. The therapist Carl Rogers (1961, 1994) argues that what people want most is unconditional positive self-regard (the feeling of being loved without strings attached). Experiences that are threatening, coercive, and judgmental undermine the ability and enthusiasm of individuals to learn. Thus, it is essential that those in positions of authority convey a fundamental respect for the people with whom they work. If a nurse is prejudiced against patients with AIDS, for example, then little will be healing or therapeutic in that nurse's relationship with them until she is genuinely able to feel respect for each patient as an individual.

Rather than acting as an authority, say humanists, the role of any educator or leader is to serve as a facilitator (Rogers, 1994). Listening—rather than talking—is the skill needed. Because the uniqueness of the individual is fundamental to the humanistic perspective, much of the learning experience is based on a direct relationship between the teacher and the learner, with instruction being tailored to the needs, self-esteem, and positive growth of each learner. Learners are the ones who choose what is to be learned. Teachers serve as resource persons whose job is to encourage learners to make wise choices. Because the central focus is on learners' perceptions, desires, and decision making, the humanistic orientation is referred to as a learner-directed approach (Snowman & McCown, 2015). Mastering information and facts is not the central purpose of the humanistic model of learning. Encouraging curiosity, enthusiasm, initiative, and responsibility is much more important and enduring and should be the primary goal of any educational effort. As an illustration, rather than inserting health education videos into television sets for patients in hospitals to view or routinely distributing lots of pamphlets and pages of small-print instructions, for example, the humanistic perspective indicates efforts should be devoted to establishing rapport and becoming emotionally attuned to patients and their family members.

Humanistic psychology stresses that feelings and emotions are the keys to learning, communication, and understanding. Humanists worry that in today's stressful society, people can easily lose touch with their feelings, which sets the stage for emotional problems and difficulties in learning (Rogers, 1961). To humanists, "Tell me how you feel" is a much more important instruction than "Tell me what you think" because thoughts and "the shoulds" may be at odds with true feelings. Humanistic principles are the foundation of self-help groups, wellness programs, and palliative care. They are also well suited to working with children and young patients undergoing separation anxiety caused by illness, surgery, and recovery (Holyoake, 1998), and to working in the areas of mental health and palliative care (Barnard, Hollingum, & Hartfiel, 2006). As in psychodynamic theory, a principal emphasis is on the healing nature of the therapeutic relationship (Pearson, 2006) and the need for health professionals to learn and grow from their healthcare experiences (Block & Billings, 1998).

The humanistic theory has its weaknesses as well. Research has not been able to substantiate some of its strongest claims, and the theory has been criticized for promoting self-centered learners who cannot take criticism or compromise. The touchy-feely approach of humanism makes some learners and educators feel truly uncomfortable. Moreover, information, facts, memorization, drill, practice, and the tedious work sometimes required to master knowledge, which humanists minimize and sometimes scorn, have been found to contribute to significant learning, knowledge building, and skill development (Gage & Berliner, 1992). To summarize, humanistic theory suggests the following principles of learning:

- Focus on the learner's desire for positive growth, subjective feelings, needs, self-concept, choices in life, and interpersonal relationships.
- The teacher's role is to assess and encourage changes in the learner's needs, self-concept, and feelings by providing support, freedom to choose, and opportunities for spontaneity and creativity.

Applying Learning Theories to Health Care

A logical question is which of these five theories best describes or explains learning—which theory, in other words, would be the most helpful to nurses interested in increasing knowledge or changing the behavior of patients, staff, or themselves? The answer to this question is that each theory contributes to understanding certain aspects of the learning process. For example, behaviorist and social learning theories emphasize external factors in the environment that promote learning, whereas cognitive, psychodynamic, and humanistic theories as well as certain features of social learning theory focus on internal psychological factors in the learning process.

In practice, psychological learning theories can be used singly or in combination to help nurses and other health professionals teach patients or themselves to acquire new information and alter behavior. As an example, patients undergoing painful procedures are first taught relaxation exercises (behaviorist) and while experiencing pain or discomfort are encouraged to employ imagery, such as thinking about a favorite, beautiful place or imagining the healthy cells gobbling up the unhealthy cells (cognitive). Staff members are highly respectful, upbeat, and emotionally supportive of each patient (humanistic) and take the time and opportunity to listen to patients discuss their fears and concerns (psychodynamic). Waiting rooms and lounge areas for patients and their families are designed to be comfortable, friendly, and pleasant to facilitate conversation and interaction, while support groups may help patients and family members learn from one another about how to cope with illness or disability and how to regulate their emotions so that their health is not further compromised (social learning).

At the same time, research indicates that some psychological learning theories are better suited to certain kinds of individuals than to others. For example, patients who are not particularly verbal may learn more effectively from behaviorist techniques, whereas curious, highly active, and self-directed persons may do better with cognitive and humanistic approaches. Moreover, some individuals learn by responding and taking action (behaviorist), whereas the route to learning for others may be through perceptions and thoughts (cognitive) or through feelings and emotions (humanistic and psychodynamic). Most people appear to benefit from demonstration and example (social learning). Also, teachers must keep in mind that some learners require external reinforcement and incentives, whereas other learners do not seem to need—and may even resent—attempts to manipulate and reinforce them.

Motor Learning

Because the majority of nurses teach motor skills to patients and their families on a frequent basis, it is important for them to explore theories and applications of motor learning in addition to theories of psychological learning. Wulf, Shea, and Lewthwaite (2010), for example, stress the importance of and need for motor skill training in medical education, and Oermann (2011), encourages nurse educators to pay attention to the current evidence on motor learning to help improve their teaching of motor skills to nursing students. Theories and variables of motor learning are useful when teaching skilled movement-related activities in a variety of settings. Patients learning to walk with crutches and family members learning to assist with ostomy care can all benefit from the application of motor learning principles. The objective of this section is to summarize selected aspects of this topic that are relevant to a wide variety of teaching and learning situations involving patients and their family members. Using theory and evidence to support and guide nurses as they teach skills can help make their instruction more effective and efficient.

Motor learning is defined as "a set of processes associated with practice or experience leading to relatively permanent changes in the capability for movement" (Schmidt & Lee, 2005, p. 302). It differs from **motor performance**, which involves attainment of a skill but not necessarily retention of that skill (Schmidt & Wrisberg, 2004). All too often, nurses tend (erroneously) to assume that performing a skill means learning a skill. For example, a nurse may demonstrate a skill to the patient, such as changing a sterile dressing, and then ask the patient to teach back the skill. If the patient is able to do so relatively accurately, it is assumed that the skill has been learned. Yet when the patient is asked to carry out the skill two days later during a home visit, the patient may not be able to perform it well. He may struggle with the order of the steps of changing the dressing, or forget how to keep the field sterile, or not be able to manipulate the bandages. As this example suggests, performance in the moment is not always an accurate reflection of learning because it can be influenced by a number of variables, and the observed ability to carry out the skill may be only temporary. Retention, which involves demonstrating a skill over time and after a period of no practice, indicates that true learning has occurred (S. B. O'Sullivan, 2007).

Stages of Motor Learning

Similar to Cronbach's concept of the learning curve, Fitts and Posner's (1967) three-stage model of motor learning is a classic approach that provides a framework for nurses to use as they organize learning strategies for patients and family members. Within the **stages of motor learning** model, the three phases of skill learning are identified as follows:

1. The cognitive stage
2. The associative stage
3. The autonomous stage

Cronbach's theory is discussed more fully in Chapter 10.

In the first (cognitive) stage, the learner works to develop an overall understanding of the skill, basically solving the problem of what is to be done. Learners must focus and pay attention in this stage. During this stage of learning, the use of specific teaching techniques and strategies is probably the most beneficial (Nicholson, 2002). Instructional strategies for nurses during this stage include the following:

- Emphasize the purpose of the skill in a context that is relevant to the learner
- Point out similarities to other learned motor skills
- Minimize distractions
- Use clear and brief instructions
- Demonstrate ideal performance of the skill

- Break down complex movements into parts, where appropriate
- Encourage the learner to state the instructions and watch the movement
- Provide some hands-on guidance but also allow for errors in performance (Kisner & Colby, 2007; S. B. O'Sullivan, 2007)

Initially, nurses can expect the performance of the skill to have many errors. Eventually, however, learners are able to carry out reasonable approximations of the skill (S. B. O'Sullivan, 2007). Rapid improvement but variable performance characterizes this stage.

The second (associative) stage of motor learning involves more reliable performance, slower gains, and fewer errors (Schmidt & Lee, 2005). The patient or student focuses on how to do the skill. The goal in this stage is to fine-tune the skill through continued practice. During this stage, better organization is seen, and the movement becomes coordinated and more accurate (S. B. O'Sullivan, 2007). Dependence on visual cues decreases, and feedback from the movement becomes more important. In this stage, nurses can continue to provide opportunities for practice, emphasizing how the movement feels and assisting learners in finding the safest and most efficient ways to carry out the skills. Helpful instructional strategies for this stage include the following:

- Increase the difficulty of the task
- Increase the level of distraction in the environment
- Encourage learners to practice independently
- Emphasize problem solving
- Decrease guidance and feedback
- Avoid hands-on guidance (Kisner & Colby, 2007)

Patients must be encouraged to self-evaluate and self-correct their performance, and in this stage, nurses should intervene only when errors appear to be consistent (S. B. O'Sullivan, 2007).

The third and final (autonomous) stage of motor learning occurs when the performance gradually improves in speed and efficiency of the performance and requires little attention and thinking about the skill (Nicholson, 2002). An advanced level of skill is achieved, and the learner can perform different tasks at the same time and under different circumstances or in a variety of environments. In this stage, learners no longer have to think about the skill. Nurses can set up progressively more difficult activities in this stage and provide more challenging situations (Kisner & Colby, 2007).

Motor Learning Variables

The variables of practice and feedback have widespread clinical applications for nurses. Gaining an understanding of these variables can assist nurses in optimizing their motor-skill teaching with patients.

PRACTICE

Practice, the repeated performance to become proficient in a skill, is the most important factor in retaining motor skills. The amount, type, and variability of practice all affect how well a skill is acquired and retained (Schmidt & Lee, 2005). Because skill in performance generally increases as a direct result of practice, staff and family members need to continuously reinforce the skills taught by nurses and other health professionals. This emphasis on reinforcement reflects behaviorist theory, as discussed previously in this chapter.

An important goal for learning new motor skills is that patients are able to transfer the learning to new situations or new tasks. For example, nurses often teach patients how to get in and out of the chair next to their hospital bed. The goal is that patients can transfer the learning to the new situations they face at home when they try to get in and out of their own kitchen and living room chairs. Researchers have noted that the more closely the demands in the practice environment resemble those in the usual environment, the better the transfer of learning will be (Schmidt & Lee, 2005; Winstein, 1991). For this reason, it is important to use a variety of chairs in the hospital that resemble chairs at home when teaching this task and not to limit practice to the chair next to the bed.

Variable practice conditions also appear to increase the individual's ability to generalize learning to new situations and seem to be particularly effective for children and adult females (Schmidt & Lee, 2005). For example, patients need to practice walking under as many different conditions as possible (e.g., in a busy corridor, in a narrow hallway, on different surfaces) to help them generalize the skill to the new conditions and environments they will face when they return home.

Nurses routinely give verbal and hands-on guidance to assist patients in performing tasks. Such guidance seems to be most effective at the beginning stages of teaching a task when the task is unfamiliar to learners (Schmidt & Lee, 2005). Too much guidance, however, can actually interfere with learning because it does not allow the learner to solve problems on his or her own. Therefore, it is important for nurses to resist the common urge to give continual direction and assistance to patients, especially once the learners are familiar with the task.

While physical practice is best for learning a motor skill, **mental practice** (imagining or visualizing the skill without body movement) can have positive effects on the performance of the skill (Dickstein & Deutsch, 2007). Patients who cannot carry out physical practice of motor skills as a result of fatigue, pain, or injury are often good candidates for the technique of mental practice alone. Patients who are too ill to exercise or get out of bed can gain a head start on learning, increase their self-efficacy, and decrease their anxiety by mentally practicing these activities. They can do so by reviewing the steps to getting out of bed with the nurse, and then imagining themselves carrying out those steps, one after the other. When possible, mental practice should be combined with physical practice to increase the rate and quality of skill learning.

FEEDBACK

Feedback plays a critical role in learning motor tasks. Feedback can be either intrinsic or extrinsic. Intrinsic (inherent or internal) feedback is the built-in sensory and perceptual information that arises when a movement is produced and can include both visual and body motion information. Extrinsic (augmented or external) feedback is information provided to the learner from an outside source (Schmidt & Wrisberg, 2004). The outside source can be the nurse, or it can be some type of machine, such as biofeedback. Extrinsic feedback adds to intrinsic feedback. Variables to consider when giving extrinsic feedback include the type, timing, and frequency of feedback. Certain types of feedback work better with specific types of skills. Generally, focusing a person's attention on the results of the movements helps learning more than when the person focuses on the details of the movements.

Nurses need to adjust the timing of feedback during the learning process. Continuous feedback occurring at the same time as the skill may be necessary in the early stages of teaching a skill to ensure safety and understanding; however, continuous feedback can interfere with learning over time. For example, suppose the nurse seeks to teach a patient how to give herself an injection. Initially, the nurse must show the patient how to hold the needle, often physically guiding the placement of the patient's hands on the needle. He also tells the patient step by step how to proceed with the injection, giving praise along the way when the patient is successful. If the nurse continues to give this level of extensive feedback each time the patient practices, it may actually slow down learning of the skill. For retention and longer term learning, learners need to self-detect and self-correct errors, so educators should use the least amount of feedback for the shortest time possible (Gentile, 2000). Nurses can often find that withholding feedback is challenging because many view giving large amounts of praise and encouragement as a way of positively supporting the patient. Nevertheless, feedback that is spaced out during practice promotes learning more effectively than does continuous feedback. The extensive use of any type of external feedback can create dependence on it, so nurses need to develop a comfort level that balances safety and support with allowing patients to problem solve, self-monitor, and self-correct when learning new motor skills.

Applying motor learning theories adds depth and breadth to the teaching skills of nurses. Although different areas of the brain are involved in motor learning as compared to psychological learning, there is considerable overlap. The combination and use of both sets of theories are necessary for the teaching and learning of motor skills. Certain aspects of some psychological theories—such as reinforcement from behaviorist theory, the gestalt and information-processing perspective from cognitive theory, modeling from social learning theory, and focusing on subjective needs and feelings of the learner from humanistic theory—are relevant to the teaching of motor skills.

Although a large body of complex research has been published in the area of motor learning, following several simple guidelines can help nurses be more effective when they teach motor skills to patients. Nurses should remember to do the following:

- Make sure patients understand the purpose of the skill and give clear guidance and assistance in the initial stages of learning.
- Practice motor skills with patients as much as possible and encourage other staff and family members to also practice skills with patients.
- Encourage mental practice prior to or along with motor practice.
- Vary the conditions of learning as much as possible.
- Within the limits of safety, decrease the amount of guidance and feedback to allow learners to problem solve, make mistakes, and self-correct errors.

Nurses who consistently apply knowledge of the three stages of motor learning and the variables of practice and feedback when teaching motor skills to patients, family members, and colleagues give themselves the best chances for successful teaching outcomes. The next section discusses common principles of learning that integrates information from all the learning theories presented in this chapter.

Common Principles of Learning

Taken together, the theories discussed in this chapter indicate that learning is a more complicated process than any one theory implies. Besides the different considerations for learning suggested by each theory, the similarities among the perspectives point to some core features of learning. The issues raised at the beginning of the chapter can be addressed by considering how the learning theories might apply to patients in the healthcare setting. Readers also can think about how the theories might apply to their own needs to acquire new knowledge or change behaviors and break bad habits.

How Does Learning Occur?

Learning takes place as individuals interact with their environment and incorporate new information or experiences with what they already know or have learned. Environmental factors that affect learning include the society's norms and values, the culture of the healthcare facility, and the particular structure of the learning situation. Role models need to be effective, learners may need reinforcement, feedback for correct and incorrect responses is required, and learners need opportunities to apply what they learned to different settings and new situations. However, the individual ultimately controls the learning process, often involving considerations of his or her developmental stage, past history (habits, cultural conditioning, socialization, childhood experiences, and conflicts), cognitive style, dynamics of self-regulation, conscious and unconscious motivations, personality (stage, conflicts, and self-concept), and emotions. Also, learners often have a preferred mode for taking in information (visual, motor, auditory, or symbolic). Although some individuals may learn best on their own, others benefit from expert guidance, social interaction, and cooperative learning.

A critical influence on whether learning occurs is the learner's motivational level. The learning theories reviewed here suggest that to learn, the individual must want to gain something (i.e., receive rewards and pleasure, meet goals and needs, master a new skill, confirm expectations, grow in positive ways, resolve conflicts), which in turn creates tension (i.e., drives or imbalances to be reduced) and the motivation to acquire information or change behavior. The relative success or failure of the learner's performance may affect future learning experiences. In some cases, previously learned information or habits may need to be replaced with more accurate information and more appropriate responses. It is, of course, easier to instill new learning than to correct past learning, which may include incorrect or incomplete information or bad habits. See Chapter 6 for more on motivation.

Which Kinds of Experiences Help or Hinder the Learning Process?

When nurses are attempting to teach learners new information or work with them to change their attitudes and behavior, the selection of learning principles and the structure of the learning experience strongly influence the course of learning. Teaching requires imagination, flexibility, and the ability to use a variety of educational methods. Teachers must know their material well and need good communication skills and the ability to motivate themselves and others. All the learning theories discussed in this chapter recognize the need to make learning a positive experience and the necessity of relating the new information to the learner's past experiences—their habits, culture, memories, and feelings about the self. The ultimate control over learning rests with the learner, but effective educators influence and guide the process so that learners advance in their knowledge, skills, perceptions, thoughts, emotional maturity, or behavior. Ignoring these considerations, of course, may hinder learning. Some obstacles to learning may involve a lack of clarity and meaningfulness in what is to be learned, neglect or harsh punishment, fear, and negative or ineffective role models. Providing inappropriate materials given the individual's ability, readiness to learn, or stage of life-cycle development creates another obstacle to learning. Moreover, individuals are unlikely to want to learn if they have had damaging socialization experiences, are deprived of stimulating environments, or lack goals and realistic expectations for themselves.

What Helps Ensure That Learning Becomes Relatively Permanent?

Four considerations assist learning in becoming permanent. First, the likelihood of learning is enhanced by organizing the learning experience, making it meaningful and pleasurable, recognizing the role of emotions in learning, and pacing the teaching session in keeping with the learner's ability to process information. Second, practicing (mentally and physically) new knowledge or skills under varied conditions strengthens learning. The third issue concerns reinforcement: Although reinforcement may or may not be necessary, some theorists have argued that it may be helpful because it serves as a signal to the individual that learning has occurred. A fourth consideration involves trying to ensure that learning will transfer beyond the immediate healthcare setting to other environments. And finally, learning cannot be assumed to be relatively lasting or permanent; it must be assessed and evaluated by the teacher soon after the learning experience has occurred as well as through follow-up measurements made at later times. What is learned from evaluating the teaching situation can then be used to improve future learning experiences for patients.

Summary

This chapter demonstrates that learning is complex. Readers may feel overwhelmed by the different perspectives, various principles of learning, and cautions. Yet, each theory highlights an important dimension that affects the overall learning process, and together the theories provide a wealth of useful options and tools to encourage learning and to change behavior in the healthcare setting. There is, of course, no single best way to approach learning, although all the theories indicate the need to be sensitive to the unique characteristics and motivations of each learner. For additional sources of information about psychological theories of learning and health care, see **Table 3–2**.

Nurses cannot be expected to know everything about the teaching and learning process. More important, perhaps, is that they can determine what needs to be known,

Table 3–2 Websites to Psychological Theories of Learning in Health Care

American Psychological Association (search for learning topics): http://www.apa.org
National Institutes of Health (search for patient education topics): http://www.nih.gov
Learning theory links (emTech.net): http://www.emtech.net/learning_theories.htm

where to find the necessary information, and how to help others benefit directly from a learning experience. Psychology and nursing work well together. Psychology has much to contribute to healthcare practice, and nursing is in a strategic position to apply psychological and motor learning theories in the clinical setting.

Review Questions

1. What are the basic principles of learning for each of the five psychological learning theories discussed in this chapter?
2. What is the role of the teacher in each of the five learning theories?
3. What contributions do the gestalt, developmental, information-processing, and social cognition approaches make to understanding the learning process?
4. What are ways that teachers can motivate learners?
5. Based on the various learning theories, what techniques are useful in helping patients remember information?
6. Using the theories of learning, what approaches can help patients break bad habits, such as smoking or lack of physical exercise?
7. What are some ways that emotions might be given more consideration in nursing and patient education?
8. In motor learning, how do the instructional strategies used during the associative stage of learning differ from those used during the cognitive stage?
9. How do the different types of practice and feedback variables affect learning?

Case Study

Suppose that the nursing unit supervisor, Mr. Locent, has asked you to set up an education class at a satellite clinic of the hospital for patients who were recently diagnosed with diabetes. Time is of the essence, and you have three 1-hour sessions planned to cover the basic information that patients need to learn for proper management of their diabetes. Mr. Locent mentioned to you that several of the patients who will be in the class are concerned about their ability to successfully manage their disease. Eileen, one of the patients, told him, "I am terrified. Learning to live with this disease is overwhelming to me. I can't imagine I will ever be able to have a normal life again. I worry that my relationships with my family and friends will suffer."

1. Describe how you will structure the educational sessions using two of the psychological learning theories discussed in this chapter. Explain why you chose each theory.
2. Judge which learning theory can best assist you in addressing the issues the patients raise about their ability to successfully manage their disease and to cope with their feelings of being overwhelmed. Why did you choose this theory?
3. What can you do to ensure that learning will become relatively permanent?

References

Allan, H. T. (2011). Using psychodynamic small group work in nurse education: Closing the theory-practice gap. *Nurse Education Today, 31*, 521–524.

Armfield, J. M., & Heaton, L. J. (2013). Management of fear and anxiety in the dental clinic: A review. *Australian Dental Journal, 58*(4), 390–407.

Bahn, D. (2001). Social learning theory: Its application to the context of nurse education. *Nurse Education Today, 21*, 110–117.

Bandura, A. (1977). *Social learning theory*. Englewood Cliffs, NJ: Prentice Hall.

Bandura, A. (2001). Social cognitive theory: An agentic perspective. *Annual Review of Psychology, 52*, 1–26.

Barnard, A., Hollingum, C., & Hartfiel, B. (2006). Going on a journey: Understanding palliative care nursing. *International Journal of Palliative Nursing, 12*, 6–12.

Beck, M. H., Cataldo, M., Slifer, K. J., Pulbrook, V., & Guhman, J. K. (2005). Teaching children with attention deficit hyperactivity disorder (ADHD) and autistic disorder (AD) how to swallow pills. *Clinical Pediatrics, 44*, 515–526.

Bethards, M. L. (2014). Applying social learning theory to the observer role in simulation. *Clinical Simulation in Nursing, 10*, e65–e69.

Bhatnagar, K. A. C., Wisniewski, L., Solomon, M., & Heinberg, L. (2013). Effectiveness and feasibility of a cognitive-behavioral group intervention for body image disturbance in women with eating disorders. *Journal of Clinical Psychology, 69*(1), 1–13.

Block, S., & Billings, J. A. (1998). Nurturing humanism through teaching palliative care. *Academic Medicine, 73*, 763–765.

Brackett, M. A., Lopes, P. N., Ivcevic, Z., Mayer, J. D., & Salovey, P. (2004). Integrating emotion and cognition: The role of emotional intelligence. In D. Y. Dai & R. J. Sternberg (Eds.), *Motivation, emotion, and cognition: Integrative perspectives on intellectual functioning and development* (pp. 175–194). Mahwah, NJ: Erlbaum.

Brunner, E., De Herdt, A., Minguet, P., Baldew, S., & Probst, M. (2013). Can cognitive behavioural therapy based strategies be integrated into physiotherapy for the prevention of chronic low back pain? A systemic review. *Disability and Rehabilitation, 35*(1), 1–10.

Bunzli, S., Gillham, D., & Esterman, A. (2011). Physiotherapy-provided operant conditioning in the management of low back pain disability: A systematic review. *Physiotherapy Research International, 16*, 4–19.

Burke, H., & Mancuso, L. (2012). Social cognitive theory, metacognition, and simulation learning in nursing education. *Journal of Nursing Education, 51*, 543–548.

Bush, G. (2006). Learning about learning: From theories to trends. *Teacher Librarian, 34*, 14–18.

Chochinov, H. M., & Breitbart, W. (Eds.). (2000). *Handbook of psychiatry in palliative medicine*. New York, NY: Oxford University Press.

Christakis, N. A., & Fowler, J. H. (2007). The spread of obesity on a large social network over 32 years. *New England Journal of Medicine, 357*, 370–379.

Christakis, N. A., & Fowler, J. H. (2008). The collective dynamics of smoking cessation in a large social network. *New England Journal of Medicine, 358*, 249–251.

Crandell, T. L., Crandell, C. H., & Vander Zanden, J. W. (2012). *Human development* (11th ed.). New York, NY: McGraw-Hill.

Dai, D. Y., & Sternberg, R. J. (Eds.). (2004). *Motivation, emotion, and cognition: Integrative perspectives on intellectual functioning and development*. Mahwah, NJ: Erlbaum.

Dickstein, R., & Deutsch, J. E. (2007). Motor imagery in physical therapist practice. *Physical Therapy, 87*(7), 942–953.

Duberstein, P. R., & Masling, J. M. (Eds.). (2000). *Psychodynamic perspectives on sickness and health*. Washington, DC: American Psychological Association.

Eccles, J. S., & Wigfield, A. (2002). Motivational beliefs, values, and goals. *Annual Review of Psychology, 53*, 109–132.

Erikson, E. (1968). *Identity: Youth and crisis*. New York, NY: Norton.

Ferguson, L., & Day, R. A. (2005). Evidence-based nursing education: Myth or reality? *Journal of Nursing Education, 44*, 107–115.

Ferns, T. (2006). Under-reporting of violent incidents against nursing staff. *Nursing Standard, 20*, 41–45.

Fitts, P. M., & Posner, M. I. (1967). *Human performance*. Belmont, CA: Brooks/Cole.

Friedrichsen, M. J., & Strang, P. M. (2003). Doctors' strategies when breaking bad news to terminally ill patients. *Journal of Palliative Medicine, 6*, 565–574.

Friedrichsen, M. J., Strang, P. M., & Carlsson, M. E. (2000). Breaking bad news in the transition from curative to palliative cancer care: Patient's view of the doctor giving the information. *Support Care Cancer, 8*, 472–478.

Gage, N. L., & Berliner, D. C. (1992). *Educational psychology* (5th ed.). Boston, MA: Houghton Mifflin.

Gage, N. L., & Berliner, D. C. (1998). *Educational psychology* (6th ed.). Boston, MA: Houghton Mifflin.

Gagné, R. M. (1985). *The conditions of learning* (4th ed.). New York, NY: Holt, Rinehart & Winston.

Gardner, H. (1978). *Developmental psychology: An introduction*. Boston, MA: Little, Brown.

Gentile, A. M. (2000). Skill acquisition: Action, movement and neuromotor processes. In J. Carr & R. Shepherd (Eds.), *Movement science: Foundations for physical therapy in rehabilitation* (pp. 111–187). Gaithersburg, MD: Aspen Publishers.

Goleman, D. (1995). *Emotional intelligence*. New York, NY: Bantam Books.

Goodwin, A. M., & Gore, V. (2000). Managing the stresses of nursing people with severe and enduring mental illness: A psychodynamic observation study of a long-stay psychiatric ward. *British Journal of Medical Psychology, 73*, 311–325.

Gorgens-Ekermans, G., & Brand, T. (2012). Emotional intelligence as a moderator in the stress-burnout relationship: A questionnaire study on nurses. *Journal of Clinical Nursing, 21*, 2275–2285.

Greene, J. D., Sommerville, R. B., Nystrom, L. E., Darley, J. M., & Cohen, J. D. (2001). An fMRI investigation of emotional engagement in moral judgment. *Science, 293*, 2105–2108.

Halpern, J. (2001). *From detached concern to empathy: Humanizing medical practice*. New York, NY: Oxford University Press.

Heaton, L. J., Leroux, B. G., Ruff, P. A., & Coldwell, S. E. (2013). Computerized dental injection fear treatment: A randomized clinical trial. *Journal of Dental Research, 92*(1), 37s–42s.

Hilgard, E. R., & Bower, G. H. (1966). *Theories of learning* (3rd ed.). New York, NY: Appleton-Century-Crofts.

Hoffman, M. L. (2000). *Empathy and moral development: Implications for caring and justice*. New York, NY: Cambridge University Press.

Holyoake, D. D. (1998). A little lady called Pandora: An exploration of philosophical traditions of humanism and existentialism in nursing ill children. *Child: Care, Health and Development, 24*, 325–336.

Hooyman, N., & Kiyak, H. A. (2011). *Social gerontology: A multidisciplinary perspective* (9th ed.). New York, NY: Pearson.

Imes, S. A., Clance, P. R., Gailis, A. T., & Atkeson, E. (2002). Mind's response to the body's betrayal: Gestalt/existential therapy for clients with chronic or life-threatening illnesses. *Journal of Clinical Psychology, 58*, 1361–1373.

Karimi, L., Leggat, S. G., Donohue, L., Farrell, G., & Couper, G. E. (2014). Emotional rescue: The role of emotional intelligence and emotional labour on well-being and job-stress among community nurses. *Journal of Advanced Nursing, 70*(1), 176–186.

Kennifer, S. L., Alexander, S. C., Pollak, K. I., Jeffreys, A. S., Olsen, M. K., Rodriguez, K. L., . . . Tulsky, J. A. (2009). Negative emotions in cancer care: Do oncologists' responses depend on severity and type of emotion? *Patient Education and Counseling, 76*, 51–56.

Kessels, R. P. C. (2003). Patients' memory of medical information. *Journal of the Royal Society of Medicine, 96*, 219–222.

Kisner, C., & Colby, L. A. (2007). *Therapeutic exercise* (5th ed.). Philadelphia, PA: F. A. Davis.

Kohler, W. (1947). *Gestalt psychology*. New York, NY: Mentor Books.

Kohler, W. (1969). *The task of gestalt psychology*. Princeton, NJ: Princeton University Press.

Kübler-Ross, E. (1969). *On death and dying*. New York, NY: Macmillan.

Lotfi-Jam, K., Carey, M., Jefford, M., Schofield, P., Charleson, C., & Aranda, S. (2008). Nonpharmacologic strategies for managing common chemotherapy adverse effects: A systematic review. *Journal of Clinical Oncology, 26*(34), 5618–5629.

Malach-Pines, A. (2000). Nurses' burnout: An existential psychodynamic perspective. *Journal of Psychosocial Nursing and Mental Health Services, 38*, 23–31.

Maslow, A. (1954). *Motivation and personality*. New York, NY: Harper & Row.

Maslow, A. (1987). *Motivation and personality* (3rd ed.). New York, NY: Harper & Row.

McCullough, L., & Andrews, S. (2001). Assimilative integration: Short-term dynamic psychotherapy for treating affect phobias. *Clinical Psychology: Science and Practice, 8*, 82–97.

Menahern, S., & Halasz, G. (2000). Parental noncompliance—a paediatric dilemma: A medical and psychodynamic perspective. *Child: Care, Health and Development, 26*, 61–72.

Murray, D. J. (1995). *Gestalt psychology and the cognitive revolution*. New York, NY: Harvester Wheatsheaf.

Nicholson, D. E. (2002). Teaching psychomotor skills. In K. F. Shepard & G. M. Jensen (Eds.), *Handbook of teaching for physical therapists* (2nd ed., pp. 387–418). Woburn, MA: Butterworth-Heinemann.

Oermann, M. H. (2011). Toward evidence-based nursing education: Deliberate practice and motor skill learning. *Journal of Nursing Education, 50*(2), 63–64.

Ormrod, J. E. (2016). *Human learning* (7th ed.). New York, NY: Pearson.

O'Sullivan, H., & McKimm, J. (2014). The role of emotion in effective clinical leadership and compassionate care. *British Journal of Hospital Medicine, 75*(5), 281–286.

O'Sullivan, S. B. (2007). Strategies to improve motor function. In S. B. O'Sullivan & T. J. Schmitz (Eds.), *Physical rehabilitation* (5th ed., pp. 471–522). Philadelphia, PA: F. A. Davis.

Papadakis, A. A., Prince, R. P. O., Jones, N. P., & Strauman, T. J. (2006). Self-regulation, rumination, and vulnerability to depression in adolescent girls. *Development and Psychopathology, 18*, 815–829.

Pearson, A. (2006). Powerful caring. *Nursing Standard, 20*(48), 20–22.

Pfeffer, J. (1985). Organizations and organizational theory. In G. Lindzey & E. Aronson (Eds.), *Handbook of social psychology: Vol. 1. Theory and method* (3rd ed., pp. 379–440). New York, NY: Random House.

Piaget, J., & Inhelder, B. (1969). *The psychology of the child* (H. Weaver, Trans.). New York, NY: Basic Books.

Piane, G. (2000). Contingency contracting and systematic desensitization for heroin addicts in methadone maintenance programs. *Journal of Psychoactive Drugs, 32*, 311–319.

Pollak, K. I., Arnold, R. M., Jeffreys, A. S., Alexander, S. C., Olsen, M. K., Abernathy, A. P., . . . Ja, T. (2007). Oncologist communication about emotions during visits with patients with advanced cancer. *Journal of Clinical Oncology, 25*, 5748–5752.

Ramesh, A., Denzil, S. B., Linda, R., Josephine, P. K., Nagpoorrnima, M., Suman Rao, P. N., & Swarna Rekha, A. (2012). Maintaining reduced noise levels in a resource-constrained neonatal intensive care unit by operant conditioning. *Indian Pediatrics, 49*, 279–282.

Rogers, C. (1961). *On becoming a person.* Boston, MA: Houghton Mifflin.

Rogers, C. (1994). *Freedom to learn* (3rd ed.). New York, NY: Merrill.

Rogers, L. Q., Matevey, C., Hopkins-Price, P., Shah, P., Dunnington, G., & Courneya, K. S. (2004). Exploring social cognitive theory constructs for promoting exercise among breast cancer patients. *Cancer Nursing, 27*, 462–473.

Ruiz-Aranda, D., Extremera, N., & Pineda-Galan, C. (2014). Emotional intelligence, life satisfaction and subjective happiness in female student health professionals: The mediating effect of perceived stress. *Journal of Psychiatric and Mental Health Nursing, 21*, 106–113.

Santrock, J. W. (2013). *Life-span development* (14th ed.). New York, NY: McGraw-Hill.

Schmidt, R. A., & Lee, T. D. (2005). *Motor control and learning: A behavioral emphasis* (4th ed.). Champaign, IL: Human Kinetics.

Schmidt, R. A., & Wrisberg, C. A. (2004). *Motor learning and performance: A problem-based learning approach* (3rd ed.). Champaign, IL: Human Kinetics.

Sherif, M., & Sherif, C. W. (1969). *Social psychology.* New York, NY: Harper & Row.

Skinner, B. F. (1974). *About behaviorism.* New York, NY: Vintage Books.

Skinner, B. F. (1989). *Recent issues in the analysis of behavior.* Columbus, OH: Merrill.

Slipp, S. (2000). Subliminal stimulation research and its implications for psychoanalytic theory and treatment. *Journal of the American Academy of Psychoanalysis, 28*, 305–320.

Snowman, J., & McCown, R. (2015). *Psychology applied to teaching* (14th ed.). Stanford, CT: Cengage Learning.

Steinke, E. E., Mosack, V., Hertzog, J., & Wright, D. W. (2012). A social-cognitive sexual counseling intervention post-MI: Development and pilot testing. *Perspectives in Psychiatric Care, 49*, 162–170.

Sternberg, R. J., & Sternberg, K. (2012). *Cognitive psychology* (6th ed.). Belmont, CA: Wadsworth Cengage Learning.

Stiles, A. S. (2005). Parenting needs, goals, and strategies of adolescent mothers. *MCN: The American Journal of Maternal/Child Nursing, 30*, 327–333.

Stockhurst, U., Steingrueber, H. J., Enck, P., & Klosterhalfen, S. (2006). Pavlovian conditioning of nausea and vomiting. *Autonomic Neuroscience, 129*, 50–57.

Stroebe, M. S., Folkman, S., Hansson, R. O., & Schut, H. (2006). The prediction of bereavement outcome: Development of an integrative risk factor framework. *Social Science & Medicine, 63*, 2440–2451.

Storey, J., Collis, M. A., & Clegg, J. (2011). A psychodynamic interpretation of staff accounts of working with people who have learning disabilities and complex needs. *British Journal of Learning Disabilities, 40*, 229–235.

Telford, K., Kralik, D., & Koch, T. (2006). Acceptance and denial: Implications for people adapting to chronic illness. Literature review. *Journal of Advanced Nursing, 55*, 457–464.

Tennant, M. (2006). *Psychology and adult learning* (3rd ed.). New York, NY: Routledge.

Vygotsky, L. S. (1986). *Thought and language.* Cambridge, MA: MIT Press.

Winstein, C. J. (1991). Designing practice for motor learning: Clinical applications. In M. J. Lister (Ed.), *Contemporary management of motor control problems: Proceedings of the II STEP conference* (pp. 65–76). Alexandria, VA: Foundation for Physical Therapy.

Wolpe, J. (1982). *The practice of behavior therapy* (3rd ed.). New York, NY: Pergamon.

Wulf, G., Shea, C., & Lewthwaite, R. (2010). Motor skill learning and performance: A review of influential factors. *Medical Education, 44*, 75–84.

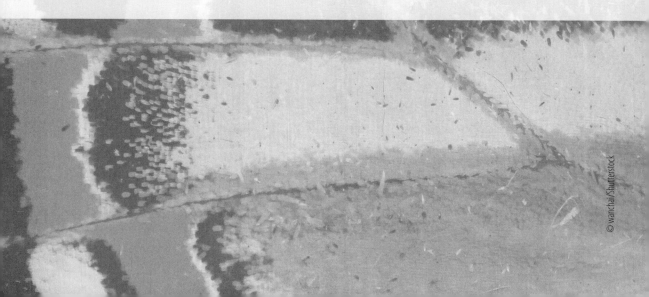

PART II

Characteristics of the Learner

Determinants of Learning

Sharon Kitchie

Chapter Highlights

- The Nurse's Role as a Teacher
- Assessment of the Learner
- Assessing Learning Needs
- Methods to Assess Learning Needs
  - *Informal Conversations*
  - *Structured Interviews*
  - *Questionnaires*
  - *Observations*
  - *Documentations*
- Readiness to Learn
  - *Physical Readiness*
  - *Emotional Readiness*
  - *Experiential Readiness*
  - *Knowledge Readiness*
- Learning Styles, Personality Types, and Intelligences
  - *Dunn and Dunn Learning Styles*
  - *Visual, Aural, Read/Write, and Kinesthetic Learning Styles*
  - *Jung and Myers-Briggs Personality Types*
  - *Kolb's Cycle of Learning*
  - *Gardner's Eight Types of Intelligence*
- Interpretation of Learning Style Models, Personality Types, and Intelligences

Key Terms

determinants of learning
learning needs
learning styles
readiness to learn

© wanchai/Shutterstock

Objectives

After completing this chapter, the reader will be able to

1. Explain the nurse's role as teacher in the learning process.
2. Identify the three components of the determinants of learning.
3. Describe the steps involved in assessing learning needs.
4. Explain methods that can be used to assess learner needs.
5. Discuss the factors that need to be assessed in each of the four types of readiness to learn.
6. Describe what is meant by learning styles.
7. Identify the similarities and differences between the major learning styles, personality types, and intelligence models.
8. Discuss the general guidelines for assessing individual learning styles.

In a variety of settings, nurses are responsible for the education of patients and their families. This learning includes self-care activities, preparations for diagnostic tests, disease management, and health promotion. Several factors make the teaching of this vital knowledge and skills challenging for the nurse in today's healthcare environment. Often, nurses have difficulty meeting patients' needs because of the time constraints of clinical practice. For example, same-day surgery and shortened lengths of stay lessen time for patient and family contact with the nurse, making it difficult to capture the teachable moments.

To meet these challenges, the nurse must know what determines how well a person learns. The **determinants of learning** include:

- Learning needs
- Readiness to learn
- Learning styles

This chapter addresses these three determinants of learning in relation to patient teaching in the practice of nursing.

The Nurse's Role as Teacher

The role of teaching others is one of the most challenging and essential interventions that a nurse performs. To do it well, the nurse must both identify the information each patient and family member needs to know and consider their readiness to learn and their styles of learning. Learning can actually occur without a teacher, but the nurse can enhance learning by serving as a facilitator. However, just providing the information alone does not guarantee that learning will occur. The nurse plays a crucial role in the learning process by doing the following:

- Assessing problems or deficits
- Providing important information and presenting it in unique and appropriate ways

- Identifying progress being made
- Giving feedback and follow-up
- Reinforcing learning in the attainment of new knowledge, skills, and attitudes
- Evaluating learners' abilities

The nurse is vital in giving support, encouragement, and direction during the process of learning. Learners may make choices on their own, without the assistance of teachers, but these choices may be limited or inappropriate. For example, the nurse can make needed changes in the home environment, such as minimizing distractions by having family members turn off the television to provide a quiet environment that will help the patient concentrate on the learning activity. The nurse can identify the best learning approaches and activities that can both support and challenge the learner based on his or her individual learning needs, readiness to learn, and learning style.

Assessment of the Learner

Assessment of patients' needs, readiness, and styles of learning is the first and most important step in patient teaching—but it is also the step most likely to be neglected. The importance of assessment of the patient may seem obvious, yet frequently, the nurse dives into teaching before addressing all of the determinants of learning. It is not unusual for patients with the same condition to be taught with the same materials in the same way. The result is that information given to the patient is neither individualized nor based on sound educational principles. Evidence suggests, however, that individualizing teaching based on prior assessment improves patient outcomes (Corbett, 2003; Frank-Bader, Beltran, & Dojlidko, 2011; Kim et al., 2004; Miaskowski et al., 2004) and satisfaction (Bakas et al., 2009; D. L. Wagner, Bear, & Davidson, 2011).

Nurses are taught that any direct physical and psychosocial care to meet the needs of patients should not be initiated unless the interventions are based on an assessment. Few would deny that this is the correct approach. The effectiveness of nursing care clearly depends on the scope, accuracy, and comprehensiveness of assessment prior to interventions. What makes assessment so significant and fundamental to the teaching process? This initial step in the process confirms the need for teaching and the approaches to be used in providing the patient with appropriate learning experiences.

Assessments do more than simply identify and prioritize information for the purposes of setting behavioral goals and objectives, planning instructional interventions, and being able to evaluate in the long run whether the learner has achieved the desired goals and objectives. Good assessments ensure that the best possible learning can occur with the least amount of stress and anxiety for the learner. Assessment prevents needless repetition of known material, saves time and energy on the part of both the learner and the teacher, and helps to establish positive communication between the two parties (Haggard, 1989). Furthermore, it increases the motivation to learn by focusing on what the patient feels is most important to know or to be able to do.

Why, then, is this first step in the teaching process so often overlooked or only partially carried out? Lack of time is the number one reason that nurses shortchange the assessment phase (Haddad, 2003; Marcum, Ridenour, Shaff, Hammons, & Taylor, 2002). Because time constraints are a major concern when carrying out patient education, nurses must become skilled in accurately conducting assessments of the three determinants of learning so as to have reserve time for actual teaching. In addition, many nurses, although expected and required by their nurse practice acts to instruct others, are unfamiliar with the principles of teaching and learning. The nurse in the role of teacher must become better acquainted and comfortable with all the elements of instructional design, but particularly with the assessment phase, because it serves as the foundation for the rest of the teaching process.

Assessment of the learner includes attending to the three determinants of learning (Haggard, 1989):

1. *Learning needs*—what the learner needs and wants to learn
2. *Readiness to learn*—when the learner is receptive to learning
3. *Learning style*—how the learner best learns

Assessing Learning Needs

Learning needs are defined as gaps in knowledge that exist between a desired level of performance and the actual level of performance (Healthcare Education Association, 1989). In other words, a learning need is the gap between what someone knows and what someone needs or wants to know. Such gaps may arise because of a lack of knowledge, attitude, or skill.

Of the three determinants of learning, nurses must identify learning needs first so they can plan appropriate and effective teaching strategies. Once nurses discover what needs to be taught, they can determine when and how learning can optimally occur. Of course, not every individual sees a need for education. Often, learners are not aware of what they do not know or want to know. Consequently, it is up to the nurse to assist learners in identifying, clarifying, and prioritizing their needs and interests. Once these aspects of the learner are determined, the information gathered can, in turn, be used to set objectives and plan appropriate and effective teaching and learning approaches for education to begin at a point suitable to the learner.

According to well-known experts in behavioral and social sciences (Bloom, 1968; Bruner, 1966; Carroll, 1963; Kessels, 2003; Ley, 1979; Skinner, 1954), most learners—90%–95% of them—can master a subject with a high degree of success if given sufficient time and appropriate support. It is the task of the nurse to help them determine what exactly needs to be learned and to identify approaches for presenting information in a way that the learner will best understand.

The following are important steps in the assessment of learning needs:

1. *Identify the learner.* Who is the audience? If the audience is one individual, is there a single need, or do many needs have to be fulfilled? Is there more than one learner? If so, are their needs the same or different? Teaching opportunities, formal or informal, must be based on accurate identification of the learner. For example, a nurse may believe that all parents of children with asthma need a formal class on potential hazards in the home. This perception may be based on the nurse's interaction with a few patients and may not be true of all families.

2. *Choose the right setting.* Establishing a trusting environment helps learners feel a sense of security in confiding information, believe their concerns are taken seriously and are considered important, and feel respected. Ensuring privacy and confidentiality is recognized as essential to establishing a trusting relationship.

3. *Collect important information about the learner.* Explore the health problems or issues that are of interest to your audience to determine the type and extent of content to be included in the teaching as well as the teaching methods and materials to be used. Patients and family members are usually the most important source of needs assessment information. Be sure to ask what is important to them, what types of social support systems are available, and how their social support system can help. Actively engaging learners in defining their own problems and needs motivates most patients because they have an investment in planning for their learning, and it allows the nurse to tailor teaching specifically to their unique circumstances. The learner is important to include as a source of information because the teacher may not always perceive the same learning needs as the patient (Burkhart, 2008; Carlson, Ivnik, Dierkhising, O'Byrne, & Vickers, 2006; Suhonen, Nenonen, Laukka, & Valimaki, 2005; Timmins, 2005; Yonaty & Kitchie, 2012). A literature search can also assist the nurse in identifying the type and extent of content to be included in teaching sessions as well as the strategies for teaching a specific population based on the analysis of needs.

4. *Involve members of the healthcare team.* Consult with other health professionals to gain insights into the needs of patients and their families. Nurses must remember to collaborate with other members of the healthcare team for a richer assessment of learning needs. This consideration is especially important because time for assessment is often limited. In addition to other health professionals, associations such as the American Heart Association, the American Diabetes Association, and the American Cancer Society are excellent sources of health information.

5. *Prioritize needs.* A list of identified needs can become endless and seemingly impossible to accomplish. Setting priorities for learning is often difficult when the nurse is faced with many learning needs in several areas. Prioritizing the identified needs helps the nurse in partnership with the patient set realistic and achievable learning goals. Nurses should prioritize learning needs based on the criteria in **Table 4–1** (Healthcare Education Association, 1989, p. 23) to foster maximum learning.

Without good assessment, a common mistake is to provide more information than the patient wants or needs. To avoid this problem, the nurse must discriminate between information that patients need to know versus information that is nice for them to know. Often, highly technical information merely serves to confuse and distract patients from the essential information they need to carry out their regimen (Hansen & Fisher, 1998; Kessels, 2003).

6. *Determine availability of educational resources.* The nurse may identify a need, but it may be useless to proceed with interventions if the proper educational resources are not available, are unrealistic to obtain, or do not match the patient's

Table 4–1   Criteria for Prioritizing Learning Needs

Mandatory: Needs that must be learned for survival or situations in which the learner's life or safety is threatened. Learning needs in this category must be met immediately. For example, a patient who has experienced a recent heart attack needs to know the signs and symptoms and when to get immediate help.
Desirable: Needs that are not life dependent but that are related to well-being or the overall ability to provide quality care in situations involving changes in institutional procedure. For example, it is important for patients who have cardiovascular disease to understand the effects of a high-fat diet on their condition.
Possible: Needs for information that is nice to know but not essential or required or situations in which the learning need is not directly related to daily activities. For example, the patient who is newly diagnosed as having diabetes mellitus most likely does not need to know about self-care issues that arise in relationship to traveling across time zones or staying in a foreign country because this information does not relate to the patient's everyday activities.

Data from Healthcare Education Association. (1985).

needs. In this case, it may be better to focus on other identified needs. For example, a patient who has asthma needs to learn how to use an inhaler and peak-flow meter. The nurse may determine that this patient learns best if the nurse first gives a demonstration of the use of the inhaler and peak-flow meter and then allows the patient the opportunity to perform a return demonstration. If the proper equipment is not available for demonstration/return demonstration at that moment, it might be better for the nurse to concentrate on teaching the signs and symptoms the patient might experience when having poor air exchange than it is to cancel the encounter altogether. Thereafter, the nurse would work immediately on obtaining the necessary equipment for future encounters.

7. *Assess the demands of the organization.* This assessment yields information that reflects the climate of the organization. What are the organization's philosophy, mission, strategic plan, and goals? The nurse should be familiar with standards of performance required in various employee categories, along with job descriptions and hospital, professional, and agency regulations. If, for example, the organization is focused on health promotion versus trauma care, then there likely will be a different educational focus or emphasis that dictates learning needs of the patients.

8. Take time-management issues into account. Because lack of time is a major barrier to the assessment process, Rankin and Stallings (2005) suggest the nurse should consider the following tips that, in the long run, are time savers:
   - Although close observation and active listening take time, it is much more efficient and effective to take the time to do a good initial assessment up front than to waste time by having to go back to discover the obstacles to learning that prevented progress in the first place.
   - Learners must be given time to offer their own thoughts about their learning needs if the nurse expects them to take charge and become actively involved in the learning process. Learners should be asked what they want to learn first, because this step allays their fears and makes it easier for them to move on to other necessary content (McNeill, 2012). This approach also shows that

the nurse cares about what the learner believes is important and, in the case of an adult, meets his or her need to be self-directed (Inott & Kennedy, 2011).

- Assessment can be conducted anytime and anywhere the nurse has contact with patients and families. With patients, many potential opportunities for assessment arise, such as when giving a bath, serving a meal, making rounds, and distributing medications.
- Informing patients ahead of time that the nurse wishes to spend time discussing problems or needs gives them advance notice to sort out their thoughts and feelings. In one large metropolitan teaching hospital, this strategy proved effective in increasing patient understanding of and satisfaction with transplant discharge information (Frank-Bader et al., 2011). Patients and their families were informed that a specific topic would be discussed on a specific day. Knowing what to expect each day allowed them to review the appropriate handouts ahead of time and prepare questions. It gave patients and family members the time they needed to identify areas of confusion or concern.
- Minimizing interruptions and distractions during planned assessment interviews allows the nurse to accomplish in 5 minutes what otherwise might have taken 15 minutes or more during an interview session that is frequently interrupted.

Methods to Assess Learning Needs

The nurse, as a teacher, must obtain information about learning needs from the patients, as well as from others who are in contact with the patients. This section describes various methods that nurses can use to assess learner needs and that should be used in combination to yield the most reliable information (Haggard, 1989).

Informal Conversations

Often learning needs are discovered during conversations that take place with other healthcare team members involved in the care of the patient and between the nurse and the patient or his or her family. The nurse must rely on active listening and open-ended questions to pick up cues and information regarding learning needs.

Structured Interviews

The structured interview is perhaps the form of needs assessment most commonly used to solicit the learner's point of view. As with the gathering of any information from a patient in the assessment phase, the nurse should strive to establish a trusting environment, use direct and open-ended questions, choose a setting that is free of distractions, and allow the learner to state what are believed to be the learning needs. It is important to remain nonjudgmental when collecting information about the learner's strengths, beliefs, and motivations. Nurses should take notes with the learner's permission so that important information is not lost. The telephone is a good tool to use for an interview if it is impossible to ask questions in person. The major drawback of a telephone interview is the inability on the part of the nurse to perceive nonverbal cues from the learner.

Interviews produce answers that may reveal uncertainties, conflicts, inconsistencies, unexpected problems, anxieties and fears, as well as the patient's current knowledge base. Examples of questions that nurse educators can ask patients as learners are as follows:

- What do you think caused your problem?
- How severe is your illness?
- What does your illness/health mean to you?
- What do you do to stay healthy?
- What results do you hope to obtain from treatments?
- What are your strengths and limitations as a learner?
- How do you learn best?

Questionnaires

Nurses can obtain learners' written responses to questions about learning needs by using survey instruments. Checklists are one of the most common forms of questionnaires. They are easy to administer, provide more privacy compared to interviews, and make it easy to summarize data. Learners seldom object to this method of obtaining information about their learning needs.

Sometimes learners may have difficulty rating themselves and may need the nurse to clarify terms or provide additional information to help them understand what is being assessed. The nurse's role is to encourage learners to make as honest a self-assessment as possible. Because checklists usually reflect what the nurse perceives as needs, a space should be provided for the patients and family members to add any other items of interest or concern. One example of a reliable and valid self-assessment tool is the Patient Learning Needs Scale (Redman, 2003). This instrument is designed to measure patients' perceptions of learning needs to manage their health care at home following a medical or surgical illness (Bubela et al., 2000; Jacobs, 2000; Polat, Celik, Erkan, & Kasali, 2014; Şendir, Büyükyılmaz, & Muşovi, 2013).

Observations

Observing health behaviors in several different time periods can help the nurse draw conclusions about established patterns of behavior. Actually watching the learner perform a task more than once is an excellent way of assessing a skill. Are all steps performed correctly? Does the learner have any difficulty with using various pieces of equipment? Does the learner require prompting? Learners may believe they can accurately perform a skill or task (e.g., walking with crutches, changing a dressing, giving an injection), but by observing the skill performance, the nurse can best determine whether additional learning may be needed.

Documentations

Initial assessments, progress notes, nursing care plans, staff notes, and discharge planning forms can provide information about the learning needs of patients. Nurses need to follow a consistent format for reviewing charts so that they review each chart in the same manner to identify learning needs based on the same information. Also, documentation by other members of the healthcare team, such as physical therapists, social workers, respiratory therapists, and nutritionists, can yield valuable insights with respect to the needs of the learner.

Readiness to Learn

Once the nurse has identified learning needs, the next step is to determine the learner's readiness to receive information. **Readiness to learn** is defined as the time when the learner demonstrates an interest in learning the information necessary to maintain optimal health. Often, nurses have noted that when a patient asks a question, the time is prime for learning. Readiness to learn occurs when the learner is receptive, willing, and able to participate in the learning process. It is the responsibility of the nurse to discover through assessment exactly when patients are ready to learn, what they need or want to learn, and how to adapt the content to fit each learner.

Assessing readiness to learn requires the nurse to understand what needs to be taught and to be skilled in collecting and verifying information. The same methods used previously to assess learning needs, including making observations, conducting interviews, gathering information from the learner as well as from other healthcare team members, and reviewing documentation, can also be used to assess readiness to learn.

No matter how important the information is or how much the nurse feels the patient needs the information, if the patient is not ready to learn, then the information will not be absorbed. If educational objectives are set by the nurse before assessing readiness to learn, then both the nurse's and the learner's time could very well be wasted because the established objectives may be beyond the readiness of the patient.

Timing—that is, the point at which teaching should take place—is very important because anything that affects physical or psychological comfort can affect a learner's ability and willingness to learn. A learner who is not receptive to information at one time may be more receptive to the same information at another time. Because the nurse often has limited contact with patients and family members as a result of short hospital stays or short visits in the outpatient setting, teaching must be brief and basic. Adults, whether they are patients or family members, are generally eager to learn when the subject of teaching is relevant and applicable to their everyday concerns.

Before teaching can begin, the nurse must find the time to first take a PEEK (Lichtenthal, 1990) at the four types of readiness to learn—physical readiness, emotional readiness, experiential readiness, and knowledge readiness. These four types of readiness to learn may be either obstacles or enhancers to learning (**Table 4–2**).

Physical Readiness

The nurse needs to consider five major components of physical readiness—measures of ability, complexity of task, environmental effects, health status, and gender—because they affect the degree or extent to which learning will occur.

Table 4–2 Take Time to Take a PEEK at the Four Types of Readiness to Learn

P = Physical Readiness
Measures of ability
Complexity of task
Environmental effects
Health status
Gender
E = Emotional Readiness
Anxiety level
Support system
Motivation
Risk-taking behavior
Frame of mind
Developmental stage
E = Experiential Readiness
Level of aspiration
Past coping mechanisms
Cultural background
Locus of control
Orientation
K = Knowledge Readiness
Present knowledge base
Cognitive ability
Learning disabilities
Learning styles

Reproduced from Lichtenthal, C. (1990, August). *A self-study model on readiness to learn*. Reprinted with permission from Cheryl Lichtenthal Harding. Unpublished manuscript.

MEASURES OF ABILITY

Ability to perform a task may require fine and/or gross motor movements using the small and large muscles of the body. Walking on crutches is a good example of a task for which a patient must have the physical ability to be ready to learn. The nurse must assess that adequate strength, flexibility, coordination, and endurance are present. In addition, for information to be accurately processed, the sense organs of seeing and hearing, in particular, must be adequately functioning. For example, if a person has a visual deficit, the nurse can make eyeglasses or a magnifying glass available so that the patient can see the lines on an insulin syringe. Creating a stimulating and accepting environment by using instructional tools and support to match learners' physical and sensory abilities encourages readiness to learn.

COMPLEXITY OF TASK

The nurse must take into account the difficulty level of the subject or task to be mastered by the learner. The more complex the task is, the more difficult it is to achieve. For example, some skills require a high degree of coordination and physical energy output. Once a skill becomes routine in nature, it is more difficult for the patient to alter it if necessary to do so, because it has become a habit. For example, if the learner has been performing a skill over a long period of time and then the procedural steps of the task change, the learner must unlearn those steps and relearn the new way. This requirement may increase the complexity of the task and put additional physical demands on the learner by lengthening the time the learner needs to adjust to doing something in a new way. Older adults, in particular, find the effort to change difficult when they are faced with information contrary to their preexisting knowledge and beliefs, and they may become confused, frustrated, or overwhelmed (Kessels, 2003).

ENVIRONMENTAL EFFECTS

An environment favorable to learning helps to hold the learner's attention and stimulate interest in learning. On the other hand, unfavorable conditions, such as extremely high levels of noise or frequent interruptions, can interfere with a learner's accuracy and precision of performance. Use of a jackhammer in the street outside the patient's home, for example, is more disruptive to the patient's ability to learn a new skill the nurse is teaching than a constant roar of traffic coming from the same street. Older adults, in particular, need more time to react and respond to stimuli. Increased inability to receive, process, and transmit information is a characteristic of aging. Environmental demands that make older persons feel rushed to perform tasks in a short time frame can overwhelm them. When an activity is self-paced, older learners respond more favorably. (See Chapter 5 for information on teaching the older adult.)

HEALTH STATUS

Assessment of the patient's health status is important to determine the amount of energy available for learning. Nurses must seriously consider a person's health status, whether well, acutely ill, or chronically ill, when assessing for readiness.

Healthy learners have energy available for learning. In such a case, readiness to learn about health-promoting behaviors is based on their perception of self-responsibility. The extent to which a patient perceives illness to potentially affect future well-being influences that person's desire to learn preventive and promotion measures. If learners perceive a threat to their quality of life, they likely will seek more information in an attempt to control the negative effects of an illness (Bubela & Galloway, 1990). This type of response behavior can best be understood by examining the health belief model and the health promotion model described in Chapter 6.

Learners who are acutely ill tend to focus their energies on the physiological and psychological demands of their illness. Learning is minimal in such persons because most of these individuals' energy is needed for the demands of the illness and gaining immediate relief. Any learning that may occur should be related to treatments, tests, and minimizing pain or other discomforts. As these patients improve and the acute phase of illness diminishes, they can then focus on learning follow-up management and how to avoid complications. Nurses must assess the readiness to learn of acutely ill patients by observing their energy levels and comfort status. Improvement in physical status usually results in being more open to learning. However, medications that cause side effects such as drowsiness, mental depression, impaired depth perception, decreased ability to concentrate, and learner fatigue also impact the patient's ability to learn. For example, giving a patient a sedative prior to a learning experience may result in less apprehension, but mental functioning and manual dexterity may be impaired.

In contrast to acute illness, chronic illness has no time limits and is of long-term duration. Models of how people deal with chronic illness also are useful as frameworks for understanding readiness to learn (Lubkin & Larsen, 2013). The physiological and psychological demands vary in chronic illness and are not always predictable. Patients may go through different stages in dealing with their illness, similar to the adjustment stages of a person experiencing a loss (Boyd, Gleit, Graham, & Whitman, 1998). If the learner is in the avoidance stage, readiness to learn likely will be limited to simple explanations because the patient's energy is concentrated on denial. Over time, energy levels stabilize and become redirected as awareness of the realities of the situation increase. Readiness to learn may be indicated by the questions the patient asks.

Exploring another perspective, Telford, Kralik, and Koch (2006) encourage health professionals to listen carefully to their patients' stories of how they actually experience the illness, rather than attempt to categorize patients into specific stages. Listening to patient stories may provide clues as to individuals' readiness to learn. Corbin and Strauss (1991) propose that chronic illness occurs in phases. Burton (2000) describes the continuous adaptation required in living with chronic illness, and Patterson (2001) suggests living with chronic illness is an ongoing and continually shifting process. It is important for nurses to understand these cycles when assessing readiness to learn, because they cannot assume that an approach that worked at one time will be just as effective at another time. The receptivity to learning and practicing of self-care measures of a person who is chronically ill is not static, but rather fluctuates over time.

GENDER

Research indicates that women are generally more receptive to medical care and take fewer risks with their health than do men (Ashton, 1999; Bertakis, Rahman, Helms, Callahan, & Robbins, 2000; Rosen, Tsai, & Downs, 2003; Stein & Nyamathi, 2000). This may be because women traditionally have taken on the role of caregivers and, therefore, are more open to health promotion teaching. In addition, women have more frequent contact with health providers while bearing and raising children. Men, by comparison, tend to be less receptive to healthcare interventions and are more likely to be risk takers with regard to health and safety issues (Harris, Jenkins, & Glaser, 2006). A good deal of this behavior is thought to be socially induced. Changes are beginning to be seen in the health-seeking behavior of men and women as a result of the increased focus on healthier lifestyles and the blending of gender roles in the home and workplace.

Emotional Readiness

Learners must be emotionally ready to learn. Like physical readiness, emotional readiness includes several factors that need to be assessed. These factors include anxiety level, support system, motivation, risk-taking behavior, frame of mind, and developmental stage.

ANXIETY LEVEL

Anxiety influences a person's ability to perform mental or physical tasks. In particular, it affects patients' ability to concentrate and retain information (Kessels, 2003; Stephenson, 2006). The level of anxiety may or may not be an obstacle to the learning of new skills. Some degree of anxiety is a motivator to learn, but anxiety that is too low or too high interferes with readiness to learn. On either end of the continuum, mild or severe anxiety may lead to inaction on the part of the learner. If anxiety is low, the individual is not driven to take steps to promote his or her health or prevent diseases. Moderate anxiety, however, drives someone to take action. As the level of anxiety increases, emotional readiness peaks and then begins to decrease in an inversely U-shaped curvilinear manner based on the Yerkes–Dodson law (Ley, 1979), as shown in **Figure 4–1**. A moderate level of anxiety is best for success in learning and is considered the optimal time for teaching.

Fear is a major contributor to anxiety and, therefore, negatively affects readiness to learn. The performance of a task in and of itself may be fear inducing to a patient because of its very nature or meaning. For example, learning self-administration of a medication by injection may produce fear for the patient because of the necessity of self-inflicted pain and the perceived danger of the needle breaking off into the skin. Fear may also lead patients to deny their illness or disability, which interferes with their ability to learn. If a situation is life threatening or overwhelming, anxiety will be high, and readiness to learn will be diminished. Although teaching may be critical for survival, learning usually can take place only if instructions are simple and are repeated over and over again. In such circumstances, families and support persons also should be educated to reinforce information and assist with caregiving responsibilities. In later stages of

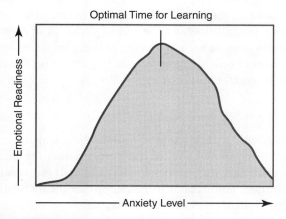

Figure 4–1 Effect of anxiety on emotional readiness to learn

adaptation, acceptance of illness or disability allows the individual to be more receptive to learning because anxiety levels are less acute.

Discovering which stressful events or major life changes the learner is experiencing gives the nurse clues about that person's emotional readiness to learn. The nurse must first identify the source and level of anxiety. High stress levels can be moderated by encouraging the patient to participate in activities such as support groups and the use of relaxation techniques such as imagery and yoga (Stephenson, 2006). After anxiety levels have been moderated and anxiety has been lessened, education is an excellent intervention to spur someone to take action when dealing with a stressful life event.

SUPPORT SYSTEM

The availability and strength of a support system also influence emotional readiness and are closely tied to how anxious an individual might feel. Members of the patient's support system who are available to assist with self-care activities at home should be present during at least some of the teaching sessions so that they can learn how to help the patient if the need arises. Kitchie (2003) suggests that families and friends are important for medication adherence among older adults who experience chronic illness. Although the nurse should not draw any conclusions about causal relationships from this type of study, the nurse's assessment benefits from incorporating questions about the learner's social network. Social support is important in buffering the effects of stressful events (Gavan, 2003; Kitchie, 2003). A strong positive support system can decrease anxiety, whereas the lack of one can increase anxiety levels.

Health professionals often act as sources of social and emotional support to clients. Epstein and Street (2007) describe the significance of fostering healing relationships with patients and responding to patients' emotions as fundamental functions of patient–clinician communication in cancer care. Street, Makoul, Arora, and Epstein (2009) identify the importance of clinicians in enhancing patients' abilities to manage emotions in one of their several recommended pathways to improved health outcomes. Beddoe (1999) describes the unique opportunity that nurses have to provide emotional support to patients. She labels this opportunity as the "reachable moment"—the time when a nurse truly connects with the client by directly meeting the individual on mutual terms. The reachable moment allows for the mutual exchange of concerns and a sharing of possible intervention options without the nurse being inhibited by prejudice or bias. When the client feels emotionally supported, the stage is set for the teachable moment, when the client is most receptive to learning.

MOTIVATION

Emotional readiness is strongly associated with motivation, which is a willingness to take action. Knowing the motivational level of the learner assists the nurse in determining when that patient is ready to learn. Assessment of emotional readiness involves determining the level of motivation, not necessarily the reasons for the motivation. A learner may be motivated to learn for many reasons, and almost any reason to learn is a valid one.

The level of motivation reflects what learners perceive as an expectation of themselves or others. Interest in informal or formal teacher–learner interactions is a cue to motivation. The patient who is ready to learn shows an interest in what the nurse is doing by demonstrating a willingness to participate or to ask questions. Prior learning experiences, whether they are past accomplishments or failures, are reflected in the current level of motivation demonstrated by the learner for accomplishing the task at hand. (See Chapter 6 for more on motivation.)

RISK-TAKING BEHAVIOR

Taking risks, at least to some extent, is part of everyday living. Indeed, many activities are done without thinking about the outcome. According to Joseph (1993), some patients, by the very nature of their personalities, take more risks than others do. The nurse can assist patients to develop strategies that help reduce the level of risk associated with their choices. If patients participate in activities that may shorten their life span rather than complying with a recommended treatment plan, for example, the nurse must be willing to teach these patients how to recognize what to do if something goes wrong.

FRAME OF MIND

Frame of mind involves concern about the here and now versus the future. If survival is of primary concern, readiness to learn will be focused on the present to meet basic human needs. With respect to information-seeking behaviors of adults, Ramanadhan and Viswanath (2006) found that a significant percentage of persons diagnosed with a serious disease, such as cancer, report that they do not seek or receive health information beyond that given by healthcare providers. Furthermore, compared to seekers of health information, nonseeker patients are more likely to come from the lowest income and education groups and are less attentive about getting health information from the media. Also, older individuals, although they gather information from a variety of sources, tend to primarily make health decisions based on information provided by the healthcare professional (Cutilli, 2010). These findings have implications for nurses when deciding on the best method for reaching various segments of the population.

Children regard life in the here and now because they are developmentally focused on what makes them happy and satisfied. This perspective affects their willingness to learn health information. In addition, their thinking is concrete rather than abstract. Adults who have reached self-actualization and those whose basic needs are met tend to plan for their future and are more ready to learn health promotion tasks.

DEVELOPMENTAL STAGE

Each task associated with human development produces a peak time for readiness to learn, known as a teachable moment (Hansen & Fisher, 1998; Hotelling, 2005; Tanner, 1989; P. S. Wagner & Ash, 1998). Unlike children, adults can build on meaningful past experiences and are strongly driven to learn information that helps them to cope better with real-life tasks. They see learning as relevant when they can apply new knowledge to help them solve immediate problems. Children, in contrast, desire to learn for learning's sake and actively seek out experiences that give them pleasure and comfort. See Chapter 5 for Erikson's nine stages of psychosocial development, which are most relevant to an individual's emotional readiness to learn.

Experiential Readiness

Experiential readiness refers to the learner's past experiences with learning and includes five elements: level of aspiration, past coping mechanisms, cultural background, locus of control, and orientation. The nurse should assess whether previous learning experiences have been positive or negative in overcoming problems or accomplishing new tasks. Someone who has had negative experiences with learning is not likely to be motivated or willing to take a risk to change behavior or acquire new behaviors.

LEVEL OF ASPIRATION

Previous failures and past successes influence the goals that learners set for themselves. Early successes are important motivators in learning future skills. Satisfaction, once achieved, elevates the level of desire, which in turn increases the probability of continued efforts to change or acquire new behavior.

PAST COPING MECHANISMS

Nurses must explore the coping mechanisms that learners have been using to understand how they have dealt with previous problems. Once these mechanisms are identified, the nurse needs to determine whether past coping strategies have been effective and, if so, whether they work well in the present learning situation.

CULTURAL BACKGROUND

Nurses' knowledge about other cultures and their sensitivity to behavioral differences between cultures are important so that they can avoid teaching in opposition to cultural beliefs. Assessment of what an illness means to the patient from the patient's cultural perspective is essential in determining readiness to learn. Remaining sensitive to cultural influences allows the nurse to bridge the gap, when necessary, between the medical healthcare culture and the patient's culture. Building on the learner's knowledge base or belief system (unless it is dangerous to well-being), rather than attempting to change it or claim it is wrong, encourages rather than dampens readiness to learn. (See Chapter 8 for more on cultural attributes.)

Language is also a part of culture and may prove to be a significant obstacle to learning if the nurse and the learner do not speak the same language fluently. Assessing whether the learner understands English well enough to be able to express herself so that others understand is the first step. Obtaining the services of a qualified interpreter is necessary if the learner and nurse do not speak the same language. Enlisting the help of someone other than a trained interpreter (such as a family member or friend) to bridge language differences may negatively influence learning, although this effect depends on such issues as the sensitivity of the topic and the need for privacy. In some instances, the patient may not want family members or associates to know about a health concern or illness.

Medical terminology in and of itself may be a foreign language to many patients, whether or not they are from another culture or their primary language is the same or different from that of the nurse. In addition, sometimes a native language does not have an equivalent word to describe the terms that are being used in the teaching situation. Differences in language compound cultural barriers. Nurses should not start teaching unless they have determined that the learner understands what they are saying and that they understand the learner's culture.

LOCUS OF CONTROL

When patients are internally motivated to learn, they have what is called an internal locus of control; that is, they are ready to learn when they feel a need to know about something. This drive to learn comes from within the learner. Usually, this type of learner indicates a need to know by asking questions. Remember that when someone asks a question, the time is prime for learning. Patients who have an external locus of control—that is, they are driven by outside forces or influences to respond—depend on the expectations and initiatives of others to get them motivated to learn. For these types of patients, the responsibility often falls on the nurse to motivate them to want to learn.

ORIENTATION

The tendency to adhere to a parochial or cosmopolitan point of view is known as orientation. Patients with a parochial orientation tend to be more close minded in their thinking, are more conservative in their approach to situations, are less willing to learn new material, and place the most trust in traditional authority figures such as the physician. This type of orientation is seen most often in people who have been raised in a small-town atmosphere or who come from sheltered neighborhoods or protective family environments. Conversely, people who exhibit a cosmopolitan orientation most likely have a more worldly perspective on life as a result of broader experiences outside their immediate spheres of influence. These individuals are more likely to be receptive to new ideas and to opportunities to learn new ways of doing things. Nurses must be careful not to stereotype individuals unfairly, but learners usually possess representative characteristics of one or the other of these two opposing orientations.

Knowledge Readiness

Knowledge readiness refers to the learner's present knowledge base, the level of learning capability, the existence of any learning disabilities, and the preferred style of learning. Nurses must assess these components to determine readiness to learn and should plan teaching accordingly.

PRESENT KNOWLEDGE BASE

How much someone already knows about a particular subject or how good that person is at performing a task is an important factor to determine before designing and implementing teaching. If nurses make the mistake of teaching material that has already been learned, they risk at the very least creating boredom and disinterest in the learner or, at the extreme, insulting the learner, which could produce resistance to further learning. The nurse must always find out what the learner knows prior to teaching and build on this knowledge base to encourage readiness to learn.

COGNITIVE ABILITY

The nurse must match the level of behavioral objectives to the ability of the learner. The learner who is capable of understanding, memorizing, recalling, or recognizing information is functioning at a lower level than the learner who demonstrates problem solving, concept formation, or application of information. For example, patients who can identify risk factors of hypertension (a low level of functioning) may struggle with generalizing this information to incorporate a low-salt diet in their lifestyle.

Individuals with limited cognitive abilities present a special challenge to the nurse and require simple explanations and step-by-step instruction with frequent repetition. Nurses should be sure to make information meaningful to them, teach at their level, and communicate in ways that they can understand. Enlisting the help of members of the patient's support system by teaching them necessary skills allows them to contribute positively to the reinforcement of self-care activities.

LEARNING AND READING DISABILITIES

Learning disabilities, which may be accompanied by low-level reading skills, are not necessarily indicative of an individual's intellectual abilities, but they do require nurses to use special or creative approaches to instruction to sustain or increase one's readiness to learn. Individuals with low literacy skills and learning disabilities may become easily discouraged unless the nurse recognizes their special needs and seeks ways to help them accommodate or overcome their problems with processing information. (See Chapter 7 on literacy and Chapter 9 on special populations.)

LEARNING STYLES

A variety of preferred styles of learning exist, and assessing how someone learns best and likes to learn helps the nurse to select appropriate teaching approaches that meet the true needs of the patients (Inott & Kennedy, 2011). Knowing the teaching methods and materials with which a learner is most comfortable or, conversely, those that the learner does not tolerate well allows the nurse to tailor teaching to meet the needs of patients with different styles of learning, thereby increasing their readiness to learn. The next section provides further information about learning styles.

Learning Styles, Personality Types, and Intelligences

Learning styles refers to the way individuals process information (Guild & Garger, 1998) and to their preferred approaches to different learning tasks (Cassidy, 2004; Furnham, 2012). Learning style models are based on the idea that certain characteristics of learning are biological in origin, whereas others are sociologically developed as a result of environmental influences. No learning style is either better or worse than another.

Recognizing that people have different approaches to learning helps the nurse create an atmosphere for learning that encourages each individual to reach his or her full potential. Understanding learning styles also can help nurses make deliberate decisions about program development and the design of their teaching (Arndt & Underwood, 1990; Chapman & Calhoun, 2006; Coffield, Moseley, Hall, & Ecclestone, 2004b; Jessee, O'Neill, & Dosch, 2006; Morse, Oberer, Dobbins, & Mitchell, 1998; Vaughn & Baker, 2008).

Determining Learning Styles

Three mechanisms to determine the different ways people learn are observation, interviews, and administration of learning style instruments. By observing the learner in action, the nurse can witness how the learner grasps information and problem solves. In an interview, the nurse can ask the learner about preferred ways of learning as well as the environment most comfortable for learning. Is group discussion or self-instruction preferable? Does the learner prefer hands-on activities or reading instructions? Simply asking the question, "How do you learn best?" can yield valuable information on this front. Once data are gathered through interview and observations, nurses can validate learning style and choose methods and materials for instruction to support a variety of learner preferences. They can then direct patients toward the ways learning is best achieved.

The identification and application of information about learning styles continue to be an emerging movement in nursing and health care. To date, researchers have defined learning styles differently, although the concepts in each definition are often overlapping. Learning style instruments can measure learning style preferences. However, since it is not always practical in a clinical setting to actually administer these instruments to every patient, the following discussion will focus on the popular theories about the different ways people learn rather than on the instruments used to measure styles of learning. These theories do not offer any single framework for teaching but do provide the nurse with a better understanding of the ways learners perceive and process information.

Dunn and Dunn Learning Styles

Dunn and Dunn (1978) identified five basic stimuli (as shown in **Figure 4–2**) that affect a person's ability to learn:

1. Environmental elements (such as sound, light, temperature, and design), which are biological in nature.
2. Emotional elements (such as motivation, persistence, responsibility, and structure), which are developmental and emerge over time as an outgrowth of experiences that have happened at home, school, play, or work.

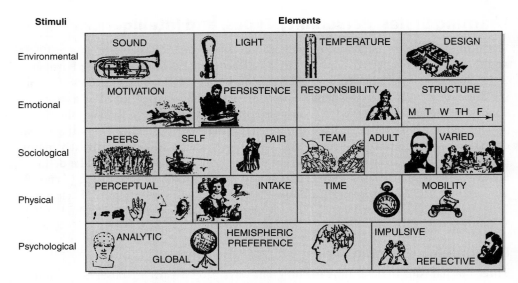

Figure 4–2 Dunn and Dunn's learning style options

Courtesy of the Association for Supervision and Curriculum Development. Dunn, R. (1983). Can students identify their own learning styles? *Educational Leadership, 40*(5), 61. Reprinted by permission of the Association for Supervision and Curriculum Development. All rights reserved.

3. Sociological patterns (such as the desire to work alone or in groups, or a combination of these two approaches), which are thought to be socioculturally based.
4. Physical elements (such as perceptual strength, intake, time of day, and mobility), which are also biological in nature and relate to the way learners function physically.
5. Psychological elements (such as the way learners process and react to information), which are also biological in nature.

Certain characteristics of Dunn and Dunn's identified stimuli are very relevant to the role of the nurse as teacher. The nurse needs to consider the following selected characteristics when assessing a patient's or family member's learning style.

THE ENVIRONMENTAL ELEMENTS

Sound. Individuals react to sound in different ways. Some learners need complete silence, others are able to block out sounds around them, and still others require sound in their environment for learning.

Light. Some learners work best under bright lights, whereas others need dim or low lighting.

Temperature. Some learners have difficulty thinking or concentrating if a room is too hot or, conversely, if it is too cold.

Design. Some learners are more relaxed and can learn better in an informal environment by being able to position themselves in a lounge chair, on the floor, on pillows, or on carpeting. Others cannot learn in an informal environment because it makes them drowsy and they require a more formal setting.

THE EMOTIONAL ELEMENTS

Motivation. Motivation, or the desire to achieve, increases when learning success increases. Unmotivated learners need short learning assignments that enhance their strengths. Motivated learners, by comparison, are eager to learn and should be told exactly what they are required to do, with resources available so that they can self-pace their learning.

Persistence. Learners differ in their preference for completing tasks in one sitting versus taking periodic breaks and returning to the task at a later time. Some patients with long attention spans can be successful learning new information in a single block of time, while those whose attention span is short need to break up the learning session and take regular breaks.

Responsibility. Responsibility involves the desire to do what the learner thinks is expected. Learners with low responsibility scores usually are nonconforming and will do something according to their own time frame and in their own way. Conversely, those who demonstrate high levels of responsibility will usually undertake to complete a task immediately and as directed. Knowing this, the nurse should give patients choices and allow them to select different ways to learn. When given appropriate choices, the nonconformist will likely be more willing to meet the nurse's expectations.

Structure. Structure refers to either the preference for receiving specific directions, guidance, or rules, or the preference for learning without structure in the learner's own way. Structure should vary in the amount and kind that is provided, depending on the learner's ability to make responsible decisions and the requirements of the task.

THE SOCIOLOGICAL ELEMENTS

Learning alone. Some people prefer to learn on their own, and therefore, self-instruction or one-to-one interaction is the best approach for learning. For those who prefer to learn with family members or friends, group discussion and role play can facilitate learning.

Presence of an authority figure. Some learners feel more comfortable when someone with authority or recognized expertise is present during learning. Others become nervous, are embarrassed to demonstrate their skills, and have trouble concentrating. Depending on the style of the learner, either one-to-one interaction or self-study may be the appropriate approach.

THE PHYSICAL ELEMENTS

Perceptual strengths. Four types of learners are distinguished in this category: (1) those with auditory preferences, who learn best while listening to verbal instruction; (2) those with visual preferences, who learn best from reading or observation; (3) those with tactile preferences, who learn best when they can underline as they read, take notes when they listen, and otherwise keep their hands busy; and (4) those with kinesthetic preferences, who absorb and retain information best when allowed to perform whole-body movement or participate in simulated or real-life experiences.

Auditory learners should be introduced to new information first by hearing about it, followed by receiving verbal feedback for reinforcement of the information. Group discussion is a teaching method best suited to this learning style. Visual learners learn more easily by viewing, watching, and observing. Simulation, video, and demonstration methods of instruction are therefore most beneficial to their learning. Tactile learners learn through touching, manipulating, and handling objects. The use of models and computer-assisted instruction is most suitable for this learning style. Kinesthetic learners learn more easily by doing and experiencing. They profit most from opportunities for role play and participating in return demonstration.

Intake. Some learners need to eat, drink, chew, or bite objects while concentrating; others prefer no intake until after they have finished learning. The nurse need not be offended if patients or family members want to eat or drink while learning.

Time of day. Some learners perform better at one time of day than another. Dunn (1995) contends that among adults, 55% are morning people and 28% work best in the evening. Many adults experience energy lows in the afternoon. School-aged children, on the other hand, have high energy levels in the late morning and early afternoon. Approximately 13% of high school students work best in the evening. This time sensitivity means that it may be easier or more difficult for a person to learn a new skill or behavior at certain times of the day than at other times. To enhance learning potential, the nurse should try to schedule teaching during the learner's best time of day.

Mobility. Mobility refers to how still the learner can sit and for how long a period of time. Some learners need to move about, whereas others can remain still for hours engaged in learning. For those who require mobility, the nurse needs to provide opportunity for movement during the teaching session.

THE PSYCHOLOGICAL ELEMENTS

Global versus analytic. Some learners are global in their thinking and learn best by first understanding an issue, problem or concept from a broad, overall perspective before focusing on the specific parts. Other learners are analytical in their thinking, like details, and process information best in a step-by-step approach to learning.

Hemispheric preference. Learners who possess right-brain preference tend to learn best in environments that have low illumination, background music, casual seating, and hands-on instructional resources. Learners with left-brain preference require the opposite type of environment, characterized by bright lighting, quiet setting, formal seating, and visual or auditory instructional resources.

Impulsivity versus reflectivity. Impulsive learners prefer opportunities to participate verbally in groups and tend to answer questions spontaneously and without consciously processing their thinking. Reflective learners seldom volunteer information unless they are asked to do so, prefer to contemplate information, and tend to be uncomfortable participating in group discussions (Dunn, 1984).

Visual, Aural, Read/Write, and Kinesthetic Learning Styles

Fleming and Mills (1992) identified four categories or preferences—visual, aural, read/write, and kinesthetic (VARK)—that seem to reflect the learning style experiences of their students. The VARK model, which is similar to the perceptual strengths stimuli of the Dunn and Dunn (1978) model, focuses on a person's preference for taking in and putting out information. Innot and Kennedy (2011) believe the VARK theory of learning styles is very conducive to patient education. According to Fleming and Mills (1992), an individual learns most effectively and comfortably by one of the following ways:

- *Visual learners*: Like information presented in the form of diagrams, flowcharts, graphs, and symbols that can be used to represent what could have been presented in words.
- *Aural learners*: Have a preference for hearing information and enjoy listening to lectures, often need directions read aloud, and prefer to discuss topics one-on-one and in study groups.
- *Read/write learners*: Like the written word, as evidenced by reading or writing, with references to additional sources of information.
- *Kinesthetic learners*: Enjoy doing hands-on activities, such as role play, return demonstration, and manipulation of objects.

Jung and Myers-Briggs Personality Types

Carl G. Jung (1921/1971), a Swiss psychiatrist, as early as 1921 developed a theory that explains personality similarities and differences by identifying attitudes of people (extraverts and introverts) along with opposite mental functions, which are the ways people perceive or prefer to take in and make use of information from the world around them. Jung proposed that people are likely to operate in a variety of ways depending on the circumstances. Despite these situational adaptations, each individual tends to develop comfortable patterns, which dictate behavior in certain predictable ways. Jung used the word *type* to identify these styles of personality, which can impact the way that people learn.

According to Jung, everyone uses these opposing perceptions to some degree when dealing with people and situations, but each person has a preference for one way of looking at the world. Individuals become more skilled in arriving at a decision in either a thinking or a feeling way and can function as extraverts at one time and as introverts at another time, but they tend to develop patterns that are most typical and comfortable.

Isabel Myers and her mother, Katherine Briggs, became convinced that Jung's theories had an application for increasing human understanding (Myers, 1980). In addition to Jung's dimensions, Myers and Briggs discovered another dimension, judgment–perception (JP) (Myers, 1987), whereby an individual comes to a conclusion about or becomes aware of something. By combining the different and opposite preferences (see **Figure 4–3**), Myers and Briggs identified 16 personality types, each with its own strengths and interests (see **Figure 4–4**), by which people can be classified.

The four pairs of opposite types are:

1. *Extraversion–introversion (E–I)*. These preferences reflect an orientation either to the outside world of people and things or to the inner world of concepts and ideas. This pair of opposite preferences describes the extent to which behavior is determined by attitudes toward the world. Jung (1921/1971) invented the terms from Latin words meaning "outward-turning" (extraversion) and

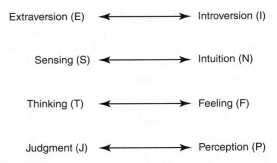

Figure 4–3   Myers-Briggs dichotomous dimensions or preferences

ISTJ	ISFJ	INFJ	INTJ
ISTP	ISFP	INFP	INTP
ESTP	ESFP	ENFP	ENTP
ESTJ	ESFJ	ENFJ	ENTJ

Figure 4–4   Myers-Briggs types

Modified and reproduced from *Introduction to Type®* 3rd edition by Isabel Briggs Myers. Copyright 1998 by Consulting Psychologists Press, Inc. All rights reserved. Further reproduction is prohibited without the Publisher's written consent.

"inward-turning" (introversion). Individuals who prefer extraversion operate comfortably and successfully by interacting with things external to themselves, such as other people, experiences, and situations. They like to clarify thoughts and ideas through talking and doing. People who operate more comfortably in an extraverted way think aloud. Individuals with a preference for introversion are more interested in the internal world of their minds, hearts, and souls. They like to brew over thoughts and actions, reflecting on them until they become more personally meaningful. Those who operate more comfortably in an intro-verted way are often thoughtful, reflective, and slow to act because they need time to translate internal thoughts to the external world. Their thoughts are well formulated before they are willing to share them with others.

2. *Sensing–intuition (S–N).* These types describe perception as coming directly through the five senses or indirectly by way of the unconscious. This pair of op-posite preferences explains how people understand what is experienced. People who prefer sensing experience the world through their senses—vision, hearing, touch, taste, and smell. They observe what is real, what is factual, and what is

actually happening. For these individuals, seeing or experiencing is believing. The sensory functions allow the individual to observe carefully, gather facts, and focus on practical actions. Conversely, those people who prefer intuition tend to read between the lines, focus on meaning, and attend to what might be. Those with intuition preferences view the world through possibilities and relationships and are tuned into subtleties of body language and tones of voice. This kind of perception leads them to examine problems and issues in creative and original ways.

3. *Thinking–feeling (T–F)*. These are the approaches used by individuals to arrive at judgments through impersonal, logical, or subjective processes. Thinking types analyze information, data, situations, and people and make decisions based on logic. They are careful and slow in the analysis of the data because accuracy and thoroughness are important to them. They trust objectivity and put faith in logical predictions and rational arguments. Thinking types explore and weigh all alternatives, and the final decision is reached impersonally, unemotionally, and carefully. For individuals with a feeling preference, the approach to decision making takes place through a subjective, perceptive, empathetic, and emotional perspective. Individuals who prefer feeling search for the effect of a decision on themselves and others. They consider alternatives and examine evidence to develop a personal reaction and commitment. They believe the decision-making process is complex and not totally objective. Circumstantial evidence is extremely important, and these individuals see the world as gray rather than black and white.

4. *Judging–perceiving (J–P)*. These are the means by which an individual comes to a conclusion about or becomes aware of something. The extremes of this continuum are a preference for judging, which is the desire to regulate and bring closure to circumstances in life, and a preference for perceiving, which is the desire to be open minded and understanding.

See **Table 4–3** for examples of how people prefer to learn based on the way they perceive and process information.

Kolb's Experiential Learning Model

Kolb's model (Kolb, 1984), represented as a cycle of learning, describes learning as a continuous process. In this model, the learner is not a blank slate, but rather approaches a topic to be learned based on past experiences, heredity, and the demands of the present environment. These factors combine to produce different orientations (modes) to learning. By understanding Kolb's theory, the nurse is better equipped to provide teaching to meet the needs of each individual's preferred style of learning. The learning cycle, which includes four modes of learning, reflects two major dimensions: perception and processing. Kolb believes that learning results from the way learners perceive information as well as how they process information.

The dimension of perception involves two opposing viewpoints: some learners perceive through concrete experience (CE mode), whereas others perceive through abstract conceptualization (AC mode). At the CE stage of the learning cycle, learners tend to rely more on feelings than on a systematic approach to problems and situations. Learners

Table 4–3 Myers-Briggs Types: Examples of Learning

Extraversion
Likes group work
Dislikes slow-paced learning
Likes action and to experience things so as to learn
Offers opinions without being asked
Asks questions to check on the expectations of the teacher
Sensing
Practical
Realistic
Observant
Learns from an orderly sequence of details
Thinking
Low need for harmony
Finds ideas and things more interesting than people
Analytical
Fair
Judging
Organized
Methodical
Work oriented
Controls the environment
Introversion
Likes quiet space
Dislikes interruptions
Likes learning that deals with thoughts and ideas
Offers opinions only when asked
Asks questions to allow understanding of the learning activity
Intuition
Always likes something new
Imaginative
Sees possibilities
Prefers the whole concept versus details
Feeling
Values harmony
More interested in people than things or ideas
Sympathetic
Accepting
Perceiving
Open ended
Flexible
Play oriented
Adapts to the environment

who fall into this category like interacting with people, benefit from specific experiences, and are sensitive to others. They learn from feeling. In contrast, at the AC stage, learners rely on logic and ideas rather than on feelings to deal with problems or situations. People who fall into this category use systematic planning and logical analysis to solve problems. They learn by thinking.

The process dimension also has two opposing orientations: Some learners process information through reflective observation (RO mode), whereas others process information through active experimentation (AE mode). At the RO stage of the learning cycle, learners rely on objectivity, careful judgment, personal thoughts, and feelings to form opinions. People who fall into this category look for the meaning of things by viewing them from different perspectives. They learn by watching and listening. At the AE stage of the learning cycle, however, learning is active, and learners like to experiment to get things done. They prefer to influence or change situations and see the results of their actions. They enjoy involvement and are risk takers. They learn by doing.

Kolb describes each learning style as a combination of the four basic learning modes (CE, AC, RO, and AE), identifying separate learning style types that best define the strengths and weaknesses of a learner. The learner predominantly demonstrates characteristics of one of four style types: (1) diverger, (2) assimilator, (3) converger, or (4) accommodator. These learning styles are discussed here as they appear in clockwise order in **Figure 4–5**, starting with the diverger.

1. The diverger combines the learning modes of CE and RO. People with this learning style are good at viewing concrete situations from many points of view. They like to observe, gather information, and gain insights rather than take action. Working in groups to generate ideas appeals to them. They place a high

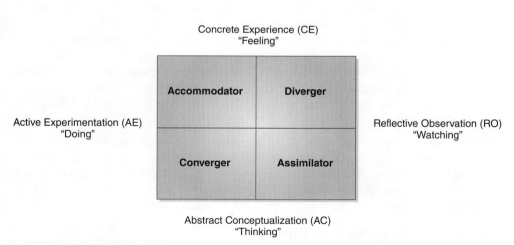

Figure 4–5   Kolb's cycle of learning

value on understanding for knowledge's sake and like to personalize learning by connecting information with something familiar in their experiences. They have active imaginations, enjoy being involved, and are sensitive to feelings. Divergent thinkers learn best, for example, through group discussions and participating in brainstorming sessions.

2. The assimilator combines the learning modes of RO and AC. People with this learning style demonstrate the ability to understand large amounts of information by putting it into concise and logical form. They are less interested in people and more focused on abstract ideas and concepts. They are good at inductive reasoning, value theory over practical application of ideas, and need time to reflect on what has been learned and how information can be integrated into their past experiences. They rely on knowledge from experts. Assimilative thinkers learn best, for example, through lecture, one-to-one instruction, and self-instruction methods with ample reading materials to support their learning.

3. The converger combines the learning modes of AC and AE. People with this learning style type find practical application for ideas and theories and have the ability to use deductive reasoning to solve problems. They like structure and factual information, and they look for specific solutions to problems. Learners with this style prefer technical tasks rather than dealing with social and interpersonal issues. Kolb claims that individuals with this learning style have skills that are important for specialist and technology careers. The convergent thinker learns best, for example, through demonstration/return demonstration methods of teaching accompanied by handouts and diagrams.

4. The accommodator combines the learning modes of AE and CE. People with this learning style learn best by hands-on experience and enjoy new and challenging situations. They act on intuition and gut feelings rather than on logic. These risk takers like to explore all possibilities and learn by experimenting with materials and objects. Accommodative thinkers are perhaps the most challenging to nurses because they demand new and exciting experiences and are willing to take risks that might endanger their safety. Role play, gaming, and computer simulations, for example, are methods of teaching most preferred by this style of learner.

Kolb believes that understanding a person's learning style, including its strengths and weaknesses, represents a major step toward increasing learning power and helping learners to get the most from their learning experiences. By using different teaching strategies to address these four learning styles, particular modes of learning can be matched, at least some of the time, with appropriate methods of teaching.

Gardner's Eight Types of Intelligence

Most models and measurement instruments on learning style focus on the adult as learner. However, children also have their own way of learning that can be assessed from the standpoint of each individual's unique pattern of growth and neurological functioning. Psychologist Howard Gardner (1983) developed a theory focused on the multiple kinds of intelligence in children. Gardner based his theory on findings from brain research, developmental work, and psychological testing. He identified seven kinds of intelligence located in different parts of the brain: (1) linguistic, (2) logical-mathematical, (3) spatial, (4) musical, (5) bodily kinesthetic, (6) interpersonal, and (7) intrapersonal. Later, Gardner (1999) identified an eighth kind of intelligence, called (8) naturalistic. Each learner possesses all eight kinds of intelligence, but in different proportions.

1. *Linguistic intelligence*: Children with a tendency to display this type of intelligence have highly developed auditory skills and think in words. They like writing, telling stories, spelling words, and reading, and they can recall names, places, and dates. These children learn best by verbalizing, hearing, or seeing words. Word games or crossword puzzles are an excellent method for helping these children to learn new material.

2. *Logical-mathematical intelligence*: The children who are strong in this intelligence explore patterns, categories, and relationships. In the adolescent years, they can think logically with a high degree of abstraction. As learners, they question many things and ask where, what, and when. A question such a learner might ask is, "If people are always supposed to be good to each other, then why do people always say they are sorry?" They can do arithmetic problems quickly in their heads, like to learn by using computers, and do experiments to test concepts they do not understand. They enjoy strategy board games such as chess and checkers.

3. *Spatial intelligence*: These children learn by images and pictures. They enjoy such activities as building blocks, jigsaw puzzles, and daydreaming. They like to draw or do other art activities, can read charts and diagrams, and learn with visual methods such as videos or photographs.

4. *Musical intelligence*: Musically intelligent children can be found singing a tune, indicating when a note is off key, playing musical instruments with ease, dancing to music, and keeping time rhythmically. They are also sensitive to sounds in the environment, such as the sound of walking on snow on a cold winter morning. Often, musically intelligent children learn best with music playing in the background.

5. *Bodily-kinesthetic intelligence*: Children with this type of intelligence learn by processing knowledge through bodily sensations, such as moving around or acting things out. It is difficult for these learners to sit still for long periods of time. They are good at athletic sports and have highly developed fine-motor coordination. Using body language to communicate and copying people's behaviors or movements come easily for this group of learners.

6. *Interpersonal intelligence*: Children with high interpersonal intelligence understand people, are able to notice others' feelings, tend to have many friends, and are gifted in social skills. They learn best in groups and gravitate toward activities that involve others in problem solving.

7. *Intrapersonal intelligence*: Children with this type of intelligence have strong personalities, prefer the inner world of feelings and ideas, and like being alone. They are very private individuals, desire a quiet area to learn, and prefer to be by themselves to learn. They tend to be self-directed and self-confident. They learn well with independent, self-paced instruction.

8. *Naturalistic intelligence*: Children with high naturalistic intelligence can distinguish and categorize objects or phenomena in nature. They enjoy subjects, shows, and stories that deal with animals or naturally occurring phenomena and are keenly aware of their surroundings and subtle changes in their environment.

Teachers may want to approach children from the perspective of these different intelligences (Armstrong, 1987). For nurses, it often can be difficult to assess the preferred learning style of a child when he or she is facing an illness or surgery. Asking some key questions of the child or parents may give the nurse some clues about how to approach the child: Which subjects does the child excel in or like best? Which kinds of hobbies does the child have? What excites this child? Which kinds of toys does the child play with? Which inner qualities does the child possess, such as courage, playfulness, curiosity, friendliness, or creativity? Which talents does the child possess?

By using Gardner's theory of the eight intelligences, the nurse can assess each child's style of learning and tailor teaching accordingly. For example, if the nurse wants to assist a child in learning about a kidney disorder, then she can use one of the following eight approaches, depending on the child's style of learning:

- *Linguistic*: Practice quizzing the child orally on the different parts of the kidney, the disease itself, and different ways to take care of himself or herself.
- *Spatial*: Have a diagram or chart that allows the child to associate different colors or shapes with concepts. Storytelling that illustrates a child with the same chronic illness can be used.
- *Kinesthetic*: Have a kidney model available that can be felt, taken apart, and manipulated. Have the child identify tactile features of the kidney or act out appropriate behavior.
- *Logical-mathematical*: Group concepts into categories, starting with simple generalizations or health behaviors. Reasoning works well in showing the child the consequences of actions.
- *Musical*: Teach self-care or the material to be learned by putting information into a song. Soft music also serves as a relaxing influence on the child.
- *Interpersonal*: Have a group of children play a card game, such as a version of Old Maid, that matches health information with medical pictures or pictures of healthcare activities and procedures.
- *Intrapersonal*: Suggest that the child become active by writing to friends, family, or local and state government officials to advocate for kidney disease research. Such learners need to research the facts and then convey their findings to others.

- *Naturalist*: Provide pet therapy, allow the child to engage in outside activities that are a form of exercise (e.g., gardening or nature walks), or offer videos that feature nature, science, or animals.

Although Gardner's theory of multiple intelligences was originally designed for use with children, several recent articles have addressed its application with adults. For example, this theory was implemented with nursing students for classroom learning (Amerson, 2006). Many teachers see the theory as simple common sense—that children (and adults) have varied talents and learn in different ways even though there is no empirical evidence supporting the multiple intelligences theory (Gardner, 2004; Waterhouse, 2006). Additional information about Gardner's theory is available at his website (www.howardgardner.com).

Interpretation of Learning Style Models, Personality Types, and Intelligences

Paying attention to different ways people learn is an important consideration in the teaching–learning process. However, caution must be used when assessing styles so as not to ignore other factors that are equally important to teaching and learning, such as readiness and capabilities to learn, educational and cultural backgrounds, and rates of learning. Learning styles, which vary from person to person, also differ from capabilities. Another caution to keep in mind is that much of the advice offered with regard to using learning styles makes intuitive sense and is logical but is not necessarily supported by empirical research (Coffield, Moseley, Hall, & Ecclestone, 2004a).

Some learning theorists advocate that learning style be matched with a similar teaching style for learners to attain an optimal level of achievement. However, research in this area is clouded by inconsistent findings (Coffield et al., 2004b). After reviewing the literature, Pashler, McDaniel, Rohrer, and Bjork (2008) concluded that sufficient evidence does not exist to justify this approach. They suggest that teachers should, instead, be more concerned with matching their instruction to the content they are teaching. Understanding learning styles helps nurses think about how to modify their teaching methods so as to best present different content and to reach the widest variety of learners.

It may be that learning occurs not so much because teacher and learner styles are a perfect match but because the teacher uses a variety of teaching approaches rather than relying on just one, so that learners feel less stressed and more confident. As a result, learners are more satisfied overall with their learning experience and hence more motivated to learn. Application of learning style theory to facilitate the teaching process allows the nurse to approach each learner holistically by recognizing that not all learners process information in precisely the same way (Arndt & Underwood, 1990; Rayner, 2007).

Research indicates that learning style preferences prevail over time, although they may change depending on the context in which learners are operating at any given moment. The concept of matching styles implies that individuals are static, which contradicts the purpose of education. Learners need to experience some discomfort before they can grow. The general guidelines below should be followed when assessing individual learning styles:

- Become familiar with the different theories and models and the various ways in which styles are classified so that it becomes easier to recognize the different approaches to learning.
- Identify key elements of a patient's learning style by observing and asking questions to verify observations. Then, provide learning choices that enable patients to operate, at least some of the time, in the style by which they prefer to learn. For example, the following questions could elicit valuable information: Do you prefer to attend group classes or one-on-one teaching with the nurse? Which do you like best, reading or viewing a video? Would you like me to demonstrate this skill first, or would you rather learn by doing while I talk you through the procedure?
- Always allow patients the opportunity to say when the teaching method is not working for them.
- Encourage patients to become aware of their learning styles as a way to increase understanding from both the nurse's and the patient's perspectives. Everyone should realize that a variety of learning modalities exist and that no one style is better than another.
- Be cautious about saying that certain teaching methods are always more effective for certain styles. Remember that everyone is unique, circumstances may alter preferences, and there are many different ways to influence learning.
- Encourage patients to expand their style ranges rather than to seek only comfortable experiences.

Nurses must exercise caution to avoid stereotyping patients as to their style. The goal should be to identify preferred styles of learning to ensure that each patient is given an equal opportunity to learn in the best or most comfortable way. Understanding how someone prefers to learn assists the nurse in choosing diverse teaching methods and instructional materials to meet the needs of all learners.

Summary

Learning is a complex concept that depends on many factors influencing a learner to change behavior or learn new behavior. This chapter stresses the importance of assessing each individual's learning needs, readiness to learn, and individual learning styles prior to planning and implementing any teaching intervention. Assessment of these determinants provides the information necessary for decision making about who and what needs to be taught, when teaching should take place, and where and how teaching should be carried out.

Identifying and prioritizing learning needs is the first step and requires the nurse to discover what the learner feels is important and wants to know, as well as what the nurse knows to be important. Once needs are established, the nurse must assess the learner's readiness to learn based on the physical, emotional, experiential, and knowledge components specific to each learner. The last determinant of learning examines individual learning styles. Assessment of learning style by way of interviewing and observing can reveal how people learn best as well as how they prefer to learn.

By accepting the diversity of needs, readiness levels, and styles among learners, the nurse can provide optimal experiences that encourage all learners to reach their full potential. Whoever the audience may be, the nurse must be able to identify and select the most appropriate teaching methods and instructional materials to facilitate learning.

Review Questions

1. What are the three determinants of learning?
2. How can patient learning needs be assessed?
3. What is meant by the term *readiness to learn*?
4. What are the four types of readiness to learn and the components of each type?
5. What is the definition of the term *learning style*?
6. Which models are available to determine someone's style of learning?
7. What are similarities and differences between the learning style models, personality types, and intelligences?

Case Study

Suppose you are a member of the interdisciplinary team working with Barbara Lund, a 36-year-old woman recovering from recent surgery for a malignant thoracic spinal cord tumor. Mrs. Lund has a supportive husband and a 2-year-old son. Mrs. Lund's husband, James, states, "I am really worried about Barbara because she was quite distressed for about 6 months prior to this surgery over the death of her father. I fear the surgery may have pushed her over the edge." Currently, 2 weeks status postresection, Mrs. Lund is beginning to ask team members questions about her prognosis and potential functional abilities. She says, "I remember my surgeon trying to explain the surgery to me, but honestly, I didn't really understand much of what he told me. I am a bit naive when it comes to anything medical." Mrs. Lund appears quite anxious about the cancer diagnosis and about how she will be able to continue caring for her son.

1. What are two methods you might use to assess Mrs. Lund's learning needs? List the advantages and disadvantages of each method.
2. Describe the criteria your team and the client will use to prioritize Mrs. Lund's learning needs. Give examples of specific learning needs that will likely be a priority.
3. Which major clues indicate Mrs. Lund's readiness to learn? Using the PEEK model, identify potential obstacles that might interfere with her readiness to learn.
4. How will knowledge of Mrs. Lund's learning preference(s) affect your team's instructional approach? Choose one learning preference for Mrs. Lund and describe the instructional approach your team will use to support this preference.

References

Amerson, R. (2006). Energizing the nursing lecture: Application of the theory of multiple intelligence learning. *Nursing Education Perspectives, 27*(4), 194–196.

Armstrong, T. (1987). *In their own way.* New York, NY: St. Martin's Press.

Arndt, M. J., & Underwood, B. (1990). Learning style theory and patient understanding. *Journal of Continuing Education in Nursing, 21*(1), 28–31.

Ashton, K. C. (1999). How men and women with heart disease seek care: The delay experience. *Progress in Cardiovascular Nursing, 14*(2), 53–60.

Bakas, T. C., Farran, C. J., Austin, J. K., Given, B. A., Johnson, E. A., & Williams, L. S. (2009). Content validity and satisfaction with a stroke caregiver intervention program. *Journal of Nursing Scholarship, 41*(4), 368–375.

Beddoe, S. S. (1999). Reachable moment. *Image: Journal of Nursing Scholarship, 31*(3), 248.

Bertakis, K. D., Rahman, A., Helms, L. J., Callahan, E. J., & Robbins, J. A. (2000). Gender differences in the utilization of health care services. *Journal of Family Practice, 49*(2), 147–152.

Bloom, B. (1968). Learning for mastery. *Instruction and curriculum, topical papers and reprints No. 1.* Durham, NC: National Laboratory for Higher Education.

Boyd, M. D., Gleit, C. J., Graham, B. A., & Whitman, N. I. (1998). *Health teaching in nursing practice: A professional model* (3rd ed.). Stamford, CT: Appleton & Lange.

Bruner, J. (1966). *Toward a theory of instruction.* Cambridge, MA: Harvard University Press.

Bubela, N., & Galloway, S. (1990). Factors influencing patients' informational needs at time of hospital discharge. *Patient Education and Counseling, 16,* 21–28.

Bubela, N., Galloway, S., McCay, E., McKibbon, A., Nagle, L., Pringle, D., . . . Shamian, J. (2000). Patient learning needs scale. Informational needs of surgical patients following discharge. *Applied Nursing Research, 13,* 12–18.

Burkhart, J. A. (2008). Training nurses to be teachers. *Journal of Continuing Education in Nursing, 39*(11), 503–510.

Burton, C. (2000). Re-thinking stroke rehabilitation: The Corbin and Strauss chronic illness trajectory framework. *Journal of Advanced Nursing, 32*(3), 595–602.

Carlson, M. L., Ivnik, M. A., Dierkhising, R. A., O'Byrne, M. M., & Vickers, K. S. (2006). A learning needs assessment of patients with COPD. *MEDSURG Nursing, 16*(4), 204–212.

Carroll, I. (1963). A model of school learning. *Teachers College Record, 64,* 723–733.

Cassidy, S. (2004). Learning styles: An overview of theories, models, and measures. *Educational Psychology, 24*(4), 419–444.

Chapman, D. M., & Calhoun, J. G. (2006). Validation of learning style measures: Implications for medical education practice. *Medical Education, 40,* 576–583.

Coffield, F., Moseley. D., Hall, E., & Ecclestone, K. (2004a). *Learning styles and pedagogy in post-16 learning: A systematic and critical review.* London, England: Learning and Skills Research Centre.

Coffield, F., Moseley, D., Hall, E., & Ecclestone, K. (2004b). *Should we be using learning styles? What research has to say about practice.* London, England: Learning and Skills Research Centre.

Corbett, C. F. (2003). A randomized pilot study of improving foot care in home health patients with diabetes. *Diabetes Educator, 29*(2), 273–282.

Corbin, J. M., & Strauss, A. (1991). A nursing model for chronic illness management based upon the trajectory framework. *Scholarly Inquiry for Nursing Practice: An International Journal, 5*(3), 155–174.

Cutilli, C. C. (2010). Seeking health information: What sources do your patients use? *Orthopaedic Nursing, 29*(3), 214–219.

Dunn, R. (1984). Learning style: State of the science. *Theory Into Practice, 23*(1), 10–19.

Dunn, R. (1995). *Strategies for educating diverse learners.* Bloomington, IN: Phi Delta Kappa.

Dunn, R., & Dunn, K. (1978). *Teaching students through their individual learning styles: A practical approach.* Reston, VA: National Association of Secondary School Principals.

Epstein, R., & Street, R. Jr. (2007). *Patient-centered communication in cancer care: Promoting healing and reducing suffering.* Publication No. 07-6225. Bethesda, MD: National Cancer Institute.

Fleming, N. D., & Mills, C. (1992). Not another inventory, rather a catalyst for reflection. *To Improve the Academy, 11,* 137–144.

Frank-Bader, M., Beltran, K., & Dojlidko, D. (2011). Improving transplant discharge education using a structured teaching approach. *Progress in Transplantation, 21*(4), 332–339.

Furnham, A. (2012). Learning styles and approaches to learning. In K. R. Harris, S. Graham, & T. Urdan (Eds.), *APA educational psychology handbook: Individual differences and cultural contextual factors* (Vol. 2, pp. 59–81). Washington, DC: American Psychological Association.

Gardner, H. (1983). *Frames of mind.* New York, NY: Basic Books.

Gardner, H. (1999). *Intelligence reframed: Multiple intelligences for the 21st century.* New York, NY: Basic Books.

Gardner, H. (2004). *Changing minds: The art and science of changing our own and other people's minds.* Boston, MA: Harvard Business School Press.

Gavan, C. S. (2003). Successful aging families: A challenge for nurses. *Holistic Nursing Practice, 17*(1), 11–18.

Guild, P. B., & Garger, S. (1998). *Marching to different drummers* (2nd ed.). Alexandria, VA: Association for Supervision and Curriculum Development.

Haddad, A. (2003). Ethics in action. Cutting corners on patient ed? *RN, 66*(7), 23–26.

Haggard, A. (1989). *Handbook of patient education.* Rockville, MD: Aspen.

Hansen, M., & Fisher, J. C. (1998). Patient-centered teaching: From theory to practice. *American Journal of Nursing, 98*(1), 56–60.

Harris, C. R., Jenkins, M., & Glaser, D. (2006). Gender differences in risk assessment: Why do women take fewer risks than men? *Judgment and Decision Making, 1*(1), 48–63.

Healthcare Education Association. (1989). *Managing hospital education.* Laguna Niguel, CA: Healthcare Education Associates.

Hotelling, B. A. (2005). Promoting wellness in Lamaze classes. *Journal of Perinatal Education, 14*(3), 45–50.

Inott, T., & Kennedy, B. B. (2011). Assessing learning styles: Practical tips for patient education. *Nursing Clinics of North America, 46*(3), 313–320.

Jacobs, V. (2000). Informational needs of surgical patients following discharge. *Applied Nursing Research, 13*(1), 12–18.

Jessee, S., O'Neill, P., & Dosch, R. (2006). Matching student personality types and learning preferences to teaching methodologies. *Journal of Dental Education, 70*(6), 644–651.

Joseph, D. H. (1993). Risk: A concept worthy of attention. *Nursing Forum, 28*(1), 12–16.

Jung, C. G. (1971). Psychological types. In *Collected works* (Vol. 6, R. F. C. Hull, Trans.). Princeton, NJ: Princeton University Press. (Originally published in German as *Psychologische Typen.* Zurich, Switzerland: Rasher Verlag, 1921)

Kessels, R. P. C. (2003). Patients' memory for medical information. *Journal of the Royal Society of Medicine, 96*(5), 219–222.

Kim, J., Dodd, M., West, C., Paul, S., Facione, N., Schumacher, K., . . . Miaskowski, C. (2004). The PRO-SELF pain control program improves patients' knowledge of cancer pain management. *Oncology Nursing Forum, 31*(6), 1137–1143.

Kitchie, S. (2003). *Rural elders with chronic disease: Place of residence, social network, social support, and medication adherence.* Doctoral dissertation, Binghamton University. Retrieved from Dissertation Abstracts International–B [Online], 64(08), 3745. (UMI No. 3102848)

Kolb, D. A. (1984). *Experiential learning: Experience as the source of learning and development*. Englewood Cliffs, NJ: Prentice Hall.

Ley, P. (1979). Memory for medical information. *British Journal of Social & Clinical Psychology, 18*(2), 245–255.

Lichtenthal, C. (1990). *A self-study model on readiness to learn*. Unpublished manuscript.

Lubkin, I. M., & Larsen, P. D. (2013). *Chronic illness: Impact and interventions* (8th ed.). Burlington, MA: Jones & Bartlett Learning.

Marcum, J., Ridenour, M., Shaff, G., Hammons, M., & Taylor, M. (2002). A study of professional nurses' perceptions of patient education. *Journal of Continuing Education in Nursing, 33*(3), 112–118.

McNeill, B. E. (2012). You teach but does your patient really learn? Basic principles to promote safe outcomes. *Tar Heel Nurse, 74*(1), 9–16.

Miaskowski, C., Dodd, M., West, C., Schumacher, K., Paul, S. M., Tripathy, D., & Koo, P. (2004). Randomized clinical trial of the effectiveness of a self-care intervention to improve cancer pain management. *Journal of Clinical Oncology, 22*(9), 1713–1720.

Morse, J. S., Oberer, J., Dobbins, J. A., & Mitchell, D. (1998). Understanding learning styles. Implications for staff development educators. *Journal of Nursing Staff Development, 14*(1), 41–46.

Myers, I. B. (1980). *Gifts differing*. Palo Alto, CA: Consulting Psychologists Press.

Myers, I. B. (1987). *Introduction to type*. Palo Alto, CA: Consulting Psychologists Press.

Pashler, H., McDaniel, M., Rohrer, D., & Bjork, R. (2008). Learning styles: Concepts and evidence. *Psychological Science in the Public Interest, 9*(3), 105–119.

Patterson, B. L. (2001). The shifting perspectives model of chronic illness. *Journal of Nursing Scholarship, 33*(1), 21–26.

Polat, S., Celik, S., Erkan H. A., & Kasali, K . (2014). Identification of learning needs of patients hospitalized at a university hospital. *Pakistan Journal of Medical Sciences, 30*(6),1253–1258.

Ramanadhan, S., & Viswanath, K. (2006). Health and the information nonseeker: A profile. *Health Communication, 20*(2), 131–139.

Rankin, S. H., & Stallings, L. D. (2005). *Patient education in health and illness* (5th ed.). Philadelphia, PA: Lippincott Williams & Wilkins.

Rayner, S. (2007). A teaching elixir, learning chimera or just fool's gold? Do learning styles matter? *Support for Learning, 22*(1), 24–30.

Redman, B. K. (2003). *Measurement tools in patient education*. New York, NY: Springer.

Rosen, A., Tsai, J., & Downs, S. (2003). Variations in risk attitude across race, gender and education. *Medical Decision Making, 23*, 511–517.

Şendir, M., Büyükyılmaz, F., & Muşovi, D. (2013). Patients' discharge information needs after total hip and knee arthroplasty: A quasi-qualitative pilot study. *Rehabilitation Nursing, 38*(5), 264–271.

Skinner, B. F. (1954). The science of learning and the art of teaching. *Harvard Educational Review, 24*, 86–97.

Stein, J. A., & Nyamathi, A. (2000). Gender differences in behavioural and psychosocial predictors of HIV testing and return for test results in a high-risk population. *AIDS Care, 12*(3), 343–356.

Stephenson, P. L. (2006). Before the teaching begins: Managing patient anxiety prior to providing education. *Clinical Journal of Oncology Nursing, 10*(2), 241–245.

Street, R., Jr., Makoul, G., Arora, N., & Epstein, R. (2009). How does communication heal? Pathways linking clinician–patient communication to health outcomes. *Patient Education and Counseling, 74*, 295–301.

Suhonen, R., Nenonen, A., Laukka, A., & Valimaki, M. (2005). Patients' informational needs and information received do not correspond in hospital. *Journal of Clinical Nursing, 14*(10), 1167–1176.

Tanner, G. (1989). A need to know. *Nursing Times, 85*(31), 54–56.

Telford, K., Kralik, D., & Koch, T. (2006). Acceptance and denial: Implications for people adapting to chronic illness. *Journal of Advanced Nursing, 55*(4), 457–464.

Timmins, F. (2005). A review of the information needs of patients with acute coronary syndromes. *Nursing in Critical Care, 10*(4), 174–183.

Vaughn, L., & Baker, R. (2008). Do different pairings of teaching styles and learning styles make a difference? Preceptor and resident perceptions. *Teaching and Learning in Medicine, 20*(3), 239–247.

Wagner, D. L., Bear, M., & Davidson, N. S. (2011). Measuring patient satisfaction with postpartum teaching methods used by nurses within the interaction model of client health behavior. *Research and Theory for Nursing Practice: An International Journal, 25*(3), 176–190.

Wagner, P. S., & Ash, K. L. (1998). Creating the teachable moment. *Journal of Nursing Education, 37*(6), 278–280.

Waterhouse, L. (2006). Multiple intelligences, the Mozart effect, and emotional intelligence: A critical review. *Educational Psychologist, 41*(4), 207–225.

Yonaty, S. A., & Kitchie, S. (2012). The educational needs of newly diagnosed stroke patients. *Journal of Neuroscience Nursing, 44*(5), E1–E9.

Developmental Stages of the Learner

Susan B. Bastable | Gina M. Myers

Chapter Highlights

- Developmental Characteristics
- The Developmental Stages of Childhood
  - *Infancy (First 12 Months of Life) and Toddlerhood (1–2 Years of Age)*
  - *Early Childhood (3–5 Years of Age)*
  - *Middle and Late Childhood (6–11 Years of Age)*
  - *Adolescence (12–19 Years of Age)*
- The Developmental Stages of Adulthood
  - *Young Adulthood (20–40 Years of Age)*
  - *Middle-Aged Adulthood (41–64 Years of Age)*
  - *Older Adulthood (65 Years of Age and Older)*
- The Role of the Family in Patient Education

Key Terms

ageism
andragogy
causality
causal thinking
conservation
crystallized intelligence
fluid intelligence
gerogogy
imaginary audience
pedagogy
personal fable
precausal thinking
syllogistic reasoning

Objectives

After completing this chapter, the reader will be able to

1. Identify the physical, cognitive, and psychosocial characteristics of learners that influence learning at various stages of growth and development.
2. Recognize the role of the nurse as teacher in assessing stage-specific learner needs according to maturational levels.
3. Determine the role of the family in patient education.
4. Discuss appropriate teaching strategies effective for learners at different developmental stages.

© Wanchai/Shutterstock

When planning, designing, implementing, and evaluating patient education, the nurse must carefully consider the characteristics of learners with respect to their developmental stage in life. The more diverse the audience, the more complex teaching will be to meet the needs of patients and their family members. Conversely, teaching a group of learners with the same characteristics will be more straightforward.

An individual's developmental stage significantly influences his or her ability to learn. To meet the health-related educational needs of learners, a developmental approach must be used. Three major factors associated with learner readiness—physical, cognitive, and psychosocial maturation—must be taken into account at each developmental period throughout the life cycle.

A deliberate attempt has been made to minimize reference to age as a criterion for learning. Research on life-span development shows that chronological age per se is not the only predictor of learning ability (Crandell, Crandell, & Vander Zanden, 2012; Santrock, 2013). At any given age, there can be a wide variation in abilities related to physical, cognitive, and psychosocial maturation. Age ranges, included after each developmental stage heading in this chapter, are intended to be used only as general guidelines; they do not imply that chronological age corresponds perfectly to developmental stage.

This chapter has specific implications for staff nurses because of the recent mandates by The Joint Commission. For healthcare agencies to meet Joint Commission accreditation requirements, teaching plans must address stage-specific competencies of the learner. In this chapter, therefore, the distinct life stages of learners are examined from the perspective of physical, cognitive, and psychosocial development. Also, this chapter emphasizes the role of the nurse in assessment of stage-specific learner needs, the role of the family in the teaching–learning process, and the teaching strategies specific to meeting the needs of learners at various developmental stages of life.

Developmental Characteristics

As noted earlier, actual chronological age is only a relative indicator of someone's physical, cognitive, and psychosocial stage of development. Unique as each individual is, however, some typical developmental trends have been identified as milestones of normal progression through the life cycle. When dealing with the teaching–learning process, it is imperative to determine the developmental stage of each learner so as to understand the cognitive, affective, and psychomotor behavioral changes that are occurring. However, other important factors, such as past experiences, physical and emotional health status, and personal motivation, as well as stress, environmental conditions, and available support systems, affect a person's ability and readiness to learn.

The major question underlying the planning for educational experiences is: When is the most appropriate or best time to teach the learner? The answer is when the learner is ready. The teachable moment, as defined by Havighurst (1976), is that point in time when the learner is most receptive to learning. Nevertheless, nurses do not always have to wait for teachable moments to occur. They can actively create opportunities by taking an interest and paying attention to the needs of the learner and use their current situation to increase awareness of the learner's need to change health behaviors (Hinkle, 2014; Lawson & Flocke, 2009).

The Developmental Stages of Childhood

Pedagogy is the art and science of helping children to learn (Knowles, 1990; Knowles, Holton, & Swanson, 2015). The different stages of childhood are divided according to what developmental theorists and educational psychologists define as specific patterns of behavior seen in particular phases of growth and development. This section reviews the teaching strategies to be used in the four stages of childhood in relation to the physical, cognitive, and psychosocial maturational levels of learners (**Table 5–1**).

Infancy (First 12 Months of Life) and Toddlerhood (1–2 Years of Age)

The field of growth and development is highly complex, and at no other time is physical, cognitive, and psychosocial maturation so changeable as during the very early years of childhood. Because of the dependency of members of this age group, the main focus of instruction for health maintenance of children is geared toward the parents, who are considered to be the primary learners rather than the very young child (Crandell et al., 2012; Palfrey et al., 2005; Santrock, 2013). However, the older toddler should not be excluded from healthcare teaching and can participate to some extent in the education process.

PHYSICAL, COGNITIVE, AND PSYCHOSOCIAL DEVELOPMENT

At no other time in life is physical maturation so rapid as during the period of development from infancy to toddlerhood (London, Ladewig, Davidson, Ball, & Bindler, 2013). Exploration of self and the environment is important in stimulating physical development (Crandell et al., 2012). Patient education must focus on teaching the parents of very young children the importance of stimulation, nutrition, the practice of safety measures to prevent illness and injury, and health promotion (Polan & Taylor, 2015).

Piaget (1951, 1952, 1976)—a noted expert in defining the key milestones in the cognitive development of children—labels the stage of infancy to toddlerhood as the *sensorimotor period*. During this stage, children learn through their senses. Motor activities promote toddlers' understanding of the world and an awareness of themselves as well as others' reactions in response to their own actions. Toddlers also have the capacity for basic reasoning, the beginnings of memory, and an elementary concept of **causality** (what causes something to happen). Also, they are oriented primarily to the here and now and have little tolerance for delayed gratification. The child who has lived with strict routines and plenty of structure has more of a grasp of time than the child who lives in an unstructured environment.

Children at this stage have short attention spans, are easily distracted, are egocentric in their thinking, and are not amenable to correction of their own ideas. Unquestionably,

Table 5–1 Stage-Appropriate Teaching Strategies

Learner	General Characteristics	Teaching Strategies	Nursing Interventions
Infancy–Toddlerhood			
Approximate age: Cognitive stage: Psychosocial stage:	Birth–2 years Sensorimotor Trust vs. mistrust (Birth–12 mo); Autonomy vs. shame and doubt (1–2 yr)	Dependent on environment Needs security Explores self and environment Natural curiosity	Orient teaching to caregiver Use repetition and imitation of information Stimulate all senses Provide physical safety and emotional security Allow play and manipulation of objects Welcome active involvement Forge alliances Encourage physical closeness Provide detailed information Answer questions and concerns Ask for information on child's strengths/limitations and likes/dislikes
Early Childhood			
Approximate age: Cognitive stage: Psychosocial stage:	3–5 years Preoperational Initiative vs. guilt	Egocentric Thinking precausal, concrete, literal Believes illness self-caused and punitive Limited sense of time Fears bodily injury Cannot generalize Animistic thinking (objects possess life or human characteristics) Centration (focus is on one characteristic of an object) Separation anxiety Motivated by curiosity Active imagination, prone to fears Play is his/her work	Use warm, calm approach Build trust Use repetition of information Allow manipulation of objects and equipment Give care with explanation Reassure not to blame self Explain procedures simply and briefly Provide safe, secure environment Use positive reinforcement Encourage questions to reveal perceptions/feelings Use simple drawings and stories Use play therapy, with dolls and puppets Stimulate senses: visual, auditory, tactile, motor Welcome active involvement Forge alliances Encourage physical closeness Provide detailed information Answer questions and concerns Ask for information on child's strengths/limitations and likes/dislikes

Middle and Late Childhood

Approximate age: 6–11 years Cognitive stage: Concrete operations Psychosocial stage: Industry vs. inferiority	More realistic and objective Understands cause and effect Deductive/inductive reasoning Wants concrete information Able to compare objects and events Variable rates of physical growth Reasons syllogistically Understands seriousness and consequences of actions Subject-centered focus Immediate orientation	Encourage independence and active participation Be honest, allay fears Use logical explanation Allow time to ask questions Use analogies to make invisible processes real Establish role models Relate care to other children's experiences; compare procedures Use subject-centered focus Use play therapy Provide group activities Use drawings, models, dolls, painting, audio– and videotapes	Welcome active involvement Forge alliances Encourage physical closeness Provide detailed information Answer questions and concerns Ask for information on child's strengths/limitations and likes/dislikes

Adolescence

Approximate age: 12–19 years Cognitive stage: Formal operations Psychosocial stage: Identity vs. role confusion	Abstract, hypothetical thinking Can build on past learning Reasons by logic and understands scientific principles Future orientation Motivated by desire for social acceptance Peer group important	Establish trust, authenticity Know their agenda Address fears/concerns about outcomes of illness Identify control focus Include in plan of care Use peers for support and influence Negotiate changes	Explore emotional and financial support Determine goals and expectations Assess stress levels Respect values and norms Determine role responsibilities and relationships
	Intense personal preoccupation, appearance extremely important (imaginary audience) Feels invulnerable, invincible/immune to natural laws (personal fable)	Focus on details Make information meaningful to life Ensure confidentiality and privacy Arrange group sessions Use audiovisuals, role play, contracts, reading materials Provide for experimentation and flexibility	Engage in 1:1 teaching without parents present, but with adolescent's permission inform family of content covered

(continued)

Table 5–1 Stage-Appropriate Teaching Strategies (*continued*)

Learner	General Characteristics	Teaching Strategies	Nursing Interventions	
Young Adulthood				
Approximate age: Cognitive stage: Psychosocial stage:	20–40 years Formal operations Intimacy vs. isolation	Autonomous Self-directed Uses personal experiences to enhance or interfere with learning Intrinsic motivation Able to analyze critically Makes decisions about personal, occupational, and social roles Competency-based learner	Use problem-centered focus Draw on meaningful experiences Focus on immediacy of application Encourage active participation Allow to set own pace, be self-directed Organize material Recognize social role Apply new knowledge through role playing and hands-on practice	Explore emotional, financial, and physical support system Assess motivational level for involvement Identify potential obstacles and stressors
Middle-Aged Adulthood				
Approximate age: Cognitive stage: Psychosocial stage:	41–64 years Formal operations Generativity vs. self-absorption and stagnation	Sense of self well-developed Concerned with physical changes At peak in career Explores alternative lifestyles Reflects on contributions to family and society	Focus on maintaining independence and reestablishing normal life patterns Assess positive and negative past experiences with learning	Explore emotional, financial, and physical support system Assess motivational level for involvement Identify potential obstacles and stressors
		Reexamines goals and values Questions achievements and successes Has confidence in abilities Desires to modify unsatisfactory aspects of life	Assess potential sources of stress caused by midlife crisis issues Provide information to coincide with life concerns and problems	

Older Adulthood

	Characteristics	Teaching Strategies
Approximate age: 65 years and over Cognitive stage: Formal operations Psychosocial stage: Ego integrity vs. despair	**Cognitive changes:** Decreased ability to think abstractly, process information Decreased short-term memory Increased reaction time Increased test anxiety Stimulus persistence (afterimage) Focuses on past life experiences	Use concrete examples Build on past life experiences Make information relevant and meaningful Present one concept at a time Allow time for processing/response (slow pace) Use repetition and reinforcement of information Avoid written exams Use verbal exchange and coaching Establish retrieval plan (use one or several clues) Encourage active involvement Keep explanations brief Use analogies to illustrate abstract information	Involve principal caregivers Encourage participation Provide resources for support (respite care) Assess coping mechanisms Provide written instructions for reinforcement Provide anticipatory problem solving (what happens if . . .)
	Sensory/motor deficits: Auditory changes Hearing loss, especially high-pitched tones, consonants (S, Z, T, F, and G), and rapid speech Visual changes Farsighted (needs glasses to read) Lenses become opaque (glare problem) Smaller pupil size (decreased visual adaptation to darkness) Decreased peripheral perception Yellowing of lenses (distorts low-tone colors: blue, green, violet) Distorted depth perception Fatigue/decreased energy levels Pathophysiology (chronic illness)	Speak slowly, distinctly Use low-pitched tones Avoid shouting Use visual aids to supplement verbal instruction Avoid glares, use soft white light Provide sufficient light Use white backgrounds and black print Use large letters and well-spaced print Avoid color coding with pastel blues, greens, purples, and yellows Increase safety precautions/provide safe environment Ensure accessibility and fit of prostheses (i.e., glasses, hearing aids) Keep sessions short Provide for frequent rest periods Allow for extra time to perform Establish realistic short-term goals	

they believe their own perceptions to be reality. Asking questions is the hallmark of this age group, and curiosity abounds as they explore places and things. They can respond to simple, step-by-step commands and obey such directives as "give Grandpa a kiss" or "go get your teddy bear" (Santrock, 2013).

Language skills increase rapidly during this period, and parents should be encouraged to talk with and listen to their child. As they progress through this phase, children begin to engage in fantasizing and make-believe play. Because they are unable to distinguish fact from fiction and have limited capacity for understanding cause and effect, disruptions in their routine during illness or hospitalizations, along with the need to separate from parents, are very stressful events for the toddler (London et al., 2013).

According to Erikson (1963), the noted authority on psychosocial development, the period of infancy is one of *trust versus mistrust*. During this time, children must work through their first major dilemma of developing a sense of trust with their primary caretaker. As the infant matures into toddlerhood, *autonomy versus shame and doubt* emerges as the central issue. During this period of psychosocial growth, toddlers must learn to balance feelings of love and hate and learn to cooperate and control willful desires (**Table 5–2**).

Children progress sequentially through accomplishing the tasks of developing basic trust in their environment to reaching increasing levels of independence. Children may have difficulty in making up their minds, and, aggravated by personal and external limits, they may express their level of frustration and feelings of ambivalence in words and behaviors, such as by engaging in temper tantrums to release tensions (Falvo, 2011). With peers, play is a parallel activity, and it is not unusual for them to end up in tears because they have not yet learned about tact, fairness, or rules of sharing (Babcock & Miller, 1994; Polan & Taylor, 2015).

Table 5–2 Erikson's Nine Stages of Psychosocial Development

Developmental Stages	Psychosocial Stages	Strengths
Infancy	Trust versus mistrust	Hope
Toddlerhood	Autonomy versus shame and doubt	Will
Early childhood	Initiative versus guilt	Purpose
Middle and late childhood	Industry versus inferiority	Competence
Adolescence	Identity versus role confusion	Fidelity
Young adulthood	Intimacy versus isolation	Love
Middle-aged adulthood	Generativity versus self-absorption and stagnation	Care
Older adulthood	Ego integrity versus despair	Wisdom
Very old age (late 80s and beyond)	Hope and faith versus despair	Wisdom and transcendence

Data from Aharoni, J. H. (1996). Strategies for teaching elders from a human development perspective. *Diabetes Educator, 22*(1), 48; and Crandell, C. H., & Vander Zanden, J. W. (2012). *Human development* (11th ed.). New York, NY: McGraw-Hill.

TEACHING STRATEGIES

Patient education for infancy through toddlerhood is usually not illness related. Time is spent teaching parents about aspects of normal development, safety, health promotion, and disease prevention. When the child is ill, the first priority before teaching is to assess the parents' and child's anxiety levels and to help them cope with their feelings of stress related to uncertainty and guilt about the cause of the illness or injury. Anxiety on the part of the child and parents can adversely affect their readiness to learn (see Chapter 4 on factors influencing readiness to learn).

Although teaching activities primarily are directed to the main caregiver(s), toddlers are capable of some degree of understanding procedures that they may experience. Therefore, it is imperative that a primary nurse is assigned to establish a relationship with the child and parents to provide consistency in the teaching–learning process and to help reduce the child's fear of strangers. Parents should be present whenever possible during teaching and learning activities to allay stress, which could be compounded by separation anxiety (London et al., 2013).

Ideally, health teaching should take place in an environment familiar to the child, such as the home or daycare center. When the child is hospitalized, the environment selected for teaching and learning sessions should be as safe and secure as possible, such as the child's bed or the playroom, to increase the child's sense of feeling protected.

Movement is an important mechanism by which toddlers communicate. Immobility tends to increase children's anxiety by restricting activity. Nursing interventions that promote children's use of gross motor abilities and that stimulate their visual, auditory, and tactile senses should be chosen whenever possible. The approach to children should be warm, honest, calm, accepting, and matter-of-fact. A smile, a warm tone of voice, a gesture of encouragement, or a word of praise goes a long way in attracting children's attention and helping them adjust to new circumstances. Fundamental to the child's response is how the parents respond to healthcare personnel and medical interventions.

The following teaching strategies are suggested to promote the child's natural desire for play and his or her need for active participation and sensory experiences.

For Short-Term Learning

- Read simple stories from books with lots of pictures.
- Use dolls and puppets to act out feelings and behaviors.
- Use simple audiotapes with music and videotapes with cartoon characters.
- Role play to bring the child's imagination closer to reality.
- Give simple, concrete, nonthreatening explanations.
- Perform procedures on a teddy bear or doll first to help the child anticipate what an experience will be like.
- Allow the child something to do—squeeze your hand, hold a Band-Aid, sing a song, cry if it hurts.
- Keep teaching sessions brief (no longer than about 5 minutes each) because of the child's short attention span.
- Cluster teaching sessions close together so that children can remember what they learned.

- Avoid analogies and explain things in straightforward and simple terms because children take their world literally and concretely.
- Pace teaching according to the child's responses and level of attention.

For Long-Term Learning

- Focus on rituals, imitation, and repetition of information to hold the child's attention.
- Use reinforcement as an opportunity for children to learn through practice.
- Use games as a way for children to learn about the world and test their ideas.
- Encourage parents to act as role models because they influence the child's development of attitudes and behaviors.

Early Childhood (3–5 Years of Age)

Preschool children's identity becomes clearer, and their world expands to involve others outside of the family. Children in this developmental category acquire new behaviors that give them more independence from their parents and allow them to care for themselves. Learning during this time period occurs through interactions with others and through mimicking or modeling the behaviors of playmates and adults (Crandell et al., 2012; Santrock, 2013).

PHYSICAL, COGNITIVE, AND PSYCHOSOCIAL DEVELOPMENT

Fine and gross motor skills become increasingly more refined and coordinated so that children are able to carry out activities of daily living with greater independence (Crandell et al., 2012; Santrock, 2013). Although their efforts are more coordinated, supervision of activities is still required because they lack judgment in carrying out the skills they have developed.

The early childhood stage of cognitive development is labeled by Piaget (1951, 1952, 1976) as the *preoperational period*. The young child continues to be self-centered and is essentially unaware of others' thoughts or the existence of others' points of view. Thinking remains literal and concrete—they believe what is seen and heard (Santrock, 2013).

Preschool children are very curious, can think intuitively, and pose questions about almost anything. They want to know the reasons, cause, and purpose for everything (the why) but are unconcerned at this point with the process (the how). Children in this cognitive stage mix fact and fiction, tend to generalize, think magically, develop imaginary playmates, and believe they can control events with their thoughts (Crandell et al., 2012; Santrock, 2013).

The young child also continues to have a limited sense of time. For children of this age, being made to wait 15 minutes before they can do something can feel like an eternity. They do, however, understand the timing of familiar events in their daily lives, such as when breakfast or dinner is eaten and when they can play or watch their favorite television program. As they begin to understand and appreciate the world around them, their attention span (ability to focus) begins to lengthen such that they can usually remain quiet long enough to listen to a song or hear a short story (Santrock, 2013).

In the preschool stage, children have an understanding of their bodies. They can name external body parts but do not understand the function of internal organs (Kotchabhakdi, 1985). Children see illness and hospitalization as a punishment for something they did wrong (London et al., 2013).

Erikson (1963) has labeled the psychosocial maturation level in early childhood as the period of *initiative versus guilt*. Children take on tasks for the sake of being involved and on the move (Table 5–2). Excess energy and a desire to dominate may lead to frustration and anger on their part. They show evidence of expanding imagination and creativity, are impulsive in their actions, and are curious about almost everything they see and do. Their growing imagination can lead to many fears—of separation, disapproval, pain, punishment, and aggression from others. Loss of body integrity is the preschool child's greatest threat, which significantly affects his or her willingness to interact with healthcare personnel (Falvo, 2011; Poster, 1983; Vulcan, 1984).

In this phase of development, children begin interacting with playmates rather than just playing alongside one another. Appropriate social behaviors demand that they learn to wait for others, give others a turn, and recognize the needs of others. Play in the mind of a child is equivalent to the work performed by adults. Play can be as equally productive as adult work and is a means for self-education of the physical and social world (Ormrod, 2012). It helps the child act out feelings and experiences so as to master fears, develop role skills, and express joys, sorrows, and hostilities. Through play, children in the preschool years also begin to share ideas and imitate parents of the same sex. Role playing is typical of this age as the child attempts to learn the responsibilities of family members and others in society (Santrock, 2013).

TEACHING STRATEGIES

The nurse's interactions with preschool children and their parents are often sporadic, usually occurring during occasional well-child visits to the pediatrician's office or when minor medical problems arise. During these interactions, the nurse should take every opportunity to teach parents about health promotion and disease and accident prevention measures, to provide guidance regarding normal growth and development, and to offer instruction about medical recommendations related to illness or disability. Parents can help the nurse in working with children in this developmental phase, and they should be included in all aspects of the educational plan and the actual teaching experience. Parents can answer questions about children's disabilities, likes and dislikes, and their favorite toys and games—all of which may affect their ability to learn (Hussey & Hirsh, 1983; Ryberg & Merrifield, 1984; Woodring, 2000).

Children's fear of pain and bodily harm is uppermost in their minds, whether they are well or ill. Because young children have fantasies and active imaginations, it is most important for the nurse to reassure them and allow them to express their fears openly (Heiney, 1991). Nurses need to choose their words carefully when describing procedures and interventions. Preschoolers are familiar with many words, but using terms such as *cut* and *knife* is frightening to them. Instead, nurses should use less threatening words such as *fix*, *sew*, and *cover up the hole*. *Band-Aids* is a much more understandable term than *dressings*, and bandages are often thought by children to have magical healing powers (Babcock & Miller, 1994).

Although the young child has begun to have increasing contact with the outside world and is usually able to interact more comfortably with others, teaching should be directed toward the significant adults in a child's life. Family members can provide support to the child, substitute as the teacher if their child is reluctant to interact with the nurse, and reinforce teaching. They are the learners who will assist the child in achieving desired health outcomes (Kaakinen, Gedaly-Duff, Coehlo, & Hanson, 2010; Whitener, Cox, & Maglich, 1998).

The following specific teaching strategies are recommended:

For Short-Term Learning

- Provide physical and visual stimuli because language ability is still limited.
- Keep teaching sessions short (no more than 15 minutes) and scheduled sequentially at close intervals so that information is not forgotten.
- Relate information needs to activities and experiences familiar to the child.
- Encourage the child to participate by choosing the instructional methods and tools, such as playing with dolls or reading a story, which promotes active involvement and helps to establish nurse–client rapport.
- Arrange small-group sessions with peers as a way to make teaching less threatening and more fun.
- Give praise and approval, through both verbal expressions and nonverbal gestures, which are real motivators for learning.
- Give rewards, such as badges or small toys, to reinforce learning skills.
- Allow the child to touch equipment and play with replicas or dolls to learn about body parts. Special kidney dolls, ostomy dolls with stomas, or orthopedic dolls with splints and tractions provide opportunities for hands-on experience.
- Use storybooks to help the child identify with particular people and situations.

For Long-Term Learning

- Enlist the help of parents to be role models of healthy habits, such as practicing safety measures and eating a balanced diet.
- Reinforce positive health behaviors and new skills learned.

Middle and Late Childhood (6–11 Years of Age)

In middle and late childhood, children have progressed in their physical, cognitive, and psychosocial skills to the point where most begin formal training in structured school systems. They approach learning with excitement of what is to come, and their minds are open to new and varied ideas. They are motivated to learn because of their natural curiosity and their desire to understand more about themselves, their bodies, the environment, and their world (Whitener et al., 1998). This stage is a period of great change for them, when attitudes, values, and perceptions of themselves, their society, and the world are shaped and expanded (Santrock, 2013).

PHYSICAL, COGNITIVE, AND PSYCHOSOCIAL DEVELOPMENT

The gross- and fine-motor abilities of school-aged children become increasingly more coordinated so that they are able to control their movements. Involvement in activities helps them to fine-tune their psychomotor skills. Physical growth during this phase is highly variable, with the rate of development differing from child to child (Crandell et al., 2012; Santrock, 2013).

Piaget (1951, 1952, 1976) labeled the cognitive development in middle and late childhood as the period of *concrete operations*. During this time, logical, rational thought processes and the ability to reason inductively and deductively develop. At this stage, they begin to use **syllogistic reasoning**—that is, they can consider two premises and draw a logical conclusion from them (Elkind, 1984; Steegen & De Neys, 2012). In addition, concepts are mastered, such as **conservation**, when they realize that a certain quantity of liquid is the same amount whether it is poured into a tall, thin glass or into a short, squat one (Snowman & McCown, 2015).

The skills of memory, decision making, insight, and problem solving are all more fully developed (Protheroe, 2007). They are able to classify objects and systems, use sarcasm, and communicate more sophisticated thoughts (Snowman & McCown, 2015). Though they can separate fantasy from reality, thinking remains quite literal, with only a vague understanding of abstractions. Early on in this phase, children are reluctant to do away with magical thinking in exchange for reality thinking. They cling to cherished beliefs, such as the existence of Santa Claus or the tooth fairy, for the fun and excitement that the fantasy provides them, even when they have information that proves contrary to their beliefs.

Children passing through elementary and middle schools have developed the ability to concentrate for extended periods, can tolerate waiting for what they want, and can generalize from experience (Crandell et al., 2012). They understand time and have some interest in the future, yet have a vague appreciation for how their actions can have implications at a later time.

As part of the shift from **precausal thinking** (preschool child unaware of what causes something) to **causal thinking**, the school-age child begins to incorporate the idea that illness is related to cause and effect and can recognize that germs create disease. Illness is thought of in terms of social consequences and role alterations, such as the realization that they will miss school and outside activities, people will feel sorry for them, and they will be unable to maintain their usual routines (Banks, 1990; Koopman, Baars, Chaplin, & Zwinderman, 2004).

Differences exist in children's reasoning skills based on their experiences with illness. Children suffering from chronic diseases have been found to have more sophisticated understanding of illness causality and body functioning than do their healthy peers (Piaget, 1976). However, the stress and anxiety resulting from having to live with a chronic illness or disability can interfere with a child's general cognitive performance (Perrin, Sayer, & Willett, 1991).

Erikson (1963) characterized school-aged children's psychosocial stage of life as *industry versus inferiority*. During this period, children begin to gain an awareness of their unique talents and the special qualities that distinguish them from one another (Table 5–2). They begin to establish their self-concept as members of a social group larger than their own nuclear family and start to compare their own family's values with those of the outside world.

With less dependency on family, they extend their intimacy to include special friends and social groups (Santrock, 2013). Relationships with peers and adults external to the home environment become important influences in their development of self-esteem and their susceptibility to social forces outside the family unit. School-aged children fear failure and being left out of groups. They worry about their inabilities and compare their own accomplishments to those of their peers.

TEACHING STRATEGIES

Woodring (2000) emphasizes the importance of following sound educational principles with the child and family, such as identifying individual learning styles, determining readiness to learn, and taking into account their learning needs and abilities to achieve positive health outcomes. Given their increased ability to comprehend information and their desire for active involvement and control of their lives, it is very important to include school-aged children in patient education efforts. The nurse must explain illness, treatment plans, and procedures in simple, logical terms in accordance with the child's level of understanding and reasoning.

Although children at this stage are able to think logically, their ability for abstract thought remains limited. Therefore, teaching should be presented in concrete terms with step-by-step instructions (Pidgeon, 1985; Whitener et al., 1998). Observe children's reactions and listen to their verbal feedback to confirm that information shared has not been misinterpreted or confused.

Parents should be informed of what their child is being taught. Teaching parents directly is encouraged so that they may be involved in fostering their child's independence, providing emotional support and physical assistance, and giving guidance regarding the child's care management. Siblings and peers should also be considered as sources of support (Hussey & Hirsh, 1983; Santrock, 2013).

Education for health maintenance, health promotion, and disease and accident prevention is most likely to occur in the school system. The school nurse, in particular, is in an excellent position to coordinate the efforts of all other providers. According to *Healthy People 2020* (U.S. Department of Health and Human Services [USDHHS], 2014b), health promotion regarding healthy eating and weight status, exercise, sleep, and prevention of injuries as well as avoidance of tobacco, alcohol, and drug use are just a few examples of objectives intended to improve the health of American children. The school nurse can play a vital role in providing education to the school-aged child to meet these goals (Leifer & Hartston, 2004) and has the opportunity to educate children not only in a group when teaching a class but also on a one-to-one basis.

The specific conditions that may come to the attention of the nurse in caring for children at this phase of development include problems such as behavioral disorders, hyperactivity, learning disorders, obesity, diabetes, asthma, and enuresis. Extensive teaching may be needed to help children and parents understand a particular condition and learn how to overcome or deal with it.

The need to sustain or bolster their self-image, self-concept, and self-esteem requires that children be invited to participate, to the extent possible, in planning for and carrying out learning activities (Snowman & McCown, 2015). Because of children's fears of falling behind in school, being separated from peer groups, and being left out of social activities, teaching must be geared toward fostering normal development despite any limitations that may be imposed by illness or disability (Falvo, 2011; Leifer & Hartston, 2004).

Children in middle and late childhood are used to the structured, direct, and formal learning in the school environment and are receptive to a similar approach when hospitalized or confined at home. The following teaching strategies are suggested when caring for children in this developmental stage of life:

For Short-Term Learning

- Allow school-aged children to take responsibility for their own health care because they are not only willing to use but also capable of using equipment with accuracy.
- Teaching sessions can be extended to last as long as 30 minutes each because school-aged children are better able to focus and retain information. However, lessons should be spread apart to allow for comprehension of large amounts of content and to provide opportunity for the practice of newly acquired skills between sessions.
- Use diagrams, models, pictures, digital media, printed materials, and computers as adjuncts to various teaching methods.
- Choose audiovisual and printed materials that show peers undergoing similar procedures or facing similar situations.
- Clarify any scientific terminology and medical jargon used.
- Use analogies as an effective means of providing information in meaningful terms, such as "Having a chest X-ray is like having your picture taken" or "White blood cells are like police cells that can attack and destroy infection."
- Use one-to-one teaching sessions as a method to individualize learning relevant to the child's own experiences.
- Provide time for clarification, validation, and reinforcement of what is being learned.
- Use group teaching sessions with others of similar age and with similar problems or needs to help children avoid feelings of isolation and to assist them in identifying with their own peers.
- Prepare children for procedures and interventions well in advance to allow them time to cope with their feelings and fears, to anticipate events, and to understand what the purpose of each procedure is, how it relates to their condition, and how much time it will take.
- Encourage participation in planning for procedures and events because active involvement helps the child to assimilate information more readily.
- Provide much-needed nurturance and support, always keeping in mind that young children are not just small adults.

For Long-Term Learning

- Help school-aged children acquire skills that they can use to assume responsibility for carrying out treatment regimens on an ongoing basis with minimal assistance.
- Assist them in learning to maintain their own well-being and prevent illnesses from occurring.

Research for the *Healthy People 2020* report suggests that lifelong health attitudes and behaviors begin in the early childhood phase of development and remain consistent into late childhood (USDHHS, 2014b).

Adolescence (12–19 Years of Age)

Adolescence marks the transition from childhood to adulthood. During this prolonged and very change-filled period of time, many adolescents and their families experience much turmoil. How adolescents think about themselves and the world significantly influences many healthcare issues facing them, from anorexia to obesity. Teenage thought and behavior give insight into the etiology of some of the major health problems of this group of learners (Elkind, 1984).

Adolescents are known to be among the nation's most at-risk populations (Ares, Kuhns, Dogra, & Karnik, 2015). Most recently, *Healthy People 2020* identified "Adolescent Health" as a new topic area, with objectives focused on interventions to promote health as well as reduce the risks associated with this population (USDHHS, 2014b). For patient education to be effective, an understanding of the characteristics of the adolescent phase of development is crucial (Ackard & Neumark-Sztainer, 2001; Michaud, Stronski, Fonseca, & MacFarlane, 2004; Ormrod, 2012).

PHYSICAL, COGNITIVE, AND PSYCHOSOCIAL DEVELOPMENT

Adolescents vary greatly in their biological, psychological, social, and cognitive development. From a physical maturation standpoint, they must adapt to rapid, dramatic, and significant bodily changes, which can temporarily result in clumsiness and poorly coordinated movement. Alterations in physical size, shape, and function of their bodies, along with the appearance and development of secondary sex characteristics, bring about a significant preoccupation with their appearance and a strong desire to express sexual urges (Crandell et al., 2012; Santrock, 2013).

Piaget (1951, 1952, 1976) termed this stage of cognitive development as the period of *formal operations*. Adolescents are capable of abstract thought and logical thinking that is both inductive and deductive. Adolescents can debate various points of view, understand cause and effect, comprehend complex explanations, imagine possibilities, and respond appropriately to multiple-step directions (Aronowitz, 2006; Crandell et al., 2012).

With the capacity for formal operational thought, teenagers can become obsessed with what others are thinking and begin to believe that everyone is focusing on the same things they are—namely, themselves and their activities. Elkind (1984) labels this belief as the **imaginary audience**, which has considerable influence over an adolescent's behavior.

The imaginary audience explains why adolescents, on the one hand, are self conscious and may feel embarrassed because they believe everyone is looking at them and, on the other hand, desire to be looked at and thought about because this attention confirms their sense of being special and unique (Crandell et al., 2012; Santrock, 2013; Snowman & McCown, 2015).

Adolescents are able to understand the concept of health and illness, the multiple causes of diseases, and the influence of variables on health status. They can also identify health behaviors, although they may reject practicing them or begin to engage in risk-taking behaviors because of the social pressures they receive from peers as well as their feelings of invincibility (Ormrod, 2012). Elkind (1984) labels this second type of social thinking as the personal fable. The **personal fable** leads adolescents to believe that they are invulnerable—other people grow old and die, but not them. Unfortunately, this leads teenagers to believe they are cloaked in an invisible shield that will protect them from bodily harm despite any risks to which they may subject themselves. They can understand implications of future outcomes, but their immediate concern is with the present. Although children in the mid- to late-adolescent period appear to be aware of the risks they take, it is important, nevertheless, to recognize that this population continues to need support and guidance (Brown, Teufel, & Birch, 2007).

Erikson (1968) has identified the psychosocial dilemma adolescents face as one of *identity versus role confusion*. Children in this age group indulge in comparing their self-image with an ideal image (Table 5–2). Adolescents find themselves in a struggle to establish their own identity, match their skills with career choices, and determine their self. They work to separate themselves from their parents so that they can emerge as more distinct individual personalities. Teenagers have a strong need for peer acceptance and peer support. Their concern over personal appearance and their need to look and act like their peers drive them to conform to the dress and behavior of this age group. This usually contradicts values of their parents' generation. Conflict, toleration, stereotyping, or alienation often characterizes the relationship between adolescents and their parents and other authority figures (Hines & Paulson, 2006).

Adolescents demand personal space, control, privacy, and confidentiality. To them, illness, injury, disability, and hospitalization mean dependency, loss of identity, a change in body image and functioning, bodily embarrassment, confinement, and separation from peers. Knowledge alone of how to protect their health and prevent disease and injury is not enough; they need coping skills for successful completion of this stage of development (Grey, Kanner, & Lacey, 1999).

TEACHING STRATEGIES

Challenges adolescents might face include chronic illness, a range of disabilities as a result of injury, or psychological problems as a result of depression or physical and/or emotional maltreatment. In addition, adolescents are considered at high risk for teen pregnancy, the effects of poverty, drug or alcohol abuse, and sexually transmitted diseases. The three leading causes of death in this age group are accidents, homicide, and suicide (Kochanek, Xu, Murphy, Minino, & Kung, 2011; London et al., 2013).

The educational needs of adolescents are broad and varied. Healthy teens have difficulty imagining themselves as sick or injured. Those with an illness or disability often comply poorly with medical regimens and continue to indulge in risk-taking behaviors. Because of their preoccupation with body image and functioning and the perceived importance of peer acceptance and support, they view health recommendations as a threat to their autonomy and sense of control.

Probably the greatest challenge to the nurse responsible for teaching the adolescent, whether healthy or ill, is to be able to develop a mutually respectful, trusting relationship (Brown et al., 2007). Adolescents are able to participate fully in all aspects of learning, but they need privacy, understanding, an honest and straightforward approach, and unqualified acceptance in the face of their fears of embarrassment and of losing independence, identity, and self-control (Ackard & Neumark-Sztainer, 2001). The existence of an imaginary audience and personal fable can contribute to the exacerbation of existing problems or cause new ones. Adolescents with disfiguring disabilities may show signs of depression and lack of will. For the first time, they look at themselves from the standpoint of others. Teenagers may fail to use contraceptives because the personal fable tells them that other people will get pregnant or get venereal disease, but not them. Teenagers with chronic illnesses may stop taking prescribed medications because they feel they can manage without them to prove to others that they are well.

The following teaching strategies are suggested when caring for adolescents:

For Short-Term Learning

- Use one-to-one instruction to ensure confidentiality of sensitive information.
- Choose peer-group discussion sessions as an effective approach to deal with health topics such as smoking, alcohol and drug use, safety measures, obesity, and teenage sexuality.
- Adolescents benefit from meeting others who have the same concerns or who have successfully dealt with problems similar to theirs.
- Use face-to-face or computer group discussion, role playing, and gaming as methods to clarify values and problem solve, which feed into the teenager's need to belong and to be actively involved. Getting groups of peers together in person or virtually can be very effective in helping teens confront health challenges and change behavior (Snowman & McCown, 2015).
- Use instructional tools, such as models, diagrams, and detailed written materials as well as different types of technology, which are comfortable approaches to learning for adolescents.
- Clarify any scientific terminology and medical jargon used.
- Allow participation in decision making. Include adolescents in formulating teaching plans related to teaching strategies and expected outcomes to meet their needs for autonomy.
- Suggest options so that they feel they have a choice about courses of action.
- Give a rationale for all that is said and done to help adolescents feel a sense of control.

- Approach them with respect, tact, openness, and flexibility to elicit their attention and encourage their involvement.
- Expect negative responses, which are common when their self-image and self-integrity are threatened.
- Avoid confrontation and acting like an authority figure. Acknowledge their thoughts and then casually suggest an alternative viewpoint or choices, such as "Yes, I can see your point, but what about the possibility of . . .?"

For Long-Term Learning

- Accept adolescents' personal fable and imaginary audience as valid.
- Acknowledge that their feelings are very real.
- Allow them the opportunity to test their own convictions.

Although much of patient education should be done directly with adolescents to respect their right to individuality, privacy, and confidentiality, teaching effectiveness may be enhanced to some extent by including their families (Brown et al., 2007). Because of the ambivalence the adolescent feels, teaching must consider the learning needs of the adolescent as well as the parents (Ackard & Neumark-Sztainer, 2001; Falvo, 2011).

The Developmental Stages of Adulthood

Andragogy, the term used by Knowles (1990) to describe his theory of adult learning, is the art and science of teaching adults. Education within this framework is more learner centered and less teacher centered; that is, instead of one party giving information to another, the power relationship between the teacher and the adult learner is more equal than in a teacher-centered framework (Curran, 2014). The concept of andragogy has served for years as a useful framework in guiding instruction for patient teaching and for continuing education of staff.

Based on emerging research and theory from a variety of disciplines, Knowles and colleagues (2015) discussed new perspectives on andragogy that have refined and strengthened the core adult learning principles that Knowles originally proposed. The following basic assumptions about Knowles's framework have major implications for planning, implementing, and evaluating teaching programs for adults as the individual matures:

1. The adult's self-concept moves from one of being a dependent personality to being an independent, self-directed human being.
2. He or she accumulates a growing reservoir of previous experience that serves as a rich resource for learning.
3. Readiness to learn becomes increasingly oriented to the developmental tasks of social roles.
4. Adults are best motivated to learn when a need arises in their life situation that will help them satisfy their desire for information.
5. Adults learn for personal fulfillment such as self-esteem or an improved quality of life.

The period of adulthood constitutes three major developmental stages—the young adult stage, the middle-aged adult stage, and the older adult stage (Table 5–1). The emphasis for adult learning revolves around differentiation of life tasks and social roles with respect to employment, family, and other activities beyond the responsibilities of home and career (Boyd, Gleit, Graham, & Whitman, 1998). The prime motivator to learn in adulthood is being able to apply knowledge and skills for the solution of immediate problems. Adults must clearly perceive the relevancy of acquiring new behaviors or changing old ones for them to be willing and eager to learn. In the beginning of any teaching–learning encounter, therefore, adults want to know how they will benefit from their efforts at learning (Knowles et al., 2015).

Typical characteristics of adult learners include being self-directed and independent in seeking information. Their past experiences form the basis for further learning, and they already have a rich resource of stored information from which to draw. They also grasp relationships quickly, in general, and they do not tolerate learning isolated facts. However, because adults already have established ideas, values, and attitudes, they also tend to be more resistant to change.

In addition, adults must overcome obstacles to learning, such as the burden of family, work, and social responsibilities, which can diminish their time, energy, and concentration for learning. Furthermore, some adults may feel too old or too out of touch with the formal learning of the school years, and if past experiences with learning were not positive, they may shy away from assuming the role of learner for fear of the risk of failure (Boyd et al., 1998). Although nurses can consider adult learners as autonomous, self-directed, and independent, these individuals often want and need structure, clear and concise specifics, and direct guidance. As such, Taylor, Marienau, and Fiddler (2000) label adults as "paradoxical" learners.

Only recently has it been recognized that learning is a lifelong process that begins at birth and does not cease until the end of life. Growth and development are a process of becoming, and learning is a key part of that process. As a person matures, learning is a significant and continuous task to maintain and enhance oneself (Knowles, 1990; Knowles et al., 2015). As the following discussion clearly reveals, there are differences in the characteristics of adult learners within the three developmental stages of adulthood.

Young Adulthood (20–40 Years of Age)

Young adulthood is a time for establishing long-term, intimate relationships with other people, choosing a lifestyle and adjusting to it, deciding on an occupation, and managing a home and family. All of these decisions lead to changes in the lives of young adults that can be a potential source of stress for them (Santrock, 2013).

PHYSICAL, COGNITIVE, AND PSYCHOSOCIAL DEVELOPMENT

During this period, physical abilities for most young adults are at their peak, and the body functions very well (Crandell et al., 2012). The cognitive capacity of young adults is fully developed, but with maturation, they continue to accumulate new knowledge and skills from an expanding reservoir of formal and informal experiences. Young adults continue in the *formal operations* stage of cognitive development (Piaget, 1951, 1952, 1976). These experiences add to their perceptions, allow them to generalize to new situations, and improve their abilities to critically analyze, problem solve, and make decisions about their personal, occupational, and social roles. Their interests for learning are oriented toward those experiences that are relevant for immediate application to problems and tasks in their daily lives (Crandell et al., 2012).

Erikson (1963) describes the young adult's stage of psychosocial development as the period of *intimacy versus isolation*. During this time, individuals work to establish trusting, satisfying, and permanent relationships with others (Table 5–2). They strive to make commitments to others in their personal, occupational, and social lives. As part of this effort, they seek to maintain the independence and self-sufficiency they worked to obtain in adolescence.

Young adults face many challenges as they take steps to control their lives. Many of the events they experience are happy and growth promoting from an emotional and social perspective, but they also can prove disappointing and psychologically draining. The new experiences and multiple decisions young adults must make regarding choices for a career, marriage, parenthood, and higher education can be quite stressful. Young adults realize that the avenues they pursue will affect their lives for years to come (Santrock, 2013).

TEACHING STRATEGIES

Young adults are generally very healthy and tend to have limited exposure to health professionals. Their contact with the healthcare system is usually for pre-employment, college, or sport physicals; for a minor episodic complaint; or for pregnancy and contraceptive care (Orshan, 2008). At the same time, young adulthood is a crucial period for the establishment of behaviors that help individuals to lead healthy lives, both physically and emotionally. Many of the choices young adults make, if not positive ones, will be difficult to change later. As Havighurst (1976) points out, this stage is full of teachable moments, and nurses must take advantage of every opportunity to promote healthy behaviors with this population (Hinkle, 2014).

The nurse as teacher must find a way of reaching and communicating with this audience about health promotion and disease prevention measures. Readiness to learn does not always require the nurse to wait for it to develop. Rather, such readiness can be actively fostered through experiences the nurse creates. Knowledge of the individual's lifestyle can provide cues to concentrate on when determining specific aspects of education for the young adult. For example, if the individual is planning marriage, then establishing healthy relationships, family planning, contraception, and parenthood are potential topics to address during teaching (Orshan, 2008).

The motivation for adults to learn comes in response to internal drives, such as need for self-esteem, a better quality of life, or job satisfaction, and in response to external motivators, such as job promotion, more money, or more time to pursue outside activities (Babcock & Miller, 1994; Crandell et al., 2012). Also, when young adults are faced with acute or chronic illnesses or disabilities, many of which may significantly alter their lifestyles, they are stimulated to learn so as to maintain their independence and return to normal life patterns. It is likely they will view an illness or disability as a serious setback to achieving their immediate or future life goals.

Because adults typically desire active participation in the educational process, whenever possible it is important for the nurse to allow them the opportunity for participation in health education decision making. They should be encouraged, as Knowles (1990) suggested, to select what to learn (objectives), how they want material to be presented (teaching methods and instructional tools), and which indicators will be used to determine the achievement of learning goals (evaluation). Also, it must be remembered that adults bring to the teaching–learning situation a variety of experiences that can serve as the foundation on which to build new learning. Consequently, it is important to draw on their personal experiences to make learning relevant, useful, and motivating. Young adults tend to be reluctant to expend the resources of time, money, and energy to learn new information, skills, and attitudes if they do not see the content of instruction as relevant to their current lives or anticipated problems (Collins, 2004; Knowles et al., 2015).

Teaching strategies must be directed at encouraging young adults to seek information that expands their knowledge base, helps them control their lives, and bolsters their self-esteem. Whether they are well or ill, young adults need to know about the opportunities available for learning. These educational opportunities must be convenient and accessible to them in terms of their lifestyle with respect to work and family responsibilities. Because they tend to be very self-directed in their approach to learning, young adults do well with written patient education materials and audiovisual tools, including computer-assisted instruction, that allow them to self-pace their learning independently. Group discussion is an attractive method for teaching and learning because it provides young adults with the opportunity to interact with others of similar age and in similar situations, such as in parenting groups, prenatal classes, exercise classes, or marital adjustment sessions.

Middle-Aged Adulthood (41–64 Years of Age)

Just as adolescence is the link between childhood and adulthood, so midlife is the transition period between young adulthood and older adulthood. During middle age, many individuals are highly accomplished in their careers, their sense of who they are is well developed, their children are grown, and they have time to share their talents, serve as mentors for others, and pursue new or latent interests. This stage is a time for them to reflect on the contributions they have made to family and society, relish in their achievements, and reexamine their goals and values.

PHYSICAL, COGNITIVE, AND PSYCHOSOCIAL DEVELOPMENT

During this stage of maturation, a number of physiological changes begin to take place. Skin and muscle tone decreases, metabolism slows down, body weight tends to increase, endurance and energy levels lessen, hormonal changes bring about a variety of symptoms, and hearing and visual acuity start to diminish. All these physical changes and others affect middle-aged adults' self-image, ability to learn, and motivation for learning about health promotion, disease prevention, and maintenance of health (Crandell et al., 2012).

The ability to learn from a cognitive standpoint remains at a steady state for middle-aged adults as they continue in Piaget's (1951, 1952, 1976) *formal operations* stage of cognitive development. For many adults, the accumulation of life experiences and their proven record of accomplishments often allow them to come to the teaching–learning situation with confidence in their abilities as learners. However, if their past experiences with learning were minimal or not positive, their motivation likely will not be at a high enough level to easily facilitate learning. Physical changes, especially with respect to hearing and vision, may impede learning as well (Santrock, 2013).

Erikson (1963) labels this psychosocial stage of adulthood as *generativity versus self-absorption and stagnation*. Midlife marks a point at which adults realize that half of their potential life has been spent. This realization may cause them to question their level of achievement and success. Middle-aged adults, in fact, may choose to modify aspects of their lives that they perceive as unsatisfactory or adopt a new lifestyle.

Developing concern for the lives of their grown children, recognizing the physical changes in themselves, dealing with the new role of being a grandparent, and taking responsibility for their own parents whose health may be failing are all factors that may cause adults in this cohort to become aware of their own mortality (Table 5–2). At this time, middle-aged adults may either feel greater motivation to follow health recommendations more closely or—just the opposite—may deny illnesses or abandon healthy practices altogether (Falvo, 2011).

The later years of middle adulthood are the phase in which productivity and contributions to society are valued. They offer an opportunity to feel a real sense of accomplishment from having cared for others—children, spouse, friends, parents, and colleagues for whom adults have served as mentors. During this time, individuals often become oriented away from self and family and toward the larger community. New social interests and leisure activities are pursued as they find more free time from family responsibilities and career demands. As they move toward their retirement years, individuals begin to plan for what they want to do after culminating their career. This transition sparks their interest in learning about financial planning, alternative lifestyles, and ways to remain healthy as they approach the later years (Crandell et al., 2012).

TEACHING STRATEGIES

When teaching members of this age group, the nurse must be aware of their potential sources of stress, the health risk factors associated with this stage of life, and the concerns typical of midlife. Stress may interfere with middle-aged adults' ability to learn or may be a motivational force for learning (Leifer & Hartston, 2004). Those who have lived healthy and productive lives are often motivated to make contact with health professionals to ensure maintenance of their healthy status. Such contacts represent an opportune time for the nurse to reach out to assist these middle-aged adults in coping with stress and maintaining optimal health status. Many need and want information related to chronic illnesses that can arise at this phase of life (Orshan, 2008).

Adult learners need to be reassured or complimented on their learning competencies. Reinforcement for learning is internalized and serves to reward them for their efforts. Teaching strategies for learning are similar to those methods and tools used for instructing the young adult learner, but the content is different to coincide with the concerns and problems specific to this group of learners.

Older Adulthood (65 Years of Age and Older)

The percentage of middle-aged adults in the United States has tripled since 1900, and in 2011, the first wave of baby boomers turned 65 years of age. Older persons constitute approximately 13% of the U.S. population now, but in the next 30 years, the number of those older than age 65 will increase to approximately 81 million Americans, or 20%. Those aged 85 and older make up the fastest-growing segment of the population in the country today, and that segment is expected to more than triple by 2050, rising to approximately 19 million (Federal Interagency Forum on Aging-Related Statistics, 2012). Some developmental experts, as Santrock (2013) points out, distinguish three categories of older adults: the young-old (65–74 years of age), the old-old (75–84 years of age), and the oldest-old (85 years and older).

Most older people suffer from at least one chronic condition, and many have multiple conditions. On the average, they are hospitalized longer than persons in other age categories and require more teaching overall to broaden their knowledge of self-care. In addition, it is approximated by the USDHHS that as of 2014, 84% of those older than 65 years of age have a high school education. These numbers have increased significantly since 1970, when only 28% of older adults had a high school diploma. However, currently only 26% have a college degree at the bachelor's level or higher (USDHHS, 2014a).

Low educational levels, sensory impairments, the disuse of literacy skills once learned, and cognitive changes in the older adult population may contribute to these individuals' decreased ability to read and comprehend written materials (Best, 2001). For these reasons, their patient education needs are generally greater and more complex than those for persons in any of the other developmental stages. In light of considerable healthcare expenditures for older people, education programs to improve their health status and reduce morbidity would be a cost-effective measure (Behm et al., 2014; Best, 2001; Mauk, 2014; Robnett & Chop, 2015).

Ageism describes prejudice against the older adult. This discrimination based on age, which exists in most segments of American society, perpetuates the negative stereotype of aging as a period of decline (Gavan, 2003). Ageism, in many respects, is similar to the discriminatory attitudes of racism and sexism (Crandell et al., 2012). It interferes with interactions between the older adult and younger age groups and must be counteracted.

Given that the aging process is universal, eventually everyone is potentially subject to this type of prejudice. New research that focuses on healthy development and positive lifestyle adaptations, rather than on illnesses and impairments in the older adult, can serve to reverse the stereotypical images of aging. Education to inform people of the significant variations that occur in the way that individuals age and education to help the older adult learn to cope with irreversible losses can combat the prejudice of ageism as well (Crandell et al., 2012).

The teaching of older persons, known as **gerogogy**, is different from teaching younger adults (andragogy) and children (pedagogy). For teaching to be effective, gerogogy must accommodate the normal physical, cognitive, and psychosocial changes that occur during this phase of growth and development (Best, 2001). Until recently, little had been written about the special learning needs of older adults that acknowledged the physiological and psychological aging changes affecting their ability to learn.

Age changes often create obstacles to learning unless nurses understand them and can adapt appropriate teaching interventions to meet the older person's needs. The following discussion of physical, cognitive, and psychosocial maturation is based on findings reported by numerous authors (Ahroni, 1996; Best, 2001; Crandell et al., 2012; Gavan, 2003; Hinkle, 2014; Mauk, 2014; Santrock, 2013; Weinrich & Boyd, 1992).

PHYSICAL, COGNITIVE, AND PSYCHOSOCIAL DEVELOPMENT

With advancing age, many physical changes occur. The senses of sight, hearing, touch, taste, and smell are usually the first areas of decreased functioning noticed by adults. Visual and auditory changes relate most closely to learning capacity. Hearing loss, which is very common beginning in the late 40s and 50s, includes diminished ability to discriminate high-pitched, high-frequency sounds. Visual changes such as cataracts, macular degeneration, reduced pupil size, decline in depth perception, and presbyopia may prevent older persons from being able to see small print, read words printed on glossy paper, or drive a car. Yellowing of the ocular lens can produce color distortions and diminished color perceptions.

Other physiological changes affect organ functioning and result in decreased cardiac output, lung performance, and metabolic rate; these changes reduce energy levels and lessen the ability to cope with stress. Nerve conduction velocity also is thought to decline by as much as 15%, influencing reflex times and muscle response rates. The interrelatedness of each body system has a total negative cumulative effect on individuals as they grow older.

Aging affects the mind as well as the body. Cognitive ability changes with age as permanent cellular alterations invariably occur in the brain itself, resulting in an actual loss of neurons, which have no regenerative powers. Physiological research has demonstrated that people have two kinds of intellectual ability—crystallized and fluid intelligence. **Crystallized intelligence** is the intelligence absorbed over a lifetime, such as vocabulary, general information, understanding social interactions, arithmetic reasoning, and ability to evaluate experiences. This kind of intelligence actually increases with experience as people age. However, it is important to understand that crystallized intelligence can be impaired by disease states, such as the dementia seen in Alzheimer's disease. **Fluid intelligence** is the capacity to perceive relationships, to reason, and to perform abstract thinking. This kind of intelligence declines as degenerative changes occur. The decline in fluid intelligence results in the following specific changes:

1. *Slower processing and reaction time.* Older persons need more time to process and react to information. However, if the factor of speed is removed from intelligence tests, older people can perform as well as younger people (Kray & Lindenberger, 2000).

2. *Persistence of stimulus (afterimage).* Older adults can confuse a previous symbol or word with a new word or symbol just introduced.

3. *Decreased short-term memory.* Older adults sometimes have difficulty remembering events or conversations that occurred just hours or days before.

4. *Increased test anxiety.* People in the older adult years are especially anxious about making mistakes when performing; when they do make an error, they become easily frustrated. Because of their anxiety, they may take an inordinate amount of time to respond to questions, particularly on tests that are written rather than verbal.

5. *Altered time perception.* For older persons, life becomes more finite and compressed. Issues of the here and now tend to be more important.

Despite the changes in cognition as a result of aging, most research supports that the ability of older adults to learn and remember remains strong if special care is taken to slow the pace of presenting information, to ensure relevance of material, and to give appropriate feedback when teaching (**Figure 5–1**).

Erikson (1963) labels the major psychosocial developmental task at this stage in life as *ego integrity versus despair*. This phase of older adulthood includes dealing with the reality of aging, the acceptance of the inevitability that all persons die, the reconciling of past failures with present and future concerns, and developing a sense of growth and

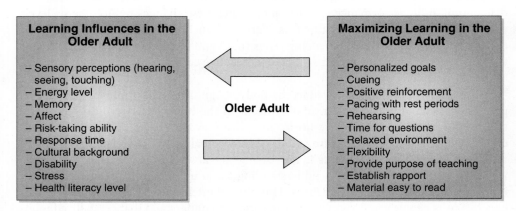

Figure 5–1 Learning in the older adult

Data from Mauk, K. L. (2014). *Gerontological nursing: Competencies for care* (3rd ed.). Burlington, MA: Jones & Bartlett Learning; Rendon, D. C., Davis, D. K., Gioiella, E. C., & Tranzillo, M. J. (1986). The right to know, the right to be taught. *Journal of Gerontological Nursing, 12*(12), 36.

purpose for those years remaining (Table 5–2). The most common psychosocial tasks of aging involve changes in lifestyle and social status as a result of the following:

- Retirement
- Illness or death of spouse, relatives, and friends
- The moving away of children, grandchildren, and friends
- Relocation to an unfamiliar environment such as an extended-care facility or senior residential living center

After Erikson's death in 1994, a ninth stage of psychosocial development, which has been labeled *hope and faith versus despair,* was published by his wife in the book *The Lifecycle Completed* (1997). It addresses those individuals reaching their late 80s and older, identifying that aging individuals have to accept the need for greater assistance as their bodies age. The goal is to find a renewed awareness of self in the midst of this need for additional care while eventually achieving a new sense of wisdom that is less materialistic and moves the individual beyond physical limitations (Crandell et al., 2012; Erikson, 1997). With aging, some individuals, particularly the oldest-old, begin to question their perception of a meaningful life—that is, the potential for further enjoyment, pleasure, and satisfaction. Depressive symptoms do increase in the oldest-old and are thought to be associated with more physical disability, more cognitive impairment, and lower socioeconomic status (Santrock, 2013).

Separate from biological aging but closely related are the many sociocultural factors that affect how older adults see themselves as competent individuals (Crandell et al., 2012; Leifer & Hartston, 2004; Santrock, 2013). The following traits regarding personal goals in life and the values associated with them are significantly related to motivation and learning:

1. *Independence.* The ability to provide for their own needs is the most important aim of the majority of older persons, regardless of their state of health. Independence gives them a sense of self-respect, pride, and self-functioning so as not to be a burden to others. Health teaching is the tool to help them maintain or regain independence.
2. *Social acceptability.* Winning approval from others is a common goal of many older adults. It is derived from health, a sense of vigor, and feeling and thinking young. Despite declining physical attributes, the older adult often has residual fitness and functioning potentials. Health teaching can help to channel these potentials.
3. *Adequacy of personal resources.* Life patterns, which include habits, physical and mental strengths, and economic situation, should be assessed to determine how to incorporate teaching to complement existing regimens and resources (financial and support systems) with new required behaviors.
4. *Coping mechanisms.* The ability to cope with change during the aging process is indicative of the person's readiness for health teaching. Positive coping mechanisms allow for self-change as older persons draw on life experiences and knowledge gained over the years. Negative coping mechanisms indicate an individual's focus on losses and show that his or her thinking is immersed in the

past. The emphasis in teaching is on exploring alternatives, determining realistic goals, and supporting large and small accomplishments.

5. *Meaning of life*. Health teaching must be directed at ways older adults can maintain optimal health so that they can derive pleasure from their leisure years.

TEACHING STRATEGIES

Understanding older persons' developmental tasks allows nurses to alter how they approach both well and ill individuals in terms of counseling, teaching, and establishing a therapeutic relationship. Decreased cognitive functioning, sensory deficits, lower energy levels, and other factors may prevent early disease detection and intervention. A decline in psychomotor performance affects the older adults' reflex responses and their ability to handle stress. Coping with simple tasks becomes more difficult. Chronic illnesses, depression, and literacy levels, particularly among the oldest-old, have implications with respect to how they care for themselves (eating, dressing, and taking medications) as well as the extent to which they understand the nature of their illnesses (Best, 2001; Katz, 1997; Mauk, 2014; Phillips, 1999).

In working with older adults, reminiscing is a beneficial approach to use to establish a therapeutic relationship. Memories can be quite powerful. Talking with older persons about their experiences can be very stimulating. Furthermore, their answers will give the nurse insight into their humanness, their abilities, and their concerns. Gavan (2003) warns that it is easy to fall into the habit of believing the myths associated with the intelligence, personality traits, motivation, and social relations of older adults.

Nurses may not even be aware of their stereotypical attitudes toward older adults. Furthermore, healthcare providers make assumptions about older clients that cause them to overlook problems that could be treatable (Gavan, 2003). To check their assumptions, nurses can think about the last time they gave instructions to an older patient and ask themselves the following questions:

- Did I talk to the family and ignore the patient when I described some aspect of care or discharge planning?
- Did I tell the older person not to worry when he or she asked a question? Did I say, "Just leave everything up to us"?
- Did I eliminate information that I normally would have given to a younger patient?
- Did I attribute a decline in cognitive functioning to the aging process without considering common underlying causes in mental deterioration, such as effects of medication interactions, fluid imbalances, poor nutrition, infection, or sensory impairments?

Remember that older people can learn, but their abilities and needs differ from those of younger persons. Because changes as a result of aging vary considerably from one individual to another, it is essential to assess each learner's physical, cognitive, and psychosocial functioning levels before developing and implementing any teaching plan. Keep in mind that older adults have an overall lower educational level of formal schooling than does the population as a whole. Also, they were raised in an era when consumerism and health education were practically nonexistent. As a result, older people may feel uncomfortable in the teaching–learning situation and may be reluctant to ask questions.

In the future, as the older population becomes more educated, these individuals will likely have an increased desire to actively participate in decision making and demand more detailed and sophisticated information. This increased participation by clients can assist in managing chronic diseases, promoting quality and safety in healthcare organizations, and ensuring effective redesign of care and treatment-related processes (Longtin et al., 2010). Further, the involvement of clients in deciding the course of their own care is an objective of *Healthy People 2020* (USDHHS, 2014b).

Health education for older persons should be directed at promoting their involvement and changing their attitudes toward learning (Ahroni, 1996; Weinrich & Boyd, 1992). They need to be made to feel important for what they once were as well as for what they are today. Interactions must be supportive, not judgmental. Interventions work best when they take place in a casual, informal atmosphere.

A recent report found that 53% of those persons older than age 65 are engaged in some type of computer use (Zickuhr & Madden, 2012). Thus, while many older adults routinely use computers, a good number do not. Assuming the client has the computer skills necessary to look up healthcare information or engage in self-education can derail learning. As the population continues to age, computer use will be more prevalent and preferred by clients who have been comfortable using technology to increase their knowledge (Mauk, 2014).

Some of the more common aging changes that affect learning and the teaching strategies specific to meeting the needs of the older adult are summarized in Table 5–1. When teaching older persons, abiding by the following specific tips can create an environment for learning that takes into account major changes in their physical, cognitive, and psychosocial functioning (Best, 2001; Crandell et al., 2012; Doak, Doak, & Root, 1996; Katz, 1997; Phillips, 1999; Robnett & Chop, 2015; Santrock, 2013; Weinrich & Boyd, 1992):

Physical Needs

1. To compensate for visual changes, teaching should be done in an environment that is brightly lit but without glare. Visual aids should include large print, well-spaced letters, and the use of primary colors. Bright colors and a visible name tag should be worn by the nurse. Use white or off-white, flat matte paper and black print for posters, diagrams, and other written materials.

    Because older adults have difficulty in discriminating certain shades of color, avoid blue, blue–green, and violet hues. Keep in mind that tasks that require recognizing different shades of color, such as test strips measuring the presence of sugar in the urine, may lead to errors because green, blue, and yellow colors may all appear gray to older persons. For patients who wear glasses, be sure they are readily accessible, lenses are clean, and frames are properly fitted.

2. To compensate for hearing losses, eliminate extraneous noise, avoid covering your mouth when speaking, directly face the learner, and speak slowly. These techniques assist the learner who may be seeking visual confirmation of what is being said.

    Low-pitched voices are heard best, but be careful not to drop your voice at the end of words or phrases. Do not shout, because the decibel level (loudness) is usually not a problem. Ask for feedback from the learner to determine whether you are speaking too softly, too fast, or not distinctly enough.

    Be alert to nonverbal cues from the audience. Participants who are having difficulty with hearing your message may try to compensate by leaning forward, turning the good ear to the speaker, or cupping their hands to their ears. Ask older persons to repeat verbal instructions to be sure they heard and interpreted correctly the entire message.

3. To compensate for musculoskeletal problems, decreased efficiency of the cardiovascular system, and reduced kidney function, keep sessions short, schedule frequent breaks to allow for use of bathroom facilities, and allow time for stretching to relieve painful, stiff joints and to stimulate circulation.

4. To compensate for any decline in central nervous system functioning and decreased metabolic rates, set aside more time for the giving and receiving of information and for the practice of psychomotor skills. Also, do not assume that older persons have the psychomotor skills necessary to handle technological equipment for self-paced learning, such as computers and mouse, ear buds instead of headsets, MP3 players, and DVD players. Be careful not to misinterpret the loss of energy and motor skills as a lack of motivation.

5. To compensate for the impact of hearing and visual changes on computer use, be sure that the speakers on the computer are working well and use headphones to block background noise (Mauk, 2014). **Table 5–3** outlines specific strategies that can assist older adults to overcome problems associated with computer use.

Cognitive Needs

1. To compensate for a decrease in fluid intelligence, provide older persons with more opportunities to process and react to information and to see relationships between concepts. Research has shown that older adults can learn anything if new information is tied to familiar concepts drawn from relevant past experiences.

    Avoid presenting long lists by dividing a series of directions for action into short, discrete, step-by-step messages and then waiting for a response after each one. Older persons also tend to confuse previous words and symbols with a new word or symbol being introduced. Nurses should wait for a response before introducing a new concept or word definition. For decreased short-term memory, coaching and repetition are very useful recall strategies. Because many older adults experience test anxiety, try to explain procedures simply and thoroughly, and provide reassurance that you are not testing them.

Table 5–3 Problems That Can Be Overcome by Older Adults Using Computers

Age Change	Effect on Computer Use	Possible Solutions
Hearing	Sound from computer may not be heard	Use earphones to enhance hearing and eliminate background noise. Speak slowly and clearly.
Vision	Vision declines, need for bifocal glasses, viewing monitor may be difficult, problems with glaucoma and light/colors	Adjust monitor's tilt to eliminate glare. Change size of font to 14. Make sure contrast is clear. Change the screen resolution to promote color perception.
Motor control tremors	May affect use of keyboard or control of mouse, may not be able to hold the mouse and consistently click correct mouse buttons	Highlight area and press Enter. Avoid double clicking.
Arthritis	May not be able to hold the mouse and consistently click correct mouse buttons	Highlight area and press Enter. Teach how to use options on keyboard.
Attention span	Problems with inability to focus and making correct inferences	Priming—introduce concept early on. Repetition is key to retention. Use cheat sheets.

Reproduced from Mauk, K. L. (2010). *Gerontological nursing: Competencies for care* (2nd ed.). Sudbury, MA: Jones & Bartlett Learning.

2. Be aware of the effects of medications and energy levels on concentration, alertness, and coordination. Try to schedule teaching sessions before or well after medications are taken and when the person is rested.

3. Be certain to ask what an individual already knows about a healthcare issue or technique before explaining it. Confirm patients' level of knowledge before beginning to teach. Basic information should be understood before progressing to more complex information.

4. Convincing older persons of the usefulness of what the nurse is teaching is only half the battle in getting them motivated. Anything that is entirely strange or that upsets established habits is likely to be significantly more difficult for older adults to learn.

5. Find out about older persons' health habits and beliefs before trying to change their ways or teach something new.

6. Arrange for brief teaching sessions because a shortened attention span (attentional narrowing) requires scheduling a series of sessions to provide sufficient time for learning. In addition, if the material is relevant and focused on the here and now, older persons are more likely to be attentive to the information being presented.

7. Take into account that the ability to think abstractly becomes more difficult with aging. Conclude each teaching session with a summary of the information presented and allow for a question-and-answer period to correct any misconceptions.

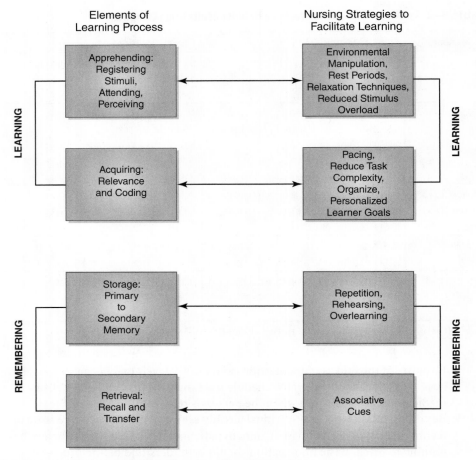

Figure 5–2 A basic gerontological teaching–learning model

Reproduced from Rendon, D. C., Davis, D. K., Gioiella, E. C., & Tranzillo, M. J. (1986). The right to know, the right to be taught. *Journal of Gerontological Nursing, 12*(12), 36.

Figure 5–2 presents strategies to meet the cognitive needs of older adults.

Psychosocial Needs

1. Assess family relationships to determine how dependent the older person is on other members for financial and emotional support. In turn, patient educators can explore the level of involvement by family members in reinforcing the lessons they are teaching and in giving assistance with self-care measures. Do family members help the older person to function independently, or do they foster dependency? With permission of the patient, include family members in teaching sessions and enlist their support.

2. Determine availability of resources, because older adults may not be able to carry out recommendations they cannot afford or lack the means to do.

3. Encourage active involvement of older adults to improve their self-esteem and to stimulate them both mentally and socially. Teaching must be directed at helping them find meaningful ways to use talents acquired over their lifetime.
4. Identify coping mechanisms. No other time in the life cycle carries with it the number of developmental tasks associated with adaptation to loss of roles, social and family contacts, and physical and cognitive capacities that this time does. Teaching must include offering constructive methods of coping.

The older person's ability to learn may be affected by the methods and materials chosen for teaching. One-to-one instruction provides a nonthreatening environment for older adults in which to meet their individual needs and goals. Group teaching also can be a beneficial approach for fostering social skills and maintaining contact with others through shared experiences. Introducing new teaching methods and tools, such as the use of computer and interactive video formats, without adequate instructions on how to operate these technical devices, may inhibit learning by increasing anxiety and frustration. Games, role playing, demonstration, and return demonstration can be used to rehearse problem-solving and psychomotor skills as long as these methods and the tools used to complement them are designed appropriately to accommodate the various developmental characteristics of this age group.

The Role of the Family in Patient Education

The role of the family is considered one of the key variables influencing positive patient care outcomes. Family caregivers provide critical emotional, physical, and social support to the patient in the midst of managing complex care regimens (Gavan, 2003; Reeber, 1992; Reinhard, Levine, & Samis, 2012). Under The Joint Commission accreditation standards, demands have been placed on healthcare organizations to show evidence of patient and family-centered care, which requires including significant others in patient education efforts (The Joint Commission, 2010). Nurses and other providers are responsible for assisting both patients and their designated support person(s) to gain the knowledge and skills necessary to meet ongoing healthcare goals, particularly the first of the *Healthy People 2020* initiatives—that is, to increase the quality and years of healthy, disease-free, and injury-free life (USDHHS, 2014b). Interdisciplinary collaboration that involves family caregivers is a major resource for ensuring continuity of client teaching about healthy lifestyles in and across healthcare settings (Reinhard et al., 2012).

Including the family members in the teaching–learning process helps to ensure that the situation is a win-win scenario for both the client and the nurse. Family role enhancement and increased knowledge on the part of the family have positive benefits for the learner as well as the nurse as teacher. Clients derive increased satisfaction and greater independence in self-care, and nurses experience increased job satisfaction and personal gratification in helping clients to reach their potentials and achieve successful outcomes (Barnes, 1995; Gavan, 2003).

Although a great deal of attention has been given to the ways in which young and adolescent families function, unfortunately minimal attention has been paid to the dynamics of the complex interactions that characterize the aging family (Gavan, 2003).

In patient education, the nurse may be tempted to teach as many family members as possible. In reality, it is difficult to coordinate the instruction of so many different people. The more individuals involved, the greater the potential for misunderstanding of instruction.

The family must make the deliberate decision as to who is the most appropriate person to take the primary responsibility as the caregiver. Then the nurse must determine how the caregiver feels about the role of providing supportive care and about learning the necessary information. The nurse also must explore what are the caregiver's learning style preferences, cognitive abilities, fears and concerns, and current knowledge of the situation (Leifer & Hartston, 2004). The caregiver needs information similar to what the patient is given to provide support, feedback, and reinforcement of self-care consistent with prescribed regimens of care. In some cases, a secondary caregiver also is identified and the same considerations in teaching must be given.

Sometimes the family members need more information than the patient to compensate for any sensory deficits or cognitive limitations the patient may have. Anticipatory teaching with family caregivers can reduce their anxiety, uncertainty, and lack of confidence. What the family is to *do* is important, but what the family is to *expect* also is essential information to be shared during the teaching–learning process (Haggard, 1989). The greatest challenge for caregivers is to develop confidence in their ability to do what is right for the patient. Education and training are the means to help them confront this challenge (Reinhard et al., 2012).

The family can be the nurse's greatest ally in preparing the patient for discharge and in helping the patient to become independent in self-care. The patient's family is perhaps the single most significant determinant of the success or failure of the education plan and achievement of successful aging (Capezuti, 2014; Gavan, 2003; Haggard, 1989). The role of the family has been stressed in each developmental section in this chapter. Table 5–1 outlines appropriate interventions for the family at different stages in the life cycle.

Summary

It is important to understand the specific and varied tasks associated with each developmental stage to individualize the approach to education in meeting the needs and desires of patients and their families. Assessment of physical, cognitive, and psychosocial maturation within each developmental period is crucial in determining the appropriate strategies to facilitate the teaching–learning process. The younger learner is, in many ways, very different from the adult learner. Issues of dependency, extent of participation, rate of and capacity for learning, and situational and emotional obstacles to learning vary significantly across the various phases of development.

Readiness to learn in children is very subject centered and highly influenced by their physical, cognitive, and psychosocial maturation. Motivation to learn in adults is very problem centered and more oriented to psychosocial tasks related to roles and expectations of work, family, and community activities. For education to be effective, the nurse must create an environment conducive to learning by presenting information at the learner's level, inviting participation and feedback, and identifying whether parental, family, and/or peer involvement is appropriate or necessary. Nurses are the main source of health information and must determine, in concert with the client, what needs to be taught, when to teach, how to teach, and who should be the focus of teaching in light of the developmental stage of the learner.

Review Questions

1. What are the seven stages of development?
2. Define *pedagogy*, *andragogy*, and *gerogogy*.
3. Who is the expert in cognitive development? What are the terms or labels used by this expert to identify the key cognitive milestones?
4. Who is the expert in psychosocial development? What are the terms or labels used by this expert to identify the key psychosocial milestones?
5. What are the specific characteristics at each stage of development that influence the ability to learn?
6. What are three main teaching strategies for each stage of development?
7. How do people you know in each stage of development compare with what you have learned about physical, cognitive, and psychosocial characteristics at the various developmental stages?
8. What is the role of the family in the teaching and learning process at each stage of development?
9. How does the role of the nurse vary when teaching individuals at different stages of development?

Case Study

Potomac University's Lillian Case Asthma Center is developing a new program that focuses on a family-centered approach to asthma management. Expected client outcomes of the program are to reduce hospitalizations and days off from work or school. You are a member of the nursing team that is developing a comprehensive, family-oriented educational program that covers important asthma topics such as pathophysiology, peak-flow meter use, and exercise. Mauricio, a member of the team, suggests, "Let's do our teaching with all the family members together in a group." Liza, another team member, states, "We should separate the family members into similar age groups for the teaching—that way, we can better keep their interest." You suggest that the team integrate Mauricio's and Liza's suggestions and plan a total of five teaching sessions, with four of the sessions grouping participants according to developmental stages and the final session grouping families together. Participants range from 6 to 50 years of age.

1. Describe how you will determine the different developmental stage groupings of the participants for the first four sessions. Explain the different age ranges, cognitive and psychosocial stages, and general characteristics of each group.

2. Choose two different developmental stage groupings and give examples of teaching strategies you will use with each group for the specific teaching sessions.
3. What are some advantages to grouping participants by developmental stages? What are some disadvantages?

References

Ackard, D. M., & Neumark-Sztainer, D. (2001). Health care information sources for adolescents: Age and gender differences on use, concerns, and needs. *Journal of Adolescent Health, 29*(3), 170–176.

Ahroni, J. H. (1996). Strategies for teaching elders from a human development perspective. *Diabetes Educator, 22*(1), 47–52.

Ares, K., Kuhns, L. M., Dogra, N., & Karnik, N. (2015). Child mental health and risk behavior over time. In B. Kirkcaldy (Ed.), *Promoting psychological wellbeing in children and families* (pp. 135–153). New York, NY: Palgrave Macmillan.

Aronowitz, T. (2006). Teaching adolescents about adolescence: Experiences from an interdisciplinary adolescent health course. *Nurse Educator, 31*(2), 84–87.

Babcock, D. E., & Miller, M. A. (1994). *Client education: Theory and practice.* St. Louis, MO: Mosby.

Banks, E. (1990). Concepts of health and sickness of preschool- and school-aged children. *Children's Health Care, 19*(1), 43–48.

Barnes, L. P. (1995). Finding the "win/win" in patient/family teaching. *MCN: The American Journal of Maternal/Child Nursing, 20*(4), 229.

Behm, L., Wilhelmson, K., Falk, K., Eklund, K., Zidén, L., & Dahlin-Ivanoff, S. (2014). Positive health outcomes following health-promoting and disease preventive interventions for independent very old persons: Long-term results of the three-armed RCT elderly persons in the risk zone. *Archives of Gerontology and Geriatrics, 58*(3), 376–383.

Best, J. T. (2001). Effective teaching for the elderly: Back to basics. *Orthopaedic Nursing, 20*(3), 46–52.

Boyd, M. D., Gleit, C. J., Graham, B. A., & Whitman, N. I. (1998). *Health teaching in nursing practice: A professional model* (3rd ed.). Norwalk, CT: Appleton & Lange.

Brown, S. L., Teufel, J. A., & Birch, D. A. (2007). Early adolescents' perceptions of health and health literacy. *Journal of School Health, 77*(1), 7–15.

Capezuti, E. (2014). It's a matter of trust: Nurses supporting family caregivers. *Geriatric Nursing, 35*, 154–155.

Collins, J. (2004). Education techniques for lifelong learners. *RadioGraphics, 24*(5), 1483–1489.

Crandell, T. L., Crandell, C. H., & Vander Zanden, J. W. (2012). *Human development* (11th ed.). New York, NY: McGraw-Hill.

Curran, M. K. (2014). Examination of the teaching styles of nursing professional development specialists, Part I: Best practices in adult learning theory, curriculum development, and knowledge transfer. *The Journal of Continuing Education in Nursing, 45*(5), 233–240.

Doak, C. C., Doak, L. G., & Root, J. H. (1996). *Teaching patients with low literacy skills* (2nd ed.). Philadelphia, PA: Lippincott.

Elkind, D. (1984). Teenage thinking: Implications for health care. *Pediatric Nursing, 10*(6), 383–385.

Erikson, E. H. (1963). *Childhood and society* (2nd ed.). New York, NY: Norton.

Erikson, E. H. (1968). *Identity: Youth and crisis*. New York, NY: Norton.

Erikson, E. (1997). *The life cycle completed* (extended version). New York, NY: Norton.

Falvo, D. (2011). *Effective patient education: A guide to increased adherence* (4th ed.). Sudbury, MA: Jones & Bartlett Learning.

Federal Interagency Forum on Aging-Related Statistics. (2012). *Older Americans 2012: Key indicators of well-being*. Washington, DC: U.S. Government Printing Office.

Gavan, C. S. (2003). Successful aging families: A challenge for nurses. *Holistic Nursing Practice, 17*(1), 11–18.

Grey, M., Kanner, S., & Lacey, K. O. (1999). Characteristics of the learner: Children and adolescents. *Diabetes Educator, 25*(6), 25–33.

Haggard, A. (1989). *Handbook of patient education*. Rockville, MD: Aspen.

Havighurst, R. (1976). Human characteristics and school learning: Essay review. *Elementary School Journal, 77*, 101–109.

Heiney, S. P. (1991). Helping children through painful procedures. *American Journal of Nursing, 91*(11), 20–24.

Hines, A. R., & Paulson, S. E. (2006). Parents' and teachers' perceptions of adolescent storm and stress: Relations with parenting and teaching styles. *Adolescence, 41*(164), 597–614.

Hinkle, J. (2014). *Brunner & Suddarth's textbook of medical-surgical nursing* (13th ed.). Philadelphia, PA: Wolters Kluwer Health/Lippincott Williams & Wilkins.

Hussey, C. G., & Hirsh, A. M. (1983). Health education for children. *Topics in Clinical Nursing, 5*(1), 22–28.

The Joint Commission. (2010). *Advancing effective communication, cultural competence, and patient- and family-centered care: A roadmap for hospitals*. Oakbrook Terrace, IL: Author. Retrieved from http://www.jointcommission.org/assets/1/6/aroadmapforhospitalsfinalversion727.pdf

Kaakinen, J. R., Gedaly-Duff, V., Coehlo, D. P., & Hanson, S. M. H. (2010). *Family health care nursing*. Philadelphia, PA: F. A. Davis.

Katz, J. R. (1997). Back to basics: Providing effective patient education. *American Journal of Nursing, 97*(5), 33–36.

Knowles, M. (1990). *The adult learner: A neglected species* (4th ed.). Houston, TX: Gulf Publishing.

Knowles, M. S., Holton, E. F., & Swanson, R. A. (2015). *The adult learner: The definitive classic in adult education and human resource development* (8th ed.). London, England: Routledge: Taylor and Francis Group.

Kochanek, K. D., Xu, J., Murphy, S. L., Minino, A. M., & Kung, H. (2011). Deaths: Final data for 2009. *National Vital Statistics Reports, 60*(3), 1–166.

Koopman, H. M., Baars, R. M., Chaplin, J., & Zwinderman, K. H. (2004). Illness through the eyes of a child: The development of children's understanding of the causes of illness. *Patient Education and Counseling, 55*(3), 363–370.

Kotchabhakdi, P. (1985). School-age children's conceptions of the heart and its function. Monograph 15. *Maternal–Child Nursing Journal, 14*(4), 203–261.

Kray, J., & Lindenberger, U. (2000). Adult age differences in task switching. *Psychology and Aging, 15*(1), 126–147.

Lawson, P. J., & Flocke, S. A. (2009). Teachable moments for health behavior change: A concept analysis. *Patient Education and Counseling, 76*(1), 25–30.

Leifer, G., & Hartston, H. (2004). *Growth and development across the lifespan: A health promotion focus*. St. Louis, MO: Saunders.

London, M. C., Ladewig, P. W., Davidson, M. C., Ball, J. W., & Bindler, R. C. (2013). *Maternal and child nursing care* (4th ed.). Upper Saddle River, NJ: Pearson.

Longtin, Y., Sax, H., Leape, L. L., Sheridan, S. E., Donaldson, L., & Pittet, D. (2010). Patient participation: Current knowledge and applicability to patient safety. *Mayo Clinic Proceedings, 85*(1), 53–62.

Mauk, K. L. (2014). *Gerontological nursing: Competencies for care* (3rd ed.). Burlington, MA: Jones & Bartlett Learning.

Michaud, P.-A., Stronski, S., Fonseca, H., & MacFarlane, A. (2004). The development and pilot-testing of a training curriculum in adolescent medicine and health. *Journal of Adolescent Health, 35*(1), 51–57.

Ormrod, J. E. (2012). *Essentials of educational psychology: Big ideas to guide effective teaching* (3rd ed.). Boston, MA: Pearson.

Orshan, S. A. (2008). *Maternity, newborn, and woman's health nursing: Comprehensive care across the lifespan*. Philadelphia, PA: Lippincott Williams & Wilkins.

Palfrey, J. S., Hauser-Cram, P., Bronson, M. B., Warfield, M. E., Sirin, S., & Chan, E. (2005). The Brookline early education project: A 25-year follow-up study of family-centered early health and development intervention. *Pediatrics, 116*(1), 144–152.

Perrin, E. C., Sayer, A. G., & Willett, J. B. (1991). Sticks and stones may break my bones . . : Reasoning about illness causality and body functioning in children who have a chronic illness. *Pediatrics, 88*(3), 608–619.

Phillips, L. D. (1999). Patient education: Understanding the process to maximize time and outcomes. *Journal of Intravenous Nursing, 22*(1), 19–35.

Piaget, J. (1951). *Judgment and reasoning in the child*. London, England: Routledge & Kegan Paul.

Piaget, J. (1952). *The origins of intelligence in children*. New York, NY: International Universities Press.

Piaget, J. (1976). *The grasp of consciousness: Action and concept in the young child*. (S. Wedgwood, Trans.). Cambridge, MA: Harvard University Press.

Pidgeon, V. (1985). Children's concepts of illness: Implications for health teaching. *Maternal–Child Nursing Journal, 14*(1), 23–35.

Polan, E., & Taylor, D. (2015). *Journey across the lifespan: Human development and health promotion* (5th ed.). Philadelphia, PA: F. A. Davis.

Poster, E. C. (1983). Stress immunization: Techniques to help children cope with hospitalization. *Maternal–Child Nursing Journal, 12*(2), 119–134.

Protheroe, N. (2007). How children learn. *Principal, 86*(5), 40–44.

Reeber, B. J. (1992). Evaluating the effects of a family education intervention. *Rehabilitation Nursing, 17*(6), 332–336.

Reinhard, S. C., Levine, C., & Samis, S. (2012). *Home alone: Family caregivers providing complex chronic care*. Washington, D. C.: AARP Public Policy Institute. Retrieved from http://www.aarp.org/ppi.

Rendon, D. C., Davis, D. K., Gioiella, E. C., & Tranzillo, M. J. (1986). The right to know, the right to be taught. *Journal of Gerontological Nursing, 12*(12), 36.

Robnett, R. H., & Chop, W. (2015). *Gerontology for the health care professional* (3rd ed.). Burlington, MA: Jones & Bartlett Learning.

Ryberg, J. W., & Merrifield, E. B. (1984). What parents want to know. *Nurse Practitioner, 9*(6), 24–32.

Santrock, J. W. (2013). *Life-span development* (14th ed.). New York, NY: McGraw-Hill.

Snowman, J., & McCown, R. (2015). *Psychology applied to teaching* (14th ed.). Stanford, CA: Wadsworth/Cengage Learning.

Steegen, S., & De Neys, W. (2012). Belief inhibition in children's reasoning: Memory-based evidence. *Journal of Experimental Child Psychology, 112*, 231–242.

Taylor, K., Marienau, C., & Fiddler, M. (2000). *Developing adult learners: Strategies for teachers and trainers*. San Francisco, CA: Jossey-Bass.

U. S. Department of Health and Human Services [USDHHS]. (2014a). *A profile of older Americans: 2014*. Administration on Aging, Administration for Community Living, U.S. Department of Health and Human Services Administration on Aging. Retrieved from http://www.aoa.acl.gov/Aging_Statistics/Profile/2014/docs/2014-Profile.pdf

U. S. Department of Health and Human Services [USDHHS]. (2014b). *Healthy People 2020*. Office of Disease Prevention and Health Promotion. Retrieved from http://www.healthypeople.gov/

Vulcan, B. (1984). Major coping behaviors of a hospitalized 3-year-old boy. *Maternal–Child Nursing Journal, 13*(2), 113–123.

Weinrich, S. P., & Boyd, M. (1992). Education in the elderly. *Journal of Gerontological Nursing, 18*(1), 15–20.

Whitener, L. M., Cox, K. R., & Maglich, S. A. (1998). Use of theory to guide nurses in the design of health messages for children. *Advances in Nursing Science, 20*(3), 21–35.

Woodring, B. C. (2000). If you have taught—have the child and family learned? *Pediatric Nursing, 26*(5), 505–509.

Zickuhr, K., & Madden, M. (2012). *Older adults and their Internet use*. Washington, DC: Pew Research Center's Internet and American Life Project. Retrieved from http://www.pewinternet.org/~/media//Files/Reports/2012/PIP_Older_adults_and_internet_use.pdf

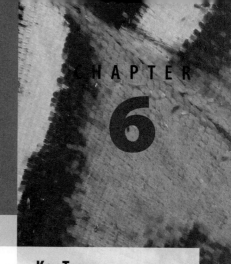

Health Behaviors of the Learner

Eleanor Richards | Pamela Gramet

Chapter Highlights

- Compliance and Adherence
  - *Noncompliance and Nonadherence*
  - *Locus of Control*
- Motivation
  - *Motivational Factors*
  - *Motivational Axioms*
  - *Assessment of Motivation*
  - *Motivational Strategies*
- Selected Models and Theories
  - *Health Belief Model*
  - *Health Promotion Model (Revised)*
  - *Self-Efficacy Theory*
  - *Stages of Change Model*
  - *Theory of Reasoned Action and Theory of Planned Behavior*
  - *Therapeutic Alliance Model*

Key Terms

adherence
compliance
health belief model
health promotion model
hierarchy of needs
locus of control
motivation
motivational axioms
motivational incentives
motivational interviewing
nonadherence
noncompliance
OARS
READS
self-efficacy theory
stages of change model
theory of planned behavior
theory of reasoned action
therapeutic alliance model

Objectives

After completing this chapter, the reader will be able to

1. Define the terms *compliance, adherence,* and *motivation* relative to behaviors of the learner.
2. Discuss compliance, adherence, and motivation concepts and theories.
3. Identify incentives and obstacles that affect motivation to learn.
4. State axioms of motivation relevant to learning.

5. Assess levels of learner motivation.
6. Outline strategies that facilitate motivation and improve compliance and adherence.
7. Explore how the selected models and theories describe, explain, or predict health behaviors.

The nurse as a teacher of patients needs to understand what drives the learner to learn and which factors promote or hinder the learning process. The terms *compliance, adherence,* and *motivation* are concepts in many health behavior models. This chapter discusses these terms as they relate to health behaviors of the learner and presents an overview of selected theories and models for consideration in the teaching–learning process.

Factors that determine health behaviors and outcomes are complex. Knowledge alone does not guarantee that the learner will engage in health-promoting behaviors or attain desired outcomes. The most well thought-out educational program or plan of care cannot achieve the prescribed goals if the learner is not understood in the context of complex factors associated with compliance, adherence, and motivation.

Compliance and Adherence

The terms compliance and adherence are often used interchangeably in the literature to refer to a patient's efforts to follow healthcare advice (Robinson, Callister, Berry, & Dearing, 2008). However, they infer different views about the healthcare provider–patient relationship. **Compliance** is defined as the "extent to which the patient's behavior (in terms of taking medications, following diets or executing other lifestyle changes) coincides with the clinical advice" (Sackett & Haynes, 1976, p. 11). According to the Merriam-Webster dictionary (2015b), compliance means "the act or process of complying to a desire, demand, proposal, or regimen or to coercion; a disposition to yield to others." Defined as such, it has an authoritative undertone. Specifically, when applied to health care, it implies that the healthcare provider or teacher is viewed as the authority, and the patient or learner is in a submissive role, passively following recommendations. Many nurses object to this hierarchical stance because they believe that patients have the right to make their own healthcare decisions and not necessarily follow predetermined courses of action set by healthcare professionals.

Adherence, according to the World Health Organization, is "the extent to which a person's behavior—taking medication, following a diet, and/or executing lifestyle changes, corresponds with agreed recommendations from a health care provider" (Sabaté, 2003, p. 3). Mihalko et al. (2004) define adherence as "level of participation achieved in a behavioral regimen once an individual has agreed to the regimen" (p. 448), and Hernshaw and Lidenmeyer (2006) describe adherence as the degree to which the patient follows the plan of care formulated in conjunction with the healthcare provider. Furthermore, the Merriam-Webster dictionary (2015a) defines adherence as "the act, action, or quality of adhering: steady or faithful attachment," suggesting the need for the patient to attach and commit to the healthcare regimen. These definitions address the need for patients to be involved in treatment decisions, which is quite different from passively following the healthcare providers' prescriptions.

During the 1990s, the terminology in the literature began to shift to adherence rather than compliance (Gardner, 2015), supporting a more inclusive and active patient role. The term adherence is seen as being more patient-centered than compliance (Vlasnik, Aliotta, & DeLor, 2005) because it supports the patient's right to choose whether or not to follow treatment recommendations.

Both compliance and adherence refer to the ability to maintain health-promoting regimens, which are determined by or in conjunction with the healthcare provider, respectively. It is possible, though, for an individual to initially comply with a regimen but not necessarily be committed to it. For example, a patient who is experiencing sleep disturbances may comply for a short period of time with medication as directed. The same patient, however, may not continue to adhere to the regimen for an extended period of time, even though the sleep disturbances continue. In this situation, there is temporary support of the plan, but no commitment to follow through. Because both compliance and adherence are terms commonly used in the measurement of health outcomes, and they are often used synonymously in the literature despite the differences in social connotations between the terms (Gardner, 2015), they will be used interchangeably in this chapter.

Noncompliance and Nonadherence

Noncompliance describes resistance of the individual to follow a predetermined regimen. It often results in blaming behavior when patient goals are not achieved (Yach, 2003) and condemns a patient's behavior as flawed for the inability to conform to treatment (Robinson et al., 2008). Ward-Collins (1998) notes that noncompliance can be a highly subjective judgmental term sometimes used synonymously with the terms *noncooperative* and *disobedient*. Helme and Harrington (2004) studied patients who were noncompliant with their diabetes regimen and found that although most people admitted their failure to comply with their healthcare plan, many offered excuses or justifications, and some denied that noncompliance had occurred. Even though in this study participants had nothing to lose by admitting their noncompliance, many felt the need to explain or deny their failure to follow orders.

There are many studies on patient noncompliance, and yet, the question of why clients are noncompliant remains largely unanswered, primarily because of the complexity of the issue. Noncompliance can be related to patient issues such as knowledge or motivation, treatment factors such as side effects, disease issues such as prognosis, lifestyle issues such as transportation, sociodemographic factors such as social and economic status, and psychosocial variables such as depression and fear (Rosner, 2006).

The expectation of total compliance in all spheres of behavior and at all times is unrealistic. At times, noncompliant behavior may be desirable and could be viewed as a necessary defensive response to stressful situations. The learner may use time-outs as the intensity of the learning situation is maintained or escalates. This mechanism of temporary withdrawal from the learning situation may actually prove beneficial. Following withdrawal, the learner could reengage, feeling renewed and ready to continue with an educational program or regimen. Viewed in this way, noncompliance is not always an obstacle to learning and does not always carry a negative connotation.

Nonadherence occurs when the patient does not follow treatment recommendations that are mutually agreed upon (Resnik, 2005). It can be intentional or unintentional and, according to the World Health Organization, can be determined by the interplay of five sets of factors or dimensions—socioeconomically related, patient related, condition related, therapy related, and healthcare team or system related (Sabaté, 2003). Patient factors that contribute to nonadherence include stress, forgetfulness, substance abuse, having multiple medical conditions, uncertainty about health beliefs and practices, and real or perceived stigma associated with the conditions of being treated (DiMatteo, 2004; Pignone & Salazar, 2014).

Locus of Control

One way to view the issue of control in the learning situation is through the concept of locus of control (Rotter, 1954) or health locus of control (Wallston, Wallston, & DeVellis, 1978). **Locus of control** refers to an individual's sense of responsibility for his or her own behavior and the extent to which motivation to take action originates from within the self (internal) or is influenced by others (external). Through objective measurement, individuals can be categorized as internals, whose health behavior is self-directed, or externals, for whom others are viewed as more powerful in influencing health outcomes. Externals believe that fate is a powerful outside force that determines life's course, whereas internals believe that they control their own destiny. For instance, an external might say, "Osteoporosis runs in my family, and it will catch up with me." An internal might say, "Although there is a history of osteoporosis in my family, I will have necessary screenings, eat an appropriate diet, and do weight bearing exercise to prevent or control this problem."

Researchers in the health professions have attempted to link locus of control with compliance, but study results in this area have been mixed. Locus of control has been linked to compliance in some therapeutic regimens but has shown no relationship in others (Epstein, Kale, & Weisshaar, 2014; Morowatisharifabad, Mahmoodabad, Baghiani-moghadam, & Tonekaboni, 2010; O'Hea et al., 2009; Porto, Machado, Martins, Galato, & Piovezan, 2014; Rosno, Steele, Johnston, & Aylward, 2008; SinJae, SugJoon, & TaeWoo, 2008; Tahar et al., 2015). Shillinger (1983) suggests that different teaching strategies are indicated for internals and externals. The literature, however, remains inconclusive as to the nature of the relationship between compliance and internals versus externals.

Motivation

Motivation is defined as "an internal state that arouses, directs, and sustains human behavior" (Glynn, Aultman, & Owens, 2005, p. 150), and as a willingness of the learner to embrace learning, with readiness as evidence of motivation (Redman, 2007). According to Kort (1987), motivation is the result of both internal and external factors and not the result of external manipulation alone. Implicit in motivation is movement in the direction of meeting a need or toward reaching a goal. Maslow (1943) developed a theory of human motivation that is still widely used in the social sciences. The major premises of Maslow's motivation theory are integrated wholeness of the individual and a hierarchy of goals. Acknowledging the complexity of the concept of motivation, Maslow noted that not all behavior is motivated and that behavior theories are not synonymous with motivation. Many determinants of behavior other than motives exist, and many motives can be involved in one behavior. Using the principles of a **hierarchy of needs**—physiological, safety, love/belonging, esteem, and self-actualization—Maslow noted the relatedness of needs, which are organized by their level of potency. Some individuals are highly motivated, whereas others are weakly motivated. When a need is fairly well satisfied, then the next potent need emerges. An example of the hierarchy of basic needs is the powerful need to satisfy hunger. This need may be met by the nurse assisting the poststroke patient with feeding. The nurse–patient interaction may also satisfy the next most potent needs, those of love/belonging and esteem. (See Chapter 3 for more on Maslow's hierarchy of needs.)

Relationships exist between motivation and learning; between motivation and behavior; and among motivation, learning, and behavior. Each theory presented in this chapter attempts to address the complex and somewhat elusive quality of motivation.

Motivational Factors

Factors that influence motivation can serve as either incentives or obstacles to achieving desired behaviors. Both creating incentives and decreasing obstacles to motivation pose a challenge for the nurse as a teacher of patients. The cognitive (thinking processes), affective (emotions and feelings), and psychomotor (skill behavior) domains as well as the social circumstances of the learner can be influenced by the teacher, who can act as either a motivational facilitator or blocker.

Motivational incentives need to be considered in the context of the individual. What may be a motivational incentive for one learner may be a motivational obstacle to another. For example, a nurse assigned to work with a woman who is elderly may be motivated to care for her when the nurse holds older adults in high regard. Another nurse may be motivationally blocked because previous experiences with older women, such as a grandmother, were unrewarding. Facilitating or blocking factors that shape motivation to learn can be classified into three major categories, which are not mutually exclusive:

1. Personal attributes, which consist of physical, developmental, and psychological components of the individual learner
2. Environmental influences, which include the surroundings and the attitudes of others
3. Learner relationship systems, such as those of significant other, family, community, and teacher–learner interaction

PERSONAL ATTRIBUTES

The factors that can shape an individual's motivation to learn include personal attributes such as:

- Developmental stage
- Age
- Gender
- Emotional readiness
- Values and beliefs
- Sensory functioning
- Cognitive ability
- Educational level
- Actual or perceived state of health
- Severity or chronicity of illness

The ability to achieve behavioral outcomes is determined by an individual's physical, emotional, and cognitive status. One's perception of the difference between the current and expected states of health can be a motivating factor in health behavior and can drive readiness to learn. Also, the learner's views about the complexity or extent of changes that are needed can shape motivation.

ENVIRONMENTAL INFLUENCES

The environment can create, promote, or detract from the ability to learn. Environmental factors that can influence the motivational level of the individual to learn include:

- Physical characteristics of the environment
- Accessibility and availability of human and material resources
- Different types of behavioral rewards

Pleasant, comfortable, and adaptable individualized surroundings, for example, can promote a state of readiness to learn. Conversely, noise, confusion, interruptions, and lack of privacy can interfere with the capacity to concentrate and to learn.

The factors of accessibility and availability of resources include physical and psychological aspects. Can the client physically access a health facility, and once there, will the healthcare personnel be psychologically available to the client? Psychological availability refers to whether the healthcare system is flexible and sensitive to patients' needs. It includes factors such as promptness of services, sociocultural competence, emotional support, and communication skills. Attitude influences the client's engagement with the healthcare system.

The manner in which the healthcare system is perceived by the client affects the client's willingness to participate in health-promoting behaviors. Behavioral rewards support learner motivation. Rewards can be external, such as praise or acknowledgment from the nurse or caretaker. Alternatively, they can be internally based, taking the form of feelings of a personal sense of fulfillment, gratification, or self-satisfaction.

RELATIONSHIP SYSTEMS

Family or significant others in the support system; cultural identity; work, school, and community roles; and teacher–learner interaction are all relationship-based factors that influence an individual's motivation. The learner exists in relationship systems. Individuals are viewed in the context of family/community/cultural systems that have lifelong effects on the choices that individuals make, including healthcare seeking and healthcare decision making.

These significant-other systems may have an even greater influence on health outcomes than commonly acknowledged, and the nurse, when in the role of teacher, needs to take into account the health-promoting use of these systems. All of these factors are forces that affect motivation and serve to facilitate or block the desire to learn.

Motivational Axioms

Axioms are premises on which an understanding of a phenomenon is based. The nurse as teacher needs to understand the premises involved in promoting motivation of the learner. **Motivational axioms** are rules that set the stage for motivation. They include (1) the state of optimal anxiety, (2) learner readiness, (3) realistic goal setting, (4) learner satisfaction/success, and (5) uncertainty reducing or uncertainty maintaining dialogue.

STATE OF OPTIMAL ANXIETY

Learning occurs best when a state of moderate anxiety exists. In this optimal state for learning, the learner's ability to observe, focus attention, learn, and adapt is operative (Peplau, 1979). Perception, concentration, abstract thinking, and information processing are enhanced. Behavior is directed at challenging learning situations. Above this optimal level, at high or severe levels of anxiety, the learner becomes increasingly self-absorbed (Shapiro, Boggs, Melamed, & Graham-Pole, 1992), and the ability to perceive the environment, concentrate, and learn is reduced. If less than the optimal level, the learner who has low anxiety is not very driven to act. Thus, a moderate state of anxiety can be comfortably managed and is known to be most effective in promoting learning (Kessels, 2003; Ley, 1979; Stephenson, 2006).

For example, a patient who has been recently diagnosed with insulin-dependent diabetes and who has a high level of anxiety will not be able to pay attention or retain information very well during instruction about insulin injections. When the nurse is able to aid the patient in reducing anxiety through techniques such as guided imagery, use of humor, words of reassurance, or relaxation tapes, the patient will respond with a higher level of focus and will be able to process and remember information better.

LEARNER READINESS

Desire to move toward a goal and readiness to learn are factors that influence motivation. Desire cannot be imposed on the learner. It can, however, be significantly influenced by external forces and be promoted by the nurse. Incentives are specific to the individual learner. An incentive for one individual can be a deterrent to another. For example, suggesting a method of weight reduction that includes physical exercise may be an incentive for one client, while totally unappealing for another. Incentives in the form of reinforcers and rewards can be tangible or intangible, external or internal.

In patient teaching, the nurse offers positive perspectives and encouragement, which shape the desired behavior toward goal attainment. By ensuring that learning is stimulating, making information relevant and accessible, and creating an environment conducive to learning, nurses can enhance motivation to learn.

REALISTIC GOALS

Goals that are within a person's grasp and possible to achieve are goals toward which an individual will work. In contrast, goals that are significantly beyond the person's reach can frustrate and discourage the learner. Setting unrealistic goals that lead to loss of valuable time can set the stage for the learner to give up.

Setting realistic goals by determining what the learner wants to change is a motivating factor. Mutual goal setting between the learner and the nurse reduces the negative effects of hidden agendas or the feeling that one has more control than another.

LEARNER SATISFACTION/SUCCESS

The learner is motivated by success. Success is self-satisfying and feeds the learner's self-esteem. When a learner feels good about step-by-step accomplishments, motivation is enhanced. Focusing on successes as a means of positive reinforcement promotes learner satisfaction and instills a sense of accomplishment.

UNCERTAINTY REDUCTION OR MAINTENANCE

Uncertainty is a common experience in the healthcare arena. Healthcare consumers and health professionals alike are often asked to make decisions about treatments and care options whose outcomes are unclear. An individual's response to this type of uncertainty may vary depending on the individual's characteristics (Politi, Han, & Col, 2007).

Uncertainty (as well as certainty) can be a motivating factor in the learning situation. Individuals may have ongoing internal dialogues that can either reduce or maintain uncertainty. Individuals carry on self-talk; they think things through. When a person wants to change a state of health, behaviors often follow a dialogue that examines uncertainty, such as, "If I stop smoking, then my chances of getting lung cancer will be reduced." When the probable outcome of health behaviors is more uncertain, behaviors may maintain uncertainty. The person might say, "I am not sure that I need this surgery because the survival rates are no different for those who had this surgery and those who did not." Some learners may maintain current behaviors, given probabilities of treatment outcomes, thereby maintaining uncertainty.

Assessment of Motivation

How does the nurse know when the learner is motivated? Redman (2001) views motivational assessment as a part of general health assessment and states that it includes such areas as level of knowledge, client skills, decision-making capacity of the individual, and screening of target populations for educational programs. The nurse can ask several questions of the learner, such as those focusing on previous attempts, curiosity, goal setting, self-care ability, stress factors, survival issues, and life situations. Motivational assessment of the learner needs to be thorough, and a number of variables need to be considered, as outlined in **Table 6–1**. This multidimensional guide allows for assessment of the level of learner motivation.

This assessment involves the judgment of the nurse because teaching–learning is a two-way process. In particular, motivation can be determined through both subjective and objective means. A subjective means of assessing level of motivation is through dialogue. By being present and using therapeutic communication skills, the nurse can obtain verbal information from the patient, such as "I really want to maintain my weight" or "I want to be able to take care of myself." Both of these statements indicate a desire with direction of movement toward a positive health outcome. Nonverbal cues also can indicate motivation, such as when the nurse sees the patient reading about healthy diets.

Measuring motivation is another aspect to be considered. Self-reports from the patient indicate the level of motivation from a subjective perspective. Behaviors that can be observed as the learner moves toward achieving preset realistic goals can serve as objective measures of motivation.

Table 6–1 Comprehensive Parameters for Motivational Assessment of the Learner

Cognitive Variables

• Capacity to learn
• Readiness to learn
  • Expressed self-determination
  • Constructive attitude
  • Expressed desire and curiosity
  • Willingness to contract for behavioral outcomes
• Facilitating beliefs

Affective Variables
• Expressions of constructive emotional state • Moderate level of anxiety
Physiological Variables
• Capacity to perform required behavior
Experiential Variables
• Previous successful experiences
Environmental Variables

• Appropriateness of physical environment
• Social support systems
  • Family
  • Group
  • Work
  • Community resources

Educator–Learner Relationship System
• Prediction of positive relationship

Motivational Strategies

Finding the spark that motivates a patient to change behavior is challenging to the nurse. The question remains, How can nurses stimulate seemingly unmotivated individuals or help motivated persons to remain engaged? As noted earlier, what motivates someone can be either internally or externally generated. Bandura (1986), for example, associates motivation with incentives. He notes, however, that intrinsic (internal) motivation, although highly appealing, is difficult to identify and maintain. Only rarely does motivation occur without extrinsic (external) influence. Green and Kreuter (1999) note that "strictly speaking we can appeal to people's motives, but we cannot motivate them" (p. 30).

Motivational strategies for the nurse as teacher are generated through the use of specific incentives. The critical question for the nurse to ask is, "Which specific behavior, under which circumstances, in which time frame, may be desired by this learner?" Strategizing begins with a systematic assessment of learner motivation, like that outlined in Table 6–1. When a variable is absent or reduced, an individual is likely to move away from a desired outcome. When considering strategies to improve learner motivation, Maslow's (1943) hierarchy of needs also can be taken into consideration. Also, an appeal can be made to the inner need for the learner to succeed, known as achievement motivation (Atkinson, 1964).

When teaching others, clearly communicating directions and expectations is critical. In addition, organizing material in a way that makes information meaningful to the learner, giving positive verbal feedback, and providing opportunities for success are motivational strategies proposed by Haggard (1989). Reducing or eliminating obstacles to be able to achieve goals is an important aspect of maintaining learner motivation.

Motivational interviewing (MI) is another motivational strategy nurses can use with patients (Droppa & Lee, 2014). It is a client-centered, directive counseling method in which clients' intrinsic motivation to change is enhanced by exploring and resolving their ambivalence toward behavior change (W. R. Miller & Rollnick, 2002). Dart (2011) states that "motivational interviewing fits perfectly into the nursing profession" (p. 23) and represents a caring, respectful tool with which to promote behavior change. MI, which is supported by evidence-based research, is an effective approach to health behavior change (Antiss, 2009).

Both as an assessment strategy and as an intervention, MI supports client self-esteem and self-efficacy through emphasis on the client's own reasons and values for change (W. R. Miller, 2004).

In this counseling approach, the nurse as teacher avoids telling a patient what he or she needs do. Rather, the interview is a collaborative venture between nurse and patient whereby a positive atmosphere is created through a partner-like relationship. The nurse guides rather than directs the patient. This approach stands in contrast to the classic relationship of expert provider and passive recipient (W. R. Miller, 2004) that is often seen in the traditional medical model. With MI, the learner has more autonomy and the nurse is less of an authority figure. **Table 6–2** includes a list of useful questions for nurses to ask patients that reinforce the guiding nature of this counseling approach.

Table 6–2 Top 10 Useful Questions in Motivational Interviewing

- Which changes would you most like to talk about?
- What have you noticed about . . . ?
- How important is it for you to change . . . ?
- How confident do you feel about changing . . . ?
- How do you see the benefits of . . . ?
- How do you see the drawbacks of . . . ?
- What will make the most sense to you . . . ?
- How might things be different if you . . . ?
- In what way . . . ?
- Where does that leave you now?

Reproduced from Rollnick, S., Butler, C. C., Kinnersley, P., Gregory, J., & Marsh, B. (2010). Competent novice: Motivational interviewing. *British Medical Journal, 340*, 1244.

Because change is ultimately the patient's responsibility, this approach encourages motivation for change to come from within, versus being imposed from the outside. Overall, MI is a form of patient empowerment, with the goal of helping patients gain control over the most important lifestyle management decisions affecting their well-being (Soderlund, Nilsen, & Kristensson, 2008). It consists of two phases: in the first phase, the nurse helps the patient enhance the internal motivation for change; in the second phase, commitment to change is strengthened (N. H. Miller, 2010; W. R. Miller & Rollick, 2002).

The five general principles of MI (Miller & Rollnick, 2002) are arranged to form the mnemonic **READS**, which helps nurses remember the key concepts of this approach. The following principles are not applied in a specific order, and all of the techniques should be used throughout the interview:

1. **R**oll with resistance
2. **E**xpress empathy
3. **A**void argumentation
4. **D**evelop discrepancy
5. **S**upport self-efficacy

Rolling with resistance refers to a strategy of acknowledging to the patient that ambivalence is natural, and, rather than oppose the resistance, the nurse "rolls" or flows with it. Resistance is expected and should not be viewed as a negative occurrence by the nurse. It can take several forms, including blaming, excusing, minimizing, arguing, challenging, interrupting, and ignoring. When the patient displays resistance, the nurse should actively involve the patient in the process of problem solving and attempt to explore the reasons behind the resistance.

Expressing empathy communicates to patients that they are understood and they are accepted as they are and where they are, which helps to facilitate change. As part of this technique, it is important that the nurse not judge, criticize, or blame the patient, but rather employ active and reflective listening skills throughout the interview to establish a therapeutic rapport with the patient.

Avoiding arguments decreases instances of confrontation, which usually make patients feel defensive. Defensiveness often leads to further resistance rather than instilling motivation for change. When the urge to argue arises, the nurse should instead change strategies to help the patient self-identify important issues and problem areas.

Developing discrepancy involves helping patients understand how their current behavior is inconsistent with their personal goals and/or values. This realization acts as a source of motivation for change by the patient. The objective is for patients, rather than the nurse, to identify why change is necessary after seeing the inconsistencies between their behaviors and their goals.

Supporting self-efficacy involves building the patient's confidence that change is possible. The nurse can do this by providing support and recognition for small steps the patient has made toward his or her goals, helping the patient set reachable goals, and demonstrating belief in the patient's ability to succeed.

In addition, the MI approach includes specific strategies that the nurse can use for building motivation to change in the early phases of treatment and continuing throughout the treatment. W. R. Miller and Rollnick (2002) suggest the mnemonic **OARS** to describe these strategies:

1. **O**pen-ended questioning
2. **A**ffirmations of the positives
3. **R**eflective listening
4. **S**ummaries of the interactions

Open-ended questions facilitate discussion between nurse and patient and encourage the patient to do most of the talking, particularly about the reasons why change is necessary or desirable. To encourage a patient-centered dialogue, the nurse should avoid closed-ended questions for which a simple "yes" or "no" answer could limit further discussion (Levensky, Forcehimes, O'Donohue, & Beitz, 2007).

Affirming the positives involves the nurse making statements that support and encourage the patient, particularly in areas where the patient may see only failure. Affirmations can take the form of complimenting efforts made by the patient, acknowledging small successes, or stating appreciation and understanding (Levensky et al., 2007). This approach promotes self-efficacy, builds rapport, and reinforces the efforts the patient is making toward change.

Reflective listening involves restating the patient's own comments in a concise manner, which demonstrates that the nurse understands what the patient is saying. The goal of this technique is to keep the conversation moving forward so the patient can see the need for change and begin to move in that direction.

Summarizing links and reinforces the information that has been discussed. It helps to build rapport with patients and demonstrates that the nurse has heard the patient. Summaries are important ways to emphasize significant parts of the discussion and to review the plan of action.

Table 6–3 provides examples of OARS questions and statements that the nurse educator might use in an MI session.

The majority of current evidence related to MI use comes primarily from studies with adults, but this technique may be particularly useful with the adolescent population

Table 6–3   Examples of OARS Questions and Statements

Open-Ended Questions
Could you share with me what has worked for you in the past when faced with a similar situation?
What are your current plans to accomplish your goal?
What do you believe you can accomplish at this time?
How do you believe it will feel to accomplish your goal?

Affirmation
You have worked very hard to get to this point.
You should be commended for all your positive efforts in meeting your goals.
It is obvious you have invested a lot into making these changes.
You have faced many challenges along the way, but you did not give up and now you are reaping the rewards.

Reflection
Previously you said you wanted to . . . but truly you are afraid of making the changes to reach that goal.
On the one hand, you are happy with your current lifestyle, but on the other hand, you realize that some changes need to be made.
You have worked on . . . in the past and have been unsuccessful and now you are afraid to try again because you could fail.
Making a change is never easy, and you realize that you will have to put forth quite a bit of effort to accomplish your goals.

Summary
Throughout our conversation you have said you would like to. . . and will accomplish this by . . . in this amount of time.
I would like to review what we talked about today.
To summarize what you just said. . .
We covered a lot today, and I would like to review what we discussed.

because its collaborative, nonconfrontational approach fits well with the developmental need for identity and autonomy that characterizes this stage of growth (Jackman, 2011).

Although study outcomes for MI are sometimes inconsistent, a number of reviews of multiple research studies have revealed statistically significant results for the use of MI in the healthcare arena (Hettema, Steele, & Miller, 2005; Lundahl, Kunz, Brownell, Tollefson, & Burke, 2010; Lundahl et al., 2013; Martins & McNeil, 2009; O'Halloran et al., 2014; Rubak, Sandbaek, Lauritzen, & Christensen, 2005; VanBuskirk & Wetherell, 2014).

Some interesting findings were that MI significantly increased patients' engagement in treatment and their intention to change, and, when MI was compared to other active treatments, the MI interventions took at least 100 fewer minutes of treatment on average yet produced equal effects (Lundahl et al., 2010). Also, another major study found as few as one MI session may be effective in enhancing readiness to change behaviors to reach health goals (VanBuskirk & Wetherell, 2014). These are particularly significant findings given that nurses have only a limited amount of time to spend with patients and need to be as efficient as possible in their interactions with patients.

MI can be a useful tool for helping nurses as teachers achieve success in one of their major roles—namely assisting patients to change negative health behaviors. Nurses need to exercise patience when learning MI, however, because this approach requires them to adjust to a new way of thinking. They need to be open minded and willing to let go of the tendency to give advice and offer expert opinions (Brobeck, Bergh, Odencrants, & Hildingh, 2011; Soderlund et al., 2008). With time and practice, nurses will also be able to let go of the "righting reflex," which is the tendency to identify a problem and solve it for the patient (Rollnick et al., 2010; Rollnick, Miller, & Butler, 2008). Instead, ideally they will use MI to empower and motivate patients to do the work themselves.

Selected Models and Theories

Compliance, adherence, and motivation are concepts relevant to health behaviors of the learner. Health behavior frameworks are blueprints and, as such, serve as tools for the nurse as teacher that can be used to maintain desired patient behaviors or promote changes (Syx, 2008). Thus, a familiarity with models and theories that describe, explain, or predict health behaviors can increase a nurse's range of health-promoting strategies when teaching patients. The principles of these models and theories can be used either to promote compliance with a health regimen or to facilitate motivation. This chapter presents an overview of the following models and theories: health belief model, health promotion model, self-efficacy theory, stages of change model, theory of reasoned action and theory of planned behavior, and therapeutic alliance model.

Health Belief Model

The original **health belief model** (HBM) was developed in the 1950s from a social psychology perspective to examine why people did not participate in health screening programs (Rosenstock, 1974). This model was modified by Becker, Drachman, and Kirscht (1974) to address compliance with therapeutic regimens.

The HBM explains and predicts health behaviors based on the clients' beliefs about the health problem and the health behavior. The model relies on the assumptions that clients are willing to participate and that they believe that health is highly valued (Becker, 1990). Both of these elements need to be present for the model to be useful in explaining health behavior. According to this model, it is possible to predict health behavior given three major interacting components: individual perceptions, modifying factors, and likelihood of action. **Figure 6–1** shows the direction and flow of these components, each of which is further divided into subcomponents:

1. *Individual perceptions*: These include the subcomponents of perceived susceptibility or perceived severity of a specific disease.
2. *Modifying factors*: These include the demographic variables, sociopsychological variables, and structural variables. These variables, in conjunction with cues to action, influence the subcomponent of perceived threat of the specific disease.
3. *Likelihood of action*: This includes the subcomponents of perceived benefits of preventive action minus perceived barriers to preventive action.

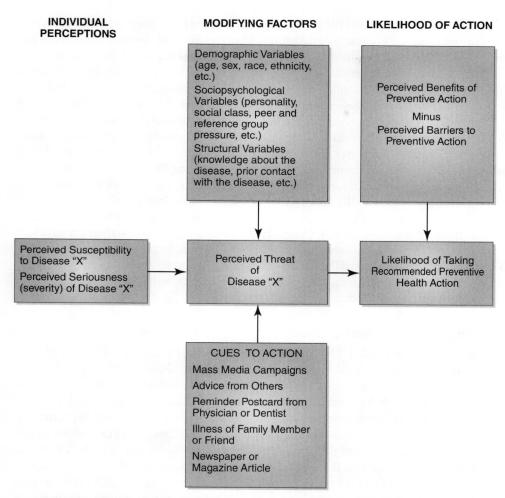

INDIVIDUAL
PERCEPTIONS

MODIFYING FACTORS

LIKELIHOOD OF ACTION

Demographic Variables
(age, sex, race, ethnicity,
etc.)
Sociopsychological
Variables (personality,
social class, peer and
reference group
pressure, etc.)
Structural Variables
(knowledge about the
disease, prior contact
with the disease, etc.)

Perceived Benefits of
Preventive Action

Minus

Perceived Barriers to
Preventive Action

Perceived Susceptibility
to Disease "X"

Perceived Seriousness
(severity) of Disease "X"

Perceived Threat
of
Disease "X"

Likelihood of Taking
Recommended Preventive
Health Action

CUES TO ACTION

Mass Media Campaigns

Advice from Others

Reminder Postcard from
Physician or Dentist

Illness of Family Member
or Friend

Newspaper or
Magazine Article

Figure 6–1 Health belief model used as a predictor of preventive health behavior

All of these components interact to predict the likelihood that the client will take recommended preventive health action.

The HBM has been the predominant model since the 1970s for explaining differences in preventive health behaviors as well as use of preventive health services (Langlie, 1977). It stands out as one of the most frequently cited and researched psychosocial models to determine health-related screening behavior (Wong et al., 2013). It has been used widely in health behavior research across disciplines, such as medicine, psychology, social behavior, and gerontology, to predict preventive health behavior and to explain sick-role behavior in acute and chronic illnesses.

Over time, research studies have supported the value of the HBM. For instance, Jachna and Forbes-Thompson (2005) studied health beliefs of clients in an assisted living facility and found that healthcare providers can influence health beliefs relative to osteoporosis, which has implications for gerontological nursing education. In China, Wang et al. (2013) successfully used a nursing intervention based on the HBM to enhance patients' health beliefs and self-efficacy toward the disease management of COPD. Turner, Kivlahan, Sloan, and Haselkorn (2007) found that this model was effective in predicting adherence to a medication regimen among patients with multiple sclerosis. Saunders, Frederick, Silverman, and Papesh (2013) determined the HBM provided an appropriate framework for examining hearing behaviors. Johnson, Mues, Mayne, and Kiblawi (2008) emphasized the need for culturally relevant screening strategies as a response to the significance of sociocultural factors influencing health-related beliefs and use of healthcare services. Findings from studies such as these, as well as from additional studies (Adams, Hall, & Fulghum, 2014; Baghianimoghadam et al., 2013), can help guide educational programs specific to high-risk populations. In a historical 10-year review of the health belief model literature, Janz and Becker (1984) found that the model strongly predicted health behaviors, with perceived barriers being the most influential factor.

Health Promotion Model (Revised)

The **health promotion model** (HPM), originally developed by Pender in 1987 and revised in 1996, has been primarily used in the discipline of nursing (Pender, 1996). The purpose of the model is to assist nurses in understanding the major determinants of health behaviors as a basis for behavioral counseling to promote healthy lifestyles (Pender, 2011). The HPM describes major components and variables that influence health-promoting behaviors (**Figure 6–2**). This model helps to provide an understanding of whether or not people choose to engage in health-promoting behaviors (Pender, Murdaugh, & Parsons, 2002) and strongly supports the partner relationship between healthcare provider and patient (Stewart, 2012). Its emphasis on helping people reach their health potential and increase their level of well-being using approach behaviors in achieving health rather than avoidance of disease behaviors distinguishes this model as focusing on health promotion rather than disease prevention.

The sequence of major components and variables is outlined as follows:

1. Individual characteristics and experiences, which consist of two variables—prior related behavior and personal factors.
2. Behavior-specific cognitions and affect, which consist of perceived benefits of action, perceived barriers to action, perceived self-efficacy, activity-related affect, interpersonal influences, and situational influences.
3. Behavioral outcome, which consists of health-promoting behavior.

The HBM and the HPM share several similarities when comparing Figures 6–1 and 6–2. Both models describe the use of factors or components that influence perceptions, but the HBM targets the likelihood of engaging in preventive health behaviors, whereas the revised HPM targets the likelihood of engaging in health promotion

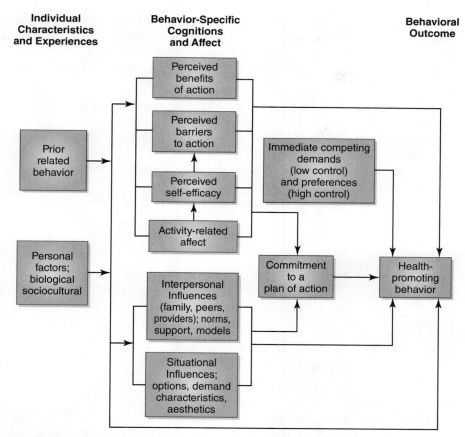

Individual Characteristics and Experiences

Behavior-Specific Cognitions and Affect

Behavioral Outcome

Perceived benefits of action

Perceived barriers to action

Perceived self-efficacy

Activity-related affect

Prior related behavior

Personal factors; biological sociocultural

Interpersonal Influences (family, peers, providers); norms, support, models

Situational Influences; options, demand characteristics, aesthetics

Immediate competing demands (low control) and preferences (high control)

Commitment to a plan of action

Health-promoting behavior

Figure 6–2 Revised health promotion model

PENDER, NOLA J., HEALTH PROMOTION IN NURSING PRACTICE, 3rd Edition, © 1996. Reprinted by permission of Pearson Education, Inc., New York, New York.

activities that lead to positive health outcomes. Support for the HPM has been demonstrated by many research studies on a number of different population groups (Buijs, Ross-Kerr, Cousins, & Wilson, 2003; Hjelm, Mufunda, Nambozi, & Kemp, 2003; Ho, Berggren, & Dahlborg-Lyckhage, 2010; Mohamadian et al., 2011; Rothman, Lourie, Brian, & Foley, 2005; Srof & Velsor-Friedrich, 2006). One conclusion that is supported by the HPM literature is that perceived self-efficacy is an important determinant of participation in health-promoting behavior and achievement of an improved health-related quality of life (Ho et al., 2010; Mohamadian et al., 2011; Srof & Velsor-Friedrich, 2006).

Self-Efficacy Theory

Self-efficacy theory is based on a person's expectations relative to a specific course of action (Bandura, 1977a, 1977b, 1986, 1997). It is a predictive theory in the sense that it deals with the belief that one is competent and capable of accomplishing a specific behavior. **Figure 6–3** shows an adaptation of Bandura's model extended to include expected outcomes based on a person's perceptions of self-efficacy.

According to Bandura (1986, 1997), self-efficacy is derived from four principal sources of information:

1. *Performance accomplishments* evidenced in self-mastery of similarly expected behaviors
2. *Vicarious experiences,* such as observing successful expected behavior through the modeling of others
3. *Verbal persuasion* by others who present realistic beliefs that the individual is capable of the expected behavior
4. *Emotional arousal* through self-judgment of physiological states of distress

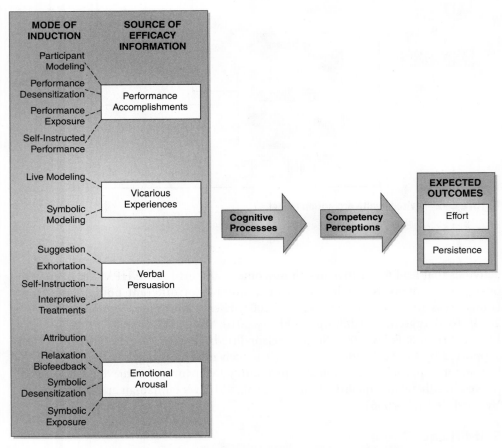

Figure 6–3 Determinants of expected outcomes using self-efficacy perceptions

Reproduced from Albert Bandura, *Social learning theory,* © 1977, p. 80. Reprinted by permission of Prentice Hall, Upper Saddle River, NJ.

Certain modes induce (influence) someone to take a specific course of action that leads to expected outcomes. Bandura (1986, 1997) notes that the most influential source of efficacy information is previous performance accomplishments.

Self-efficacy has proved useful in predicting participation in healthy behaviors by employees in a physical activity program (Kaewthummanukul & Brown, 2006) and by women in cervical cancer screening (Tung, Lu, & Cook, 2010). Self-efficacy also has been linked with positive self-care behaviors in older women (Callaghan, 2005), memory improvement in older adults (West, Bagwell, & Dark-Freudeman, 2008), self-management of hypertension and diabetes mellitus (Jang & Yoo, 2012), healthy eating in university students and staff (Strachan & Brawley, 2009), and patient recovery for postacute injury (Connolly, Aitkin, & Tower, 2014).

The use of self-efficacy theory by the nurse is particularly relevant in developing educational programs. The behavior-specific predictions of this theory can be used for understanding the likelihood of individuals participating in existing or future educational programs. Educational strategies such as modeling, demonstration, and verbal reinforcement parallel modes of self-efficacy induction.

Stages of Change Model

Another model that sheds light on the phenomenon of health behaviors of the learner is the **stages of change model**, also known as the trans-theoretical model (TTM) of behavioral change (Prochaska & DiClemente, 1982). This model (**Table 6–4**) was developed around addictive and problem behaviors. Prochaska (1996) notes that it encompasses six distinct time-related stages of change:

1. *Precontemplation*: Individuals have no current intention of changing. Strategies involve simple observations, confrontation, or consciousness raising.
2. *Contemplation*: Individuals accept or realize that they have a problem and begin to think seriously about changing it. Strategies involve increased consciousness raising.
3. *Preparation*: Individuals are planning to take action within the time frame of 1 month. Strategies include a firm and detailed plan for action.
4. *Action*: There is overt/visible modification of behavior. This is the busiest stage, and strategies include commitment to the change, self-reward, countering (substitute behaviors), creating a friendly environment, and supportive relationships.

Table 6–4 Six Stages of Change

- Precontemplation
- Contemplation
- Preparation
- Action
- Maintenance
- Termination

5. *Maintenance*: Maintenance is a difficult stage to achieve and may last 6 months to a lifetime. There are common challenges to this stage, including overconfidence, daily temptation, and relapse self-blame. The strategies in this stage are the same for the action stage.
6. *Termination*: This stage occurs when the problem no longer presents any temptation. However, some experts note that termination does not occur; instead, maintenance simply becomes less vigilant.

The extent to which people are motivated and ready to change is seen as an important element of concept in this model. It is useful in health care to stage the client's intentions and behaviors for change as well as to determine those strategies that will enable completion of the specific stage. More recent use of the stages of change model in health research has focused on its value in health promotion and the processes by which people decide to change (or not to change) behaviors.

The stages of change model has been used to investigate health behaviors, such as using sun protection (Prentice-Dunn, McMath & Cramer, 2009), managing weight loss (Mastellos, Gunn, Felix, Car, & Majeed, 2014), and exercising (Lowther, Mutrie, & Scott, 2007). Also, it has been used as a method of outcome evaluation in continuing education for nurses (Randhawa, 2012). This popular model can be used with children and adults, which has implications for a variety of settings.

Theory of Reasoned Action and Theory of Planned Behavior

The **theory of reasoned action** (TRA) is concerned with predicting and understanding any form of human behavior within a social context (Ajzen & Fishbein, 1980). It is based on the idea that humans behave in a rational way that is consistent with their beliefs (Fishbein, 2008). This theory suggests that a person's behavior can be predicted by examining the individual's attitudes about the behavior as well as the individual's beliefs about how others might respond to the behavior. For example, when using this theory to predict how a client might respond to a weight-reduction plan, it would be vital not only to consider the client's beliefs about food and exercise but also to examine what the client thinks about how the people around him would view his attempts to lose weight. It is important to note that reasoned action in this theory is not emotion free but rather based on beliefs that are influenced by emotion and mood (Fishbein, 2008). According to this theory (**Figure 6–4**), specific behavior is determined by (1) beliefs, attitude toward the behavior, and intention; and (2) motivation to comply with influential persons (known as referents), subjective norms, and intention. The person's intention to perform can be measured by relative weights of attitude and subjective norms.

As the TRA began to be applied in the social sciences, Ajzen and other researchers realized the theory had several limitations (Godin & Kok, 1996). One of the strongest limitations was use of the theory with people who felt they had little power over their behaviors. To remedy this, in 1985, Ajzen proposed a new model—the **theory of planned behavior** (TPB). The TPB added a third element to the TRA model—the concept of perceived behavioral control (Ajzen, 1991). See **Figure 6–5**.

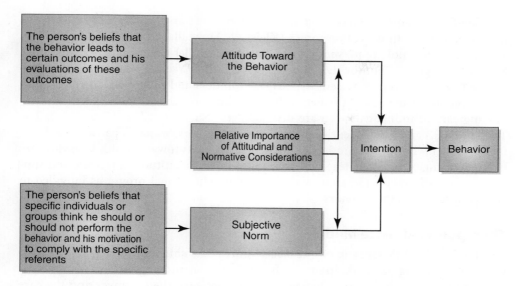

Note: Arrows indicate the direction of influence.

Figure 6–4   Theory of reasoned action: Factors determining a person's behavior

Reproduced from Ajzen, I., & Fishbein, M. *Understanding attitudes and predicting social behavior*, © 1980, p. 8. Reprinted by permission of Prentice Hall, Upper Saddle River, NJ.

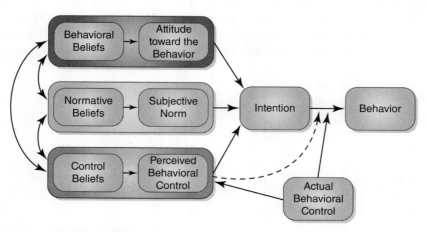

Figure 6–5   Theory of planned behavior

Reprinted from *Organizational Behavior and Human Decision Processes, 50*(2), Ajzen, I., The theory of planned behavior, p. 182, Copyright 1991, with permission from Elsevier.

The TRA and the TPB have been used to determine nurses' attitudes toward teaching particular health education topics (Kleier, 2004; Mullan & Westwood, 2010), as a framework in smoking prevention and intention studies (Hanson, 2005; McGahee, Kemp, & Tingen, 2000), for designing interventions to reduce heterosexual risk behavior (Tyson, Covey, & Rosenthal, 2014), to understand intentions to receive human papillomavirus vaccine (Fisher, Kohut, Salisbury, & Salvadori, 2013), and to study nursing care of individuals who are drug addicts (Natan, Beyil, & Neta, 2009). The TRA and TPB are useful theories in predicting behaviors, which is particularly helpful for nurses who want to understand whether attitudes toward health behaviors are likely to change. Nurses as teachers need to take beliefs, attitudinal factors, and subjective norms into consideration when designing educational programs intended to change specific health behaviors.

Therapeutic Alliance Model

Barofsky's (1978) **therapeutic alliance model** addresses a shift in power from the provider to a learning partnership in which collaboration and negotiation with the patient are keys. A therapeutic alliance is formed between the caregiver and the care receiver in which the participants are viewed as having equal power. The patient is viewed as active and responsible, with an outcome expectation of self-care. The shift toward self-determination and control over one's own life is fundamental to this model.

The therapeutic alliance model uses the components of compliance, adherence, and alliance (**Figure 6–6**). According to Barofsky (1978), change is needed in the way nurses and patients interact. The nurse–patient relationship must change from coercion in compliance and from conforming in adherence to collaboration in alliance. The power in the relationship between the participants is equalized by alliance. The role of the patient is neither passive nor rebellious, but rather active and responsible. The expected outcome is neither compliant dependence nor adherent

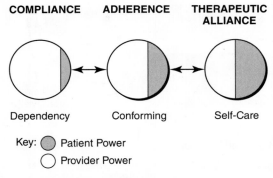

Figure 6–6 Continuum of the therapeutic alliance model

conformity, but responsible self-care as a result of a coalliance between the nurse and the patient.

This interpersonal model is appropriate for teaching because it shifts the focus from the patient as a passive-dependent learner to the patient as an active learner. It serves as a guide to refocus education efforts on collaboration rather than on compliance. The nurse as teacher and the patient as learner form an alliance with the goal of self-care. It must be noted that the technique of MI, as presented earlier, may be combined with the therapeutic alliance model. Duran (2003) points out that successful MI takes place in an atmosphere in which the client feels understood and respected and is collaborative in nature, with the highest priority placed on the client's autonomy and freedom of choice.

The significance of the therapeutic alliance between caregiver and patient as it relates to adherence has been studied in patients with mental health issues (Byrne & Deane, 2011; Jaeger, Weißaupt, Flammer, & Steinert, 2014; Sylvia et al., 2013). Del Re, Flückiger, Horvath, Symonds, and Wampold (2012) found that therapist behavior in the alliance partnership is more important than patient behavior in achieving the goal of improved outcomes. The therapeutic alliance also has been studied relative to weight gain in patients with anorexia nervosa (Bourion-Bedes et al., 2013; Brown, Mountford, & Waller, 2013), although its impact has been mixed.

Summary

This chapter includes a discussion of the concepts of compliance, adherence, and motivation; assessment of the level of learner motivation; identification of incentives and obstacles that affect motivation; and discussion of axioms of motivation relevant to learning. Strategies that facilitate health behaviors of the learner are outlined, and selected theories and models that influence compliance and motivation are presented. When people are motivated and know that they can make a difference in their own lives, the foundation is set for change in health behaviors.

Review Questions

1. How are the terms *compliance*, *adherence*, and *motivation* defined?
2. How do the terms defined in question 1 relate to one another?
3. What are the three major motivational factors?
4. Which axioms (premises) are involved in promoting motivation of the learner?
5. What are the six parameters for a comprehensive motivational assessment of the learner?
6. What are the five general principles of MI?
7. What are the basic concepts particular to each model or theory?

Case Study

"Keeping our employees healthy is not only the right thing to do, it is good for the bottom line." With this statement and a directive from the chief nursing officer, Marie De-Santis, RN, PhD, the staff in the Office of Human Resources at Longwood Skilled Nursing Facility developed a "Let's Get Healthy" initiative for its 500 employees. Weight Watchers, a smoking cessation program, and yoga classes were brought on site and offered free of charge to all employees. Nicotine patches were offered at 50% of cost, and gym memberships were provided at a significant reduction in price. The cafeteria began offering healthy, low-calorie meals, and a walking club was started to support staff who chose to exercise before and after work or during lunch hours. Staff who were willing to submit an individual health plan and agreed to participate in one or more of the facility's available health programs were offered a 10% discount on their health premiums.

One year after the start of Let's Get Healthy, the initiative is in trouble. Although it initially met with a great deal of enthusiasm, staff compliance has declined. Attendance at Weight Watchers and smoking cessation classes is episodic, and yoga classes were canceled because of lack of interest. Anecdotal information suggests that although the facility has renewed gym memberships for approximately 20% of the staff, few are actually using them on a regular basis. Convinced that Let's Get Healthy is a good idea, Longwood has hired a health educator to evaluate the program and make recommendations for improvement.

1. Using one of the identified models and theories of adherence (health belief model, revised health promotion model, self-efficacy theory, stages of change model, theory of reasoned action and theory of planned behavior, or therapeutic alliance model), provide a possible explanation for why the staff members at Longwood Skilled Nursing Facility are not participating in the Let's Get Healthy campaign.
2. Which motivational strategies did the human resources staff use in Let's Get Healthy? Why do you think these strategies did not work?
3. Do you think that if a health education campaign were offered in conjunction with the Let's Get Healthy program, the results would have been different?

References

Adams, A., Hall, M., & Fulghum. J. (2014). Utilizing the health belief model to assess vaccine acceptance of patients on hemodialysis. *Nephrology Nursing Journal, 41*(4), 393–406.

Adherence (Def. 1, 2). (2015a). *Merriam-Webster Dictionary.* Retrieved from http://www.merriamwebster.com/dictionary/adherence

Ajzen, I. (1991). The theory of planned behavior. *Organizational Behavior and Human Decision Processes, 50*(2), 179–211.

Ajzen, I., & Fishbein, M. (1980). *Understanding attitudes and predicting social behavior.* Englewood Cliffs, NJ: Prentice Hall.

Antiss, T. (2009). Motivational interviewing in primary care. *Journal of Clinical Psychology in Medical Settings, 16,* 87–93.

Atkinson, J. W. (1964). *An introduction to motivation*. Princeton, NJ: Van Nostrand.

Baghianimoghadam, M. H., Shogafard, G., Sanati, H. R., Baghianimoghadam, B., Mazloomy, S. S., & Askarshahi, M. (2013). Application of the health belief model in promotion of self-care in heart failure patients. *Acta Medica Iranica, 51*(1), 52–58.

Bandura, A. (1977a). Self-efficacy: Toward a unifying theory of behavioral change. *Psychological Review, 84*(2), 191–215.

Bandura, A. (1977b). *Social learning theory*. Englewood Cliffs, NJ: Prentice Hall.

Bandura, A. (1986). *Social foundations of thought and action: A social cognitive theory*. Englewood Cliffs, NJ: Prentice Hall.

Bandura, A. (1997). *Self-efficacy: The exercise of control*. New York, NY: W. H. Freeman.

Barofsky, I. (1978). Compliance, adherence and the therapeutic alliance: Steps in the development of self-care. *Social Science & Medicine, 12*(5), 369–376.

Becker, M. (1990). Theoretical models of adherence and strategies for improving adherence. In S. A. Shumaker, E. B. Schron, & J. K. Ockene (Eds.), *The handbook of human health behavior* (pp. 5–43). New York, NY: Springer.

Becker, M. W., Drachman, R. H., & Kirscht, J. P. (1974). A new approach to explaining sickrole behavior in low-income populations. *American Journal of Public Health, 64*(3), 205–216.

Bourion-Bedes, S., Baumann, C., Kermarrec, S., Ligier, F., Feillet, F., Bonnemains, C., . . . Kabuth, B. (2013). Prognostic value of early therapeutic alliance in weight recovery: A prospective cohort of 108 adolescents with anorexia nervosa. *Journal of Adolescent Health, 52*, 344–350.

Brobeck, E., Bergh, H., Odencrants, S., & Hildingh, C. (2011). Primary healthcare nurses' experiences with motivational interviewing in health promotion practice. *Journal of Clinical Nursing, 20*, 3322–3330.

Brown, A., Mountford, V., & Waller, G. (2013). Therapeutic alliance and weight gain during cognitive behavioural therapy for anorexia nervosa. *Behaviour Research and Therapy, 51*, 216–220.

Buijs, R., Ross-Kerr, J., Cousins, S., & Wilson, D. (2003). Promoting participation: Evaluation of a health promotion program for low income seniors. *Journal of Community Health Nursing, 20*(2), 93–107.

Byrne, M. K., & Deane, F. P. (2011). Enhancing patient adherence: Outcomes of medication alliance training on therapeutic alliance, insight, adherence, and psychopathology with mental health patients. *International Journal of Mental Health Nursing, 20*, 284–295.

Callaghan, D. (2005). Health behaviors, self-efficacy, self-care and basic conditioning factors in older adults. *Journal of Community Health Nursing, 22*(3), 169–178.

Compliance (Def. 1a, 2). (2015b). *Merriam-Webster Dictionary*. Retrieved from http://www.merriam-webster.com/dictionary/compliance

Connolly, F. R., Aitkin, L. M., & Tower, M. (2014). An integrative review of self-efficacy and patient recovery post acute injury. *Journal of Advanced Nursing, 70*(4), 714–728.

Dart, M. (2011). *Motivational interviewing in nursing practice: Empowering the patient*. Sudbury, MA: Jones & Bartlett Learning.

Del Re, A. C., Flückiger, C., Horvath, A. O., Symonds, D., & Wampold, B. E. (2012). Therapist effects in the therapeutic alliance–outcome relationship: A restricted-maximum likelihood meta-analysis. *Clinical Psychology Review, 32*, 642–649.

DiMatteo, M. R. (2004). Social support and patient adherence to medical treatment: A meta-analysis. *Health Psychology, 23*(2), 207–218.

Droppa, M., & Lee, H. (2014). Motivational interviewing: A journey to improve health. *Nursing, 44*(3), 40–46.

Duran, L. S. (2003). Motivating health: Strategies for the nurse practitioner. *Journal of the American Academy of Nurse Practitioners, 15*(5), 200–203.

Epstein, F. R., Kale, P. P., & Weisshaar, D. M. (2014). Association between the chance locus of control belief with self-reported occasional nonadherence after heart transplantation: A pilot study. *Transplantation, 98*(1), 4.

Fishbein, M. (2008). A reasoned action approach to health promotion. *Medical Decision Making, 28*, 834–844.

Fisher, W. A., Kohut, T., Salisbury, C. M., & Salvadori, M. I. (2013). Understanding human papillomavirus vaccination intentions: Comparative utility of the theory of reasoned action and the theory of planned behavior in vaccine target age women and men. *Journal of Sexual Medicine, 10*, 2455–2464.

Gardner, C. L. (2015). Adherence: A concept analysis. *International Journal of Nursing Knowledge, 26* (2), 96–101.

Glynn, S. M., Aultman, L. P., & Owens, A. M. (2005). Motivation to learn in general education programs. *The Journal of General Education, 54*(2), 150–170.

Godin, G., & Kok, G. (1996). The theory of planned behavior: A review of its applications to health-related behaviors. *American Journal of Health Promotion, 11*(2), 87–98.

Green, L. W., & Kreuter, M. W. (1999). *Health promotion planning: An educational and ecological approach* (3rd ed.). Mountain View, CA: Mayfield.

Haggard, A. (1989). *Handbook of patient education.* Rockville, MD: Aspen.

Hanson, M. S. (2005). An examination of ethnic differences in cigarette smoking intention among female teenagers. *Journal of the American Academy of Nurse Practitioners, 17*(4), 149–155.

Helme, D. W., & Harrington, N. G. (2004). Patient accounts for noncompliance with diabetes self-care regimens and physician compliance-gaining response. *Patient Education and Counseling, 55*, 281–292.

Hernshaw, H., & Lidenmeyer, A. (2006).What do we mean by adherence to treatment and advice for living with diabetes? A review of the literature on definitions and measurements. *Diabetic Medicine, 23*(7), 720–728.

Hettema, J., Steele, J., & Miller, W. R. (2005). Motivational interviewing. *Annual Review of Clinical Psychology, 1*, 91–111.

Hjelm, K., Mufunda, E., Nambozi, G., & Kemp, J. (2003). Preparing nurses to face the pandemic of diabetes mellitus: A literature review. *Journal of Advanced Nursing, 41*(5), 424–434.

Ho, A. Y., Berggren, B., & Dahlborg-Lyckhage, E. (2010). Diabetes empowerment related to Pender's health promotion model: A meta-synthesis. *Nursing & Health Sciences, 12*, 259–267.

Jachna, C. M., & Forbes-Thompson, S. (2005). Osteoporosis: Health beliefs and barriers to treatment in an assisted living facility. *Journal of Gerontological Nursing, 31*(1), 24–30.

Jackman, K. (2011). Motivational interviewing with adolescents: An advanced practice nursing intervention for psychiatric settings. *Journal of Child and Adolescent Psychiatric Nursing, 25*, 4–8.

Jaeger, S., Weißaupt, S., Flammer, E., & Steinert, T. (2014). Control beliefs, therapeutic relationship, and adherence in schizophrenia outpatients: A cross-sectional study. *American Journal of Health Behavior, 38*(6), 914–923.

Jang, Y., & Yoo, H. (2012). Self-management programs based on the social cognitive theory for Koreans with chronic disease: A systematic review. *Contemporary Nurse, 40*(2), 147–159.

Janz, N. K., & Becker, M. H. (1984). The health belief model: A decade later. *Health Education Quarterly, 11*(1), 1–47.

Johnson, C. E., Mues, K. E., Mayne, S. L., & Kiblawi, A. N. (2008). Cervical cancer screening among immigrants and ethnic minorities: A systematic review using the health belief model. *Journal of Lower Genital Tract Disease, 12*(3), 232–241.

Kaewthummanukul, T., & Brown, K. C. (2006). Determinants of employee participation in physical activity: A review of the literature. *American Association of Occupational Health Nurses Journal, 54*(6), 249–261.

Kessels, R. P. C. (2003). Patients' memory for medical information. *Journal of the Royal Society of Medicine, 96*, 219–222.

Kleier, J. A. (2004). Nurse practitioners' behavior regarding testicular self-examination. *Journal of the American Academy of Nurse Practitioners, 16*(5), 206–208, 210, 212.

Kort, M. (1987). Motivation: The challenge for today's health promoter. *Canadian Nurse, 83*(9), 16–18.

Langlie, J. K. (1977). Social networks, health beliefs, and preventive health behavior. *Journal of Health and Social Behavior, 18*, 244–260.

Levensky, E. R., Forcehimes, A., O'Donohue, W. T., & Beitz, K. (2007). Motivational interviewing: An evidence based approach to counseling helps patients follow treatment recommendations. *American Journal of Nursing, 107*(10), 50–58.

Ley, P. (1979). Memory for medical information. *British Journal of Social and Clinical Psychology, 18*, 245–255.

Lowther, M., Mutrie, N., & Scott, E. M. (2007). Identifying key processes of exercise behavior change associated with movement through the stages of exercise behaviour change. *Journal of Health Psychology, 12*, 261–271.

Lundahl, B. W., Kunz, C., Brownell, C., Tollefson, D., & Burke, B. L. (2010). A meta-analysis of motivational interviewing: Twenty-five years of empirical studies. *Research on Social Work Practice, 20*(2), 137–160.

Lundahl, B., Moleni, T., Burke, T., Butters, R., Tollefson, D., Butler, C., & Rollnick, S. (2013). Motivational interviewing in medical care settings: A systematic review and meta-analysis of randomized controlled trials. *Patient Education and Counseling, 93*, 157–168.

Martins, R. K., & McNeil, D. W. (2009). Review of motivational interviewing in promoting health behaviors. *Clinical Psychology Review, 29*, 283–293.

Maslow, A. H. (1943). A theory of human motivation. *Psychological Review, 50*(4), 371–396.

Mastellos, N., Gunn, L. H., Felix, L. M., Car, J., & Majeed, A. (2014). Transtheoretical model stages of change for dietary and physical exercise modification in weight loss management for overweight and obese adults (Review). *Cochrane Database of Systematic Reviews, 2*, 1–87, Art. No.: CD008066. doi: 10.1002/14651858.CD008066.pub3

McGahee, T. W., Kemp, V., & Tingen, M. (2000). A theoretical model for smoking prevention studies in preteen children. *Pediatric Nursing, 26*(2), 135–138, 141.

Mihalko, S. L., Brenes, G. A., Farmer, D. F., Katula, J. A., Balkrishnan, R., & Bowen, D. J. (2004). Challenges and innovations in enhancing adherence. *Controlled Clinical Trials, 25*, 447–457.

Miller, N. H. (2010). Motivational interviewing as a prelude to coaching in healthcare settings. *Journal of Cardiovascular Nursing, 25*(3), 247–251.

Miller, W. R. (2004). Motivational interviewing in service to health promotion. *American Journal of Health Promotion, 18*, A1–A10.

Miller, W. R., & Rollnick, S. (2002). *Motivational interviewing: Preparing people for change* (2nd ed.). New York, NY: Guilford Press.

Mohamadian, H., Eftekhar, H., Rahimi, A., Mohamad, H. T., Shojaiezade, D., & Montazeri, A. (2011). Predicting health-related quality of life by using a health promotion model among Iranian adolescent girls: A structural equation modeling approach. *Nursing & Health Sciences, 13*, 141–148.

Morowatisharifabad, M. A., Mahmoodabad, S. S., Baghianimoghadam, M. H., & Tonekaboni, N. R. (2010). Relationships between locus of control and adherence to diabetes regimen in a sample of Iranians. *International Journal of Diabetes in Developing Countries, 30*(1), 27–32.

Mullan, B., & Westwood, J. (2010). The application of the theory of reasoned action to school nurses' behaviour. *Journal of Research in Nursing, 15*(3), 261–271.

Natan, M. B., Beyil, V., & Neta, O. (2009). Nurses' perception of the quality of care they provide to hospitalized drug addicts: Testing the theory of reasoned action. *International Journal of Nursing Practice, 15*, 566–573.

O'Halloran, P. D., Blackstock, F., Shields, N., Holland, A., Iles, R. Kingsley, M., . . . Taylor, N. F. (2014). Motivational interviewing to increase physical activity in people with chronic health conditions: A systematic review and meta-analysis. *Clinical Rehabilitation, 28*(12), 1160–1171.

O'Hea, E. L., Moon, S., Grothe, K. B., Boudreaux, E., Bodenlos, J. S., Wallston, K., & Brantley, P. J. (2009). The interaction of locus of control, self-efficacy, and outcome expectancy in relation to HbA1c in medically underserved individuals with type 2 diabetes. *Journal of Behavioral Medicine, 32*, 106–117.

Pender, N. (1996). *Health promotion in nursing practice* (3rd ed.). Upper Saddle River, NJ: Pearson Education.

Pender, N. J. (2011). *The health promotion model manual.* Retrieved from http://deepblue.lib.umich.edu/handle/2027.42/85350

Pender, N. J., Murdaugh, C. L., & Parsons, M. A. (2002). *Health promotion in nursing practice* (4th ed.). Upper Saddle River, NJ: Prentice Hall.

Peplau, H. E. (1979). *The psychotherapy of Hildegard E. Peplau.* Madison, WI: Atwood.

Pignone, M., & Salazar, R. (2014). Disease prevention and health promotion. In S. J. McFee & M. A. Papadakis (Eds.), *Lange 2014 current medical diagnosis & treatment* (53rd ed., pp. 1–2). New York, NY: McGraw-Hill Medical.

Politi, M. C., Han, K. J., & Col, N. F. (2007). Communicating the uncertainty of harms and benefits of medical interventions. *Medical Decision Making, 27*, 681–695.

Porto, T. M., Machado, D. C., Martins, R. O., Galato, D., & Piovezan, A. P. (2014). Locus of pain control associated with medication adherence behaviors among patients after an orthopedic procedure. *Patient Preference and Adherence, 8*, 991–995.

Prentice-Dunn, S., McMath, B. F., & Cramer, R. J. (2009). Protection motivation theory and change in sun protective behavior. *Journal of Health Behavior, 14*, 297–305.

Prochaska, J. O. (1996, September). *Just do it isn't enough: Change comes in stages.* Tufts University Special Report Diet & Nutrition Letter.

Prochaska, J. O., & DiClemente, C. C. (1982). Trans theoretical therapy: Towards a more integrative model of change. *Psychotherapy: Theory, Research & Practice, 19*(3), 276–288.

Randhawa, S. (2012). Using the transtheoretical model for outcome evaluation in continuing education. *Journal of Continuing Education in Nursing, 43*(4), 148–149.

Redman, B. K. (2001). *The practice of patient education* (9th ed.). St. Louis, MO: Mosby.

Redman, B. K. (2007). *The practice of patient education: A case study approach* (10th ed.). St. Louis, MO: Mosby.

Resnik, D. B. (2005). The patient's duty to adhere to prescribed treatment: An ethical analysis. *Journal of Medicine and Philosophy, 30*, 167–188.

Robinson, J. H., Callister, L. C., Berry, J. A., & Dearing, K. A. (2008). Patient-centered care and adherence: Definitions and applications to improve outcomes. *Journal of the American Academy of Nurse Practitioners, 20*, 600–607.

Rollnick, S., Butler, C. C., Kinnersley, P., Gregory, J., & Marsh, B. (2010). Competent novice: Motivational interviewing. *British Medical Journal, 340*, 1242–1245.

Rollnick, S., Miller, W. R., & Butler, C. C. (2008). *Motivational interviewing in health care: Helping patients change behavior.* New York, NY: Guilford Press.

Rosenstock, I. M. (1974). Historical origins of the health belief model. In M. H. Becker (Ed.), *The health belief model and personal health behavior* (p. 328). Thorofare, NJ: Slack.

Rosner, F. (2006). Patient noncompliance: Causes and symptoms. *Mount Sinai Journal of Medicine, 73*, 553–559.

Rosno, E. A., Steele, R. G., Johnson, C. A., & Aylward, B. S. (2008). Parental locus of control: Associations to adherence and outcomes in treatment of pediatric overweight. *Children's Health Care, 37*(2), 126–144.

Rothman, N. L., Lourie, R. J., Brian, D., & Foley, M. (2005).Temple health connection: A successful collaborative model of community-based primary health care. *Journal of Cultural Diversity, 12*(4), 145–151.

Rotter, J. B. (1954). *Social learning theory and clinical psychology.* Englewood Cliffs, NJ: Prentice Hall.

Rubak, S., Sandbaek, A., Lauritzen, T., & Christensen, B. (2005). Motivational interviewing: A systematic review and meta-analysis. *British Journal of General Practice, 55*, 305–312.

Sabaté, E. (Ed.). (2003). *Adherence to long-term therapies: Evidence for action.* Retrieved from http://www.who.int/chp/knowledge/publications/adherence_report/en/

Sackett, D. L., & Hayes, R. B. (1976). *Compliance with therapeutic regimens.* Baltimore, MD: The Johns Hopkins University Press.

Saunders, G. H., Frederick, M. T., Silverman, S., & Papesh, M. (2013). Application of the health belief model: Development of the hearing beliefs questionnaire (HBQ) and its associations with hearing health behaviors. *International Journal of Audiology, 52*, 558–567.

Shapiro, D. E., Boggs, S. R., Melamed, B. G., & Graham-Pole, J. (1992). The effect of varied physician affect on recall, anxiety, and perceptions in women at risk for breast cancer: An analogue study. *Health Psychology, 11*(1), 61–66.

Shillinger, F. (1983). Locus of control: Implications for nursing practice. *Image: Journal of Nursing Scholarship, 15*(2), 58–63.

SinJae, L., SugJoon, A., & TaeWoo, K. (2008). Patient compliance and locus of control in orthodontic treatment: A prospective study. *American Journal of Orthodontics and Dentofacial Orthopedics, 133*(3), 354–358.

Soderlund, L. L., Nilsen, P., & Kristensson, M. (2008). Learning motivational interviewing: Exploring primary health care nurses' training and counseling experiences. *Health Education Journal, 67*(2), 102–109.

Srof, B. J., & Velsor-Friedrich, B. (2006). Health promotion in adolescents: A review of Pender's health promotion model. *Nursing Science Quarterly, 19*(4), 366–373.

Stephenson, P. L. (2006). Before the teaching begins: Managing patient anxiety prior to providing education. *Clinical Journal of Oncology Nursing, 10*(2), 241–245.

Stewart, M. N. (2012). *Patient literacy: The medagogy model.* New York, NY: McGraw-Hill Companies, Inc.

Strachan, S. M., & Brawley, L. R. (2009). Healthy-eater identity and self-efficacy predict healthy eating: A prospective view. *Journal of Health Psychology, 14*, 684–695.

Sylvia, L. G., Hay, A., Ostacher, M. J., Miklowitz, D. J., Nierenberg, A. A., Thase, M. E., . . . Perlis, R. H. (2013). Association between therapeutic alliance, care satisfaction, and pharmacological adherence in bipolar disorder. *Journal of Clinical Psychopharmacology, 33*(3), 343–350.

Syx, R. (2008). The practice of patient education: The theoretical perspective. *Orthopaedic Nursing, 27*(1), 50–56.

Tahar, M., Bayat, Z. F., Zandi, K. N., Ghasemi, E., Abredari, H., Karimy, M., & Abedi, A. R. (2015). Correlation between compliance regimens with health locus of control in patients with hypertension. *Medical Journal of the Islamic Republic of Iran, 29*(194), 1–4.

Tung, W., Lu, M., & Cook, D. (2010). Cervical cancer screening among Taiwanese women: A transtheoretical approach. *Oncology Nursing Forum, 37*(4), E288–E294.

Turner, A. P., Kivlahan, T. R., Sloan, A. P., & Haselkorn, J. K. (2007). Predicting ongoing adherence to disease modifying therapies in multiple sclerosis: Utility of the health beliefs model. *Multiple Sclerosis Journal, 13,*1146–1152.

Tyson, M., Covey, J., & Rosenthal, H. E. (2014). Theory of planned behavior interventions for reducing heterosexual risk behaviors: A meta-analysis. *Health Psychology, 33*(12), 1454–1467.

VanBuskirk, K. A., & Wetherell, J. L. (2014). Motivational interviewing with primary care populations: A systematic review and meta-analysis. *Journal of Behavioral Medicine, 37,* 768–780.

Vlasnik, J. J., Aliotta, S. L., & DeLor, B. (2005). Medication adherence: Factors influencing compliance with prescribed medication plans. *Case Manager, 16*(2), 47.

Wallston, K. A., Wallston, B. S., & DeVellis, R. (1978, Spring). Development of the multidimensional health locus of control (MHLC) scales. *Health Education Monographs,* 160–170.

Wang, Y., Zang, X., Bai, J., Liu, S., Zhao, Y., & Zhang, Q. (2013). Effect of a health belief model–based nursing intervention on Chinese patients with moderate to severe chronic obstructive pulmonary disease: A randomised controlled trial. *Journal of Clinical Nursing, 23,* 1342–1353.

Ward-Collins, D. (1998). Noncompliant: Isn't there a better way to say it? *American Journal of Nursing, 98*(5), 17–31.

West, R. L., Bagwell, D. K., & Dark-Freudeman, A. (2008). Self-efficacy and memory aging: The impact of memory intervention based on self-efficacy. *Aging, Neuropsychology and Cognition, 15,* 302–329.

Wong, R. K., Wong, M. L., Chan, Y. H., Feng, Z., Wai, C. T., & Yeoh, K. G. (2013). Gender differences in predictors of colorectal cancer screening uptake: A national cross-sectional study based on the health belief model. *BMC Public Health, 13,* 677.

Yach, D. S. (2003). *Adherence to long-term therapies: Evidence for action.* Geneva, Switzerland: World Health Organization.

Literacy in the Adult Patient Population

Susan B. Bastable | Gina M. Myers

Chapter Highlights

- Definition of Terms
  - *Literacy Relative to Oral Instruction*
  - *Literacy Relative to Computer Instruction*
- Scope and Incidence of the Problem
- Trends Associated With Literacy Problems
- Those at Risk
- Myths, Stereotypes, and Assumptions
- Assessment: Clues to Look for
- Impact of Illiteracy on Motivation and Compliance
- Ethical, Financial, and Legal Concerns
- Readability of PEMs
- Methods to Measure Literacy Levels of PEMs
  - *Flesch-Kincaid Scale*
  - *Fog Index*
  - *Fry Readability Graph—Extended*
  - *SMOG Formula*
  - *Computerized Readability Software Programs*
- Tests to Measure Comprehension of PEMs
  - *Cloze Test*
  - *Listening Test*
- Tests to Measure General Reading Skills and Health Literacy Skills of Patients
  - *WRAT*
  - *REALM*
  - *TOFHLA*

Key Terms

comprehension
cueing
e-health literacy
functional illiteracy
health literacy
illiterate
literacy
literate
low literacy
numeracy
readability
reading
tailoring

© wanchai/Shutterstock

- *NVS*
- *eHealth Literacy Scale*
- *Literacy Assessment for Diabetes*
- *SAM*
■ Simplifying the Readability of PEMs
■ Strategies to Promote Health Literacy

Objectives

After completing this chapter, the reader will be able to

1. Define the terms *literacy, illiteracy, health literacy, low literacy, functional illiteracy, reading, readability, comprehension*, and *numeracy*.

2. Identify the magnitude of the literacy problem in the United States.

3. Describe the characteristics of those individuals at risk for having difficulty with reading and comprehension of written and oral language.

4. Discuss common myths and assumptions about people with illiteracy.

5. Identify clues that are indicators of reading and writing deficiencies.

6. Assess the impact of illiteracy and low literacy on patient motivation and compliance with healthcare regimens.

7. Recognize the role of the nurse as a teacher in the assessment of patients' literacy skills.

8. Use specific formulas and tests to critically analyze the readability and comprehension levels of printed materials and the reading skills of patients.

9. Describe specific guidelines for writing effective education materials.

10. Outline various teaching strategies useful in educating patients with low literacy skills.

Adult illiteracy continues to be a major problem in the United States despite public and private efforts at all levels to address the issue. Today, the fact remains that many individuals do not possess the basic literacy abilities required to function effectively in a technologically complex society. Many adult citizens have difficulty reading and comprehending information well enough to be able to perform such common tasks as filling out job and insurance applications, interpreting bus schedules and road signs, completing tax forms, applying for a driver's license, registering to vote, and ordering from a restaurant menu (Weiss, 2003).

In 1992, the U.S. Department of Education conducted the National Adult Literacy Survey (NALS), which revealed a shockingly high level of illiteracy in the country

(Weiss, 2003; Weiss et al., 2005; Zarcadoolas, Pleasant, & Greer, 2006). Since then, awareness about illiteracy in the United States—once thought previously to be a problem mainly confined to developing countries—has taken on new meaning (Lasater & Mehler, 1998; Schwartzberg, VanGeest, & Wang, 2004).

Particularly since the turn of the century, nursing and other health professions literature has focused significant attention on the effects of patient illiteracy on healthcare delivery and health outcomes. Today, the emphasis is on health literacy—that is, the extent to which Americans can read and understand health information well enough to function successfully in a healthcare environment and make appropriate decisions for themselves.

Although more research needs to be done on the causes and effects associated with poor health literacy as well as the methods available to screen and teach patients, much has been learned about the magnitude and consequences of the health literacy problem (Friedman & Hoffman-Goetz, 2008; Gazmararian, Curran, Parker, Bernhardt, & DeBuono, 2005; Paasche-Orlow & Wolf, 2007a; Pignone, DeWalt, Sheridan, Berkman, & Lohr, 2005). *Healthy People 2010* and *Healthy People 2020* both identified limited health literacy as one of the nation's top public health agenda concerns (U.S. Department of Health and Human Services [USDHHS], 2000, 2014a). In 2006, several agencies of the USDHHS joined forces to establish a health literacy work group. In the fall of 2010, this highly diverse work group released the *National Action Plan to Improve Health Literacy*, also known as the NAP or simply referred to as the "Action Plan" (Baur, 2011).

The NAP was created to provide guidance to organizations, professionals, policy makers, communities, individuals, and families in identifying actions to take to improve the widespread problem of limited health literacy facing not only the United States but other countries worldwide (USDHHS, 2010). The NAP is not just a report on the state of the problem—it is an urgent request to identify, select, and use strategies that have the greatest potential to produce effective, measurable improvements in health literacy (Speros, 2011).

By focusing on health literacy issues and working together, nurses can improve the accessibility, quality, and safety of health care provided, reduce costs, and improve the health and quality of life for millions of people in the United States. The Action Plan highlights seven goals that will improve health literacy (USDHHS, 2010).

These goals, such as developing and distributing health information that is accurate, readable, and culturally appropriate as well as sharing interventions that could improve health literacy of patients, cannot be achieved by a single group or organization. Instead, meeting the goals of the NAP will require close collaboration between health professionals and communities to meet the needs of specific populations with low health literacy (Clancy, 2011).

What must be of particular concern to the healthcare industry are the numbers of consumers who are illiterate, functionally illiterate, or low literate. People who cannot read or who are poor readers with limited comprehension skills have much higher medical costs, increased number of hospitalizations and readmissions, greater risk of death, and more perceived physical and psychosocial problems than do literate persons (Baker, Parker, Williams, & Clark, 1998; Baker, Williams, Parker, Gazmararian, & Nurss, 1999;

DeWalt, Berkman, Sheridan, Lohr, & Pignone, 2004; Eichler, Wieser, & Brügger, 2009; McNaughton et al., 2015; Parnell, 2014; Sudore, Yaffe, et al., 2006; Weiss, 2003; Weiss et al., 2005). Patients are expected to assume greater responsibility for self-care and health promotion, which requires increased knowledge and skills. If people with low literacy abilities cannot fully benefit from the type and amount of information they are typically given, they cannot be expected to maintain health and manage independently. The result is a significant negative impact on the cost of health care and the quality of life (Dickens & Piano, 2013; Kogut, 2004; Levy & Royne, 2009; Pignone et al., 2005; M. V. Williams, Davis, Parker, & Weiss, 2002; Wood, Kettinger, & Lessick, 2007).

Traditionally, healthcare professionals have relied heavily on printed education materials (PEMs) as a low-cost and fast way to communicate health messages. An assumption was made that the written materials commonly distributed to patients were sufficient to ensure informed consent for tests and procedures, to promote compliance with treatment regimens, and to guarantee adherence to discharge instructions. Only recently have healthcare providers begun to recognize that the scientific and technical terminology used in printed teaching materials is poorly understood by the majority of people (Ache, 2009; Adkins, Elkins, & Singh, 2001; Morrow, Weiner, Steinley, Young, & Murray, 2007). Kessels (2003) points out that 40% to 80% of medical information provided by health professionals is forgotten immediately, not just because medical terminology is too difficult to understand, but also because delivery of too much information leads to poor recall. Furthermore, half of the information that is remembered is remembered incorrectly. Unless education materials are written at a level and style appropriate for patients, they cannot be expected to be able or willing to accept responsibility for self-care. Even though illiteracy and low literacy are quite prevalent in the U.S. population, problems with literacy frequently continue to go undiagnosed (C. C. Doak, Doak, & Root, 1996; Zarcadoolas et al., 2006).

This chapter examines the magnitude of the literacy problem, the myths associated with it, and the factors that influence literacy levels. It emphasizes the important role that nurses play in assessing patients' literacy skills and the effects of reading and health illiteracy on the well-being of the public. In addition, the formulas and tests used to evaluate readability of printed information and to assess patients' comprehension and reading skills are reviewed, specific guidelines are put forth for writing effective health education materials, and teaching strategies are recommended as a means for breaking down the barriers of illiteracy.

Definition of Terms

For many years, there was no clear agreement of what it meant to be literate in U.S. society. A literate person was loosely described as someone who possessed socially required and expected reading and writing abilities, such as being able to sign his or her name and read and write a simple sentence. Over time, performance on reading tests in school became the conventional method to measure grade-level achievement.

Because it is difficult, if not impossible, to measure reading abilities on a population-wide basis, the U.S. Bureau of the Census continues to this day to use the number of years of schooling attended to define literacy levels (Giorgianni, 1998). This method has been found to be an inadequate predictor of reading ability (Chew, Bradley, & Boyko, 2004; C. C. Doak et al., 1996; Weiss, 2003; Winslow, 2001).

In the United States, the term literacy is generally defined as the ability to read and speak English (Andrus & Roth, 2002). The 1992 NALS survey defined **literacy** as "the ability to use printed and written information to function in society, to achieve one's goals, and to develop one's knowledge and potential" (National Center for Education Statistics, 1993, p. 6). NALS categorized literacy into three general kinds of tasks (National Center for Education Statistics, 1993):

- Prose tasks, which measure reading comprehension and the ability to extract themes from newspapers, magazines, poems, and books
- Document tasks, which assess the ability of readers to interpret documents such as insurance reports, consent forms, and transportation schedules
- Quantitative tasks, which assess the ability to work with numerical information embedded in written material, such as computing restaurant bills, figuring out taxes, interpreting paycheck stubs, or calculating calories on a nutrition checklist

Most recently the NAP defined literacy as a set of reading, writing, math, speech, and comprehension skills and further adds that **numeracy** is a part of literacy, which refers to the ability to understand basic mathematical concepts. Overwhelmingly, those persons with limited literacy also have limited skills in numeracy (Andrus & Roth, 2002; C. C. Doak et al., 1996; Fisher, 1999; M. V. Williams et al., 1995).

Although no precise cut-off point defines the difference between literacy and illiteracy, the commonly accepted working definition of what is meant by **literate** is the ability to write and to read, understand, and interpret information written at the eighth-grade level or above. On the other end of the continuum, **illiterate** is defined as being unable to read or write at all or having reading and writing skills at the fourth-grade level or below.

Low literacy, also termed *marginally literate* or *marginally illiterate*, refers to the ability of adults to read, write, and comprehend information between the fifth- and eighth-grade levels of difficulty. Persons with low literacy have trouble using commonly printed and written information to meet their everyday needs, such as reading a TV schedule, taking a telephone message, or filling out a relatively simple application form (C. C. Doak et al., 1996).

Functional illiteracy means that adults lack the basic reading, writing, and comprehension skills that are needed to operate effectively in today's society. People who are functionally illiterate have very limited competency to perform the tasks of everyday life (Giorgianni, 1998; M. V. Williams, Baker, Parker, & Nurss, 1998). They do not read well enough to understand and interpret what they have read or use the information as it was intended (C. C. Doak et al., 1996). For example, someone who is functionally illiterate may be able to read the simple words on a label of a can of soup that directs him or her to "Pour soup into pan. Add one can water. Heat until hot." However, he or she cannot understand the meaning and sequence of the words to carry through with these directions.

Although an individual may have poor reading skills, this does not necessarily imply a lack of intelligence. Low literacy or illiteracy cannot be equated with IQ level. A person can be illiterate or low literate, yet intellectually be within at least normal IQ range (C. C. Doak et al., 1996).

Health literacy is defined by the Patient Protection and Affordable Care Act of 2010, Title V, as the "degree to which an individual has the capacity to obtain, communicate, process, and understand basic health information and services to make appropriate health decisions" (Centers for Disease Control and Prevention [CDC], 2015, para 1). A health-literate individual must be able to read a medication label and then figure out the correct dose and frequency of taking the medication. He or she must be able to fill out health insurance forms, know when to vaccinate his or her child or have a mammogram, or give informed consent for a lifesaving procedure. Although literacy and health literacy are closely related, they are different concepts. Health literacy is complex, such that even those people with strong reading and writing skills, high levels of education, and affluence can face challenges with health literacy. In fact, 45% of high school graduates have limited health literacy skills (USDHHS, 2010).

The CDC (2015) outlines the following common health literacy challenges facing many people:

1. They are not familiar with medical terms or how their bodies work.
2. They have to interpret or calculate numbers or risks that could have health and safety consequences.
3. They are scared and confused when diagnosed with a serious illness.
4. They have health conditions that require high levels of complicated self-care instructions.
5. They are voting on a critical local issue affecting the community's health and are relying on unfamiliar technical information.

Because of multiple factors, health literacy level cannot be determined from stereotypes, generalizations, or assumptions, or by simply looking at a patient. Furthermore, health literacy levels change over time with education, aging, social interactions, language, culture, and life experiences with health and disease (Baker, 2006; Speros, 2011, Volandes, 2007). Yet, given the widespread adoption of the managed care model and the Affordable Care Act, individuals will be required to take more responsibility for self-care and symptom management; health literacy is becoming an important determinant of health status. Poor health literacy may lead to serious negative consequences, such as increased illness and death, when a person is unable to read and comprehend instructions for medications, follow-up appointments, diet, procedures, and other regimens. Patients cannot be expected to be compliant, independent, and self-directed in navigating the healthcare system if they do not have the ability to follow basic instructions (Bennett, Chen, Soroui, & White, 2009; Davis et al., 2006). Further, low health literacy can result in more emergency department visits and hospital admissions. It also affects use of preventive services such as mammography and flu vaccination and lessens the likelihood a person will take medications or follow health instructions correctly (Berkman, Sheridan, Donahue, Halpern, & Crotty, 2011).

Reading, readability, and *comprehension* also are terms frequently used when determining levels of literacy. Fisher (1999) defines **reading** or word recognition as "the process of transforming letters into words and being able to pronounce them correctly" (p. 57). **Readability** is defined as the ease with which written or printed information can be read. It is based on a measure of several different elements within a given text of information (Hasselkus, 2009). **Comprehension**, in comparison, is the degree to which individuals understand what they have read (Fisher, 1999; Koo, Krass, & Aslani, 2005). It is the ability to grasp the meaning of a message—to get the gist of it. Nurses can determine whether comprehension of health instruction has occurred by noting whether patients are able to demonstrate correctly or recall in their own words the message that was received.

The ability to read does not, by itself, guarantee reading comprehension. Understanding the written word is affected by the amount, clarity, and complexity of the information presented. If the elements of logic, language, and experience in health instruction match with and are culturally appropriate to the patients' background, the message likely will be clear and relevant to them (C. C. Doak et al., 1996). On the other hand, a mismatch will likely make the message confusing, beyond understanding, and useless to the individual. Illness, medication, treatment, or disruptive life situations, all of which may cause stress and anxiety, have been found to interfere significantly with comprehension (Kessels, 2003; Stephenson, 2006). Readability and comprehension, therefore, are particularly complex activities involving many variables with respect to both the reader and the actual written material (C. C. Doak et al., 1996; Fisher, 1999). Both of these activities are commonly determined by using one or more measurement formulas (see the later discussions of measurement tools in this chapter).

Literacy Relative to Oral Instruction

To date, very little attention has been paid to the role of oral communication in the assessment of illiteracy. Certainly, inability to comprehend the spoken word or oral instruction above the level of understanding simple words, phrases, and slang words should be considered an important element in the definition or assessment of literacy. Often health information is provided verbally, and many patients prefer to learn in a face-to-face encounter (Morrow et al., 2007). However, oral instruction alone is not a very successful method of teaching. "Written information is better remembered and leads to better treatment adherence" (Kessels, 2003, p. 221).

Literacy Relative to Computer Instruction

Computer literacy has emerged as an increasingly popular concern and an important dimension of the literacy issue. Patients who are well educated and career oriented are likely to own a computer and be computer literate, whereas those with limited resources, literacy skills, and technological know-how are being left behind (Kerka, 2003; Zarcadoolas et al., 2006). As healthcare organizations and agencies continue to invest more resources in computer technology and software programs for educational purposes, computer literacy in the overall patient population must be addressed.

Computers not only are used to convey instructional messages, but they also serve as valuable tools for accessing a wide array of additional sources of health information. The opportunity to expand patients' knowledge base through telecommunications and virtual resources requires nurses in the role of teacher to attend to computer literacy levels of their audiences. In the same way that they now recognize the negative effects that illiteracy and low literacy have had on patients' understanding of healthcare information when printed materials are relied upon, nurses must begin to advocate for computer literacy in the public they serve (C. C. Doak et al., 1996; Moore, Bias, Prentice, Fletcher, & Vaughn, 2009).

Since 2000, the concept of e-health and informatics has grown globally to encompass use of the Internet and other virtual resources for the delivery of patient education and organization of care (Pagliari et al., 2005). Thus e-health literacy must be an additional concern to the nurse. Norman and Skinner (2006b) define **e-health literacy** as "the ability to seek, find, understand, and appraise health information from electronic sources and apply the knowledge gained to addressing or solving a health problem" (para 6). These authors draw attention to the knowledge and complex skill set that is often taken for granted when people interact with technology to access and share information. Nurses now must focus their attention on learning and usability issues, whether it be in an acute care setting or at the population health level. E-health tools include digital resources designed to help patients, consumers, and caregivers find health information, store and manage their personal health information, make decisions, and manage their health (CDC, 2009). Undertaking an assessment of not only health literacy but also e-health literacy is an important action the nurse can take to determine whether the use of technology will be useful or useless to the patient's understanding of health information (Collins, Currie, Bakken, Vawdrey, & Stone, 2012).

Scope and Incidence of the Problem

Literacy has been termed the "silent epidemic," the "silent barrier," the "silent disability," and "the dirty little secret" (Conlin & Schumann, 2002; L. G. Doak & Doak, 1987; Kefalides, 1999; Wedgeworth, 2007). Based on available statistics over the past 20 years, it is clear that the United States has significant literacy problems (Kogut, 2004). In fact, this country ranked only in the middle among a list of industrialized nations on most measures of adult literacy.

The 1992 NALS, considered to be the first highly accurate and detailed profile on the condition of English-language literacy in the United States, revealed surprising statistics. Based on the findings from this assessment of literacy skills in three areas (prose, document, and quantitative), literacy abilities were categorized into five levels, with level 1 being the lowest and level 5 being the highest. Some 21% to 23% (approximately 40–44 million) of the 191 million adults in the country at that time scored in the lowest level of the three skill areas. They were considered to be functionally illiterate. Another 25% to 28%, or approximately 50 million adults, scored in the level 2 category; that is, they were considered to have low literacy skills. Thus, the number of illiterate and low-literate adults in the United States was conservatively estimated to be approximately

90–94 million in total. This indicates that roughly half of the U.S. adult population had deficiencies in reading, writing, and math skills (Fisher, 1999; Weiss, 2003). The researchers found that those individuals with poor literacy skills (levels 1 and 2) were more often from minority populations and lower socioeconomic groups, and they had poorer health status (Andrus & Roth, 2002; Fisher, 1999; Weiss, 2003).

In 2003, building on the NALS of 10 years earlier, the National Assessment of Adult Literacy (NAAL) became the first study to identify the literacy of America's adults in the 21st century. New, more sensitive instruments were designed to enhance measurement of the literacy abilities of the least literate adults. Most important, this evaluation included a health literacy component to assess adults' understanding of health-related materials and forms (National Center for Education Statistics, 2006).

The NAAL categorized literacy skills into four levels, and the findings revealed the following percentages and total numbers: below basic, 14% (30 million); basic, 29% (63 million); intermediate, 44% (95 million); and proficient, 13% (28 million). Of the overall 216 million adults in the U.S. population in 2003, 43% (93 million) fell into the lowest two categories (National Center for Education Statistics, 2006).

The average score results indicated no significant change in prose and document literacy and only a slight increase in quantitative literacy between 1992 and 2003. However, a higher percentage of several population groups, such as those who did not graduate from high school, Hispanics, and those older than 65 years of age, fell into the below basic level of prose literacy (Kutner, Greenberg, Jin, & Paulsen, 2006). The NAAL's Health Literacy Report specifically found that 36% (47 million) of adults had basic or below basic health literacy and that older adults (65 years and older) had the lowest health literacy levels (Baer, Kutner, & Sabatini, 2009; National Center for Education Statistics, 2006).

In 2004, the Institute of Medicine (IOM), the Agency for Healthcare Research and Quality (AHRQ), and the American Medical Association issued their own reports on the status of health literacy in the United States. All three reports revealed that as many as 50% of all American adults lack the basic reading and numerical skills essential to function adequately in the healthcare environment (Aldridge, 2004; IOM, 2004; Schwartzberg et al., 2004; Weiss et al., 2005).

Limited literacy leads to poor health outcomes. In fact, literacy skills are "a stronger predictor of an individual's health status than income, employment status, education level, and racial or ethnic group" (Weiss, 2007, p. 13). Individuals with limited literacy skills are less knowledgeable about their health problems and have higher hospitalization rates, more emergency department visits, higher healthcare costs, less healthy behaviors, and poorer health status (Eichler et al., 2009; Weiss, 2007; Weiss et al., 2005; Wood, 2005). McNaughton et al. (2015) found that acute heart failure patients with low health literacy scores were at higher risk for death after hospital discharge.

The rates of illiteracy and low literacy in general and health literacy in particular continue to pose a major threat to many segments of society. This problem is expected to grow worse in light of the many forces operating in the United States and worldwide unless specific measures are taken to curb the tide. To be literate 100 years ago meant that people could read and write their own name. Today, being literate means that one is able to learn new skills, think critically, problem solve, and apply general knowledge to various situations (Weiss, 2003).

Trends Associated With Literacy Problems

The trend toward an increased proportion of Americans having literacy levels that are inadequate for active participation in this advanced society is the result of factors such as the following (Baur, 2011; Gazmararian et al., 1999; Giorgianni, 1998; Hayes, 2000; Hirsch, 2001; Kogut, 2004; Weiss, 2007):

- An increase in the number of immigrants
- The aging of the population
- The increasing amount and complexity of information
- The increasing sophistication of technology
- More people living in poverty
- Changes in policies and funding for public education
- Disparities between minority versus nonminority populations

Levels of literacy are often seen as indicators of the well-being of individuals, and the literacy problem has larger implications for the social and economic status of the country as a whole (Kogut, 2004). Low levels of literacy have been associated with marginal productivity, high unemployment, minimum earnings, high costs of health care, and high rates of welfare dependency (Andrus & Roth, 2002; Eichler et al., 2009; Giorgianni, 1998; Winslow, 2001; Ziegler, 1998).

In addition, illiteracy contributes to many of the grave social issues confronting the United States today, such as homelessness, teen pregnancy, unemployment, delinquency, crime, and drug abuse (Fleener & Scholl, 1992; Kogut, 2004). Deficiencies in basic literacy skills become compounded and create devastating cumulative effects on individuals, which produces a social burden that is extremely costly for the American people. Illiteracy and low literacy are not necessarily the reasons for these problems, but the high correlation between literacy levels and social problems is a marker for disconnectedness from society in general (Kogut, 2004; USDHHS, 2011).

Those at Risk

Illiteracy has been described "as an invisible handicap that affects all classes, ethnic groups, and ages" (Fleener & Scholl, 1992, p. 740). Illiteracy knows no boundaries and exists among persons of every race and ethnic background, socioeconomic class, and age category (Duffy & Snyder, 1999; Parnell, 2014; Weiss, 2003). It is true, however, that illiteracy is rare in the higher socioeconomic classes, for example, and that certain segments of the U.S. population are more likely to be affected than others by lack of literacy skills.

According to many research studies (Cole, 2000; Hayes, 2000; Kogut, 2004; Montalto & Spiegler, 2001; Nath, Sylvester, Yasek, & Gunel, 2001; Rothman et al., 2004;

Schillinger et al., 2002; Schultz, 2002; Weiss, 2007; M. V. Williams et al., 1998; Winslow, 2001; Wood, 2005), populations that have been identified as having poorer reading and comprehension skills than the average American include the following:

- Those who are economically disadvantaged
- Older adults
- Immigrants (particularly illegal ones)
- Those with English as a second language
- Racial minorities
- High school dropouts
- Those who are unemployed
- Prisoners
- Inner-city and rural residents
- Those with poor health status resulting from chronic mental and physical problems
- Those on Medicaid

Of course, not every member of an at-risk population suffers from low literacy. Further, some people do not fall into an "at risk" category, yet still lack literacy skills (Baur, 2011; Weiss, 2007).

Statistics indicate that 34 million Americans are presently living in poverty and that nearly half (43%) of all adults with low literacy live in poverty (Darling, 2004). Although those who are disadvantaged represent many diverse cultural and ethnic groups, including millions of poor Caucasians, one third of disadvantaged people in this country are minorities, and a larger percentage of minorities fall into the disadvantaged category (Giorgianni, 1998; Weiss et al., 2005).

In the 21st century, the major growth in the U.S. population is predicted to come from the ranks of minority groups. By 2050, 53% of the people in the United States are projected to belong to a racial or ethnic minority, and one in five will be foreign born (Passel & Cohn, 2008). The U.S. Bureau of the Census reported that almost 40 million immigrants reside in this country, more than quadruple the number in 1970, with more than half of those individuals living in California, New York, Florida, and Texas. One third of the foreign-born population has arrived since 2000, 62% of immigrant families have children, and 30% of immigrants do not have a high school diploma (Grieco et al., 2012; U.S. Census Bureau, 2012). Of the 1100 community-based adult literacy programs supported by ProLiteracy (2012), 86% teach English as a second language (ESL).

Also, many minority and economically disadvantaged people, as well as the prison population—which has the highest concentration of adult illiteracy (Duffy & Snyder, 1999; "The U.S. Illiteracy Rate," 2013)—do not benefit from mainstream health education activities, which often fail to reach them. Many lack enough reading ability to make good use of written health education materials. Moreover, while the majority of PEMs are written in English, fluency in verbal skills in another language does not guarantee functional literacy in that native language (Horner, Surratt, & Juliusson, 2000). Areas with the highest percentage of minorities and the highest rates of poverty and immigration also have the highest percentage of functionally illiterate people. When these people need medical care, they tend to require more resources, have longer hospital stays, and have a greater number of readmissions (Levy & Royne, 2009; Weiss, 2007).

Among Americans older than 65 years of age, two out of five adults (approximately 40%) are considered functionally illiterate (Davidhizar & Brownson, 1999; Gazmararian et al., 1999; M. V. Williams et al., 2002). In 2010, the population of older adults totaled approximately 40 million (more than 13% of the total U.S. population), and individuals older than 85 years of age make up the fastest-growing age group in the country (Greenberg, 2011). At the turn of the century, the oldest-old numbered 4.2 million people, but it is projected that by 2050 that number could reach 19 million. Children born today can expect to live to be 80 years old. Statistics indicate that the U.S. population is growing older as people live longer. By 2030, it is expected that the 65-and-older population will double from its size at the beginning of the 21st century (Crandell, Crandell, & Vander Zanden, 2012; Federal Interagency Forum on Aging-Related Statistics, 2012).

As time goes on, members of the older population will be more educated and demand more services. In 1960, only 20% of older people were high school graduates; in 2014, 84% were educated at the high school level (USDHHS, 2014b). However, the information explosion and rapid technological advances may cause them to fall behind. Today, the illiteracy problem in the aged is caused by the facts that not only did these individuals have less education in the past, but their reading skills have also declined over time because of disuse. If a person does not use a skill, he or she loses that skill. Reading ability can deteriorate over time if not exercised regularly (Brownson, 1998).

In addition, cognition and some types of intellectual functioning are affected by aging (Crandell et al., 2012; Kessels, 2003; Santrock, 2013). The majority of older people have some degree of cognitive changes and sensory impairments, such as vision and hearing loss. On the average, 28% of people aged 65 to 74 and 38% of those older than 75 years of age have serious hearing impairment; women fare better than men in this regard (Crandell et al., 2012). Along with these normal physiological changes, many older adults suffer from chronic diseases, and large numbers are taking prescribed medications. All of these conditions can interfere with the ability to learn or can negatively affect thought processes, which contributes to the high incidence of illiteracy in this population group (Sudore, Yaffe et al., 2006).

Cultural diversity, although not considered to be directly related to illiteracy, may also serve as a barrier to effective patient education. According to Davidhizar and Brownson (1999), most adults with illiteracy problems in the United States are Caucasian, native-born, English-speaking individuals, which is a claim supported by the NAAL's 2003 statistics. However, when examining the proportion of the population that has poor literacy skills, minority ethnic groups are at a disproportionately higher risk (Andrus & Roth, 2002).

When nurses and other healthcare providers communicate with patients from cultures different from their own, it is important for them to be aware that their patients may not be fluent in English. Furthermore, even if people speak the English language, the meanings of words and their understanding of facts may vary significantly based on life experiences, family background, and culture of origin, especially if English is the patient's second language (Purnell, 2013). In conversation, an individual must be able to understand subtle meanings of words, voice tones, and the context (slang, terminology, or customs) in which the message is being delivered.

Purnell (2013) stresses the importance of assessing other elements of verbal and nonverbal communication, such as emotional tone of speech, gestures, eye contact, touch, voice volume, and stance, between persons of different cultures that may affect the interpretation of behavior and the true meaning of information being received or sent. Nurses must be aware of these potential barriers to communication when interacting with patients from other cultures whose literacy skills may be limited. Given the increasing diversity of the U.S. population, most currently available written materials are considered inadequate based on the literacy level of minority groups and the fact that the majority of written materials are available only in English.

Thus, individuals with less education; low-income, older adults; racial minorities; and people for whom English is a second language are likely to have more difficulty with reading and comprehending written materials as well as with understanding oral instruction (Winslow, 2001). This profile is not intended to stereotype people who are illiterate, but rather to give a broad picture of who most likely lacks literacy skills. When carrying out assessments on their patient populations, it is essential that nurses and other healthcare providers be aware of those susceptible to having literacy problems.

Myths, Stereotypes, and Assumptions

Rarely do people voluntarily admit that they are illiterate. Illiteracy carries a stigma that creates feelings of shame, inadequacy, fear, and low self-esteem (Paasche-Orlow & Wolf, 2007b; Weiss, 2007; M. V. Williams et al., 2002; Wolf et al., 2007). Most individuals with poor literacy skills have learned that it is dangerous to reveal their illiteracy because of fear that others, such as family, strangers, friends, or employers, would consider them dumb or incapable of functioning responsibly. In fact, the majority of people with literacy problems have never told their spouse or children of their disability (Quirk, 2000; M. V. Williams et al., 2002).

People also tend to underreport their limited reading abilities because of embarrassment or lack of insight about the extent of their limitation. The NALS report revealed that the majority of adults performing at the two lowest levels of literacy skill describe themselves as competent in being able to read and/or write English (Ad Hoc Committee on Health Literacy, 1999). Because self-reporting is so unreliable and because illiteracy and low literacy are so common, many experts suggest that all patients should be screened to identify those who have reading difficulty to determine the extent of their impairment (Andrus & Roth, 2002; Weiss, 2007; Weiss et al., 2005). Nurses must recognize that many patients would approach such testing reluctantly and be fearful of having their literacy report recorded in their health record (Paasche-Orlow & Wolf, 2007b; Wolf et al., 2007).

Most people with limited literacy abilities are masters at concealment. Typically, they are ashamed of their limitation and attempt to hide the problem in clever ways. Many have discovered ways to function quite well in society without being able to read by memorizing signs and instructions, making intelligent guesses, or finding employment opportunities that are not heavily dependent on reading and writing skills.

An important thing to remember is that many myths about illiteracy exist. It is very easy for healthcare providers to fall into the trap of labeling someone as illiterate or, for that matter, assuming that they are literate based on stereotypical images. Some of the most common myths about people who struggle with literacy skills are outlined in **Table 7–1** (Andrus & Roth, 2002; C. C. Doak et al., 1996; Weiss, 2007; M. V. Williams et al., 2002; Winslow, 2001).

Assessment: Clues to Look for

So the question remains: How does one recognize an illiterate person? Identifying illiteracy is not easy because there is no stereotypical pattern. It is easily overlooked because illiteracy has no particular face, age, socioeconomic status, or nationality (Cole, 2000; Hayes, 2000). Nurses, because of their role with healthcare consumers, are in an ideal position to determine the literacy levels of individuals (Cutilli, 2005; Monsivais & Reynolds, 2003). Because of the prevalence of illiteracy, nurses must never assume that a patient is literate. Because people with illiteracy or marginal literacy skills often have had many years of practice in disguising the problem, they may go to elaborate lengths to hide it. In so many instances when someone does not fit the stereotypical image, nurses and other health professionals have never even considered the possibility that an illiteracy problem exists.

Overlooking the problem has the potential for grave consequences in treatment outcomes and has resulted in frustration for both patients and caregivers (Cole, 2000;

Table 7–1 Myths and Truths about Those Who Struggle With Literacy

Myth	Truth
They are intellectually slow learners or incapable of learning at all.	Many have average or above-average IQs.
They can be recognized by their appearance.	Appearance alone is an unreliable basis for judgment; some very articulate, well-dressed people have no visible signs of a literacy disability.
The number of years of schooling completed correlates with literacy skills.	Grade-level achievement does not correspond well to reading ability. The number of years of schooling completed overestimates reading levels by four to five grade levels.
Most are foreign born, poor, and of ethnic or racial minority.	They come from very diverse backgrounds and the majority are white, native-born Americans.
Most will freely admit that they do not know how to read or do not understand.	Most try to hide their reading deficiencies and will go to great lengths to avoid discovery, even when directly asked about their possible limitations.

Weiss, 2007). If healthcare providers become aware of a patient's literacy problem, they must convey sensitivity and maintain confidentiality to prevent increased feelings of shame (Quirk, 2000). During assessment, the nurse should take note of the following clues that patients with illiteracy or low literacy may demonstrate (Andrus & Roth, 2002; Carol, 2007; Davis, Michielutte, Askov, Williams, & Weiss, 1998; Weiss, 2007):

- Reacting to complex learning situations by withdrawal, complete avoidance, or being repeatedly noncompliant
- Using the excuse that they were too busy, too tired, too sick, or too sedated with medication to maintain their attention span when given a booklet or instruction sheet to read
- Claiming that they just did not feel like reading, that they gave the information to their spouse to take home, or that they lost, forgot, or broke their glasses
- Surrounding themselves with books, magazines, and newspapers to give the impression they are able to read
- Insisting on taking the information home to read or having a family member or friend with them when written information is presented
- Asking you to read the information for them with the excuse that their eyes are bothersome, they lack interest, or they do not have the energy to learn
- Showing nervousness as a result of feeling stressed by the threat of the possibility of getting caught or having to confess to illiteracy
- Acting confused, talking out of context, or holding reading materials upside down
- Showing a great deal of frustration and restlessness when attempting to read, often mouthing words aloud (vocalization) or silently (subvocalization), substituting words they cannot decipher (decode) with meaningless words, pointing to words or phrases on a page, pronouncing words incorrectly, or exhibiting facial signs of bewilderment or defeat
- Standing in a location clearly designated for authorized personnel only
- Listening and watching very attentively to observe and memorize how things work
- Demonstrating difficulty with following instructions about relatively simple activities such as breathing exercises or operating the TV, electric bed, call light, and other simple equipment, even when the operating instructions are clearly printed on them
- Failing to ask any questions about the information they received
- Turning in registration forms or health questionnaires that are incomplete, illegible, or blank
- Revealing a discrepancy between what is understood by listening and what is understood by reading
- Missing appointments or failing to follow up with referrals
- Not taking medications as prescribed

These clues from the patient in the form of puzzled looks, inappropriate behaviors, excuses, or irrelevant statements may give the nurse the intuitive feeling that the message being communicated has been neither received nor understood. Not only do illiterate people become confused and frustrated in their attempts to deal with the complex system of health care, which is so dependent on written and verbal information, but they also become stressed in their efforts to cover up their disability.

Nurses, in turn, can feel frustrated when persons who have undiagnosed literacy problems seem at face value to be unmotivated and noncompliant in following self-care instructions. Many times, nurses wonder why patients make caregiving so difficult for themselves as well as for the provider. It is not unusual for nurses to conclude, "He's too proud to take advice," "She's in denial," or "He's just being stubborn—it's a control issue." Nurses in their role as teachers must go beyond their own assumptions, look beyond a patient's appearance and behavior, and conduct a thorough initial assessment to uncover the possibility that a literacy problem exists. An awareness of this possibility and good skills at observation are key to diagnosing illiteracy or low literacy in learners. Early diagnosis enables nurses to intervene appropriately to avoid disservice to those who should not be blamed, but rather supported and encouraged.

Impact of Illiteracy on Motivation and Compliance

In addition to the fact that poor literacy skills affect the ability to read as well as to understand and interpret the meaning of written and verbal instructions, a person with illiteracy or low literacy struggles with other significant interrelated limitations with communication that can negatively influence healthcare teaching (C. C. Doak, Doak, Friedell, & Meade, 1998; Kalichman, Ramachandran, & Catz, 1999). The person's organization of thought, perception, vocabulary and language/fluency development, and problem-solving skills are adversely affected, too (Fleener & Scholl, 1992; Giorgianni, 1998).

People with poor reading skills have difficulty analyzing instructions, taking in and organizing new information, and coming up with questions (Giorgianni, 1998). They may be reluctant to ask questions because they do not even know what to ask or they are afraid others will think of them as ignorant or lacking in intelligence. Even when questioned about their understanding, persons with low literacy skills will most likely claim that they understood the information even when they did not (Davis et al., 2006; C. C. Doak et al., 1996; McCormack, Bann, Uhrig, Berkman, & Rudd, 2009; Sudore, Landefeld, et al., 2006; Walfish & Ducey, 2007).

Most nurses can recount a situation in which a patient failed to follow advice because he or she did not understand the instructions that were given. For example, a young pregnant girl prescribed antiemetic suppositories to control her nausea had no relief of symptoms. Questioning by the nurse revealed that she was swallowing the medication (Hussey & Guilliland, 1989). Obviously, not only did she not understand how to take the medicine, but also she likely had never seen a suppository and was not even able to read or understand the word. She did not ask what it was, probably because she did not know what to ask in the first place, and she may have been reluctant to question the treatment out of fear that she would be regarded as stupid.

People with poor literacy skills may also think in only concrete, specific, and literal terms. An example of this limitation is the diabetic patient whose glucose levels were out of control even when the patient insisted he was taking his insulin as he was taught—by injecting the orange and then eating the fruit (Hussey & Guilliland, 1989).

The person with limited literacy also may experience difficulty handling large amounts of information. Older adults, in particular, who need to take several different medications at various times and in different dosages, may either become confused with the schedule or ignore the instruction. If asked to change their daily medication routine, a great deal of retraining may be needed to convince them of the benefits of the new regimen (Kessels, 2003).

Another major factor in noncompliance is a lack of adequate and specific instructions about prescribed treatment regimens. Unfortunately, poor literacy skills are seldom assessed by healthcare personnel when, for example, teaching a patient about medications. Literacy problems tend to limit the patient's ability to understand the many instructions regarding medication labels, dosage scheduling, adverse reactions, drug interactions, and complications (Davis et al., 2006; Elliot, 2007; Mauk, 2014; M. V. Williams et al., 2002). No wonder those who lack the required vocabulary, organized thinking skills, and ability to formulate questions, and who also receive inadequate instruction, become confused and easily frustrated to the point of taking medications incorrectly or refusing to take them at all.

Thus illiteracy, functional illiteracy, and low literacy significantly affect both motivation and compliance levels. What is often mistaken for noncompliance is, instead, the simple inability to comply. Although almost half of the adult population is functionally illiterate, this statistic is overlooked by many healthcare professionals as being a major factor in noncompliance with prescribed regimens, follow-up appointments, and measures to prevent medical complications (Andrus & Roth, 2002; C. C. Doak et al., 1996; Weiss, 2007; M. V. Williams et al., 2002).

A number of studies have correlated literacy levels with noncompliance (C. C. Doak et al., 1998; Kalichman et al., 1999; Mayeaux et al., 1996; Weiss, 2007). Individuals who have both poor literacy skills and inadequate language skills often have difficulty following instructions and providing accurate and complete health histories, which are vital to the delivery of good health care. The burden of illiteracy leads patients into noncompliance not because they do not want to comply, but rather because they are unable to do so (Hayes, 2000; D. M. Williams, Counselman, & Caggiano, 1996).

Ethical, Financial, and Legal Concerns

Printed materials are distributed primarily by nurses and other health professionals and are the major sources of information for patients participating in health programs in many settings. Unfortunately, many of these sources fail to take into account the educational level, preexisting knowledge base, cultural influences, language barriers, or socioeconomic backgrounds of persons with limited literacy skills.

Unless patients are competent in reading and comprehending the literature given to them, these tools are useless as adjuncts for health education. They are neither a cost-effective nor a time-efficient means for teaching and learning. Materials that are widely distributed, but not fully understood, pose not only a health hazard for patients but also an ethical, financial, and legal liability for healthcare providers (Ad Hoc Committee on Health Literacy, 1999; French & Larrabee, 1999; Gazmararian et al., 2005; Giorgianni, 1998; Ryhanen, Johansson, Salo, Salantera, & Leino-Kilpi, 2008; Schultz, 2002; Vallance, Taylor, & LaVallee, 2008). Health education cannot be considered to have taken place if the written information that has been distributed to patients does not enhance their knowledge and requisite skills necessary for self-care (Fisher, 1999; Weiss, 2007; Winslow, 2001).

Initial standards for health education put forth in 1993 by the Joint Commission on Accreditation of Healthcare Organizations (JCAHO)—now known as The Joint Commission—remain the current standard, requiring "the patient and/or, when appropriate, his/her significant other(s) [be] provided with education that can enhance their knowledge, skills, and those behaviors necessary to fully benefit from the health care interventions provided by the organization" (JCAHO, 1993, p. 1030). In 1996, JCAHO identified additional standards necessary for patient care to meet accreditation mandates. Not only is patient and family (or significant other) instruction required, but education must be provided by all relevant members of the interdisciplinary healthcare team, with special consideration being given to the patient's literacy level, educational level, and language. All patients must have an assessment of their readiness to learn and identification of any obstacles to learning (Weiss, 2003).

Education relevant to a person's healthcare needs must be understandable and culturally appropriate to the patient and/or significant others. Therefore, PEMs must be written in ways that are culturally relevant and assist patients in comprehending their health needs and problems to undertake self-care regimens involving medications, diet, exercise therapies, and use of medical equipment (Fisher, 1999; Weiss, 2007).

Furthermore, the federally mandated Patient's Bill of Rights has established the rights of patients to receive complete and current information regarding their diagnoses, treatments, and prognoses in terms they can understand (Duffy & Snyder, 1999). The reading levels of PEMs must match the patients' reading abilities, and vice versa. Trends in the current healthcare system in the United States have hindered the professional ability of nurses to provide needed information to ensure self-care that is both safe and effective. Patient education has assumed an even more vital role in assisting patients to independently manage their own healthcare needs given the following factors:

- Early discharge
- Decreased reimbursement for direct care
- Increased emphasis on delivery of care in the community and home setting
- Greater demands on nursing personnel in all settings
- Increased technological complexity of treatment
- Assumption by caregivers that printed information is an adequate substitute for direct instruction of patients

These constraints do not allow for sufficient opportunities for patients in the home or various healthcare settings to receive the necessary education they need for self-management. Consequently, professional nurses are relying to a greater extent than ever before on PEMs to supplement their teaching (Horner et al., 2000; Vanderhoff, 2005). Thus, the burden has fallen on nurses to safeguard the lives of their patients by becoming better, more effective communicators of written health information (Wood, 2005).

The potential for misinterpretation of instructions not only can adversely affect treatment but also raises serious concerns about the ethical and legal implications with respect to professional responsibility and liability when information is written at a level incomprehensible to many patients (French & Larrabee, 1999; Weiss, 2007). A properly informed consumer is not only a legal concern in health care today but an ethical one as well.

Readability of PEMs

A substantial body of evidence in the literature indicates that a significant gap exists between patients' reading and comprehension levels and the level of reading difficulty of PEMs (Andrus & Roth, 2002; Ryan et al., 2014; Vallance et al., 2008; Weiss, 2007; Wilson, 2009; Winslow, 2001). Healthcare providers are beginning to recognize that the reams of written materials relied on by so many of them to convey health information to consumers are essentially useless to those with illiteracy and low literacy problems. For example, look at the following text on information about colonoscopy:

> Your naicisyhp has dednemmocer that you have a ypocsonoloc. A ypoc-sonoloc is a test for noloc recnac. It sevlovni gnitresni a elbixelf gniweiv epocs into your mutcer. You must drink a laiceps diuqil the thgin erofeb the noitani-maxe to naelc out your noloc.

Does this passage make sense, or are you confused? The words probably appear unreadable, much like what written teaching instructions look like to someone who cannot read (Weiss, 2003).

Many researchers have assessed specific population groups in a variety of healthcare settings based on the ability of patients to meet the literacy demands of written materials related to their care. Their findings revealed the following information:

- Emergency department instructional materials (average 10th-grade readability) are written at a level of difficulty out of the readable range for most patients (Duffy & Snyder, 1999; Lerner, Jehle, Janicke, & Moscati, 2000; D. M. Williams et al., 1996).
- A significant mismatch exists between the reading ability of older adults and the readability levels of documents essential to their gaining access to health-related services offered through local, state, and federal government programs (Winslow, 2001).
- A large discrepancy exists between patients' average reading comprehension levels and the readability demand of PEMs used in ambulatory care and home care settings (Ache, 2009; Lerner et al., 2000; Schillinger et al., 2002; Walfish & Ducey, 2007; Wood, 2005).

- Standard consent forms used in hospitals, private physician offices, and clinics require high school to college-level reading comprehension (C. C. Doak et al., 1998; Paasche-Orlow, Taylor, & Brancati, 2003; Sudore, Landefeld, et al., 2006).
- Physicians' letters to their patients required an average of 16th- to 17th-grade reading ability; likewise, health articles in newspapers ranged from 12th- to 14th-grade level (Conlin & Schumann, 2002).
- The reading grade levels of 15 psychotropic medication handouts for patient education ranged from 12th to 14th grade, well above the 5th-grade level recommended by the National Cancer Institute guidelines (Myers & Shepard-White, 2004).

As these examples demonstrate, most health education literature is written above the eighth-grade level, with the average level falling between the 10th and 12th grades. Many PEMs exceed this upper range, even though the average reading level of adults falls at the eighth-grade level. Millions of people in the population read at considerably lower levels and need materials written at the fifth-grade level or lower (Bastable, Chojnowski, Goldberg, McGurl, & Riegel, 2005; Brownson, 1998; Davis, Williams, Marin, Parker, & Glass, 2002; C. C. Doak et al., 1998). Furthermore, people typically read at least two grade levels below their highest level of schooling and prefer materials that are written below their literacy abilities. In fact, contrary to popular belief, good readers prefer simplified PEMs when ill because of low energy and concentration levels, and even when well because of the demands of their busy schedules (Giorgianni, 1998; Lasater & Mehler, 1998; Winslow, 2001).

The conclusion to be drawn is that complex and lengthy PEMs serve no useful teaching purpose if consumers of health care are unable to understand them or unwilling to read them. Literacy levels of patients compared with literacy demands of PEMs, whether in hospital or community-based settings, are an important factor in the ability of patients to follow treatment regimens and avoid relapse of their illness. The Internet is an excellent resource for nurses in the role of teacher to locate easy-to-read PEMs.

Methods to Measure Literacy Levels of PEMs

Because nurses rely heavily on PEMs to convey necessary information to their patients, the usefulness and effectiveness of these materials must be determined. To objectively evaluate the difficulty of written materials, two basic measurement methods exist: formulas and tests. Various formulas measure readability of PEMs and are based on finding the average length of sentences and words (vocabulary difficulty) to determine the grade level at which they are written. Standardized tests, which measure actual comprehension and reading skills, involve readers' responses to instructional materials or the ability to decode and pronounce words to determine their grade level.

Readability formulas are mathematical equations that measure literacy levels of PEMs by determining the correlation between an author's style of writing and a reader's ability to identify words as printed symbols within a context (C. C. Doak et al., 1996). Most of them provide fairly accurate grade-level estimates, give or take one grade level of error. In many respects, a readability formula is like a reading test, except that it does not test people but rather written material (Fry, 1977).

The first guideline to remember is that readability formulas should not be the only tool used for assessing PEMs. The second rule is to select readability formulas that have been validated in the reader population for whom the PEM is intended. Several formulas are geared to specific types of materials or population groups. Because so many readability formulas are available for assessment of reading levels of PEMs, only those that are relatively simple to work with, that are accepted as reliable and valid, and that are in widespread use have been chosen for review here.

Flesch-Kincaid Scale

This formula was developed to measure readability of materials between fifth grade and college level. It has been used for more than 50 years to assess news reports, adult education materials, and government publications. The Flesch-Kincaid formula is based on a count of two basic language elements: average sentence length (in words) of selected samples and average word length (measured as syllables per 100 words of sample). The reading ease score is calculated by combining these two variables (Flesch, 1948; Spadaro, 1983; Spadaro, Robinson, & Smith, 1980).

Fog Index

The Fog index developed by Gunning (1968) is appropriate for use in determining the readability of materials from fourth grade to college level. It is calculated based on average sentence length and the percentage of multisyllabic words in a 100-word passage. The Fog index is considered one of the simpler methods because it is based on a short sample of words (100), it does not require counting syllables of all words, and the rules are easy to follow (Spadaro, 1983; Spadaro et al., 1980).

Fry Readability Graph—Extended

The Fry formula tests readability of materials (especially books, pamphlets, and brochures) at the level of first grade through college (C. C. Doak et al., 1996). A series of simple rules can be applied to plot two language elements—the number of syllables and the number of sentences in three 100-word selections (Fry, 1968, 1977; Spadaro et al., 1980).

SMOG Formula

This formula, developed by McLaughlin (1969), is recommended not only because it offers relatively easy computation (simple and fast) but also because it is one of the most valid tests of readability. The SMOG formula measures readability of PEMs from fourth grade to college level based on the number of multisyllabic words within a set number of sentences (C. C. Doak et al., 1996). It evaluates the readability grade level of PEMs to within 1.5 grades of accuracy (Myers & Shepard-White, 2004). Thus, when using the SMOG formula to calculate the grade level of material, the SMOG results are usually about two grades higher than the grade levels calculated by the other methods (Spadaro, 1983). The SMOG formula has been used extensively to judge grade-level readability of patient education materials. It is one of the most popular measurement tools because of its reputation for reading-level accuracy, its simple directions, and its speed of use, which is a particularly important factor if computerized resources for analysis of test samples are not available (Meade & Smith, 1991). See **Appendix 7–A** for how to use the SMOG formula.

C. C. Doak et al. (1996) state that it is critically important to determine the readability of all written materials at the time they are drafted or adopted by using one or more of the many available formulas. These authors believe that you cannot afford to "fly blind" by using health materials that are untested for readability difficulty. Pretesting PEMs before distribution enables the nurse to be sure they fit the literacy level of the audience for which they are intended. It is imperative that the formulas used to measure grade-level readability of PEMs are appropriate for the type of material being tested (**Table 7–2**).

Computerized Readability Software Programs

Computerized programs have greatly facilitated the use of readability formulas. Some software programs are capable of applying a number of formulas to analyze one text selection. In addition, some packages are able to identify difficult words in written passages that may not be understood by patients. Dozens of user-friendly, menu-driven commercial software packages can automatically calculate reading levels as well as provide advice on how to simplify text (Aldridge, 2004; C. C. Doak et al., 1996).

Computerized assessment of readability is fast and easy, and it provides a high degree of reliability, especially when several formulas are used. Determining readability by computer programs rather than doing so manually is also more accurate in calculating reading levels. This is because it eliminates human error in scoring and because entire articles, pamphlets, or books can be scanned (Duffy & Snyder, 1999). It is advisable,

Table 7–2 Appropriate Readability Formula Choice

Formula	Selection Shorter Than 300 Words	Selection Longer Than 300 Words	Entire Piece	Grade Level
Flesch-Kincaid formula	Yes	Yes	Yes	5 to college
Fog index	Yes (minimum of 100 words)	Yes	Yes	4 to college
Fry graph	Not recommended	Yes	Yes	1 to college
SMOG formula	Yes	Yes	Yes	4 to college

Data from Spadero, D. C., Robinson, L. A., & Smith, L. T. (1980). Assessing readability of patient information materials. *American Journal of Hospital Pharmacy, 37,* 215–221; Doak, C. C., Doak, L. G., & Root, J. H. (1996). *Teaching patients with low literacy skills* (2nd ed.). Philadelphia, PA: Lippincott.

however, to use several different formulas and software programs when calculating estimates to get an average level of readability.

Tests to Measure Comprehension of PEMs

A number of standardized tests have proved reliable and valid in measuring a reader's understanding of information—a relatively new concept in health education (C. C. Doak et al., 1996). Measuring how well someone comprehends the content of health education materials is essential from the standpoint of making sure patients are able to assume self-care as well as protecting the health professional from legal liability. The two most popular standardized methods to measure comprehension of written materials are the cloze test and the listening test. These tests can be used to assess how much someone understands from reading or listening to a passage of text.

Cloze Test

This test (derived from the term *closure*) has been specifically recommended for assessing understanding of health education literature. Although it takes more time and resources to perform than do readability formulas, the cloze test has been validated for use in assessing the reading difficulty of medical literature. This procedure is not a formula that provides a school grade-type level of readability like the formulas already described, but rather is an assessment that takes into consideration the context of a written passage (C. C. Doak et al., 1996).

The cloze test should be used only with those individuals whose reading skills are at sixth-grade level or higher (approximately level 1 on the NALS scale); otherwise, it is likely that the test will prove too difficult (C. C. Doak et al., 1996). The reader may or may not be familiar with the material being tested. The procedure for designing the cloze test is to systematically delete every fifth word from a portion of a text. The reader is asked to fill in the blanks with the exact word replacements. One point is scored for every missing word guessed correctly by the reader. The final cloze score is the total number of blanks filled in correctly by the reader. To be successful, the reader must demonstrate sensitivity to clues related to grammar and vocabulary. How well the reader is able to fill in the blanks with appropriate words indicates how well the material has been comprehended (Dale & Chall, 1978; C. C. Doak et al., 1996). A score for the cloze test is obtained by dividing the number of exact word replacements by the total number of blanks. A score of 60% or better indicates that the passage was sufficiently understood by the patient. A score of 40% to 59% indicates a moderate level of difficulty, where supplemental teaching is required for the patient to understand the message. A score of less than 40% indicates the material is too difficult and is not suitable to be used for teaching (C. C. Doak et al., 1996).

Because the cloze test determines the learners' ability to understand what they have read, be sure to be honest about the purpose of the test. You might state that it is important for patients to understand what they are to do when on their own after discharge, so the nurse in the role of teacher wants to be sure they understand the written instructions they will need to follow. C. C. Doak, Doak, and Root (1985) found that most people are willing to participate in this testing activity. They suggest that the following guidelines should be used in preparing participants for the cloze test:

1. Encourage participants to read through the entire test passage before attempting to fill in the blanks.
2. Tell them that only one word should be written in each blank.
3. Let them know that it is okay to guess but that they should try to fill in every blank as accurately as possible.
4. Reassure them that spelling errors are okay just as long as the word they have put in the blank can be recognized.
5. Explain to them that this exercise is not a timed test. (If readers struggle to complete the test, tell them not to worry, that it is not necessary for them to fill in all the blanks, and set the test aside to go on to something else less frustrating or less threatening.)

Listening Test

Unlike the cloze test, which may be too difficult for patients who read below the sixth-grade level—that is, for those persons who likely lack fluency and read with hesitancy—the listening test is a good approach to determining what a low-literate person understands and remembers when listening (C. C. Doak et al., 1996). The procedure for administering the listening test is to select a passage from an instructional material that takes about 3 minutes to read aloud and is written at approximately the fifth-grade level. Formulate 5 to 10 short questions relevant to the content of the passage by selecting key points of the text. Read the passage to the person at a normal rate. Ask the listener the questions orally and record the answers (C. C. Doak et al., 1996). To determine the percentage score, divide the number of questions answered correctly by the total number of questions. The instructional material will be appropriate for the patient's comprehension level if the score is in the range of 75% to 89% (some additional assistance when teaching the material may be necessary for full comprehension). A score of 90% or higher indicates that the material is easy for the patient and can be fully comprehended independently. A score of less than 75% means that the material is too difficult, and simpler instructional material will need to be used when teaching the individual. Doak et al. (1996) provide an example of a sample listening test passage and questions to measure comprehension.

Tests to Measure General Reading Skills and Health Literacy Skills of Patients

The four most popular standardized methods to measure reading and health literacy skills are the Wide Range Achievement Test (WRAT), the Rapid Estimate of Adult Literacy in Medicine (REALM), the Test of Functional Health Literacy in Adults (TOFHLA), and the Newest Vital Sign (NVS). In addition, the eHealth Literacy Scale assesses patient comfort in using the Internet and technology to obtain health information. The Literacy Assessment for Diabetes is an instrument specific to patients with diabetes. The Suitability Assessment of Materials (SAM) assesses how appropriate instructional materials are for the intended audience of patients.

WRAT

The WRAT is a word recognition screening test that takes 5 minutes to administer. It is used to assess a learner's ability to recognize and pronounce a list of words out of context as a criterion for measuring reading skills.

Although it does not test other aspects of reading such as vocabulary and comprehension of text material, this test is nevertheless useful for determining an appropriate level of instruction and for establishing a patient's level of literacy. As designed, the WRAT should be used only to test people whose native language is English. It tests on two levels: Level I is designed for testing children 5 to 12 years of age, and Level II is intended for testing persons older than age 12. The WRAT consists of a graduated list of 42 words, starting with the most easy and ending with the most difficult. The individual administering the test listens carefully to the patient's responses. Next to those words that are mispronounced, a checkmark should be placed. When five words are mispronounced, indicating that the patient has reached his or her limit, the test is stopped. To score the test, the number of words missed or not tried is subtracted from the total list of words on the master score sheet to get a raw score. A table of raw scores is then used to find the equivalent grade rating. For more information on this test, see Doak et al. (1996), Davis et al. (1998), and Quirk (2000).

REALM

The REALM test has advantages over the WRAT and other word tests because it measures a patient's ability to read medical and health-related vocabulary, it takes less time to administer, the scoring is simpler, and the test is well received by most patients (Davis et al., 1998; Duffy & Snyder, 1999; Foltz & Sullivan, 1998). Although it has established validity, REALM offers less precision than other word tests (Hayes, 2000). The raw score is converted to a range of grade levels rather than an exact grade level, but this result correlates well with the WRAT reading scores.

A list of 66 medical and health-related words are arranged in 3 columns of 22 words each, beginning with short, easy words such as *fat, flu, pill,* and *dose,* and ending with more difficult words such as *anemia, obesity, osteoporosis,* and *impetigo.* Patients are asked to begin at the top of the first column and read down, pronouncing all the words that they can from the 3 lists. The total number of words pronounced correctly is the patient's raw score, which is converted to a grade ranging from third grade and below to ninth grade and above (Schultz, 2002; Weiss, 2003).

TOFHLA

The TOFHLA was developed in the mid-1990s for measuring patients' health literacy skills using actual hospital materials, such as prescription labels, appointment slips, and informed consent documents. The test consists of two parts: reading comprehension and numeracy. It has demonstrated reliability and validity, requires approximately

20 minutes to administer, and is available in a Spanish version (TOFHLA-S) as well as an English version (Parker, Baker, Williams, & Nurss, 1995; Quirk, 2000; M. V. Williams et al., 1995).

NVS

The NVS is a tool recently developed to identify those at risk for low health literacy. It is available in both English and Spanish versions and is easy and inexpensive to administer, taking as little as 3 minutes from start to finish (Johnson & Weiss, 2008; Welch, VanGeest, & Caskey, 2011). Patients are asked to look at an ice cream label and answer questions in relation to the label (Collins et al., 2012; Weiss, 2007). Each correct answer gives them one point. Patients are placed into one of three categories related to their literacy level: likelihood of limited literacy; possibility of limited literacy; and adequate literacy (Johnson & Weiss, 2008). It is suggested that the tool be administered while the nurse is obtaining vital signs. More information on this tool can be found free of charge at http://www.pfizerhealthliteracy.com/physicians-providers/NewestVitalSign .aspx. See Appendix 7–A.

eHealth Literacy Scale

The eHealth Literacy Scale, which was designed by Norman and Skinner (2006a), is one of only a few tools available to determine a patient's ability to find and navigate electronic health information. It consists of eight items that collectively measure patients' comfort level and perceived ability to address their health problems by finding and using electronic health information. This scale offers a way to assess whether a patient would be a good candidate to engage in e-health materials (Collins et al., 2012).

Literacy Assessment for Diabetes

The Literacy Assessment for Diabetes was specifically developed in 2001 to measure word recognition in adult patients with diabetes (Nath et al., 2001). It consists of three word lists presented in ascending order of difficulty. The majority of terms are at the fourth-grade reading level, but the remaining words range from 6th- through 16th-grade levels. The Literacy Assessment for Diabetes can be administered in 3 minutes or less.

SAM

In addition to using formulas and tests to measure readability, comprehension, and reading skills, C. C. Doak et al. (1996) designed the SAM instrument to rapidly and systematically assess the suitability of instructional materials for a given population of learners. Not only can the SAM tool be used with print material and illustrations, but it has also been applied to videotaped and audiotaped instructions.

The SAM instrument yields a numerical (percentage) score, with materials tested falling into one of three categories: superior, adequate, or not suitable. The SAM instrument can assess the content, literacy demand, graphics, layout and typography, learning stimulation and motivation, and cultural appropriateness of instructional materials being developed or already in use (L. G. Doak & Doak, 2010).

Simplifying the Readability of PEMs

Even though printed materials are the most commonly used form of media, as currently written, they remain the least effective means for reaching a large proportion of the adult population who have marginal literacy skills (Monsivais & Reynolds, 2003; Ryan et al., 2014). Despite the well-documented potential of written materials to increase knowledge, compliance, and satisfaction with care, PEMs are often too difficult for even motivated patients to read. Agarwal, Hansberry, Sabourin, Tomei, & Prestigiacomo (2013) studied online patient education materials from 16 specialties. Readability assessments found all materials to be well over the sixth-grade reading level. What the nurse in the role of teacher must strive to achieve when designing or selecting health-based literature is a good and proper fit between the material and the reader (Winslow, 2001).

Certainly the best solution for improving the overall comprehension and reading skills of patients would be to strengthen their basic general education, but this process would require decades to accomplish. What is needed now are ways in which to write or rewrite educational materials to match the current comprehension and reading skills of learners. Nathaniel Hawthorne was once reported to have said, "Easy reading is damned hard writing" (Pichert & Elam, 1985, p. 181). He was correct in his perception that clear and concise writing is a task that takes effort and practice. It is possible, though, to reduce the disparity between the literacy demand of written instructional materials and the actual reading level of patients. This requires attention to some basic linguistic, motivational, organizational, and content principles. *Linguistics* refers to the type of language and grammatical style used. *Motivation principles* focus on those elements that stimulate the reader, such as relevance and appeal of the material. *Organizational factors* deal with layout and clarity. *Content principles* relate to load and concept density of information (Bernier, 1993; Wood et al., 2007).

Prior to writing or rewriting a text for easier reading, some preliminary planning steps need to be taken to ensure that the final written material will be geared to the target audience (Davis et al., 1998; C. C. Doak et al., 1996; Kessels, 2003):

1. *Decide what the patient should do or know.* In other words, what is the purpose of the instruction? Which outcomes do you hope learners will achieve?
2. *Choose information that is relevant and needed by the patient to achieve the behavioral objectives.* Limit or cut out altogether extraneous and nice-to-know information such as the history or detailed physiological processes of a disease. Include only survival skills and essential main ideas of who, what, where, and when, with new information related to what the reader already knows. Remember: A person does not have to know how an engine works to drive a car.

3. *Select other media to supplement the written information*. This could include pictures, demonstrations, models, audiotapes or CDs, and videotapes or DVDs. Even poor readers will benefit from written material if it is combined with other forms of delivering a message. Consider the field of advertising, for example. Advertisers get their message across with relatively few words that are often combined with strong, action-packed visuals.

4. *Organize topics into chunks that follow a logical sequence*. Prioritize to present the most important information first. If topics are of equal importance, proceed from the more general as a basis on which to build to the more specific. Begin with a statement of purpose. In a list of items, place key facts at the top and bottom because readers best remember information presented first and last in a series.

5. *Determine the preferred reading level of the material*. If the readers have been tested, preferably write two to four grades below their reading grade-level score. If the audience has not been tested, the group is likely to display a wide range of reading skills. When in doubt, write instructional materials at the fifth-grade level, which is the lowest common denominator, keeping in mind that the average reading level of the population is approximately eighth grade, that more than 20% read below the fifth-grade level, and that fewer than 50% read above the 10th-grade level.

6. *Consider developing two sets of instructions to cover a wide range of reading skills*. One set can be at a higher grade level and one at a lower grade level, and patients can select the one they prefer. Once the reading grade level of a piece of written material is determined, it should be printed on the back of the document in coded form as, for example, RL = 7 (reading level = seventh grade), for easy reference.

The literature contains numerous references related to techniques for writing effective educational materials (Aldridge, 2004; Andrus & Roth, 2002; Buxton, 1999; C. C. Doak et al., 1996, 1998; L. G. Doak & Doak, 2010; Duffy & Snyder, 1999; Horner et al., 2000; Mayer & Rushton, 2002; Monsivais & Reynolds, 2003; Pignone et al., 2005; Weiss, 2007).

The strategies described in this section are specific with regard to simplifying written health information for patients with low literacy skills. The key factor in accommodating low-literate readers is to write in plain, familiar language using an easy visual format. The following general guidelines outline some basic linguistic, motivational, organizational, and content principles to adhere to when writing effective PEMs:

1. Write in a conversational style using the personal pronoun *you* and the possessive pronoun *your*. Use an active voice in the present tense rather than a passive voice in the past or future tense. The message is more personalized, more imperative, more interesting, and easier to understand if instruction is written as "Take your medicine . . ." instead of "Medicine should be taken . . ." This rule is considered to be the most important technique to reduce the level of reading difficulty and to improve comprehension of what is read. Directly addressing

the reader through personal words and sentences engages the reader. For example:

Less Effective

People who sunburn easily and have fair skin with red or blond hair are most prone to develop skin cancer. The amount of time spent in the sun affects a person's risk of skin cancer.[1]

More Effective

If you sunburn easily and have fair skin with red or blond hair, you are more likely to get skin cancer. How much time you spend in the sun affects your risk of skin cancer.

2. Use short words and common vocabulary words with only one or two syllables as much as possible. Rely on sight words, known as high-frequency words, which are recognized by almost everyone. The key is to choose words that sound familiar and natural and are easy to read and understand, such as *shot* rather than *injection, doctor* rather than *physician*, and *use* instead of *utilize*. Avoid compound words, such as *lifesaver*, and words with prefixes or suffixes, such as *reoccur* or *emptying*, that create multisyllable words.

   Also, try to avoid technical words and medical terms, and substitute common, nontechnical, lay terms such as *stroke* instead of *cardiovascular accident*. Select substitutions carefully because they may have a different meaning for some people than for others. For example, if the word *medicine* is replaced with the word *drug*, the latter may be interpreted as the illegal variety. Using modest words is not considered talking down to patients; it is considered talking to them at a more comfortable level.

3. Spell out words rather than using abbreviations or acronyms. *That is* should be used instead of *i.e.* and *for example* instead of *e.g.* Abbreviations for the months of the year (such as *Sept.*) or the days of the week (such as *Wed.*) are a real problem for patients with limited vocabulary. Also do not use acronyms, such as CVA or NPO, unless these medical abbreviations are clearly defined beforehand in the text.

4. Organize information into chunks, which improves recall. Also, use numbers sparingly and only when absolutely necessary. Statistics are usually meaningless and are another source of confusion for the low-literate reader. Limit the number of items in any list to no more than seven. People have a difficult time remembering more than seven consecutive items (Baddeley, 1994).

5. Keep sentences short, preferably not longer than 20 words and fewer if possible, because they are easier to read and understand for patients with short-term memories. Avoid use of commas, colons, or dashes that result in long, complex sentences that turn off the reader. Titles also should be short and convey the purpose and meaning of the material that follows.

---

[1] American Cancer Society. (1985). *Fry now, pay later* (No. 2611).

6. Clearly define any technical or unfamiliar words by using parentheses that include simple terms after difficult words—for example, "bacteria (germ)." A glossary of terms is a helpful tool, but spell out terms phonetically (by how they sound), immediately following the unfamiliar word within the text—for example, "Alzheimer's (pronounced Alts-hi-merz)." If a new vocabulary word needs to be introduced, such as the medical term *hypertension*, it should be used and repeated frequently or simplified to the term *high blood pressure* (Byrne & Edeani, 1984; Spees, 1991). Technical words should be taught to the reader prior to introducing the instructional material to increase reader comprehension (Standal, 1981).

7. Use words consistently throughout the text and avoid interchanging words. For example, if discussing diet, continue to use the word *diet* rather than substituting other terms for it, such as *meal plan, menu, food schedule,* and *dietary prescription*, which merely confuse readers and can lead to misunderstanding of instruction.

8. Avoid value judgment words with many interpretations, such as *excessive, regularly,* and *frequently*. How much pain or bleeding is excessive? How often is regularly or frequently? Use exact terms to describe what you mean by using, for example, a scale of 1–5 or explaining frequency in terms of minutes, hours, or days. For example, instead of saying "drink milk frequently," you should be more specific by stating "drink three full glasses of milk every day."

9. Put the most important information first by prioritizing the need-to-know information. Place essential messages up front and get rid of extraneous details.

10. Use advance organizers (topic headings or headers) and subheadings. They clue the reader as to what is going to be presented and help focus the reader's attention on the message.

11. Limit the use of connectives such as *however, consequently, even though,* and *in spite of* that lengthen sentences and make them more complex.

12. Make the first sentence of a paragraph the topic sentence, and, if possible, make the first word the topic of the sentence. For example:

Less Effective

Even though overexposure to the sun is the leading cause, it isn't necessary to give up the outdoors in order to reduce your chances of developing skin cancer.[2]

More Effective

Enjoying the outdoors is still possible if you take steps to reduce your risk of skin cancer when in the sun.

or

You can reduce your chance of skin cancer even when enjoying the outdoors.

---

[2] American Cancer Society. (1985). *Fry now, pay later* (No. 2611).

13. Reduce concept density by limiting each paragraph to a simple message or action and include only one idea per sentence.

14. Keep density of words low by not exceeding 30 to 40 characters (letters) per line (count each space between words as one character). Note: The number of words in each line is dependent on the size of the font.

15. Allow for plenty of white space in margins, and use generous spacing between paragraphs and double spacing within paragraphs to reduce density. Pages that are not crowded seem less overwhelming to the reader with low literacy skills.

16. Keep right margins unjustified because the jagged right margins help the reader distinguish one line from another. In this way, the eye does not have to adjust to different spacing between letters and words as it does with justified type.

17. Design layouts that encourage eye movement from left to right, as in normal reading. In simple drawings and diagrams, use arrows or circles that give direction to the reader.

18. Select a simple type style (serif, Times New Roman, or Courier) and a large font (14 or 16 point size) in the body of the text for ease of reading and to increase motivation to read. A sans serif font (which does not have the little hooks at the top and bottom of letters) or other type of clean style should be used only for titles to give style to the page. Avoid *italics*, *fancy lettering,* and ALL CAPITAL letters. Low-literate readers are not fluent with the alphabet and need to look at each letter to recognize a word. To help poor readers decode words in titles, headings, and subheadings, use uppercase and lowercase letters, which provide reading cues given by tall and short letters on the type line. Avoid using a large stylized letter to begin a new paragraph, such as in this example:

    *T*his looks attractive, but it is confusing to a poor reader who cannot decode the word minus the first letter.

19. Highlight important ideas or key terms with **bold type** or <u>underlining.</u>

20. If using color, use it consistently throughout the text to emphasize key points or to organize topics. Color, if applied appropriately, attracts the reader. Bright, bold colors are more eye-catching and easier to read than light, pastel colors.

21. Create a simple cover page with a short title (ideally one to four words in length) that clearly and succinctly states the topic to be addressed.

22. Limit the entire length of a document—the shorter, the better. It should be long enough just to cover the essential, need-to-know information. Too many pages with nice-to-know information will turn off even the most eager and capable reader.

23. Select paper on which the typeface is easy to read. Black print on white paper is most easily read and most inexpensive. Dull (rather than high gloss) finishes reduce the glare of light. Appearance must match the informal tone of your message.

24. Use bold line drawings and simple, realistic pictures and diagrams. Basic visuals aid the reader to better understand the text information. Use cartoons carefully because they can make the message seem less important or less believable.

Graphic designs that are strictly decorative should never be used because they are distracting and confusing. Also, never overlay words on a background design because it makes reading the letters of the words very difficult. Only illustrations that enhance understanding of the text and that relate specifically to the message should be included.

The visuals should clearly show only those actions that you want the reader to do and remember. Avoid cultural bias.

Use simple subtitles and captions for each picture. Also, be sure drawings are recognizable to the audience. For instance, if you draw a picture of the lungs, be certain they are within the outline of the person's body to accurately depict the location of the organs. The person with low literacy may not know what he or she is looking at if the lungs are not put in context with the body's torso.

25. Include a summary section to review what has already been presented. Ask for feedback after patients have read your instructions. Either have readers explain the information in their own words or have them demonstrate the desired behavior. If learners can do so correctly, it is a good indication that the information is understood. Avoid asking questions such as "Do you understand?" because you are likely to get only a "yes" or "no" answer.

26. Put the reading level (RL) on the back of the PEM for future reference (e.g., sixth-grade level would be RL = 6).

27. Determine readability, reading skills, and comprehension by applying a selection of formulas described in this chapter. (See Appendix 7–A)

It does not take a great deal of effort to improve the readability and comprehension level of instructional materials. (**Table 7–3** provides a summary of tips.) The benefits are significant in terms of compliance and quality of care when marginally literate patients are given PEMs that effectively communicate messages they can read and understand.

Always remember to test any new materials before printing and distributing them. Not only will this effort save the cost of printing handouts that might not be useful, but patients will have the opportunity to participate in the evaluation process. As L. G. Doak and C. C. Doak (1987) so aptly point out, "With so much to be gained, the investments of a little time and thoughtful attention to the materials provided to patients can pay back dividends too important to ignore" (p. 8).

Strategies to Promote Health Literacy

Working with patients who are illiterate and low literate requires more than just designing simple-to-read instructional literature. It also calls for using alternative and innovative teaching strategies to break down the barriers of illiteracy. Using techniques to improve communication with patients has the potential to greatly enhance their understanding (Mayeaux et al., 1996; Weiss, 2007).

Teaching patients with poor reading skills does not have to be viewed as a problem, but rather can be seen as a challenge (Dunn, Buckwalter, Weinstein, & Palti, 1985).

Table 7–3 Formatting Checklist for Easy-to-Read Written Materials

General Content
• Limit content to one or two key objectives. Don't provide too much information or try to cover everything at once.
• Limit content to what patients really need to know. Avoid information overload.
• Use only words that are well known to individuals without medical training.
• Make certain content is appropriate for age and culture of the target audience.

Text Construction
• Write at or below the fifth-grade level.
• Use one- or two-syllable words.
• Use short paragraphs.
• Use active voice.
• Avoid all but the most simple tables and graphs. Clear explanations (legends) should be placed next to the table or graph, and also in the text.

Fonts and Type Styles
• Use large font (minimum 12 point) with serifs. (Serif text has the little horizontal lines that you see in this text at the bottoms of letters like f, x, n, and others. This text, on the other hand, is sans serif.)
• Don't use more than two or three font styles on a page. Consistency in appearance is important.
• Use upper and lowercase text. ALL UPPERCASE TEXT IS HARD TO READ.

Layout
• Ensure a good amount of empty space on the page. Don't clutter the page with a lot of words or pictures.
• Use headings and subheadings to separate blocks of text.
• Bulleted lists are preferable to blocks or text in paragraphs.
• Illustrations are useful if they show simple, easy-to-recognize objects. Images of people, places, and things should be age appropriate and culturally appropriate to the target audience. Avoid complex diagrams.

Reproduced from Weiss BD. *Help patients understand: A Manual for clinicians*. 2nd ed. Chicago: American Medical Association and American Medical Association Foundation; 2007.

Many literate and highly motivated patients also can benefit from some of these same teaching strategies.

Many authors (Austin, Matlock, Dunn, Kesler, & Brown, 1995; Davis et al., 2002; C. C. Doak et al., 1998; Houts et al., 1998; Hyde & Kautz, 2014; Kessels, 2003; Lerner et al., 2000; Mayeaux et al., 1996; Pignone et al., 2005; Rothman et al., 2004; Ryan et al., 2014; Schultz, 2002; Webber, Higgins, & Baker, 2001; Weiss, 2007; Winslow, 2001) suggest the following tips as useful strategies for the nurse to use when in the role of teacher:

1. *Establish a trusting relationship (partnership) before beginning the teaching–learning process.* Start by getting to know the patients to reduce their anxiety. Because many poor readers have a history of being defensive, the nurse must attempt to overcome their defense mechanisms. Focus on patients' strengths, be open and honest about what specifically needs to be learned, and build up their confidence in their ability to perform self-care activities. Encourage family and friends to help reinforce the patients' self-confidence.

2. *Use the smallest amount of information possible to accomplish the predetermined behavioral objectives.* Stick to the essentials by focusing on the need-to-know rather than nice-to-know information. Prioritize information by selecting only one or two concepts to present and discuss in any one session. Explain what you are going to teach before giving any new information. Remember, patients with poor comprehension and reading skills are easily overwhelmed. Therefore, keep teaching sessions short, limiting them to no more than 15 to 20 minutes each.

3. *Make points of information as vivid and explicit as possible.* Explain information in simple, concrete terms using everyday language and personal examples relevant to the patient's background. For example, a sign reading "NOTHING BY MOUTH" or, worse yet, "NPO" should be changed to "Do not eat or drink anything" (remember to avoid using all-capital letters and abbreviations). Visual aids, such as signs and pictures (pictographs), should be large with readable print and contain only one or two messages. Underlining, highlighting, color coding, arrows, and common international symbols can be used effectively to give directions and draw attention to important information.

4. *Teach one step at a time.* Teaching information in small amounts (chunks) helps to reduce anxiety and confusion and gives enough time for patients to understand each item and ask questions before proceeding to the next unit of information. The pacing of instruction allows for more adequate time between sessions for learners to absorb information.

5. *Use multiple teaching methods and tools requiring fewer literacy skills.* Oral instruction, which contains cues such as tone, gestures, and expressions, should be used first. Next follow up with resources such as simple lists, pictures, audiotapes, videotapes, and interactive computer programs. These media forms can be sent home with the patient to reinforce health messages.

6. *Allow patients the chance to restate information in their own words and to demonstrate any procedures being taught (teach-back or tell-back).* Encouraging learners to explain something in their own words is a patient-centered approach to learning and can reveal gaps in knowledge or misconceptions of information. Return demonstration, hands-on practice, role playing real-life situations, and sharing personal stories in dialogue form are communication modes that provide you with feedback as to the patient's level of functioning (Fidyk, Ventura, & Green, 2014; Kemp, Floyd, McCord-Duncan, & Lang, 2008; Hyde & Kautz, 2014).

7. *Elicit feedback by asking questions and making statements appropriately.* Avoid asking questions that will elicit only a "yes" or "no" response, because patients will likely answer that they understand so as to not appear dumb or ignorant. Instead, use open-ended statements, such as "Tell me what you understand about . . . ," to obtain feedback from them to verify their comprehension. Encouraging patients to repeat instructions in their own words or physically demonstrate an activity is an effective approach to verifying what they really understand (Chew et al., 2004).

8. *Keep motivation high*. People with limited literacy may feel like failures when they cannot work through a problem. Reassure them that it is normal to have trouble with new information and that they are doing well and encourage them to keep trying. Recognize any progress they make, even if it is small. Rewards—not punishments—are excellent motivators to maintain a learner's interest and willingness to learn.

9. *Coordinate procedures to fit into everyday routines*. A way to facilitate learning is to simplify information by using the principles of tailoring and cueing. **Tailoring** refers to coordinating recommended regimens into the daily schedules of patients rather than forcing them to adjust their lifestyles to these regimens imposed on them. Tailoring allows new tasks to be associated with old behaviors. For example, coordinating a medication schedule to a patient's mealtimes does not drastically alter everyday lifestyle and tends to increase motivation and compliance. **Cueing** focuses on the appropriate combination of time and situation using prompts and reminders to get a person to perform a routine task. For example, placing medications where they best can be seen on a frequent basis or keeping a simple chart to check off each time a pill is taken serves as a reminder to comply with taking medications as prescribed.

10. *Use repetition to reinforce information*. Repetition, at appropriate intervals, is a key strategy to use with patients who have low literacy. Review information often and set aside time to remind learners of what has already been learned and to prepare them for what is to follow. Repetition, in the form of saying the same thing in different ways, is one of the most powerful tools to increase understanding.

All of these teaching strategies are especially well suited to the individual needs of people with low literacy skills. Creating an open, trusting, and accepting environment that makes it all right for the patient to say, "I don't understand," is the cornerstone of effective communication (Cole, 2000). It is always a challenge to teach patients who, because of illness or a threat to their well-being, may be anxious, frightened, depressed, in denial, or in pain. Teaching patients is even more of a special challenge in today's healthcare environment, when varying degrees of literacy in a significant portion of the adult population interferes with their ability to understand information vital to their health and welfare.

Summary

The prevalence of functional illiteracy and low literacy is a major problem in the adult population of this country. Nurses in the role of teachers and interpreters of health information must always be alert to the potentially limited capacity of patients to grasp the meaning of written and oral instruction. Nurses need to know how to identify patients with literacy problems, assess their needs, and choose appropriate interventions that help those with poor reading and comprehension skills to better and more safely care for themselves. An awareness of the effects that literacy levels have on motivation and compliance with self-management regimens is key to understanding the barriers to communication between nurses and patients.

The first half of this chapter focused on defining literacy terms, the scope of the illiteracy problem, the populations at risk, myths and stereotypes associated with poor literacy skills, and the assessment of literacy levels. The remainder of the chapter examined the readability of printed education materials (PEMs), the measurement tools available to test for readability of PEMs as well as the comprehension and reading skills of patients, guidelines for writing effective education materials, and specific teaching strategies to be used to match the logic, language, and experience of low literate patients.

Written materials are an important source of health information to reinforce and complement other methods and tools of instruction. PEMs are the most cost-effective and time-efficient means to communicate health messages. However, a large gap exists between the reading skills of patients and the readability level of current written instructional aids. Unless this gap is narrowed, printed sources of information will serve no useful purpose for adults who suffer with illiteracy and low literacy.

Removing the barriers to communication between patients and healthcare providers offers an ideal opportunity for nurses to improve the quality of care delivered to consumers. It is their mandated responsibility to teach in understandable terms so that patients can fully benefit from interventions to enhance their health and well-being.

Review Questions

1. What are the definitions of the terms *literacy, illiteracy, low literacy, functional illiteracy*, and *health literacy*? How are literacy and health literacy different?
2. Approximately how many Americans are considered to be illiterate or functionally illiterate? What percentage of the U.S. population does this number represent?
3. Why are the rates of low literacy and illiteracy suspected to be on the rise in the United States?
4. Why is the number of years of schooling a poor indicator of someone's literacy level?
5. Which segments of the U.S. population are more likely to be at risk for having poor reading and comprehension skills?
6. Why are problems with low literacy and functional illiteracy greater in older adults than in younger age groups?
7. What are three common myths about people who are illiterate?
8. What are the clues that patients who are illiterate may demonstrate?
9. How does illiteracy or low literacy affect a person's level of motivation and compliance?
10. How does relying on printed educational material pose an ethical or legal liability for nurses?

11. Which measurement tools are used specifically to test readability, comprehension, reading, and health literacy skills?
12. What are the 27 general guidelines to simplify written educational materials?
13. What are 10 teaching strategies that can be used by nurses to make health information more understandable for patients with poor reading and comprehension skills?

Case Study

As an institution committed to serving the community, Smithfield University Hospital has agreed to provide healthcare services to the women and children living in the Elias Domestic Violence Shelter (EDVS), located 5 miles from the hospital. These services include a special weekly clinic held at the shelter as well as in-hospital services as needed. It is anticipated that all units in the hospital will participate in the program.

EDVS is a 32-bed shelter for women and children seeking refuge from violence in their homes. The residents represent the highest-risk segment of the domestic violence population. The violence they have experienced is severe, and they have very limited social and material resources. Women and children come to the shelter because they have nowhere else to go. Only a few of the women are employed, and the majority of them have not completed high school. Their healthcare needs range from emergency services to acute and preventive physical and mental health services. Several of the women and children have chronic conditions. The residents are a transient population, and their contact with healthcare services is limited and infrequent. Health education is an important component of the care they receive from the nursing staff, who strive to teach them to care for themselves and their children.

1. Which risk factors suggest that this population may have low literacy and inadequate health literacy skills?
2. As the nurse providing education, how would you assess the reading and comprehension levels of the residents? Which clues will you look for?
3. Select a teaching strategy you would use with this population. Explain why this strategy would work when teaching groups with mixed literacy levels.
4. How will you evaluate the learning that has taken place as a result of your instruction?

References

Ache, K. A. (2009). Are end of life patient education materials readable? *Palliative Medicine, 23*, 545–548.

Ad Hoc Committee on Health Literacy for the Council on Scientific Affairs, American Medical Association. (1999). Health literacy: Report of the Council on Scientific Affairs. *Journal of the American Medical Association, 281*(6), 552–557.

Adkins, A. D., Elkins, E. N., & Singh, N. N. (2001). Readability of NIMH easy to read patient education materials. *Journal of Child and Family Studies, 10*, 279–285.

Agarwal, N., Hansberry, D. R., Sabourin, V., Tomei, K. L., & Prestigiacomo, C. J. (2013). Research letter: A comparative analysis of the quality of patient education materials from medical specialists. *JAMA Internal Medicine, 173*(13), 1257–1259.

Aldridge, M. D. (2004). Writing and designing readable patient education materials. *Nephrology Nursing Journal, 31*(4), 373–377.

Andrus, M. R., & Roth, M. T. (2002). Health literacy: A review. *Pharmacotherapy, 22*(3), 282–302.

Austin, P. E., Matlock, R., Dunn, K. A., Kesler, C., & Brown, C. K. (1995). Discharge instructions: Do illustrations help our patients understand them? *Annals of Emergency Medicine, 25*(3), 317–320.

Baddeley, A. (1994). The magical number seven: Still magic after all these years? *Psychological Review, 101*(2), 353–356.

Baer, J., Kutner, M., & Sabatini, J. (2009). *Basic reading skills and the literacy of America's least literate adults: Results from the 2003 National Assessment of Adult Literacy (NALS) Supplemental Studies* (NCES 2009-481). Washington, DC: National Center for Education Statistics, Institute of Education Sciences, U.S. Department of Education.

Baker, D. W. (2006). The meaning and measure of health literacy. *Journal of General Internal Medicine, 21*, 878–883.

Baker, D. W., Parker, R. M., Williams, M. V., & Clark, W. S. (1998). Health literacy and the risk of hospital admission. *Journal of General Internal Medicine, 13*, 791–798.

Baker, D. W., Williams, M. V., Parker, R. M., Gazmararian, J. A., & Nurss, J. (1999). Development of a brief test to measure functional health literacy. *Patient Education and Counseling, 38*, 33–42.

Bastable, L. C., Chojnowski, D., Goldberg, L., McGurl, P., & Riegel, B. (2005, September). *Comparing heart failure patient literacy levels with available educational materials.* Poster presentation at the Heart Failure Society of America, 9th Annual Scientific Conference, Boca Raton, FL.

Baur, C. (2011). Calling the nation to act: Implementing the national action plan to improve health literacy. *Nursing Outlook, 59*, 63–69.

Bennett, I. M., Chen, J., Soroui, J., & White, S. (2009). The contribution of health literacy to disparities in self-rated health status and preventative health behaviors in older adults. *Annals of Family Medicine, 7*, 204–211.

Berkman, N. D., Sheridan, S. L., Donahue, K. E., Halpern, D. J., & Crotty, K. (2011). Low health literacy and health outcomes: An updated systematic review. *Annals of Internal Medicine, 155*(2), 97–107.

Bernier, M. J. (1993). Developing and evaluating printed education materials: A prescriptive model for quality. *Orthopaedic Nursing, 12*(6), 39–46.

Brownson, K. (1998). Education handouts: Are we wasting our time? *Journal for Nurses in Staff Development, 14*(4), 176–182.

Buxton, T. (1999). Effective ways to improve health education materials. *Journal of Health Education, 30*(1), 47–50, 61.

Byrne, T., & Edeani, D. (1984). Knowledge of medical terminology among hospital patients. *Nursing Research, 33*(3), 178–181.

Carol, P. (2007). Health literacy: A critical patient safety tool. *RT, The Journal for Respiratory Care Practitioners, 20*(7), 36–39.

Centers for Disease Control and Prevention (CDC). (2009). *Improving health literacy for older adults: Expert panel report 2009.* Atlanta, GA: U.S. Department of Health and Human Services. Retrieved from http://www.cdc.gov/healthliteracy/Learn/Resources.html

Centers for Disease Control and Prevention (CDC). (2015). *Learn about health literacy*. Retrieved from http://www.cdc.gov/healthliteracy/Learn/index.html

Chew, L. D., Bradley, K. A., & Boyko, E. J. (2004). Brief questions to identify patients with inadequate health literacy. *Family Medicine, 36*(8), 588–594.

Clancy, C. (2011). *Health literacy research in action: Empowering patients and improving health care quality*. Agency for Healthcare Research and Quality (AHRQ). Retrieved from http://www.nap.edu/read/13016/Chapter/7

Cole, M. R. (2000). The high risk of low literacy. *Nursing Spectrum, 13*(10), 16–17.

Collins, S. A., Currie, L. M., Bakken, S., Vawdrey, D. K., & Stone, P. W. (2012). Health literacy screening instruments for eHealth applications: A systematic review. *Journal of Biomedical Informatics, 45*, 598–607.

Conlin, K. K., & Schumann, L. (2002). Literacy in the health care system: A study on open heart surgery patients. *Journal of the American Academy of Nurse Practitioners, 14*(1), 38–42.

Crandell, T. L., Crandell, C. H., & Vander Zanden, J. W. (2012). *Human development* (10th ed.). New York, NY: McGraw-Hill.

Cutilli, C. C. (2005). Do your patients understand? Determining your patient's health literacy skills. *Orthopaedic Nursing, 24*(5), 372–377.

Dale, E., & Chall, J. S. (1978). The cloze procedure: Measuring the readability of selected patient education materials. *Health Education, 9*, 8–10.

Darling, S. (2004, Spring). Family literacy: Meeting the needs of at-risk families. *Phi Kappa Phi Forum*, 18–21.

Davidhizar, R. E., & Brownson, K. (1999). Literacy, cultural diversity, and client education. *Health Care Manager, 18*(1), 39–47.

Davis, T. C., Michielutte, R., Askov, E. N., Williams, M. V., & Weiss, B. D. (1998). Practical assessment of adult literacy in health care. *Health Education & Behavior, 25*(5), 613–624.

Davis, T. C., Williams, M. V., Marin, E., Parker, R. M., & Glass, J. (2002). Health literacy and cancer communication. *CA: A Cancer Journal for Clinicians, 52*(3), 134–151.

Davis, T. C., Wolf, M. S., Bass, P. F., Middlebrook, M., Kennen, E., Baker, D. W., . . . Parker, R. (2006). Low literacy impairs comprehension of prescription drug warning labels. *Journal of General Internal Medicine, 21*, 847–851.

DeWalt, D. A., Berkman, N. D., Sheridan, S., Lohr, N., & Pignone, M. P. (2004). Literacy and health outcomes: A systematic review of the literature. *Journal of General Internal Medicine, 19*, 1228–1239.

Dickens, C., & Piano, M. R. (2013). Health literacy and nursing: An update. *American Journal of Nursing, 113*(6), 52–58.

Doak, C. C., Doak, L. G., Friedell, G. H., & Meade, C. D. (1998). Improving comprehension for cancer patients with low literacy skills: Strategies for clinicians. *CA: A Cancer Journal for Clinicians, 48*(3), 151–162.

Doak, C. C., Doak, L. G., & Root, J. H. (1985). *Teaching patients with low literacy skills*. Philadelphia, PA: Lippincott.

Doak, C. C., Doak, L. G., & Root, J. H. (1996). *Teaching patients with low literacy skills* (2nd ed.). Philadelphia, PA: Lippincott.

Doak, L. G., & Doak, C. C. (1987, July/August). Lowering the silent barriers to compliance for patients with low literacy skills. *Promoting Health*, 6–8.

Doak, L. G., & Doak, C. C. (2010). Writing for readers with a wide range of reading skills. *American Medical Writers Association Journal, 25*(4), 149–154.

Duffy, M. M., & Snyder, K. (1999). Can ED patients read your patient education materials? *Journal of Emergency Nursing, 25*(4), 294–297.

Dunn, M. M., Buckwalter, K. C., Weinstein, L. B., & Palti, H. (1985). Teaching the illiterate client does not have to be a problem. *Family & Community Health, 8*(3), 76–80.

Eichler, K., Wieser, S., & Brügger, U. (2009). The cost of limited health literacy: A systematic review. *International Journal of Public Health, 54*, 313–324.

Elliot, V. S. (2007). *Literacy advocates call for drug label uniformity.* Retrieved from http://www.ama-assn.org/amednews/2007/11/19/hlsc1119.htm

Federal Interagency Forum on Aging-Related Statistics. (2012). *Older Americans 2012: Key indicators of well-being.* Washington, DC: U.S. Government Printing Office.

Fidyk, L., Ventura, K., & Green, K. (2014). Teaching nurses how to teach. *Journal of Nurses in Professional Development, 30*(5), 248–253.

Fisher, E. (1999). Low literacy levels in adults: Implications for patient education. *Journal of Continuing Education in Nursing, 30*(2), 56–61.

Fleener, F. T., & Scholl, J. F. (1992). Academic characteristics of self-identified illiterates. *Perceptual and Motor Skills, 74*(3), 739–744.

Flesch, R. (1948). A new readability yardstick. *Journal of Applied Psychology, 32*(3), 221–233.

Foltz, A., & Sullivan, J. (1998). Get real: Clinical testing of patients' reading abilities. *Cancer Nursing, 21*(3), 162–166.

French, K. S., & Larrabee, J. H. (1999). Relationships among educational material readability, client literacy, perceived beneficence, and perceived quality. *Journal of Nursing Care Quality, 13*(6), 68–82.

Friedman, D. B., & Hoffman-Goetz, L. (2008). Literacy and health literacy as defined in cancer education research: A systematic review. *Health Education Journal, 67*, 285–304.

Fry, E. (1968). A readability formula that saves time. *Journal of Reading, 11*, 513–516, 575–579.

Fry, E. (1977). Fry's readability graph: Clarifications, validity, and extension to level 17. *Journal of Reading, 21*, 242–252.

Gazmararian, J. A., Baker, D. W., Williams, M. V., Parker, R. M., Scott, T. L., Green, D. C., . . . Koplan, J. P. (1999). Health literacy among Medicare enrollees in a managed care organization. *Journal of the American Medical Association, 281*(6), 545–551.

Gazmararian, J. A., Curran, J. W., Parker, R. M., Bernhardt, J. M., & DeBuono, B. A. (2005). Public health literacy in America: An ethical perspective. *American Journal of Preventive Medicine, 28*(3), 317–322.

Giorgianni, S. J. (Ed.). (1998). Perspectives on health care and biomedical research: Responding to the challenge of health literacy. *Pfizer Journal, 2*(1), 1–37.

Greenberg, S. (2011). *A profile of older Americans: 2011.* Administration on Aging, U.S. Department of Health and Human Services Administration on Aging. Retrieved from http://www.aoa.gov/aging_statistics/Profile/2011/docs/2011profile.pdf

Grieco, E. M., Acosta, A. D., de la Cruz, D. P., Gambino, C., Gryn, T., Larsen, L. J., . . . Walters, N. P. (2012). *Foreign born population.* Retrieved from http://www.census.gov/prod/2012pubs/acs-19.pdf

Gunning, R. (1968). The Fog index after 20 years. *Journal of Business Communication, 6*, 3–13.

Hasselkus, A. (2009). Health literacy in clinical practice. *ASHA Leader, 14*(1), 28–29.

Hayes, K. S. (2000). Literacy for health information of adult patients and caregivers in a rural emergency department. *Clinical Excellence for Nurse Practitioners, 4*(1), 35–40.

Hirsch, E. D. (2001). Overcoming the language gap. *American Educator, 4*, 6–7.

Horner, S. D., Surratt, D., & Juliusson, S. (2000). Improving readability of patient education materials. *Journal of Community Health Nursing, 17*(1), 15–23.

Houts, P. S., Bachrach, R., Witmer, J. T., Tringali, C. A., Bucher, J. A., & Localio, R. A. (1998). Using pictographs to enhance recall of spoken medical instructions. *Patient Education and Counseling, 35*, 83–88.

Hussey, L. C., & Guilliland, K. (1989). Compliance, low literacy, and locus of control. *Nursing Clinics of North America, 24*(3), 605–611.

Hyde, Y. M., & Kautz, D. D. (2014). Enhancing health promotion during rehabilitation through information-giving, partnership building, and teach-back. *Rehabilitation Nursing, 39*, 178–182.

Institute of Medicine (IOM). (2004). IOM report calls for national effort to improve health literacy. Retrieved from http://www8.nationalacademies.org/onpinews/newsitem.aspx?RecordID=10883

Johnson, K., & Weiss, B. D. (2008). How long does it take to assess health literacy skills in clinical practice? *Journal of the American Board of Family Medicine, 21*(3), 211–214.

Joint Commission on Accreditation of Healthcare Organizations (JCAHO). (1993). *Accreditation manuals for hospitals—1993*. Chicago, IL: Author.

Kalichman, S. C., Ramachandran, B., & Catz, S. (1999). Adherence to combination antiretroviral therapies in HIV patients of low health literacy. *Journal of General Internal Medicine, 14*, 267–273.

Kefalides, P. T. (1999). Illiteracy: The silent barrier to health care. *Annals of Internal Medicine, 130*(4), 333–336.

Kemp, E. C., Floyd, M. R., McCord-Duncan, E., & Lang, F. (2008). Patients prefer the method of "tell-back-collaborative inquiry" to assess understanding of medical information. *JABFM, 21*(1), 24–30.

Kerka, S. (2003). Health literacy beyond basic skills. *ERIC Digest*, ED478948.

Kessels, R. P. C. (2003). Patients' memory for medical information. *Journal of the Royal Society of Medicine, 96*, 219–222.

Kogut, B. H. (2004, Spring). Why adult literacy matters. *Phi Kappa Phi Forum*, 26–28.

Koo, M. M., Krass, I., & Aslani, P. (2005). Patient characteristics influencing evaluation of written medicine information: Lessons for patient education. *Annals of Pharmacotherapy, 39*(9), 1434–1440.

Kutner, M., Greenberg, E., Jin, Y., & Paulsen, C. (2006, September). The health literacy of America's adults: Results from the 2003 National Assessment of Adult Literacy. Retrieved from http://nces.ed.gov/pubsearch/pubsinfo.asp?pubid=2006483

Lasater, L., & Mehler, P. S. (1998). The illiterate patient: Screening and management. *Hospital Practice, 33*(4), 163–165, 169–170.

Lerner, E. B., Jehle, D. V. K., Janicke, D. M., & Moscati, R. M. (2000). Medical communication: Do our patients understand? *American Journal of Emergency Medicine, 18*(7), 764–766.

Levy, M., & Royne, M. (2009). The impact of consumers' health literacy on public health. *Journal of Consumer Affairs, 43*, 367–372.

Mauk, K. L. (2014). *Gerontological nursing: Competencies for care* (3rd ed.). Burlington, MA: Jones & Bartlett Learning.

Mayeaux, E. J., Murphy, P. W., Arnold, C., Davis, T. C., Jackson, R. H., & Sentell, T. (1996). Improving patient education for patients with low literacy skills. *American Family Physician, 53*(1), 205–211.

Mayer, G. G., & Rushton, N. (2002). Writing easy-to-read teaching aids. *Nursing 2002, 32*(3), 48–49.

McCormack, L., Bann, C., Uhrig, J., Berkman, N., & Rudd, R. (2009). Health insurance literacy of older adults. *Journal of Consumer Affairs, 43*, 223–247.

McLaughlin, G. H. (1969). SMOG—grading: A new readability formula. *Journal of Reading, 12*, 639–646.

McNaughton, C. D., Cawthon, C., Kripalani, S., Liu, D., Storrow, A. B., & Rournie, C. L. (2015). Health literacy and mortality: A cohort study of patients hospitalized for acute heart failure. *Journal of the American Heart Association, 4*, 1–9.

Meade, C. D., & Smith, C. F. (1991). Readability formulas: Cautions and criteria. *Patient Education and Counseling, 17*, 153–158.

Monsivais, D., & Reynolds, A. (2003). Developing and evaluating patient education materials. *Journal of Continuing Education in Nursing, 34*(4), 172–176.

Montalto, N. J., & Spiegler, G. E. (2001). Functional health literacy in adults in a rural community health center. *West Virginia Medical Journal, 97*(2), 111–114.

Moore, M., Bias, R. G., Prentice, K., Fletcher, R., & Vaughn, T. (2009). Web usability testing with a Hispanic medically underserved population. *Journal of the Medical Library Association, 97*(2), 114–121.

Morrow, D. G., Weiner, M., Steinley, D., Young, J., & Murray, M. D. (2007). Patients' health literacy and experience with instructions: Influence preferences for heart failure medication instructions. *Journal of Aging and Health, 19*, 575–592.

Myers, R. E., & Shepard-White, F. (2004). Evaluation of adequacy of reading level and readability of psychotropic medication handouts. *Journal of the American Psychiatric Nurses Association, 10*, 55–59.

Nath, C. R., Sylvester, S. T., Yasek, V., & Gunel, E. (2001). Development and validation of a literacy assessment tool for persons with diabetes. *Diabetes Educator, 27*(6), 857–864.

National Center for Education Statistics. (1993). *Adult literacy in America: National Adult Literacy Survey*. Washington, DC: U.S. Department of Education.

National Center for Education Statistics. (2006). National Assessment of Adult Literacy (NAAL): Health literacy component. Retrieved from http://nces.ed.gov/NAAL/index.asp?file=highlights/healthliteracyfactsheet.asp

Norman, C., & Skinner, H. (2006a). eHEALS: The eHealth Literacy Scale. *Journal of Medical Internet Research, 8*, e27.

Norman, C., & Skinner, H. (2006b). eHealth literacy: Essential skills for consumer health in a networked world. *Journal of Medical Internet Research, 8*, e9.

Paasche-Orlow, M. K., Taylor, H. A., & Brancati, F. L. (2003). Readability standards for informed-consent forms as compared with actual readability. *New England Journal of Medicine, 348*(8), 721–726.

Paasche-Orlow, M. K., & Wolf, M. (2007a). The causal pathway linking health literacy to health outcomes. *American Journal of Health Behavior, 31*, S19–S26.

Paasche-Orlow, M. K., & Wolf, M. (2007b). Evidence does not support clinical screening of literacy. *Journal of General Internal Medicine, 23*, 100–102.

Pagliari, C., Sloan, D., Gregor, P., Sullivan, F., Detmer, D., Kahan, J.P., . . . MacGillivray, S. (2005). What is ehealth? A scoping exercise to map the field. *Journal of Medical Internet Research, 7*(1). Retrieved from http://www.jmir.org/2005/1/e9

Parker, R., Baker, D., Williams, M., & Nurss, J. (1995). The Test of Functional Health Literacy in Adults (TOFHLA): A new instrument for measuring patients' literacy skills. *Journal of General Internal Medicine, 10*, 537–545.

Parnell, T. A. (2014). *Health literacy in nursing: Providing person-centered care*. New York, NY: *Springer Publishing Company*.

Passel, J. S., & Cohn, D. (2008). U.S. population projections 2005–2050. Pew Research Center. Retrieved from http://pewhispanic.org/files/reports/85.pdf

Pichert, J. W., & Elam, P. (1985). Readability formulas may mislead you. *Patient Education and Counseling, 7*, 181–191.

Pignone, B. D., DeWalt, D. A., Sheridan, S., Berkman, N., & Lohr, K. W. (2005). Interventions to improve health outcomes for patients with low literacy. *Journal of Internal Medicine, 20*, 185–192.

ProLiteracy. (2012). *ProLiteracy international programs update: Literacy at the heart of social change.* Syracuse, NY: Author.

Purnell, L. D. (2013). *Transcultural health care: A culturally competent approach* (4th ed.). Philadelphia, PA: F. A. Davis.

Quirk, P. A. (2000). Screening for literacy and readability: Implications for the advanced practice nurse. *Clinical Nurse Specialist, 14*(1), 26–32.

Rothman, R. L., DeWalt, D. A., Malone, R., Bryant, B., Shintani, A., Crigler, B., . . . Pignone, M. (2004). Influence of patient literacy on the effectiveness of a primary care-based diabetes disease management program. *Journal of the American Medical Association, 292*(14), 1711–1716.

Ryan, L., Logsdon, M. C., McGill, S., Stikes, R., Senior, B., . . . Davis, D. W. (2014). Evaluation of printed health materials for use by low-education families. *Journal of Nursing Scholarship, 46*(4), 218–228.

Ryhanen, A. M., Johansson, V. H., Salo, S., Salantera, S., & Leino-Kilpi, H. (2008). Evaluation of written patient educational materials in the field of diagnostic imaging. *Radiography, 15*, e1–e5.

Santrock, J. W. (2013). *Life-span development* (14th ed.). New York, NY: McGraw-Hill.

Schillinger, D., Grumbach, K., Piette, J., Wang, F., Osmond, D., Daher, C., . . . Bindman, A. B. (2002). Association of health literacy with diabetes outcomes. *Journal of the American Medical Association, 288*(4), 475–482.

Schultz, M. (2002). Low literacy skills needn't hinder care. *RN, 65*(4), 45–48.

Schwartzberg, J., VanGeest, J., & Wang, C. (Eds.). (2004). *Understanding health literacy: Inspirations for medicine and public health.* Chicago, IL: American Medical Association Press.

Spadaro, D. C. (1983). Assessing readability of patient information materials. *Pediatric Nursing, 9*(4), 274–278.

Spadaro, D. C., Robinson, L. A., & Smith, L. T. (1980). Assessing readability of patient information materials. *American Journal of Hospital Pharmacy, 37*, 215–221.

Spees, C. M. (1991). Knowledge of medical terminology among clients and families. *Image: Journal of Nursing Scholarship, 23*(4), 225–229.

Speros, C. I. (2011). Promoting health literacy: A nursing imperative. *Nursing Clinics of North America, 46*(3), 321–333.

Standal, T. C. (1981). How to use readability formulas more effectively. *Social Education, 45*, 183–186.

Stephenson, P. L. (2006). Before teaching begins. Managing patient anxiety prior to providing education. *Clinical Journal of Oncology Nursing, 10*(2), 241–245.

Sudore, R., Landefeld, S., Williams, B., Barnes, D., Lindquist, K., & Schillinger, D. (2006). Use of modified informed consent process among vulnerable patients: A descriptive study. *Journal of General Internal Medicine, 21*, 867–873.

Sudore, R. L., Yaffe, K., Satterfield, S., Harris, T. B., Mehta, K. M., Simonsick, E. M., . . . Schillinger, D. (2006). Limited literacy and mortality in the elderly. *Journal of General Internal Medicine, 21*, 806–812.

The U.S. illiteracy rate hasn't changed in 10 years. (2013, September 6). *The Huffington Post.* Retrieved from http://www.huffingtonpost.com/2013/09/06/illiteracy-rate_n_3880355.html

U.S. Census Bureau. (2012). Census Bureau reports foreign-born households are larger, include more children and grandparents. Retrieved from https://www.census.gov/newsroom/releases/archives/foreignborn_population/cb12-79.html

U.S. Department of Health and Human Services. (2011, April). *HHS Action Plan to Reduce Racial and Ethnic Health Disparities*. Retrieved from http://www.minorityhealth.hhs.gov/npa/files/plans/hhs/hhs_plan_complete.pdf

U.S. Department of Health and Human Services. (2014a). *Healthy People 2020*. Office of Disease Prevention and Health Promotion. Retrieved from http://www.healthypeople.gov/.

U. S. Department of Health and Human Services. (2014b). *A profile of older Americans: 2014*. Administration on Aging, Administration for Community Living, U.S. Department of Health and Human Services. Retrieved from http://www.aoa.acl.gov/Aging_Statistics/Profile/2014/docs/2014-Profile.pdf

U.S. Department of Health and Human Services. Office of Disease Prevention and Health Promotion. (2000). *Healthy People 2010*. Washington, DC: Author. Retrieved from http://www.healthypeople.gov/

U.S. Department of Health and Human Services, Office of Disease Prevention and Health Promotion. (2010). *National action plan to improve health literacy*. Washington, DC: Author. Retrieved from http://www.dhh.state.la.us/assets/docs/GovCouncil/MinHealth/Health_Literacy_Action_Plan.pdf

Vallance, J. K., Taylor, L. M., & LaVallee, C. (2008). Suitability and readability assessment of educational print resources related to physical activity: Implications and recommendations for practice. *Patient Education and Counseling, 72*, 342–349.

Vanderhoff, M. (2005). Patient education and health literacy. *PT: The Magazine of Physical Therapy, 13*(9) 42–46.

Volandes, A. (2007). Health literacy, health inequality and a just healthcare system. *American Journal of Bioethics, 7*(11), 5–8.

Walfish, S., & Ducey, B. B. (2007). Readability levels of Health Insurance Portability and Accountability Act notices of privacy practices used by psychologists in clinical practice. *Professional Psychology: Research and Practice, 38*, 203–207.

Webber, D., Higgins, L., & Baker, V. (2001). Enhancing recall of information from a patient education booklet: A trial using cardiomyopathy patients. *Patient Education and Counseling, 44*, 263–270.

Wedgeworth, R. (2007). *Fundraising letter*. Syracuse, NY: ProLiteracy Worldwide.

Weiss, B. D. (2003). *Health literacy: A manual for clinicians*. Chicago, IL: American Medical Association & American Medical Association Foundation.

Weiss, B. D. (2007). *Health literacy: A manual for clinicians* (2nd ed.). Chicago, IL: American Medical Association & American Medical Association Foundation.

Weiss, B. D., Mays, M. Z., Martz, W., Castro, K. M., DeWalt, D. A., Pignone, M. A., . . . Hale, F. A. (2005). Quick assessment of literacy in primary care. *Annals of Family Medicine, 3*(8), 514–522.

Welch, V. L., VanGeest, J. B., & Caskey, R. (2011). Time, costs, and clinical utilization of screening for health literacy: A case study using the newest vital sign (NVS) instrument. *Journal of the American Board of Family Medicine, 24*(3), 281–289.

Williams, D. M., Counselman, F. L., & Caggiano, C. D. (1996). Emergency department discharge instructions and patient literacy: A problem of disparity. *American Journal of Emergency Medicine, 14*(1), 19–22.

Williams, M. V., Baker, D. W., Parker, R. M., & Nurss, J. R. (1998). Relationship of functional health literacy to patients' knowledge of their chronic disease. *Archives of Internal Medicine, 158*, 166–172.

Williams, M. V., Davis, T., Parker, R. M., & Weiss, B. D. (2002). The role of health literacy in patient–physician communication. *Family Medicine, 34*(5), 383–389.

Williams, M. V., Parker, R. M., Baker, D. W., Parikh, W. S., Pitkin, K., Coates, W. C., & Nurss, J. R. (1995). Inadequate functional health literacy among patients at two public hospitals. *Journal of the American Medical Association, 274*(21), 1677–1682.

Wilson, M. (2009). Readability and patient education materials used for low-income populations. *Clinical Nurse Specialist, 23*, 33–40.

Winslow, E. H. (2001). Patient education materials: Can patients read them, or are they ending up in the trash? *American Journal of Nursing, 101*(10), 33–38.

Wolf, M. S., Williams, M. V., Parerk, R. M., Parikh, N. S., Nowlan, A. W., & Baker, D. W. (2007). Patients' shame and attitudes toward discussing the results of literacy screening. *Journal of Health Communication, 12*, 1–12.

Wood, F. G. (2005). Health literacy in a rural clinic. *Journal of Rural Nursing and Health Care, 5*(1). Retrieved from http://rnojournal.binghamton.edu/index.php/RNO/article/view/187

Wood, M. R., Kettinger, C. A., & Lessick, M. (2007). Knowledge is power: How nurses can promote health literacy. *Nursing for Women's Health, 11*(2), 180–188.

Zarcadoolas, C., Pleasant, A. F., & Greer, D. J. (2006). *Advancing health literacy: A framework for understanding and action.* San Francisco, CA: Jossey-Bass.

Ziegler, J. (1998). How literacy drives up health care costs. *Business & Health, 16*(4), 53–54.

APPENDIX 7-A

Tests to Measure Readability and Comprehension and Tools to Assess Instructional Materials

How to Use the SMOG Formula

Passages with 30 Sentences or More

Count 10 consecutive sentences near the beginning, 10 consecutive sentences from the middle, and 10 consecutive sentences from the end of the selection to be assessed. A sentence is any independent unit of thought punctuated by a period, question mark, or exclamation point. If a sentence has a colon or semicolon, consider each part before and after that punctuation as a separate sentence.

From the 30 randomly selected sentences, count the words containing three or more syllables (polysyllabic), including repetitions. Abbreviated words should be read in their full form to determine their syllable count (e.g., *Sept.* = *September* = three syllables). Letters or numerals in a string beginning or ending with a space or punctuation mark

Table 7A-1 SMOG Conversion Table for Passages with 30 Sentences or More

Word Count	Grade Level
0–2	4
3–6	5
7–12	6
13–20	7
21–30	8
31–42	9
43–56	10
57–72	11
73–90	12
91–110	13
111–132	14
133–156	15
157–182	16
183–210	17
211–240	18

Developed by Harold C. McGraw, Office of Educational Research, Baltimore County Public Schools, Towson, MD. In U.S. Department of Health and Human Services, National Institutes of Health, National Cancer Institute. (2004). Making health communication programs work: A planner's guide. Retrieved from http://www.cancer.gov/publications/health-communication/pink-book.pdf.

should be counted if, when read aloud in context, at least three syllables can be distinguished. For example, "1984" is read as "nineteen eighty-four" and has 5 syllables. Do not count words ending in *-ed* or *-es* if the ending makes the word have a third syllable. Hyphenated words are counted as one word. Proper nouns should be counted.

Approximate the reading grade level from the SMOG conversion table (**Table 7A–1**) or calculate the reading grade level by estimating the nearest perfect square root of the number of words with three or more syllables and then adding a constant of 3 to the square root. For example, if the total number of polysyllabic words was 53, the nearest perfect square would be 49. The square root of 49 would be 7. By adding a constant of 3, the reading level would be 10th grade (Doak, Doak, & Root, 1996).

Figure 7A–1 is an example of how to count all the words containing three or more syllables in a set of 10 sentences taken from one of the many pamphlets designed and distributed by the National Cancer Institute. In Figure 7A–1, there are 20 words with three or more syllables. Note that the word *United* is not counted as a three-syllable word because only the *-ed* ending makes it polysyllabic (see rule 2). For this passage of 10 sentences, the conversion number is 3 using the conversion table (**Table 7A–2**) for passages with fewer than 30 sentences. That is, 10 sentences × 3 (conversion number) = 60, which falls at the 11th-grade level on Table 7A–1 as per the rules in the next section for passages shorter than 30 sentences.

[1]**Mastectomy: A Treatment for Breast Cancer**

[2]You've been diagnosed as having breast cancer and your doctor has recommended a mastectomy.

[3]If you're like most women, you probably have many concerns about this treatment for breast cancer.

[4]Surgery of any kind is a frightening experience, but surgery for breast cancer raises special concerns.

[5]You may be wondering if the surgery will cure your cancer, how you'll feel after surgery—and how you're going to look.

[6]It's not unusual to think about these things. [7]More than 100,000 women in the United States will have mastectomies this year. [8]Each of them will have personal concerns about the impact of the surgery on her life.

[9]This booklet is designed to ease some of your fears by letting you know what to expect—from the time you enter the hospital to your recovery at home. [10]It may also help the special people in your life who are concerned about your well-being.

Figure 7A–1 Example of counting words with three or more syllables

Reproduced from National Cancer Institute of the National Institutes of Health, Public Health Service, U.S. Department of Health and Human Services, pamphlet entitled Mastectomy: A Treatment for Breast Cancer (1987, p. 1).

Table 7A–2 SMOG Conversion for Passages with Fewer than 30 Sentences

Number of Sentences in Sample Material	Conversion Number
29	1.03
28	1.07
27	1.1
26	1.15
25	1.2
24	1.25
23	1.3
22	1.36
21	1.43
20	1.5
19	1.58
18	1.67
17	1.76
16	1.87
15	2.0
14	2.14
13	2.3
12	2.5
11	2.7
10	3

Passages with Fewer than 30 Sentences

1. Count the number of sentences in the material and the number of words containing three or more syllables.
2. In the left hand column of Table 7A-2, locate the number of sentences. Then in the column opposite, locate the conversion number.
3. Multiply the word count found in step 1 by the conversion number identified in step 2. Locate this number in Table 7A–1 to obtain the corresponding grade level.

Example: If the material is 25 sentences long and 15 words of three or more syllables were counted in this material, the conversion number in Table 7A–2 for 25 sentences is 1.2. Multiply the word count of 15 by 1.2 to get 18. For the word count of 18, the grade level in Table 7A–1 is 7. Therefore, the material is at a seventh-grade reading level.

Guidelines for Writing and Evaluating Printed Education Materials

To reduce reading level and increase reading ease, do the following:

1. Write in conversational style with an active voice in the present tense using the second person pronoun *you* or *your*.
2. Use short, simple vocabulary of one- or two-syllable words; avoid multisyllabic words.
3. Spell out words rather than using abbreviations or acronyms, unless they are familiar to the reader or defined.
4. Organize information into chunks or series of numbered and bulleted lists; use statistics sparingly. A question-and-answer format is an interactive approach to presenting single units of information.
5. Keep sentences short (20 words maximum); avoid complex grammatical sentence structures that contain colons, semicolons, commas, and dashes.
6. Focus on familiar terms; avoid technical jargon and medical terminology; define or spell out difficult words phonetically; include a glossary if "medicalese" is necessary.
7. Use words consistently (repetition) throughout text; avoid synonyms.
8. Use exact terms; avoid value-judgment words with many interpretations.
9. Put the most important information first by prioritizing the need to know.
10. Use advance organizers to cue the reader about the topic being presented.
11. Limit the use of connective words that lengthen and make sentences more complex.
12. Make the first sentence of a paragraph the topic sentence.
13. Reduce concept density by including only one idea per sentence and limiting each paragraph to a single message or action.
14. Keep the density of words low (do not exceed 30–40 characters per line).
15. Provide adequate white space for margins and between lines and paragraphs (use double spacing).
16. Justify left margins and keep right margins unjustified.
17. Use arrows or numbers that give direction and organization to layouts.
18. Select large print (minimum of 12-point font, ideally 14- to 16-point font size) and simple style type (serif); avoid *italics*, all CAPITAL letters, and *fancy lettering*.
19. Rely on bold print or underlining to emphasize key points or words.
20. Attract attention with consistent use of appealing colors to highlight and organize topics.
21. Use a simple, short title that clearly indicates the subject being presented.
22. Keep the length of the document short; avoid including details and extraneous information.
23. Avoid glossy paper to reduce glare; rely on bold primary colors (not pastels) and black print on white paper for an older audience.
24. Use simple, realistic illustrations that convey the intended message; never superimpose typed words on a background design.

25. Include a summary at the end to review key points of information.
26. Put reading grade level (RGL) on the back of the tool for future reference.
27. Determine readability, comprehension, and reading skills by applying at least two formulas or tests.

Readability Formulas	Comprehension Tests	Reading Skills Tests
1. SMOG	1. Cloze procedure	1. WRAT
2. Fog	2. Listening test	2. REALM
3. Fry		3. TOFHLA

Newest Vital Sign

How to Use the Newest Vital Sign

ADMINISTERING THE NEWEST VITAL SIGN

A nurse (or other trained clinic staff) is the preferred administrator of the Newest Vital Sign. Administer at the same time that other vital signs are being taken.

ASK THE PATIENT TO PARTICIPATE

A useful way to ask the patient is an explanation similar to this:

> We are asking our patients to help us learn how well patients can understand the medical information that doctors and nurses give them. Would you be willing to help us by looking at some health information and then answering a few questions about that information? Your answers will help our doctors and nurses learn how to provide medical information in ways that patients will understand. It will only take about 3 minutes.

HAND THE NUTRITION LABEL TO THE PATIENT

The patient can and should retain the nutrition label throughout administration of the Newest Vital Sign. The patient can refer to the label as often as desired. See **Figure 7A–2a**.

ASK THE QUESTIONS

Start asking the six questions, one by one, giving the patient as much time as needed to refer to the nutrition label to answer the questions found on the Score Sheet. See **Figure 7A–2b**.

There is no maximum time allowed to answer the questions. The average time needed to complete all six questions is about 3 minutes. However, if a patient is still struggling with the first or second question after 2 or 3 minutes, the likelihood is that the patient has limited literacy, and you can stop the assessment.

ASK THE QUESTIONS IN SEQUENCE

Continue even if the patient gets the first few questions wrong. However, if question 5 is answered incorrectly, do not ask question 6.

Figure 7A–2a Label on ice cream container

Nutrition Facts		
Serving Size		½ cup
Servings per container		4
Amount per serving		
Calories 250	Fat Cal	120
		%DV
Total Fat 13g		20%
Sat Fat 9g		40%
Cholesterol 28mg		12%
Sodium 55mg		2%
Total Carbohydrate 30g		12%
Dietary Fiber 2g		
Sugars 23g		
Protein 4g		8%

*Percentage Daily Values (DV) are based on a 2,000 calorie diet. Your daily values may be higher or lower depending on your calorie needs.

Ingredients: Cream, Skim Milk, Liquid Sugar, Water, Egg Yolks, Brown Sugar, Milkfat, Peanut Oil, Sugar, Butter, Salt, Carrageenan, Vanilla Extract.

You can stop asking questions if a patient gets the first four correct. With four correct responses, the patient almost certainly has adequate literacy.

DO NOT PROMPT PATIENTS WHO ARE UNABLE TO ANSWER A QUESTION

Prompting may jeopardize the accuracy of the test. Just say, "Well, then, let's go on to the next question."

DO NOT SHOW THE SCORE SHEET TO PATIENTS

If they ask to see it, tell them that "I can't show it to you because it contains the answers, and showing you the answers spoils the whole point of asking you the questions."

DO NOT TELL PATIENTS IF THEY HAVE ANSWERED CORRECTLY OR INCORRECTLY

If patients ask, say something like: "I can't show you the answers until you are finished, but for now you are doing fine. Now let's go on to the next question."

Figure 7A–2b Score sheet for the Newest Vital Sign questions and answers

Questions and Answers		
READ TO SUBJECT: This information is on the back of a container of a pint of ice cream (see food label).	**Answer Correct?**	
1. If you eat the entire container, how many calories will you eat? **Answer:** *1000 is the only correct answer.*	yes	no
2. If you are allowed to eat 60 grams of carbohydrates as a snack, how much ice cream could you have? **Answer:** *Any of the following is correct: 1 cup (or any amount up to 1 cup), half the container, or two servings. Note: If patient answers "two servings," ask "How much ice cream would that be if you were to measure to it into a bowl?"*		
3. Your doctor advises you to reduce the amount of saturated fat in your diet. You usually have 42 g of saturated fat each day, which includes one serving of ice cream. If you stop eating ice cream, how many grams of saturated fat would you be consuming each day? **Answer:** *33 is the only correct answer.*		
4. If you usually eat 2500 calories in a day, what percentage of your daily value of calories will you be eating if you eat one serving? **Answer:** *10% is the only correct answer.*		
READ TO SUBJECT: **Pretend that you are allergic to the following substances: penicillin, peanuts, latex gloves, and bee stings.**		
5. Is it safe for you to eat this ice cream? **Answer:** *No*		
6. Ask only if the patient responds "no" to question 5: Why not? **Answer:** *Because it has peanut oil.*		
Number of correct answers:		

SCORE BY GIVING ONE POINT FOR EACH CORRECT ANSWER

There is a maximum of six points. See Figure 7A–2b. The score indicates the following:

0–1 suggests high likelihood (50% or more) of limited literacy.
2–3 indicates the possibility of limited literacy.
4–6 almost always indicates adequate literacy.

Record the NVS score in the patient's medical record, preferably near other vital sign measures (Pfizer, 2011).

References

Doak, C. C., Doak, L. G., & Root, J. H. (1996). *Teaching patients with low literacy skills* (2nd ed.). Philadelphia, PA: Lippincott.

Pfizer. (2011). *Implementation guide for the Newest Vital Sign.* Retrieved from http://www.pfizerhealthliteracy.com/asset/pdf/NVS_Eng/files/nvs_flipbook_english_final.pdf

Gender, Socioeconomic, and Cultural Attributes of the Learner

Susan B. Bastable | Deborah L. Sopczyk

Chapter Highlights

Key Terms

acculturation
assimilation
cultural awareness
cultural competence
cultural diversity
cultural relativism
culture
ethnic group
ethnocentrism
gender bias
gender gap
gender-related cognitive abilities
gender-related personality behaviors
ideology
poverty cycle
primary characteristics of culture
religiosity
secondary characteristics of culture
socioeconomic status
spirituality
stereotyping
subculture
transcultural
worldview

Objectives

After completing this chapter, the reader will be able to

1. Identify gender-related characteristics in the learner based on social and hereditary influences on brain functioning, cognitive abilities, and personality traits.
2. Recognize the influence of socioeconomics in determining health status and health behaviors.

© wanchai/Shutterstock

3. Define the various terms associated with diversity.

4. Examine cultural assessment from the perspective of different models of care.

5. Distinguish between the beliefs and customs of the four predominant ethnic (subcultural) groups in the United States.

6. Suggest teaching strategies specific to the needs of learners belonging to each of the four ethnic (subcultural) groups.

7. Examine ways in which transcultural nursing can serve as a framework for meeting the learning needs of various ethnic populations.

8. Identify the meaning of stereotyping, the risks involved, and ways to avoid stereotypical behavior.

Gender, socioeconomic level, and cultural background have a significant influence on a learner's willingness and ability to respond to and make use of the teaching–learning situation. These three factors also play a role in how patients experience health and illness and their expectations of the nurse (Core, 2008). Understanding diversity, particularly those variations among learners related to gender, socioeconomics, and culture, is of major importance when designing and implementing education programs to meet the needs of an increasingly unique population of learners.

This chapter explores how individuals respond differently to healthcare interventions through examination of gender-related variations resulting from heredity or social conditioning that affects how the brain functions for learning. In addition, the influence of environment on the learner from a socioeconomic viewpoint is examined. Consideration is also given to the significant effects that cultural norms have on the behaviors of learners from the perspective of the four major ethnic (subcultural) groups in the United States. Models for cultural assessment and the planning of care are highlighted as well. Finally, this chapter outlines ways to prepare nurses for diversity care and to deal with the issue of stereotyping.

Gender Characteristics

Most of the information on gender variations with respect to learning is found in the educational psychology and neuroscience literature. The nursing literature, however, contains relatively little information about this subject from a teaching–learning perspective. It is clear that characteristics of male and female orientations do affect learning. Therefore, these findings need to be considered more closely and applied to patient education in nursing practice.

Two well-established facts exist with respect to gender. First, individual differences within a group of males or females are usually greater than differences between groups of males versus groups of females. Second, studies that compare the sexes seldom are able to separate genetic differences from environmental influences on behavior (Crandell, Crandell, & Vander Zanden, 2012; Santrock, 2013).

A gap in knowledge remains about what the sexes would be like if humans were not subject to behavioral conditioning. No person can survive outside a social setting, and, therefore, individuals begin to be shaped by their environment right from birth. For example, our U.S. culture exposes girls and boys, respectively, to pink and blue blankets in the nursery, dolls and trucks in preschool, ballet and basketball in the elementary grades, and cheerleading and football in high school. These social influences continue to affect the sexes throughout the life span.

Of course, men and women *are* different. But questions remain: How different or the same are they when it comes to learning, and to what can the differences and similarities be attributed? Biological and behavioral scientists have, to date, been unable to determine the exact impact that genetics and environment have on the brain. Opinions are rampant, and research findings are still inconclusive.

However, the fact remains that there are gender differences as to how males and females act, react, and perform in situations affecting every aspect of life (Cahill, 2006; Thompson, 2010). As Cahill believes, the issue of gender influences is much too important to be ignored or marginalized. He further points out that the National Academy of Sciences reports "sex does matter in ways that we did not expect. Undoubtedly, it matters in ways that we have not yet begun to imagine" (p. 7).

For example, when it comes to human relationships, intuitively, women tend to pick up subtle tones of voice and facial expressions, whereas men tend to be less sensitive to these communication cues (Thompson, 2010). In navigation, women tend to have difficulty finding their way, whereas men seem to have a better sense of direction. In cognition, females tend to excel in languages and verbalization, yet men are likely to demonstrate stronger spatial abilities and interest in mathematical problem solving. Scientists are beginning to believe that gender differences have as much to do with the biology of the brain as with the way people are raised (Baron-Cohen, 2005; Gorman, 1992; C. J. Wilson & Auger, 2013). The debate, then, is not whether human development is influenced by nature or nurture, but how much influence heredity and environment have on shaping the abilities and personalities of men and women (Eliot, 2009; McLeod, 2007; Sincero, 2012). Kimura (1999) and Larkin (2013), for example, have reported on the many different patterns of behavior and cognition between men and women that are thought to reflect varying hormonal influences on brain development.

Some would argue that these examples are representative of stereotyping. Nevertheless, as generalizations, these statements seem to hold some truth. Neuroscientists have begun to detect both structural and functional differences in the brains of males and females. These early findings have led to an upsurge in neuroscience research into the mental lives of men and women (Baron-Cohen, 2005; Larkin, 2013).

Neurobiologists are just at the dawn of understanding how the human brain works, including exactly which types of sensory input wire the brain and how that input affects it. Scientists suspect that cognitive abilities operate much like sensory ones in that they are stimulated by those activities and experiences to which a person is exposed right from birth. Circuits in different regions of the brain are thought to mature at different stages of development. These circuits represent critical windows of opportunity at different ages for the learning of math, music, language, and emotion.

Brain development is much more sensitive to life experiences than once believed (Begley, 1996; Hancock, 1996). A baby's brain is like "a work in progress, trillions of neurons waiting to be wired . . . to be woven into the intricate tapestry of the mind" (Begley, 1996, pp. 55–56). Some of the neurons of the brain have been hardwired by genes, but trillions more have almost limitless potential and are waiting to be connected by the influence of environment. The first 3 years of life, scientists have realized, are crucial in the development of the mind. The wiring of the brain—a process both of nature and of nurture, dubbed the "dual sculptors"—forms the connections that determine the ability to learn and the interest for learning different types of skills (Harrigan, 2007; Nash, 1997).

Thanks to modern technology, imaging machines are revolutionizing the field of neuroscience. Functional magnetic resonance imaging (fMRI) and positron emission tomography (PET) are being used to observe human brains in the very acts of thinking, feeling, and remembering (Kawamura, Midorikawa, & Kezuka, 2000; Monastersky, 2001; Speck et al., 2000; Yee et al., 2000). Amazing discoveries through brain scanning have been made, such as where the emotion of love is located in the brain. Although machines can measure the brain's blood flow that supports nerve activity, no machines have been developed to date that can read or interpret a person's thoughts. The field of brain scanning still has far to go, but experts consider its potential to be incredible.

The trend in current studies is to focus on how separate parts of the brain interact while performing different tasks rather than focusing on only isolated regions of the brain associated with certain tasks (Monastersky, 2001). Researchers have already reported that men and women use different clusters of neurons when they read than when their brains are less active. For example, Kawamura et al. (2000) focused on the center in the brain of a male patient for reading and writing music, which is located in the cerebrum. They concluded that the left side of the brain is involved in this type of task, just as it is for the ability to read and write language. Also, neuroimaging studies have found that gender makes a difference in how the brain is connected (Gong, He, & Evans, 2011).

In addition, gender differences in the level of brain activity during working memory—an important component for performing many higher functions—have been examined with fMRI. For example, in a study of verbal working memory by Speck et al. (2000), the amount of brain activity was found to increase with task difficulty. Interestingly, male subjects demonstrated more right-sided hemispheric dominance, whereas females showed more left-sided hemispheric dominance. Females, though, demonstrated higher accuracy and slightly slower reaction times in doing the tasks than did males. The results revealed significant gender differences in the brain's organization for working memory.

In general, the brains of men and women seem to operate differently. Studies have revealed that women use more of their brains when thinking sad thoughts. When men and women subjects were asked to recall sad memories, the front of the limbic system in the brain of women glowed with activity eight times more than in men. Also, although men and women have been able to perform equally well in math problems, tests indicate that they seem to use the temporal lobes of the brain differently to figure out problems. Also, men and women use different parts of their brains to figure out rhymes. These study results are just a few examples of early yet interesting findings from research that are beginning to show that male and female identity is a creation of both nature and nurture. Along with genetics, life experiences and the choices men and women make over the course of a lifetime help to mold personal characteristics and determine gender differences in the very way the sexes think, sense, and respond (Begley, Murr, & Rogers, 1995).

In comparing how men and women feel, act, process information, and perform on cognitive and psychological tests, scientists have been able to identify some gender differences in the actual brain chemistry and structure of humans (**Table 8–1**). Most structural differences that have been uncovered are relatively small, as measured statistically, but quite significant (Cahill, 2014).

Table 8–1 Gender Differences in Brain Structure

	Men	Women
Temporal Lobe		
Regions of the cerebral cortex help to control hearing, memory, and a person's sense of self and time.	In cognitively normal men, a small region of the temporal lobe has approximately 10% fewer neurons than it does in women.	More neurons are located in the temporal region where language, melodies, and speech tones are understood.
Corpus Callosum		
The main bridge between the left and right brain contains a bundle of neurons that carry messages between the two brain hemispheres.	This part of the brain in men takes up less volume than a woman's does, which suggests less communication between the two brain hemispheres.	The back portion of the callosum in women is bigger than that in men, which may explain why women use both sides of their brains for language.
Amygdala		
This is the part of the brain that processes fear, triggers action, and signals danger.	In males, this part of the brain is larger and has testosterone receptors that heighten aggressive responses to compete and fight.	Women's hormone receptors in this part of the brain lead them to seek safety and connections within a group.
Prefrontal Cortex		
Along with the subdivision area known as the straight gyrus, this area of the brain is involved in social cognition and interpersonal awareness.	The straight gyrus in men is smaller, which reduces their social awareness and empathy.	The straight gyrus is 10% larger in women and correlates with their increased social perceptions and sensitive nurturing.
Anterior Commissure		
This collection of nerve cells, smaller than the corpus callosum, also connects the brain's two hemispheres.	The commissure in men is smaller than in women, even though men's brains are, on average, larger in size than women's brains.	The commissure in women is larger than it is in men, which may be a reason why their cerebral hemispheres seem to work together on tasks from language to emotional responses.

(continued)

Table 8–1 Gender Differences in Brain Structure (*continued*)

	Men	Women
Hippocampus		
This area of the brain is the center for memory and emotion.	Males have more specifically organized but fewer neuron connections and so take longer to process emotional information.	Females have a higher density of and more activity in neural connections that allow them to absorb more sensory and emotional information.
Brain Hemispheres		
The left side of the brain controls language, and the right side of the brain is the seat of emotion.	The right hemisphere of men's brains tends to be dominant.	Women tend to use their brains more holistically, calling on both hemispheres simultaneously.
Brain Size		
Total brain size is approximately 3 pounds.	Men's brains, on average, are larger than women's.	Women have smaller brains, on average, than men because the anatomic structure of their entire bodies is smaller. However, they have more neurons than men (an overall 11%) crammed into the cerebral cortex.

Data from Begley, S., Murr, A., & Rogers, A. (1995, March 27). Gray matters. *Newsweek*, 51; Eliot, L. (2009). Girl brain, boy brain? *Scientific American*. Retrieved from http://www.scientific american.com/article/girl-brain-boy-brain /; O'Brien, G. (2007). *Understanding ourselves: Gender differences in the brain*. Retrieved from http://www.columbiaconsult.com/pubs/V52_fall07.html; Jantz, G. L. (2014, February 27). *Brain differences between genders*. Retrieved from http://www.psychologytoday.com.

This comparison in brain structure variations seems to account better for psychological gender than simple biological sex differences (Eliot, 2009; Ruigrok et al., 2014). In fact, the gap in differences between adult women and men is larger than between girls and boys. This suggests that if differences between the sexes appear early in life, they are likely to be biological in nature, and those gender differences that appear later in adulthood development are shaped by the environment as a result of social learning (Eliot, 2009).

Nevertheless, a great deal of overlap exists in terms of how the brains of the two sexes work. Otherwise, "women could never read maps and men would always be left-handed. That flexibility within the sexes reveals just how complex a puzzle gender actually is, requiring pieces from biology, sociology, and culture" (Gorman, 1992, p. 44).

With respect to brain functioning, a mixture of the factors of heredity and environment likely accounts for gender characteristics. Nevertheless, even the largest differences in **gender-related cognitive abilities** are not as significant as, for example, the disparity found between male and female height. The following is a comparison of cognitive abilities between females and males in the United States based on developmental and educational psychology findings in Crandell et al. (2012), Santrock (2013), Snowman & McCown (2015), and Baron-Cohen (2005).

Cognitive Abilities
GENERAL INTELLIGENCE

Various studies have not yielded consistent findings on whether males and females differ in general intelligence. If any gender differences do exist, they seem to be attributed to patterns of ability rather than to IQ (intelligence quotient). When mean differences have been noted, they have proved small (Kimura, 1999). However, what is well documented is the strong correlation between IQ and heredity (Santrock, 2013). On IQ tests during preschool years, girls score higher; in high school, boys score higher on these tests. These differences may be due to higher dropout rates in high school for low-ability boys and gender identity formation in adolescence. Thus overall no dramatic differences between the sexes have been found on measures of general intelligence (Crandell et al., 2012).

VERBAL ABILITY

Girls learn to talk, form sentences, and use a variety of words earlier than boys. In addition, girls speak more clearly, read earlier, and do consistently better on tests of spelling and grammar. Originally, researchers believed females performed verbally at a higher level than males, but recent research has questioned this early superiority of females. On tests of verbal reasoning, verbal comprehension, and vocabulary, the findings are not consistent. The conclusion is that no significant gender differences in verbal ability exist.

MATHEMATICAL ABILITY

During the preschool years, there appear to be no gender-related differences in ability to do mathematics. By the end of elementary school, however, boys show signs of excelling in mathematical reasoning, and the differences in math abilities of boys relative to girls become even greater in high school. Recent studies reveal that any male superiority may be related to the way math is traditionally taught—as a competitive individual activity rather than as a cooperative group learning endeavor. Women have been shown to have higher level of math anxiety, using up working memory resources in the brain, leading to underperformance on math tests (Ganley & Vasilyeva, 2014).

SPATIAL ABILITY

The ability to recognize a figure when it is rotated, to detect a shape embedded in another figure, or to accurately replicate a three-dimensional object has consistently been found to be better among males than among females. Of all possible gender-related differences in cognitive activity, the spatial ability of males is consistently better than that of females and probably has a genetic origin. A number of research findings have shown that men do perform better on spatial tasks than women (Gur et al., 2000). However, the magnitude of this sex difference is still quite small (only about 5% variation) in spatial ability.

Interestingly, women surpass men in the ability to recognize and later recall the location of objects in a complex, random pattern (Kimura, 1999). Scientists have reasoned that historically, men may have developed strong spatial skills so as to be successful hunters, whereas women may have needed other types of visual skills so as to excel as gatherers of nearby sources of food (Gorman, 1992).

PROBLEM SOLVING

The complex concepts of problem solving, creativity, and analysis, when examined, have led to mixed findings regarding gender differences in these skills. Men tend to try new approaches in problem solving and are more likely to be more focused on important cues and common features in certain learning tasks. Males also show more curiosity and are significantly less conservative than women in risk-taking situations. In the area of human relations, however, women perform better at problem solving than do men.

SCHOOL ACHIEVEMENT

Without exception, girls get better grades on average than boys, particularly at the elementary school level. Scholastic performance of girls is more stable and less fluctuating than that of boys.

Although no compelling evidence proves significant gender-linked differences in the areas of cognitive functioning, except in spatial ability, some findings do reveal sex differences when it comes to personality characteristics of males and females in the United States. Evidence reported by Crandell et al. (2012), Santrock (2013), and Snowman & McCown (2015) substantiates the following summary findings unless otherwise noted.

Personality Traits

Most of the observed **gender-related personality behaviors** are thought to be largely determined by culture but are, to some extent, a result of mutual interaction between environment and heredity.

AGGRESSION

Males of all ages and in most cultures are generally more aggressive than females (Baron-Cohen, 2005). The role of the gender-specific hormone testosterone has been cited as a possible cause of the more aggressive behavior demonstrated by males (Kimura, 1999). However, anthropologists, psychologists, sociologists, and scientists in other fields continue to disagree about whether aggression is biologically based or environmentally influenced. Nevertheless, male and female roles differ widely in most cultures, with males usually being more dominant, assertive, active, hostile, and destructive.

CONFORMITY AND DEPENDENCE

Females have been found generally to be more conforming and more influenced by suggestion. The gender biases of some studies have left these findings open to suspicion, however.

EMOTIONAL ADJUSTMENT

The emotional stability of the sexes is approximately the same in childhood, but differences do arise in how emotional reactions are displayed. Research has revealed many differences in the way males and females "detect, process, and express" emotion (Thompson, 2010, p 1). For example, a study of 55 cultures found that women tend to be more emotional, better perceive verbal and visual emotional cues, and respond with greater sadness and more anxiety than men. On the other hand, men are more likely to be less extroverted and conscientious, react to stress by showing an increase in blood pressure, and experience love and anger less intensely than women. These differences may be a result of cultural stereotyping and heredity. Nevertheless, emotional reactions of women have a direct effect on their physical and mental health. Women tend to be at greater risk for depression, anxiety, and mood disorders, and men are at greater risk for hypertension, substance abuse, and antisocial behavior (Larkin, 2013).

Thus, evidence indicates that adolescent girls and adult females have more neurotic symptoms than males. However, this tendency may reflect how society defines mental health in ways that coincide with male roles. In addition, tests to measure mental health usually have been designed by men and, therefore, may be biased against females.

VALUES AND LIFE GOALS

In the past, men have tended to show greater interest in scientific, mathematical, mechanical, and physically active occupations as well as to express stronger economic and political values. Women have tended to choose literary, social service, and clerical occupations and to express stronger aesthetic, social sense, and religious values. These differences have become smaller over time, however, as women have begun to think differently about themselves, women have more freely pursued career and interest pathways, and society has begun to take a more equal-opportunity viewpoint for both sexes.

ACHIEVEMENT ORIENTATION

Females are more likely to express achievement motivation in social skills and social relations, whereas men are more likely to try to succeed in intellectual or competitive activities. This difference is thought to reflect sex-role expectations that are strongly communicated at very early ages.

The behavioral and biological differences between males and females, known as the **gender gap,** are well documented. Also well documented is **gender bias,** "a preconceived notion about the abilities of women and men that prevented individuals from pursuing their own interests and achieving their potentials" (Santrock, 2006, p. 66). How do these differences between the genders relate to the healthcare needs of individuals and the process of engaging them in patient education?

With respect to gender differences and aging, as suggested by current life-span mortality rates, white females have a life expectancy of approximately 80 years compared to approximately 73 years for white males. Also, men have higher mortality rates for each of the 10 leading causes of death (U.S. Department of Health and Human Services

[USDHHS], 2009). However, more needs to be understood about women's health, because for years their health issues have been underrepresented in research studies. Fortunately, this trend has changed within the last 2 to 3 decades, and significant evidence is beginning to surface about the physical and mental health status of females (DeCola, 2012; Dignam, 2000; USDHHS, 2012).

One point that is known is that women are likely to seek health care more often than men do (U.S. Census Bureau, 2012a). It is suspected that one of the reasons women have more contact with the healthcare system is that they traditionally have tended to be the primary caretakers of their children, who need pediatric services. In addition, during their childbearing years, women seek health services for care surrounding pregnancy and childbirth (Smith, 2006). However, other variables—such as sociodemographics and health status—come into play and also account for gender differences in the use of healthcare services (Bertakis, Azari, Helms, Callahan, & Robbins, 2000).

Perhaps the reason that men tend not to rely as much as women on care from health providers is the sex-role expectation by our society that men should be stronger. They also have a tendency to be risk takers and to think of themselves as more independent. Although men are less likely to pursue routine health care for purposes of health and safety promotion and disease and accident prevention, they typically face a greater number of health hazards, such as a higher incidence of automobile accidents, use of drugs and alcohol, suicide, heart disease, and participation in dangerous occupations. Furthermore, men are less likely to notice symptoms or report them to physicians (Courtenay, 2000).

Sexual Orientation and Gender Identity

The exact number of lesbian, gay, bisexual, transgender, and queer/questioning (LGBTQ) individuals in the United States and around the world is unknown; however, this population is estimated to include more than 8 million people in this country alone (Fenway Institute, 2010a). This number is based on U.S. Census data and represents a very conservative estimate of the LGBTQ population. Although the U.S. Census does gather information on same-sex couples, it does not ask questions about sexual orientation or gender identity (Gates, 2013). Therefore, single gays and lesbians are not identified in U.S. Census data, nor are members of the transgender community. Because of hesitancy on the part of many members of the LGBTQ population to disclose their sexual preference and/or gender identity, underrepresentation is always an issue.

When considering gender and the social and other factors that influence the unique learning styles and educational needs of men and women, it is important to include the LGBTQ community. The LGBTQ population represents a distinct cultural group whose needs are often overlooked by nurses and other health professionals (American Medical Student Association, 2015). Although members of the LGBTQ population have many of the same health problems as the general population, disparities do exist, and as a group, their health outcomes are worse than those of the heterosexual community (Centers for Disease Control and Prevention [CDC], 2010; Krehely, 2009).

Three main problems contribute to the health disparities experienced by the LG-BTQ population:

1. The social stigma associated with being LGBTQ creates undue stress and contributes to negative health behavior patterns. For example, research has identified increased rates of tobacco, alcohol, and drug use among the LGBTQ population as well as a high incidence of depression, anxiety, suicide, and other mental health problems (Livingston et al., 2015; Woodiel & Cowdery, 2014).

2. Structural barriers decrease access to health care for people who are LGBTQ (Mayer et al., 2008). For example, unemployment in the LGBTQ community resulting from job discrimination and lack of insurance benefits for same-sex domestic partners have led to a higher than average number of people without health insurance coverage (Gonzales, 2014; Krehely, 2009).

3. Lack of culturally appropriate care for the LGBTQ community results in limited or ineffective use of healthcare services. For example, in an attempt to avoid negative interactions with healthcare providers, LGBTQ patients—particularly bisexual men and women—are often reluctant to disclose their sexual preference or gender identity. Without this vital piece of information, nurses and other health professionals are unable to provide comprehensive care. Other members of the LGBTQ community simply avoid seeking health care unless absolutely necessary. As a result, they may not take advantage of preventive services or receive early treatment for serious health problems (Durso & Meyer, 2012; McRae, Ochsner, Mauss, Gabrieli, & Gross, 2008).

TEACHING STRATEGIES

Davidson, Trudeau, van Roosmalen, Stewart, and Kirkland (2006) describe gender as a "multifaceted construct" (p. 731) that includes a number of modifiable attributes that influence health outcomes and health education. These attributes include personality, social supports, coping skills, values, and health-related behaviors. When planning teaching strategies, nurses must be aware of the extent to which attributes such as these, as well as heredity-related characteristics of the genders, affect health-seeking behaviors and influence individual health needs. As stated previously, in some areas males and females display different orientations and learning styles (Severiens & Ten Dam, 1994, 1997; Wehrwein, Lujan, & DiCarlo, 2007). The precise differences seem to depend on interests and past experiences in the biological and social roles of men and women in American society.

Women and men are part of different social cultures, too. They use different symbols, belief systems, and ways to express themselves, much in the same manner that different ethnic groups exhibit distinct cultures. In the future, these gender differences may become less pronounced as the sex roles become more blended. Language and symbols are also very important to the LGBTQ community. The most commonly employed symbols of the LGBTQ community are the pink triangle and the rainbow pride flag. These symbols, which are used by this community as a show of pride and unity, are often displayed in healthcare settings as a sign of welcome to LGBTQ patients (Woodiel & Cowdery, 2014).

It is also important that nurses become familiar with the labels, terms, and phrases preferred by the LGBTQ community and use them appropriately in conversation and in preparing teaching materials. Language and culture continually change, so the nurse must work toward remaining current. For example, although the word *queer* was once considered derogatory, in recent years, many within the LGBTQ community have embraced the term and use it proudly.

When serving in the role of patient educator, nurses must create an environment that is welcoming to all men and women regardless of lifestyle. Patients, particularly those living alternative lifestyles, look for subtle clues to determine whether the nurse will accept them without judgment (Woodiel & Cowdery, 2014). For example, a women's or children's health clinic that displays photos of only traditional families may give the message that nontraditional families are not welcome. Brochures on LGBTQ health issues and unisex bathrooms are all strategies that give a welcoming message to a diverse patient base.

When working with men and women, it is important that the nurse avoid making assumptions about family structure, sexual preference, or lifestyle. Many families in the 21st century are structured differently from families in years past. For example, more men are assuming primary responsibility for child care. The nurse should never assume that a client is heterosexual, even if that person is or has been married to a member of the opposite sex, as almost half of self-identified lesbians have been or are currently married to men (Fenway Institute, 2010b). Likewise, the nurse should not assume that when a patient refers to a spouse that he or she is talking about a member of the opposite sex. As more and more states are legalizing same sex marriage, the LGBTQ community is using the term husband or wife rather than partner.

To complete an accurate assessment of each individual, the nurse should take every opportunity to gather accurate information from the patient. Admission or intake forms are often designed for the traditional family. Patients are often not given an opportunity to identify a same-sex domestic partner. Transgender patients are usually forced to select either male or female. By adjusting the forms to be more inclusive, the nurse not only creates a welcoming environment but also offers an opportunity for the patient to share important information. Nurses also must be knowledgeable about gender-related health disparities and are encouraged to include this information when educating patients. They also are encouraged to use versatile teaching-style strategies so as not to perpetuate stereotypical approaches to teaching and learning with the two genders.

Socioeconomic Characteristics

Socioeconomic status (SES), in addition to gender characteristics, influences the teaching–learning process. SES is considered to be the single most important determinant of both physical and mental health in our society (Crimmins & Saito, 2001; Meyer, Castro-Schilo, & Agular-Gaxiola, 2014; Singh-Manoux, Ferrie, Lynch, & Marmot, 2005). Socioeconomic class is an aspect of diversity that must be addressed in the context of education and in the process of teaching and learning.

Social and economic levels of individuals have been found to be significant variables affecting health status, literacy levels, and health behaviors (Crimmins & Saito, 2001;

Monden, van Lenthe, & Mackenbach, 2006). Over 46 million Americans (about 15% of the total population) live in poverty (U.S. Census Bureau, 2015a). Poverty is defined as an income of $24,250 per year, for a family of four (U.S. Census Bureau, 2015b; USD-HHS, 2015b).

Disadvantaged people—those with low incomes, low educational levels, or social deprivation—come from many different ethnic groups, including millions of poor white people (USDHHS, 2012). SES takes into account the variables of educational level, family income, and family structure (Crandell et al., 2012). Collectively, all of these variables influence health beliefs, health practices, and readiness to learn (Darling, 2004; Mackenbach et al., 2003).

Although many educators, psychologists, and sociologists have recognized that a cause-and-effect relationship exists among low SES, low cognitive ability, and poor quality of health and life, they are hard pressed to suggest solutions for breaking this cycle (Batty, Deary, & Macintyre, 2006). Likewise, nurses well recognize that patients belonging to lower social classes have higher rates of illness, more severe illnesses, and reduced rates of life expectancy (Mackenbach et al., 2003). People with low SES, as measured by indicators such as income, education, and occupation, have increased rates of morbidity and mortality compared to those with higher SES (USDHHS, 2012).

A significant relationship exists between SES and health status. Individuals who have higher incomes and are better educated live longer and healthier lives than those who are of low income and poorly educated (Crimmins & Saito, 2001; Rognerud & Zahl, 2005). Thus the level of socioeconomic well-being is a strong indicator of health outcomes. **Figure 8–1** illustrates the relationship between SES and health status. In turn, health

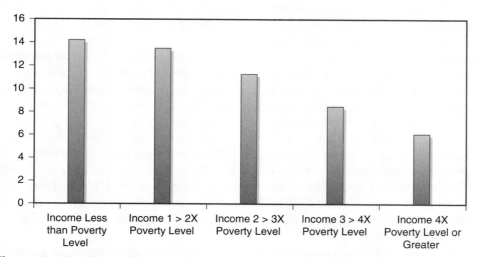

Figure 8–1 Percentage of persons with perceived fair to poor health status by income level

U.S. Census Bureau. (2010). Retrieved from http://2010.census.gov/2010census/

status affects SES (Elstad & Krokstad, 2003). As such, people with good health tend to move up in the social hierarchy, whereas those with poor health move downward.

These findings raise serious questions about health differences among people of the United States as a result of unequal access to health care due to SES. These unfortunate health trends are costly to society in general and to the healthcare system in particular. Although harmful health-related behaviors and less access to medical care have been found to contribute to higher morbidity and mortality rates, there is newer but still limited research on the effect SES has on a disability-free life or active life expectancy (Crimmins & Saito, 2001; Mackenbach et al., 2003).

Crandell et al. (2012) and Santrock (2013) explain that many factors, including poor health care, limited resources, family stress, discrimination, and low-paying jobs, maintain the cycle by which generation after generation is born into poverty. In addition, rates of illiteracy and low literacy have been linked to poorer health status, high unemployment, low earnings, and high rates of welfare dependency, all of which are common measures of a society's economic well-being (Giorgianni, 1998; Weiss, 2003).

Whatever the factors that keep particular groups from achieving at higher levels, these groups are likely to remain on the lower end of the occupational structure. This continuous circle of entrapment has been coined the **poverty cycle** and is described as a phenomenon whereby poor families become trapped in poverty for generations because of economic, social, and geographical factors that perpetuate new cycles and a seemingly endless continuation of being impoverished (Christian Reformed Church in North America, n.d.; "Poverty cycle," n.d.).

The lower socioeconomic class has been studied by social scientists more than other economic classes. This research focus probably arises because the health views of this group of individuals deviate the most from the viewpoints of the health professionals who care for them. People from the lower social stratum have been characterized as being indifferent to the symptoms of illness until poor health interferes with their lifestyle and independence. Their view of life is one of a sense of powerlessness, meaninglessness, and isolation from middle-class knowledge of health and the need for preventive measures, such as vaccination for their children (Lipman, Offord, & Boyle, 1994; Maholmes & King, 2012; USDHHS, 2012; Winkleby, Jatulis, Frank, & Fortmann, 1992).

The high cost of health care may well be a major factor affecting health practices of people in the lower socioeconomic classes. Lack of health insurance remains an important factor influencing health status in the United States, particularly among the poor. However, the Affordable Care Act, which was signed into law in 2010, is beginning to show an impact on access to health care for all Americans. Whereas the number of Americans without health insurance was over 17% in recent years (O'Hara & Caswell, 2012), the National Health Interview Survey conducted in 2014 revealed that this number has dropped to around 13%. Of those adults under 65 years of age, 17.7% were covered by a public health insurance plan and 67.3% with a private plan (Ward, Clarke, Freeman, & Schiller, 2015).

Just as SES can have a negative effect on illness, so, too, can illness have devastating implications for a person's socioeconomic well-being (Elstad & Krokstad, 2003).

A catastrophic or chronic illness can lead to unemployment, enforced social isolation, and a strain on social support systems (Lindholm, Burstrom, & Diderichsen, 2001; Mulligan, 2004). Without the socioeconomic means to decrease these threats to their well-being, individuals in poverty may be powerless to improve their situation.

These multiple losses burden the individual, their families, and the healthcare system. Low-income groups are especially affected by changes in federal and state assistance in the form of Medicare and Medicaid. The high costs associated with illness that result in overuse of the healthcare system have resulted in increased interest on the part of the public and healthcare providers to control costs (Carpenter, 2011). Today, more emphasis is being given to keeping people well by efforts aimed at health promotion, health maintenance, and disease prevention.

Teaching Strategies

The current trends in health care, as a result of these economic concerns, are directed toward teaching individuals how to attain and maintain health. The nurse plays a key role in educating the consumer about avoiding health risks, reducing illness episodes, establishing healthful environmental conditions, and accessing healthcare services. Patient education by nurses for those individuals who are socially and economically deprived has the potential to yield short-term benefits in meeting these individuals' immediate healthcare needs. However, more research must be done to determine whether teaching can ensure the long-term benefits of helping deprived people develop the skills needed to reach and sustain independence in self-care management (Adams, 2010; Gronning, Rannestad, Skomsvoll, Rygg, & Steinsbekk, 2014; Niedermann, Fransen, Knols, & Uebelhart, 2004).

Nurses must be aware of the likely effects of low SES on an individual's ability to learn as a result of less than average cognitive functioning, poor academic achievement, low literacy, high susceptibility to illness, and inadequate social support systems. Low-income people are at greater risk for these factors, all of which can interfere with learning. Stress hormones caused by poverty, for example, have been shown to "poison the brain for a lifetime" (Krugman, 2008). However, nurses cannot assume that everyone at the poverty or near-poverty level is equally influenced by these threats to their well-being. To avoid stereotyping, it is essential that each individual or family be assessed to determine their particular strengths and weaknesses for learning. In this way, teaching strategies unique to particular circumstances can be designed to assist socioeconomically deprived individuals in meeting their needs for health care.

Nevertheless, it is well documented that individuals with literacy problems, poor educational backgrounds, and low academic achievement are likely to have low self-esteem, feelings of helplessness and hopelessness, and low expectations. Also, they tend to think in concrete terms, to focus more on satisfying immediate needs, to have a more external locus of control, and to have decreased attention spans. They often have difficulty in problem solving and in analyzing and summarizing large amounts of information. The nurse will most likely have to rely on specific teaching methods and tools similar to those identified as appropriate for intervening with patients who have low literacy abilities.

Cultural Characteristics

The racial makeup of the United States continues to undergo change. At the beginning of the 21st century, the composition of this nation's population was approximately 71.3% white and 28.7% minority. By 2012, minority representation in the country grew to 37%. It is anticipated that the minority population will continue to grow and more than double in the next 50 years. By 2043, it is projected that there will be no majority group in the United States and that by 2060, minority groups will constitute 57% (241.3 million people) of the U.S. population (U.S. Census Bureau, 2012b).

To keep pace with a society that is becoming increasingly more culturally diverse, nurses need to have sound knowledge of the cultural values and beliefs of specific ethnic groups as well as be aware of individual practices and preferences (Price & Cortis, 2000; Purnell, 2013). Lack of cultural sensitivity by nurses and other healthcare professionals has the potential to waste millions of dollars through misuse of healthcare services and misdiagnosis of health problems with tragic and dangerous consequences. Furthermore, cultural sensitivity may serve to reduce the racial and ethnic bias perceived by culturally diverse patients in healthcare settings and minimize the alienation of large numbers of people (Benjamins & Whitman, 2014; Nguyen & Mills, 2015).

Underrepresented ethnic groups are beginning to demand culturally relevant health care that respects their cultural rights and incorporates their specific beliefs and practices into the care they receive. This expectation is in direct conflict with the unicultural, Western, biomedical paradigm taught in many nursing and other healthcare provider programs across the country (Purnell, 2013).

Definition of Terms

Before examining the major ethnic (subcultural) groups within the United States, it is important to define the following terms, as identified by Purnell (2013), that are commonly used in addressing the subject of culture:

Acculturation: A willingness to adapt or "to modify one's own culture as a result of contact with another culture" (p. 481).

Assimilation: The willingness of an individual or group "to gradually adopt and incorporate characteristics of the prevailing culture" (p. 481).

Cultural awareness: Recognizing and appreciating "the external signs of diversity" in other ethnic groups, such as their art, music, dress, and physical features (p. 482).

Cultural competence: Possessing the "knowledge, abilities, and skills to deliver care congruent with the patient's cultural beliefs and practices" (p. 7).

Cultural diversity: A term used to describe the variety of cultures that exist within society.

Cultural relativism: "The belief that the behaviors and practices of people should be judged only from the context of their cultural system" (p. 482).

Culture: "The totality of socially transmitted behavioral patterns, arts, beliefs, values, customs, lifeways, and all other products of human work and thought characteristic of a population of people that guide their worldview and decision making. These patterns may be explicit or implicit, are primarily learned and transmitted within the family, and are shared by the majority of the cultures" (p. 482).

Ethnic group: Also referred to as a *subculture*; a population of "people who have experiences different from those of the dominant culture" (p. 483).

Ethnocentrism: "The tendency of human beings to think that [their] own ways of thinking, acting, and believing are the only right, proper, and natural ones and to believe that those who differ greatly are strange, bizarre, or unenlightened" (p. 483).

Ideology: "The thoughts, attitudes, and beliefs that reflect the social needs and desires of an individual or ethnocultural group" (p. 484).

Subculture: A group of people "who have had different experiences from the dominant culture by status, ethnic background, residence, religion, education, or other factors that functionally unify the group and act collectively on each other" (p. 486).

Transcultural: "Making comparisons for similarities and differences between cultures" (p. 8).

Worldview: "The way individuals or groups of people look at the universe to form values about their lives and the world around them" (p. 487).[1]

Assessment Models for the Delivery of Culturally Sensitive Care

Given increases in immigration and the birth rates of minority populations in the United States as well as the significant increased geographical mobility of people around the globe, the U.S. system of health care and this country's educational institutions must respond by shifting from a dominant, monocultural, ethnocentric focus to a more multicultural, transcultural focus (Narayan, 2003).

Leininger (1994), a proponent of transcultural nursing, posed a question that remains relevant today: How can nurses competently respond to and effectively care for people from diverse cultures who act, speak, and behave in ways different than their own? Studies indicate that nurses are often unaware of the complex factors influencing patients' responses to health care.

The Purnell model for cultural competence represents a popular organizing framework for understanding the complex phenomena of culture and ethnicity. This framework "provides a comprehensive, systematic, and concise" approach that can assist health professionals to provide "holistic, culturally competent" (Purnell, 2013, p. 15) care when teaching patients in a variety of practice settings.

Purnell (2013) has proposed that a number of factors influence an individual's identification with an ethnic group. These factors may be distinguished as primary and secondary characteristics of culture. **Primary characteristics of culture** include nationality, race, color, gender, age, and religious affiliation. **Secondary characteristics of culture** include many of a person's attributes that are addressed in this text, such as SES, physical characteristics, educational status, occupational status, and place of residence (urban versus rural). These two major characteristics affect one's belief system and view of the world.

---

[1] *Transcultural health care: A culturally competent approach* (4th ed.) by Purnell, Larry D., & Paulanka, Betty J. (2013). Reproduced with permission of F.A. Davis in the format Republish in a book via Copyright Clearance Center.

The Purnell model, depicted in a circle format, includes the layers of the following concepts:

1. Global society (outermost sphere)
2. Community (second sphere)
3. Family (third sphere)
4. Individual (innermost sphere)

The interior of the circle is cut into 12 equally sized, pie-shaped wedges that represent cultural domains that should be assessed when planning to deliver patient education in any setting:

1. Communication (e.g., dominant language and nonverbal expressions and cues)
2. Family roles and organization (e.g., head of household, gender roles, developmental tasks, social status, alternative lifestyles, roles of older adults)
3. Workforce issues (e.g., language barriers, autonomy, acculturation)
4. Biocultural ecology (e.g., heredity, biological variations, genetics)
5. High-risk behaviors (e.g., smoking, alcoholism, physical activity, safety practices)
6. Nutrition (e.g., common foods, rituals, deficiencies, limitations)
7. Pregnancy (e.g., fertility, practices, views toward childbearing, beliefs about pregnancy, birthing practices)
8. Death rituals (e.g., views of death, bereavement, burial practices)
9. Spirituality (e.g., religious beliefs and practices, meaning of life, use of prayer)
10. Healthcare practices (e.g., traditions, responsibility for health, pain control, sick role, medication use)
11. Healthcare practitioners (e.g., folk practitioners, gender issues, perceptions of providers)
12. Overview/heritage (e.g., origins, economics, education, occupation, economics)

Purnell has also identified 19 assumptions upon which the model is based, the following of which are most relevant to this chapter:

- One culture is not better than another—they are just different.
- The primary and secondary characteristics of culture determine the degree to which one varies from the dominant culture.
- Culture has a powerful influence on one's interpretation of and responses to health care.
- Each individual has the right to be respected for his or her uniqueness and cultural heritage.
- Prejudices and biases can be minimized with cultural understanding.
- Caregivers who intervene in a culturally competent manner improve the care of patients and their health outcomes.
- Cultural differences often require adaptations to standard professional practices.

Other models for conducting a nursing assessment have also been proposed (Shen, 2015). Giger and Davidhizar's transcultural assessment model was first developed in 1988 to teach nursing students how to provide appropriate care to culturally diverse patients (Giger & Davidhizar, 2004). This model includes six cultural phenomena (Giger, 2013;

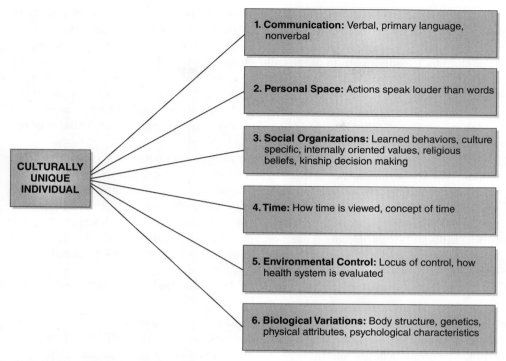

Figure 8–2 Six cultural phenomena

Adapted from Giger, J. N., & Davidhizar, R. E. (2004). *Transcultural nursing: Assessment and intervention* (4th ed.). St. Louis, MO: Mosby-Year Book.

Giger & Davidhizar, 2004) that serve as a framework to design and deliver culturally sensitive care: (1) communication, (2) personal space, (3) social organization, (4) time, (5) environmental control, and (6) biological variations (**Figure 8–2**).

Another model, the nurse–client negotiations model, was developed in the mid-1980s for the purpose of cultural assessment and planning for care of culturally diverse people. Although it is approximately 30 years old, this model remains relevant. It recognizes differences that exist between what the nurse and patient think about health, illness, and treatments and attempts to bridge the gap between the scientific perspectives of the nurse and the cultural beliefs (known as popular perspectives) of the patient (J. M. Anderson, 1990).

The nurse–client negotiations model serves as a framework to attend to the culture of the nurse as well as the culture of the patient. In addition to the professional culture, each nurse has his or her own personal beliefs and values, which may operate without the nurse being fully aware of them. These beliefs and values may influence nurses' interactions with patients and families.

Explanations of the same phenomena may yield different interpretations based on the cultural perspective of the layperson or the professional. For example, putting lightweight covers on a patient may be interpreted by family members as placing their loved one at risk for getting a chill, whereas the nurse may use this technique to reduce a fever. As another example, a Jehovah's Witness family considers a blood transfusion for their child to be contamination of the child's body, whereas the nurse and other health-care team members believe the transfusion is a life-saving treatment (J. M. Anderson, 1987). The important aspect of the nurse–client negotiations model is that it can open lines of communication between the nurse and the patient/family. It helps each party understand how the other interprets or values a problem or practice such that they respect one another's goals.

Negotiation implies a mutual exchange of information between the nurse and the patient. The nurse should begin this negotiation by learning from the patients about their understanding of their situation, their interpretations of illness and symptoms, the symbolic meanings they attach to an event, and their notions about treatment. The goal is to actively involve patients in the learning process so as to help them acquire healthy coping skills and styles of living. Together, nurse and patient then need to work out how the popular and scientific perspectives can be combined to achieve goals related to the individual patient's needs and interests (J. M. Anderson, 1990).

General areas to assess when first meeting the patient include the following:

1. The patient's perceptions of health and illness
2. His or her use of traditional remedies and folk practitioners
3. The patient's perceptions of nurses, hospitals, and the care delivery system
4. His or her beliefs about the role of family and family member relationships
5. His or her perceptions of and need for emotional support (J. M. Anderson, 1987; Jezewski, 1993)

According to J. M. Anderson (1990) and Narayan (2003), the following questions can be used as a means for understanding the patient's perspectives or viewpoints. The answers then serve as the basis for negotiation:

- What do you think caused your problem?
- Why do you think the problem started when it did?
- Which major problems does your illness cause you?
- How has being sick affected you?
- How severe do you think your illness is? Do you see it as having a short- or long-term course?
- Which kinds of treatments do you think you should receive?
- What are the most important results you hope to obtain from your treatments?
- What do you fear most about your illness?

Nurses who are competent in cultural assessment and negotiation likely will be the most successful at designing and implementing culturally effective patient education. They also will be able to assist their colleagues in working with patients who may be considered uncooperative or noncompliant. Using active listening skills to understand patients' perspectives and using the universal skills of establishing rapport with them can help nurses to identify potential areas of cultural conflict and select teaching interventions that minimize such conflict (Campinha-Bacote, 2011). Labeling of patient behaviors, which may stem from cultural beliefs and practices, can negatively influence nurse–patient interactions (J. M. Anderson, 1987, 1990; Gutierrez & Rogoff, 2003).

Nurses must remember one very important thing when conducting cultural assessments: They must be especially careful not to avoid stereotyping patients based on their ethnic heritage. Just because someone belongs to a particular subculture does not necessarily mean that the person adheres to all the beliefs, values, customs, and practices of that ethnic group. Nurses should never assume a patient's learning needs or preferences for treatment will be like those of others who share the same ethnicity. Knowledge of different cultures should serve only as background cues for gathering additional information about individual variations through assessment.

General Assessment and Teaching Interventions

Given that culture affects the way someone perceives a health problem and understands its course and possible treatment options, it is essential to carry out a thorough assessment prior to establishing a plan of action for short- and long-term behavioral change. Different cultural backgrounds not only create different attitudes and reactions to illness but also can influence how people express themselves, both verbally and nonverbally, which may prove difficult to interpret. For example, asking a patient to explain what he or she believes to be the cause of a problem will help to reveal whether the patient thinks it is due to a spiritual intervention, a hex, an imbalance in nature, or some other culturally based belief. The nurse should accept the patient's explanation (most likely reflecting the beliefs of the support system as well) in a nonjudgmental manner.

Culture also guides the way an ill person is defined and treated. For example, some cultures believe that once the symptoms disappear, illness is no longer present. This belief can be problematic for individuals with an acute illness, such as a streptococcal infection, when a 1- or 2-day course of antibiotic therapy relieves the soreness in the throat. This belief also can pose a problem for the individual with a chronic disease that often has periods of remission or exacerbation.

In addition, readiness to learn must be assessed from the standpoint of a person's culture. Behavior change may be context specific for some patients and their family members; that is, they will adhere to a recommended medical regimen while in the hospital, but then fail to follow through with the guidelines once they return home. Also, the nurse must not assume that the values adhered to by professionals are equally important or cherished by the patient and family. Consideration, too, must be given to specific cultural influences that may hinder readiness to learn, such as perceptions of time, financial barriers, and environmental variables. Finally, the patient needs to believe that new behaviors are not only possible but also beneficial for behavioral change to be maintained over the long term (Kessels, 2003).

Providing culture-specific programs and teaching interventions for children and adults from minority groups is both a practical and ethical need in the U.S. healthcare system. To adequately serve patients in a multiethnic society, attention must be focused on identifying cross-cultural barriers and delivering culturally effective health education. Studies have clearly shown that health outcomes are improved when education is appropriately given in the context of the individual (Bailey et al., 2009; Hawthorne, Robles, Cannings-John, & Edwards, 2008; Vidaeff, Kerrigan, & Monga, 2015).

The following specific guidelines for assessment should be used regardless of the particular cultural orientation of the patient (J. M. Anderson, 1987; Uzundede, 2006):

1. Identify the patient's primary language. Assess his or her ability to understand, read, and speak the language of the nurse.
2. Observe the interactions between the patient and his or her family. Determine who makes the decisions, how decisions are made, who is the primary caregiver, which type of care is given, and which foods and other objects are important.
3. Listen to the patient. Find out what the person wants, how his or her wants differ from what the family wants, and how they differ from what you think is appropriate.
4. Consider the patient's communication abilities and patterns. Note, for example, manners of speaking (rate of speech, expressions used) and nonverbal cues that can enhance or hinder understanding. Also, be aware of your own nonverbal behaviors that may be acceptable or unacceptable to the patient and family.
5. Explore customs or taboos. Observe behaviors and clarify beliefs and practices that may interfere with care or treatment.
6. Become oriented to the individual's and family's sense of time and time frames.
7. Determine which communication approaches are appropriate with respect to what is the most comfortable way to address the patient and family. Find the symbolic objects and activities that provide comfort and security.
8. Assess the patient's religious practices and determine how his or her religious beliefs influence perceptions of illness and treatment.

These guidelines will assist in the exchange of information between the nurse and patient. The teacher/learner role is a mutual one in which the nurse is both teacher and learner and the patient is also both learner and teacher. The goal of negotiation is to arrive at ways of working together to solve a problem or to determine a course of action (J. M. Anderson, 1987, 1990). The nurse must recognize that each person is an individual and that differences exist within and between ethnic and racial groups.

Another useful framework for patient teaching is the LEARN model that emphasizes ways to improve cross-cultural communication between patients and healthcare providers. These guidelines are as follows (Berlin & Fowkes, 1983):

L—*Listen* with sympathy and understanding to the patient's perception of the problem
E—*Explain* your perceptions of the problem
A—*Acknowledge* and discuss the differences and similarities
R—*Recommend* approaches to treatment
N—*Negotiate* agreement

Use of Interpreters

When the nurse does not speak the same language as the patient, it is necessary to secure the assistance of an interpreter. Interpreters may be family members or friends, other healthcare staff, or professional interpreters. For many reasons, the use of family or friends as interpreters is not as desirable as using professionally trained individuals for nurse–patient interactions.

Research has shown that ad hoc interpreters (e.g., family, friends, nonclinical hospital employees) are much more likely to make a clinically significant error in interpretation than professional interpreters (Flores, Abreu, Barone, Bachur, & Lin, 2012; "LEP Patients," 2012). Family members and friends may not be sufficiently fluent to assume the role of interpreter, or they may choose to omit portions of the content they believe to be unnecessary or unacceptable. Finally, the presence of family members or friends may inhibit communication with the nurse and violate the patient's right to privacy and confidentiality (Baker, Parker, Williams, Coates, & Pitkin, 1996; Poss & Rangel, 1995; Schenker, Lo, Ettinger, & Fernandez, 2008).

Ideally, professionally trained interpreters will be used for assessment, teaching, and other important interactions. Interpreters can convey messages verbatim, and they work under an established code of ethics and confidentiality. When determining whether a healthcare interpreter is required, the nurse should consider how critical and complex the teaching situation is, the degree to which the nurse can be understood by the client, the patient's preferences, and the availability of resources (Schenker et al., 2008).

If a bilingual person is not available to facilitate communication, telephone interpreting services, such as Certified Language International, provide professional interpreters in more than 200 languages on a 24-hours-a-day, 7-days-a-week basis. These services are certified by The Joint Commission and other accrediting bodies, are approved by the Department of Human Services, and are HIPAA (Health Insurance Portability and Accountability Act) compliant. Also, iPhones and iPads now have translation software apps, known as Vocre and My Language Pro, that will instantly translate voice or text into many different languages to connect people in the world so language is no longer a major barrier (http://www.vocre.com; https://itunes.apple.com/US/app/voice-text-translator-speak/id323470584?mt=8).

When not using an interpreter, the nurse can use the following strategies when teaching clients who are partially fluent in English (Poss & Rangel, 1995; Stanislav, 2006).

- Speak slowly and distinctly and allow twice as much time for the teaching session.
- Use simple sentences, relying on an active rather than a passive voice.
- Avoid technical terms (e.g., use *heart* rather than *cardiac*, or *stomach* rather than *gastric*).
- Also avoid medical jargon (e.g., use *blood pressure* rather than *BP*) and idioms (e.g., *it's just red tape you have to go through* or *I heard it straight from the horse's mouth*).
- Organize instructional material in a logical order.
- Do not make assumptions that the patient understands what has been said. Ask patients to explain what they heard by using the teach-back approach or request a return demonstration.

The Four Major Subcultural Ethnic Groups

The U.S. Census Bureau (2011a) defines the major minority ethnic groups in this country as follows: Black/African American (of African, Haitian, and Dominican Republic descents), Hispanic/Latino (of Mexican, Cuban, Puerto Rican, and other Latin descents), Asian/Pacific Islander (of Japanese, Chinese, Filipino, Korean, Vietnamese, Hawaiian, Guamanian, Samoan, and Asian Indian descents), and American Indian/Alaska Native (descendants of hundreds of tribes of Native Americans and of Eskimo descent).

Given the fact that there are many ethnic groups (subcultures) in the United States, and hundreds worldwide, it is impossible to address the cultural characteristics of each one of them. Instead, this section reviews the beliefs and health practices of the four major subcultures in this country as identified by the U.S. Census Bureau. Based on the latest 2010 census data available (a full national census is conducted every 10 years), these groups account for approximately one third (34.09%) of the total U.S. population. The Hispanic/Latino and Asian/Pacific Islander groups are the fastest growing ethnic subcultures in this country (U.S. Census Bureau, 2011b).

One of the most important roles of the nurse is to serve as an advocate for patients. To do so effectively, nurses must be aware of the customs, beliefs, and lifestyles of the diverse populations they serve.

The number of registered nurses (RNs) who are from the four ethnic minority subcultures as compared to the dominant white culture are highly underrepresented in the U.S. workforce (see **Figure 8–3**). If the ethnic profile of RNs is to more closely mirror the ethnic percentages of people in this country, then a concerted effort has to be made to attract and retain culturally diverse nursing students to provide culturally appropriate and sensitive health care for better health outcomes (Muronda, 2015).

In addition to information provided here on the four major ethnic groups, libraries and the World Wide Web provide an array of resources that describe the beliefs and practices of particular tribes or subcultures specifically not addressed.

Hispanic/Latino Culture

According to the U.S. Census Bureau, the Hispanic/Latino group is the largest and the fastest growing subculture in the United States. As of the last full census survey in 2010, there were approximately 50.5 million people of Hispanic/Latino origin in this country, an increase of 43% since the start of the 21st century. Due to immigration and a high birth rate, members of this group represented 16% of the total population in the United States (U.S. Census Bureau, 2011a).

Hispanic or Latino Americans derive from diverse origins. Members of this heterogeneous group of Americans with varied backgrounds in culture and heritage are of Latin American or Spanish origin and use Spanish (or a related dialect) as their dominant language. Those of Mexican heritage account for the largest number of people (approximately 60%) of this subculture, followed by Puerto Ricans, Central and South Americans, and Cuban Americans.

Hispanic/Latino Americans are found in every state but are concentrated in just nine states. California and Texas together are home to half of the Hispanic population,

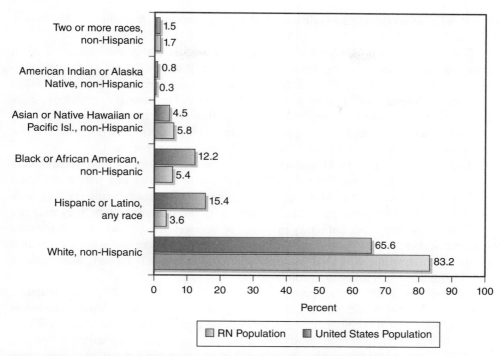

Figure 8–3 **Distribution of registered nurses and the U.S. population by racial/ethnic background in 2008**

U.S. Department of Health and Human Services, Health Resources Services Administration. (2010, September). *The registered nurse population: Findings from the 2008 National Sample Survey of Registered Nurses.*

but other large concentrations are found in New York, New Jersey, Florida, Illinois, Arizona, New Mexico, and Colorado (U.S. Census Bureau, 2010b). Nurses who practice in the Southwestern states are most likely to encounter patients of Mexican heritage, those practicing in the Northeast states will most likely be caregivers of patients of Puerto Rican heritage, and nurses in Florida will deliver care to a large number of Cuban Americans. While Hispanic Americans have many common characteristics, each subgroup has unique characteristics.

The people of Hispanic heritage have particular healthcare needs that must be addressed. They are disproportionately affected by certain cancers, alcoholism, drug abuse, obesity, hypertension, diabetes, adolescent pregnancy, tuberculosis, dental disease, and human immunodeficiency virus (HIV)/acquired immune deficiency syndrome (AIDS). Homicide, AIDS, and perinatal conditions rank in the top 10 as causes of mortality of Hispanic/Latino Americans. Hispanics are less likely to receive preventive care, often lack health insurance, and have less access to health care than whites living in the United States (CDC, 2011; Chen, Bustamante, & Tom, 2015; Fernandez & Hebert, 2000;

Hebert & Fernandez, 2000; Hosseini, 2015; Pacquiao, Archeval, & Shelley, 2000; Purnell, 2013; USDHHS, 2012).

Fluency in Spanish as a foreign language for nurses is highly recommended when delivering care to this growing, underserved, culturally diverse ethnic group. Spanish-speaking people represent 62% of all non-English-speaking persons in the United States (U.S. Census Bureau, 2010b). In proportion to their share of the nation's population, those of Hispanic heritage are underrepresented in the professional nursing workforce. Only 3.6% of all graduates of basic nursing programs are of Hispanic descent (Figure 8–3)—far too few to satisfy the increasing need for Hispanic healthcare professionals.

Access to health care by Hispanics is limited both by choice and by unavailability of health services. Only one fifth of all Puerto Rican Americans, one fourth of Cuban Americans, and one third of Mexican Americans see a physician during the course of a year. Even when Hispanic people have access to the healthcare system, they may not receive the care they need. Difficulty in obtaining services, dissatisfaction with the care provided, and inability to afford the rising costs of medical care are major factors that discourage them from using the healthcare system (Fernandez & Hebert, 2000; Juckett, 2013; Purnell, 2013; Whittemore, 2007).

Approximately 25% of Hispanic families live below the poverty line. Hispanic Americans, along with African Americans, are approximately twice as likely to be below the poverty level than members of other subcultural groups in the United States (CDC, 2011). Their general economic disadvantage leaves little disposable income for paying out-of-pocket expenses for health care. When they do seek a regular source of care, many people in this minority group rely on public health facilities, hospital outpatient clinics, and emergency rooms (Kaplan & Inguanzo, 2011; Purnell, 2013; Wright & Newman-Ginger, 2010). Also, they are very accepting of health care being delivered in their homes, where they feel a sense of control, stability, and security (Pacquiao et al., 2000).

The health beliefs of Hispanic people also affect their decisions to seek traditional care. Many studies dating from the 1940s to the current day on Hispanic health beliefs and practices stress the existence of folklore practices, such as this group's use of herbs, teas, home remedies, and over-the-counter drugs for treating symptoms of acute and chronic illnesses. In addition, Hispanic/Latino Americans place a high degree of reliance on health healers, known as *curanderos* or *espiritistas*, for health advice and treatment (Fernandez & Hebert, 2000; Purnell, 2013). In addition to being culturally appropriate, these health healers are more likely to speak Spanish than traditional healthcare providers, and their services can be obtained at lower cost (Titus, 2014).

Illnesses of Mexican Americans as a Hispanic subgroup can be organized into the following categories (Caudle, 1993; Juckett, 2013; Markides & Coreil, 1986; Purnell, 2013):

1. Diseases of hot and cold, believed to be due to an imbalanced intake of foods or ingestion of foods at extreme opposites in temperature. In addition, cold air is thought to lead to joint pain, and a cold womb results in barrenness in women. Heating or chilling is the traditional cure for parts of the body afflicted by disease.
2. Diseases of dislocation of internal organs, cured by massage or physical manipulation of body parts.

3. Diseases of magical origin, caused by *mal ojo*, or evil eye, a disorder of infants and children as a result of a woman's looking admiringly at someone else's child without touching the child, resulting in crying, fitful sleep, diarrhea, vomiting, and fever.
4. Diseases of emotional origin, attributed to sudden or prolonged terror called *susto*.
5. Folk-defined diseases, such as *latido*.
6. Standard scientific diseases.

The overall health status of Hispanic Americans can be determined by examining key health indicators of infant mortality, life expectancy, and mortality from cardiovascular disease and cancer and measures of functional health. Research findings indicate that the health of people of Hispanic heritage is much closer to that of white Americans than to that of African Americans, even though the Hispanic and black populations share similar socioeconomic conditions. Concerning the incidence of diabetes and infectious and parasitic diseases, however, Hispanic people are clearly at a disadvantage in relation to white people. Possible explanations for the relative advantages and disadvantages in health status of Hispanic Americans involve such factors as the following (Purnell, 2013):

- Cultural practices favor reproductive success.
- Early pregnancies and high fertility rates contribute to low breast cancer incidence but increased cervical cancer rates.
- Dietary habits are linked to low cancer rates but a high prevalence of obesity and diabetes.
- Genetic heritage.
- Extended family support reduces the need for psychiatric services.
- Low SES contributes to increased infectious and parasitic diseases.

Alcoholism also represents a serious health problem for many Hispanic Americans. Chronic liver disease and cirrhosis are among the leading causes of death for this population (CDC, 2012). Furthermore, as the Hispanic population becomes more acculturated, certain risk factors for cardiovascular disease and certain cancers are expected to play larger roles in this group (Markides & Coreil, 1986; Purnell, 2013).

Today, the literature disagrees about the extent and frequency to which Hispanic people use home remedies and folk practices. In the southwestern United States, the Hispanic population has been found to use herbs and other home remedies to treat illness episodes at twice the proportion reported in the total U.S. population. Other studies claim that the use of folk practitioners has declined and practically disappeared in some Hispanic subgroups (Purnell, 2013).

Knowing where people get their health information can provide clues to nurses as to how to best teach particular population groups. For example, Mexican Americans, like other Latin American groups, tend to rely on family as the primary source of credible health information. Therefore, when teaching a patient, health information should be shared with significant others within the family unit (Eggenberger, Grassley, & Restrepo, 2006; Purnell, 2013).

Because the family is the center of Hispanic people's lives, the extended family serves as the single most important source of social support. This culture is characterized by a pattern of respect and obedience to elders as well as a pattern of male dominance. The focus of patient education by nurses, therefore, needs to be on the family rather than on the individual. It is likely, for example, that a woman would be reluctant to make a decision about her or her child's health care without consulting her husband first (Purnell, 2013).

Gender and family member roles are changing, however, as more Hispanic women take jobs outside the home. Also, children tend to pick up the English language more quickly than their parents and often end up in the powerful position of acting as interpreters for their adult relatives. The heavy reliance on family has been linked to this minority group's low utilization of healthcare services. In addition, levels of education correlate highly with access to health care. The less education members within a household have, the poorer the family's health status and access to health care (Purnell, 2013; USDHHS, 2012). Hispanic Americans are more likely than the general U.S. population to read English below the basic health literacy level and to have lower educational attainment than non-Hispanic whites (National Center for Education Statistics, 2006).

TEACHING STRATEGIES

Only approximately 40% of the Hispanic population has completed 4 years of high school or more, and only 10% have completed college, as compared with approximately 80% and 20%, respectively, of the non-Hispanic population (Pew Research Center, 2010). Both the educational level and the primary language of Hispanic patients need to be taken into consideration when selecting instructional materials (National Center for Education Statistics, 2006). Sophisticated teaching methods, such as self-instruction and simulation, and instructional tools, such as computer resources and high literacy print materials, likely would be inappropriate for those who have minimal levels of education.

The age of the population also can affect health and patient education efforts. According to the U.S. Census Bureau (2009), the Hispanic population is young as a total group (34% of this group is younger than 18 years of age). Thus the school system is an important setting for educating members of the Hispanic community. For Hispanic students, education programs in the school system on alcohol and drug abuse and on cardiovascular disease risk reduction have proved successful when the following criteria were met by the nurse in the role of patient educator:

- Cultural beliefs were observed.
- An individual accepted and respected by the group was the one to introduce the nurse.
- Family members were included.
- The community was encouraged to take responsibility for resolving the health problems discussed.

Morbidity, mortality, and risk factor data also provide clues to the areas in which patient education efforts should be directed. As mentioned earlier, Hispanic people have higher rates of diabetes, AIDS, obesity, alcohol-related illnesses, and mortality from homicide compared to the general population. All of these topics should be targeted for educational efforts at disease prevention and health promotion (Caudle, 1993; CDC, 2012). The following general suggestions are useful when designing and implementing education programs for Hispanic Americans (Caudle, 1993; Fernandez & Hebert 2000; Hebert & Fernandez, 2000; Pacquiao et al., 2000; Purnell, 2013):

1. Identify the Hispanic American subgroups (e.g., Mexican, Cuban, and Puerto Rican) in the community whose needs differ in terms of health beliefs, language, and general health status. Design education programs that can be targeted to meet their distinct ethnic needs.

2. Be alert to individual differences within subgroups as to age, years of education, income levels, job status, and degree of acculturation.

3. Take into account special health needs with respect to incidences of diseases and risk factors to which they are vulnerable—breast cancer in women (Borrayo, 2004), diabetes, AIDS, obesity, alcohol-related illnesses, homicide, and accidental injuries.

4. Recognize the importance of family in supporting one another, so be sure to direct education efforts to include all interested members and remember that decision making typically rests with the male and elder authority figures in homes where tradition is strong.

5. Provide adequate space for teaching to accommodate family members who typically accompany patients seeking health care.

6. Be aware of the importance of the Roman Catholic religion in their lives when dealing with such issues as contraception, abortion, and family planning.

7. Demonstrate cultural sensitivity to health beliefs by respecting and taking time to learn about their ethnic values and beliefs.

8. Consider other care practices, such as home remedies that they might be using before entering or while within the healthcare system.

9. Be aware of the modesty felt by some women and girls, who may be particularly uncomfortable in talking about sexual issues in mixed company.

10. Display warmth, friendliness, and tactfulness when developing relationships because they expect nurses and other health providers to be informal and interested in their lives.

11. Determine whether Spanish is the language by which the patient best communicates, but remember that even though speaking Spanish may be preferred, the patient and family members are not always literate in reading their own native language.

12. Speak slowly and distinctly, avoiding the use of technical words and slang if the patient has limited proficiency in the English language.

13. Do not assume that a nod of the head or a smile indicates understanding of what has been said. Members of this heritage respect authority and, therefore, it is not uncommon for them to display nonverbal cues that may be misleading or misinterpreted by the nurse. Ask patients to repeat in their own words what they have been told using the teach-back method to determine their level of understanding (Weiss, 2003).

14. If interpreters are used, be sure they speak the dialect of the learner and that they interpret instructions rather than just translate them verbatim, so that the real meaning gets conveyed. Also, be sure to talk to the patient, not to the interpreter. If an interpreter is not available, use a telephone interpreting service.
15. Provide written and audiovisual materials in Spanish that reflect linguistic appropriateness and cultural sensitivity (Borrayo, 2004).

As listed previously, nurses must take into account the cultural beliefs and health and education needs of Hispanic Americans. By extending themselves to Hispanics in a culturally sensitive manner, nurses have the opportunity to effectively and efficiently address the needs of this rapidly growing segment of the U.S. population (Borrayo, 2004).

Black/African American Culture

According to the most recent census survey, members of the black/African American culture make up the second largest ethnic group in the United States. Currently, black Americans constitute 14% of the nation's population. The majority of this ethnic population resides in the South (54%), and approximately 19% live in the Midwest, 18% in the Northeast, and 9% in the West. The greatest concentration resides in large metropolitan areas (U.S. Census Bureau, 2010a).

The cultural origins and heritage of black Americans are quite diverse. Their roots are mainly from Africa and the Caribbean Islands. They speak a variety of languages, including French, Spanish, African dialects, and various forms of English. Depending on the age cohort group to which they belong, African Americans may prefer to identify themselves differently as a racial group. For example, the youngest generation often refers to themselves by the term *African American*, while middle-aged and older members of this ethnic group usually prefer the term *black* or *black American*. Each designation is politically correct according to the U.S. Census Bureau's identification of this ethnic group as black/African American. However, because the diversity of cultural heritage varies within the many black subgroups, nurses and other providers need to be aware of ethnic differences in cultural beliefs, customs, and traditions between these groups (Purnell, 2013).

Unfortunately, African Americans have suffered a long history of inequality in educational opportunity. They were victims of school segregation and inferior facilities until a 1954 U.S. Supreme Court decision, *Brown v. Board of Education of Topeka*, outlawed the separation of blacks and whites in the public school systems. However, this educational deprivation has had long-term consequences, such as unequal access to higher paying and higher status job opportunities, which has led to low wages and a disproportionate number (approximately 23%) of African Americans living at or below the poverty level (U.S. Census Bureau, 2010a).

Poverty and low educational attainment also have had major consequences for the black American community in terms of social and medical issues. Although black families place a high value on education, which they see as a means to raise their standard of living by being able to secure better jobs and a higher social status, there continues to be a greater than average high school dropout rate among blacks, and many individuals remain poorly educated with accompanying literacy problems (Purnell, 2013). Despite the fact that fewer African Americans have a college degree than white Americans, one promising trend is that recently the number of black workers in the labor force earning a college degree (25%) is growing more quickly than ever before in history (U.S. Department of Labor, 2012). Nevertheless, low educational levels and socioeconomic deprivation that have persisted and continue to persist in the black community are strongly correlated with higher incidence of disease, poor nutrition, lower survival rates, and a decreased quality of life in general (Purnell, 2013; Rognerud & Zahl, 2005).

Also, increased exposure to hazardous working conditions in low-paying, manual labor jobs has resulted in a greater incidence of occupation-related diseases and illnesses among this population. In addition, the majority of blacks reside in inner-city areas where exposure to violence and pollution puts them at greater risk for disease, disability, and death. The average life span of black Americans is shorter than that of white Americans due to the high death rates of blacks from cancer, cardiovascular disease, cirrhosis, diabetes, accidents, homicides, and infant mortality (R. M. Anderson et al., 2000; Dignam, 2000; Forrester, 2000; Holt, Kyles, Wiehagen, & Casey, 2003; Keyserling et al., 2000; Mackenbach, Cavelaars, Kunst, Groenhof, & EU Working Group on Socioeconomic Inequalities in Health, 2000; Monden et al., 2006; Rognerud & Zahl, 2005; Samuel-Hodge et al., 2006; Yanek, Becker, Moy, Gettelsohn, & Koffman, 2001). Also, blacks are at higher risk for drug and alcohol abuse, drug addiction, teenaged pregnancy, and sexually transmitted diseases (Purnell, 2013).

Purnell (2013) reported findings indicating that African Americans are pessimistic about human relationships and that their belief system emphasizes three major themes:

1. The world is a hostile and dangerous place to live.
2. The individual is vulnerable to attack from external forces.
3. The individual is considered helpless, with few internal resources with which to combat adversity.

Because many African Americans tend to be suspicious of Western ethnocentric medical providers, they often seek the assistance of nurses and physicians only when absolutely necessary (Purnell, 2013). Figure 8–3 shows that not enough RNs from this ethnic group are represented in the nursing workforce in proportion to the number of blacks in the U.S. population. This mistrust of blacks toward traditional U.S. health care is believed to stem from centuries of discrimination and unethical research practices, such as the infamous Tuskegee syphilis study (L. D. Wilson, 2011). Instead, folk practitioners are held in high esteem by this population and are sought after for the culturally sensitive care they provide.

Common to the black culture is the concept of extended family, consisting of several households, with the older adults often taking the leadership role within the family constellation. Respect for elders and ancestors is greatly valued. Older adults are held in high regard because living a long life indicates that the individual had more opportunities to acquire greater experience and knowledge. Decision making regarding healthcare issues is, therefore, often left to the elders. Family ties are especially strong between grandchildren and grandparents, such that it is not unusual for grandmothers to want to stay at the hospital bedside when their grandchildren are ill. This extended family network provides emotional, physical, and financial support to members during times of illness and other crises (Forrester, 2000; Purnell, 2013).

Single parenting within the African American culture is an accepted position without stigma attached to it. In 2011, approximately 67% of black or African American children were being raised in a single-parent family, as compared to 25% of white children and 42% of Hispanic or Latino children (National Kids Count Program, 2011). Becoming a mother at a young age, although not highly desirable or condoned by black women, is met with a fairly high level of tolerance in this cultural group (Purnell, 2013). In fact, black women do not perceive negative sanctions within their culture if they do not meet the ideal norm of getting an education or job prior to marriage and children. Relatives are supportive of one another if help is needed with childrearing.

Spirituality and religiosity are very much a prominent cultural component of this ethnic group's community. These aspects are a central and defining feature of African American life, serving as a source of hope, renewal, liberation, and unity among its members. **Spirituality** is defined as a belief in a higher power, a sacred force that exists in all things. **Religiosity** is defined as an individual's level of adherence to beliefs and ritualistic practices associated with religious institutions (Holt, Clark, & Kreuter, 2003; Mattis, 2000; Mattis & Jagers, 2001; Puchalski & Romer, 2000).

Both spirituality and religion often play a role in the development and maintenance of social relationships throughout the human life span. Blacks, more so than whites, turn to religion to cope with health challenges. Additionally, as trusted resources in the community, African American blacks are turning more and more to their churches for support in times of illness, as well as for health education and other health promotion activities (Collins, 2015; Hayes, 2015).

Religious practices also have been found to influence health beliefs and positively influence health status and outcomes in the African American community (Newlin, Knafl, & Melkus, 2002). These strong religious values and beliefs by individuals may extend to their feelings about illness and health. A majority of black Americans find inner strength from their trust in God. Some believe that whatever happens is God's will. This belief has led to the perception that black Americans have a fatalistic view of life (Purnell, 2013) and are governed by a relatively strong external locus of control (Holt, Clark, & Kreuter, 2003).

A traditional folk practice, known as *voodoo*, consists of beliefs about good or evil spirits inhabiting the world. One belief is that a religious leader or voodoo doctor has the power to appease or release hostile spirits. Illness, or disharmony, is thought to be caused by evil spirits because a person failed to follow religious rules or the dictates of ancestors. Curative measures involve finding the cause of an illness—a hex or a spell placed on a person by another or the breaking of a taboo—and then finding someone with magical healing powers or witchcraft to rid the afflicted individual of the evil spirit(s). Some black American families also continue to practice home remedies such as the use of mustard plasters, taking of herbal medicines and teas, and wearing of amulets to cure or ward off a variety of illnesses and afflictions (Purnell, 2013).

TEACHING STRATEGIES

In a review of articles published from 2005 to 2010, Weekes (2012) found that health literacy had a notable impact on health outcomes among African Americans. Specifically, health literacy influenced their understanding of diseases, their feelings of self-efficacy, their perceived susceptibility to illness, and their adherence to medical protocols and medication regimens. This literature review highlights the important role of health literacy when nurses carry out patient education in various healthcare settings.

In teaching black Americans preventive and promotion measures as well as when caring for them during illnesses, the nurse must explore the patients' value systems and cultural beliefs. Generally, any folk practices or traditional beliefs should be respected, allowed (if they are not harmful), and incorporated into the recommended treatment or healthcare interventions used by Western medicine. The following list offers more specific points for nurses to consider to be sure they render culturally appropriate care for black Americans (Forrester, 2000; Purnell, 2013). Members of this minority population group tend to:

- Express feelings openly to family and friends, but they are much more private about family matters when in the company of strangers.
- Prefer being greeted in a formal manner by using their surnames when outside their circle of family and friends, which demonstrates respect and pride for their family heritage.
- Feel comfortable with less personal space and use humor, joking, and teasing to reduce stress and tension.
- Be oriented more to the present than the past or future and, thus, are likely to be relaxed about specific time frames. As a result, appointments will usually be kept, but they may be late, which requires health providers to be flexible with scheduling.
- Live in a traditional family structure that is matriarchal with a high percentage of households run by a female single parent. Women play a dominant role in decision making, and grandmothers are often involved in providing economic support and child care for their grandchildren, so nurses must recognize the importance of sharing health information directly with them.

Diabetes and hypertension continue to be the most serious health problems for African Americans, with higher morbidity and mortality rates from these diseases than in other Americans (Samuel-Hodge et al., 2006; Yanek et al., 2001). Also, as stated previously, blacks are at higher risk for being victims of violence, accidents, disabilities, and cancer (Forrester, 2000; Purnell, 2013). Obesity is another major problem among black Americans. Food to them is a symbol of health and wealth, and a higher than ideal body weight is viewed positively by members of this ethnic group.

Nurses must concentrate on disease prevention measures; institute early screening for high blood pressure, cancer, and diabetes, as well as screening for signs and symptoms of other diseases common in this population; and provide culturally appropriate health education to improve the overall health status of black Americans (Bailey, Erwin, & Belin, 2000; Powe, Daniels, Finnie, & Thompson, 2005). Their strong family ties encourage black individuals to be treated by the family before seeking care from nurses and other health professionals. This cultural practice may be a factor contributing to the delay or failure of blacks to seek treatment for diseases at the early stages of illness.

Due to economic factors, black Americans are likely to have less ready access to healthcare services. Identified barriers to black Americans seeking the health care they need include lack of culturally relevant care, perceptions of racial discrimination, and a general distrust of both healthcare professionals and the healthcare system. Establishing a trusting relationship, therefore, is an essential first step to be taken by nurses if blacks are to receive and accept the health services they require and deserve. Recognizing their unique responses to health and illness based on their spiritual and religious foundations, their strong family ties, and other traditional beliefs is essential if therapeutic interventions developed by the healthcare team are to be successful. Efforts to recruit more blacks into the nursing profession would most assuredly help to reduce some of the barriers to caring for this population of Americans.

Asian/Pacific Islander Culture

People from Asian countries and the Pacific Islands constitute the third major ethnic subcultural group in the United States. Although Japanese and Chinese immigrants settled in the United States in the early 1900s, many Southeast Asians came as refugees to the United States after World War II, the Korean War, the fall of South Vietnam, and the chaos in the governments of Laos and Cambodia. To a large extent, they have settled on the West Coast, particularly in the San Francisco Bay area of California and in Washington state (U.S. Census Bureau, 2010c; Villanueva & Lipat, 2000; Young, McCormick, & Vitaliano, 2002). Also, the states of New York, New Jersey, and Texas have experienced a large influx of Asian peoples, particularly from China, the Philippines, and Japan. As of 2010, more than 17.3 million Asian/Pacific Islanders (5.6% of the total U.S. population) live in the country (U.S. Census Bureau, 2010c).

Although Asian/Pacific Islander people have been classified as a single ethnic group, their beliefs and practices are not the same because a wide variety of cultural, religious, and language backgrounds are represented. Some similarities exist among members of this group, but there are also many differences (Purnell, 2013). By understanding the basic beliefs of the Asian/Pacific Islander people, nurses can be better prepared to understand and accept their cultural differences and varied behavior patterns (Villanueva & Lipat, 2000; Young et al., 2002). Figure 8–3 indicates that the supply of registered nurses of Asian/Pacific Islander descent had grown to 5.8% in 2008 (from 3.1% in 2004) and is close in proportion (although not necessarily in geographic distribution) to the population of this ethnic group in the United States.

The major philosophical orientation of the Asian/Pacific Islander people is a blend of four philosophies—Buddhism, Confucianism, Taoism, and phi. Four common values are strongly reflected in all of these philosophies:

1. Male authority and dominance
2. Saving face (behavior as a result of a sense of pride)
3. Strong family ties
4. Respect for parents, elders, teachers, and other authority figures

The following is a brief review of the beliefs and healthcare practices of the Asian/ Pacific Islander people (Pang, 2007; Purnell, 2013).

BUDDHISM

The fundamental belief underlying Buddhism is that all existence is suffering. The continuation of life, and therefore suffering, arises from desires and passions. According to the Buddhist philosophy, humans are not limited to a single existence terminating in death; instead, everyone is reincarnated. Cambodians, who are particularly strongly influenced by the Buddhist philosophy, strive to accumulate religious merits or good deeds to ensure a better life to come. Sharing, donating, being generous, and being kind are all ways to accumulate merits. They adhere to a deep belief in *karma*, whereby things done in this existence will help or hinder them to reach nirvana, a place free of pain and suffering.

CONFUCIANISM

Moral values and beliefs are heavily influenced by Confucian philosophy, which focuses on the moral aspects of one's personality. Two predominant moral qualities are humaneness (the attitude that is shown toward others) and a sense of moral duty and obligation (attitudes that persons display toward themselves). The principles that guide the social behavior of people who adhere to Confucianism are described as follows.

Patterns of Authority

The following five relationships run from inferior (No. 1) to superior (No. 5) to form a pattern of obligation and authority in the family as well as in social and political realms:

1. Son (child) to father
2. Wife to husband
3. Younger brother to older brother
4. Friend to friend
5. Subject to ruler

These patterns of authority and obligation influence decision making and social interactions. For example, a friend is to regard a friend as a younger or older brother. Women's subservience to men is reflected in a woman's behavior to always seek the advice of her husband when making decisions. This authority needs to be respected by nursing staff when, for instance, a woman refuses to choose a contraceptive method until she asks for her husband's advice and permission.

Man in Harmony With the Universe

In the Confucian system, people are seen as being between heaven and earth, and life has to be in harmony with the universe. An example of this principle is when an Asian responds passively to new information, accepting it rather than actively seeking to clarify it. Therefore it is important for the nurse to ask the patient for an explanation of the information taught to determine if it was understood.

Ancestor Worship

Concern for the moral order of relationships is reflected in a deep reverence for tradition and rituals. Great emphasis is placed on funerals, the procedures for mourning, and the group sharing of a meal with the dead.

TAOISM

The Tao philosophy has its roots in the belief of two opposing magical forces in nature, the negative (yin) and the positive (yang), which affect the course of all material and spiritual life. The basic concepts of Chinese philosophy—namely, the beliefs in *tao* (the way of nature) and *yin and yang* (the principle of balance)—stress that human achievement in harmony with nature should be accomplished through nonaction.

Common also is the idea that good health depends on the balance between hot and cold. Equilibrium of hot and cold elements, it is thought, produces good health. Thus drugs, natural elements, and foods are classified as either hot or cold. It is believed that sickness can be caused by eating too much hot or cold food. Hot foods include meats, sweets, and spices; cold foods include rice and vegetables.

Illness is believed to result from an imbalance in the forces of nature. Ill health is believed to be a curse from heaven, with mental illness being the worst possible curse, because the individual was irresponsible in not obtaining the right amount of rest, food, and work. The Chinese people believe in strong family ties, respect for elders, and the authority of men as the head of the household. As a consequence, sons are highly valued.

PHI

Phi worship is a belief in the spirits of dead relatives or the spirits of animals and nature. Phi ranges from bad to good. If a place has a strong phi, the individual must make an offering before doing anything in that place, such as building a house or tilling the land. If someone violates a rule of order, an atmosphere of bad phi can result in illness or death. Redemption can be sought from a phi priest as a hope of getting relief from suffering. Offerings are made and special rites are performed to rid the person of a bad phi.

Worshipers of this philosophy respect elders and avoid conflict by doing things in a pleasant manner. Those who adhere to the phi philosophy are hospitable and generous. They show respect to others by the way a person is addressed, and they tend to prize hard work and ambition.

The Asian/Pacific Islander culture values harmony in life and a balance of nature. Shame is something to be avoided, families are the center of life, elders are respected, and ancestors are worshiped and remembered. Children are highly valued because they carry on the family name and are expected to care for aging parents. The woman's role is one of subservience throughout her entire life—she will follow the advice of parents while unmarried, the husband's advice while married, and the children's advice when widowed. For people of this ethnic group, marked cultural differences confront them when they live in the United States with respect to ways of life, ways of thinking, values orientation, social structure, and family interactions (Chao, 1994; Young et al., 2002).

Children may adapt quickly to this environment, but the older generations tend to have difficulty acculturating.

The medical practices of Asian/Pacific Islanders, like their other unique cultural practices, differ significantly from Western ways. The health-seeking behaviors of immigrants tend to be crisis oriented, following the pattern in their homelands where medical care was not readily available. They are likely to seek health care only when seriously ill. Reinforcement is needed to encourage them to come for follow-up visits after an initial encounter with the healthcare system. Sometimes they are viewed by practitioners as noncompliant when they do not do exactly what is expected of them, when they withdraw from follow-up treatments, or when they do not keep scheduled appointments.

Asian people make great use of herbal remedies to treat various ills, such as fevers, diarrhea, and coughs. Dermabrasion—a practice often misunderstood by U.S. healthcare providers—is a home remedy implemented to cure a wide variety of problems such as headaches, cold symptoms, fever, and chills. In their traditional healthcare system, Asian individuals rely on folk medicines from healers, sorcerers, and monks.

Western medicine is thought to be "shots that cure," and Asian patients expect to get some form of medicine (injections or pills) whenever they seek medical help in the United States. If no medication is prescribed, the person may feel that care is inadequate unless an explanation is given.

Common to many Southeast Asians is the idea that illnesses, just like foods, are classified as hot and cold. This belief coincides with the yin and yang philosophy of the principle of balance. If a disease is considered hot in origin, then giving cold foods is believed to be the proper treatment.

Conflict and fear are the most likely responses to laboratory tests and having blood drawn. Many members of this ethnic group believe that removing blood makes the body weak and that blood is not replenished. Fear of surgery may result from the conviction that souls inhabit the body and may be released. Another major fear is the loss of privacy leading to extreme embarrassment and humiliation.

TEACHING STRATEGIES

Among Asian/Pacific Islanders, respect is automatically given to most healthcare providers who are seen as knowledgeable. Asians are sensitive and formal, so using a nonthreatening approach is necessary before caring for them. They must be given permission to ask a question but are not offended by questions from others. Language barriers are usually the first and biggest obstacles to overcome in working with people of Asian/Pacific Islander descent.

One particular characteristic to be noted of the Japanese subculture is a childlike dependency known as *amae*. This dependent behavior continues through adulthood but is especially evident when people are ill. Awareness of this common behavior pattern will allow nurses to approach patients of Japanese heritage in a culturally relevant and tolerant manner (Hisama, 2000).

Asian/Pacific Islanders' approach to learning involves repetition and rote memorization of information. The learning style of Asians is essentially passive—no personal opinions, no confrontations, no challenges, and no outward disagreements. Nurses should be aware that in the Asians' wish to save face for themselves and others, they avoid being disruptive and will agree to what is said.

Decision making, however, is a family affair. Family members, especially the male authority figure, must be included in identifying the best solution for a situation. Asians are easily shamed, so patients must be reassured and told what is considered acceptable behavior by Western moral and legal standards. Nods of the head do not necessarily mean agreement or understanding. Questions need to be asked in several ways to confirm that they understand any instructional messages given.

When working with members of this Asian/Pacific Islander culture, nurses must remember that education is most effective when it is a two-way process. Patients and their families need to be aware of the beliefs and practices of American culture, and, in turn, the nurse needs to recognize the challenges created by the cultural beliefs and practices of this ethnic group. This mutual understanding will strengthen the therapeutic relationship between the nurse and the patient to create an emotional environment that is appropriate for learning to take place (Park, Chesla, Rehm, & Chun, 2011).

American Indian/Alaska Native Culture

The U.S. Census Bureau (2010b) has identified more than 5.2 million people (almost 1.7% of the U.S. population) who are members of the American Indian/Alaska Native ethnic group (Norris, Vines, & Hoeffel, 2011). More than 500 distinct tribes of American Indians and Alaska Natives exist, including Eskimo and Aleut tribes (Lowe & Struthers, 2001). The largest of these tribes is the Cherokee. Other tribes of significant size are the Navaho, Sioux, Chippewa, Choctaw, Pueblo, and the Latin American Indian. These tribes reside primarily in the northwestern, central, and southwestern regions of the United States (Norris et al., 2011). The term *Native American* will be used throughout this section of the chapter to include both the American Indian and Native Alaska people.

Approximately half of the members of this ethnic group are eligible for health services provided by the federal government. The Indian Health Service of the United States Public Health Service maintains responsibility for providing health care to them (Mail, McKay, & Katz, 1989; Sequist, Cullen, & Acton, 2011; USDHHS, 2015a). Figure 8–3 clearly indicates that proportionately there are fewer RNs of Native American heritage to provide culturally appropriate care for the people belonging to this population group.

The current challenge to nurses is to integrate Western medicine with traditional non-Western tribal folk medicine to provide cross-cultural health education to Native Americans in reservation-based communities across the nation. To do so, nurses must understand contemporary cultural patterns that set this ethnic group apart from non-Native Americans, including their theories of what causes various diseases and the associated treatments (Cantore, 2001; Lowe & Struthers, 2001; Mail et al., 1989). It is also essential for nurses to become focused on a more ethnomedical orientation. This means understanding the nature and consequences of illness problems and therapeutic interventions from the ethnic group's perspective, rather than adhering to the biomedical orientation of defining diseases and treatment options from only a Western perspective.

The Native American concept of health and illness incorporates the relationship of humans with their universe. Differences in beliefs, however, may be found among the various Native American tribes in the United States. The following are major characteristics associated with this ethnic group as addressed by Purnell (2013), Lowe and Struthers (2001), Harding (1998), Scharnberg (2007), Joho and Ormsby (2000), Portman and Garrett (2006), and Cantore (2001).

1. A spiritual attachment to the land and harmony with nature
2. An intimacy of religion and medicine
3. Emphasis on strong ties to an extended family network, including immediate family, other relatives, and the entire tribe
4. The view that children are an asset, not a liability
5. A belief that supernatural powers exist in both animate and inanimate objects
6. A desire to remain distinct and avoid acculturation, thereby retaining one's own culture and language
7. A lack of materialism, lack of time consciousness, and a desire to share with others

These common characteristics can easily be overlooked by the nurse when care is being provided to patients of this ethnic group. To some extent, Anglo-American culture and Western healthcare practices have been integrated into the Native American way of life. However, these seven characteristics still predominate today to set this subculture apart as a unique entity.

Native Americans see a close connection between religion and health. When a family member becomes ill, witchcraft is still perceived by some tribes as the real cause of illness. In traditional societies, witchcraft functions to supply answers to perplexing or disturbing questions. It also explains personal insecurities, intragroup tensions, fears, and anxieties.

Some Native American tribes still practice witchcraft but tend to deny it as a reality because of the negative stereotype and stigma attached to it by outsiders. Nevertheless, the intimacy between religion and medicine persists and is exhibited in the form of "sing" prayers and ceremonial cure practices. However, few nurses would think of providing space and privacy for several relatives to be able to conduct a ceremony for a hospitalized family member.

Also, some Native American tribal beliefs require incorporating the medicine man (shaman) into the system of care given to patients. The central and formal aspects of Native American medicine are ceremonial, embracing the notion of a supernatural power. Although the ceremonies vary from tribe to tribe, the ideas of causation and cure are common to all Native Americans. The rituals performed are based on the signs and symptoms of an illness. In some instances, family members also conduct these rituals. Cornmeal, from the sacred food of corn, is an item that is frequently used in a variety of curative ceremonies. Herbal remedies have for generations served native healers as their pharmacopoeia. The nurse must demonstrate legitimate respect for such ritualistic symbols and ceremonial activities.

To be without a family of many relatives is to be considered really poor in the Native American world. The family and tribe are of utmost importance, which is a belief that children learn from infancy. It is not unusual for many family members—sometimes large groups of 10 to 15 people—to arrive at the hospital and camp out on the hospital grounds to be with their sick relative. Talking is unnecessary, but simply being there is highly important for everyone concerned.

Grandmothers, in particular, are of great importance to a sick child, and they frequently must give permission for a child to be hospitalized and treated. The Native American kinship system allows for a child to have several sets of grandparents, aunts, uncles, cousins, brothers, and sisters. Sometimes a number of women substitute as a mother figure for a child, which may cause role confusion for the healthcare provider.

Children are given a great deal of freedom and independence to learn from their decisions and live with the consequences of their actions. They tend not to be seen as very competitive or assertive because to call attention to oneself is interpreted by Native Americans as showy and inappropriate. They may appear spoiled, but in fact they are taught self-care and respect for others at a very early age. Children are doted on by family members, and, in turn, they have high regard for their elders. In fact, the older adults in Native American communities are highly respected and looked to for advice and counsel.

Another characteristic of Native Americans is that they generally are not very future oriented; they take one day at a time and do not feel they have control over their own destiny. Time is seen as existing on a continuum with no beginning and no end. Native Americans tend not to live by clocks and schedules. In fact, many of their homes do not have clocks, and family members eat meals and do other activities when they please.

Members of this ethnic group tend to be casual in their approach to life. This lack of time consciousness and pressure is a crucial factor when a prescribed regimen calls for the patient to follow a medication, exercise, or dietary schedule. Inattention to time, in addition, can interfere with Native Americans keeping scheduled appointments, although lack of funds rather than time seems to be the main cause of missed appointments.

Another aspect of time is reflected in Native Americans' belief that death is a part of the life cycle. Their grief processes are culturally very different. Funerals are accompanied by large feasts and the sharing of gifts with relatives of the deceased. The outward signs of grieving may differ from tribe to tribe; some tribes believe that death and passage to the afterlife should be celebrated, while others believe that tears ease the passage to the afterlife, so mourning is expected. Life after death is viewed as an opportunity to join the world of long-ago ancestors. Native Americans' view of death is closely related to their opinion about the appropriate disposal of amputated limbs. Because diabetes is so prevalent in the Native American population (O'Connell, Yi, Wilson, Manson, & Acton, 2010), it is important to know that they usually want to reclaim an amputated body part for proper burial.

Sharing is another core value of Native Americans. The concept of "being" is fundamental, and there is little stress on achievement or material wealth. Individuals are valued much more highly than material goods. Overall, Native Americans are a proud, sensitive, cooperative, passive people, devoted to tribe and family, and willing to share possessions and self with others. They are very vulnerable when it comes to their pride and dignity, and they can be easily offended by insensitive caregivers.

In terms of human relationships, Native Americans believe that to look someone in the eye is considered disrespectful. Some tribes feel that looking into the eyes of another person reveals and may even steal someone's soul. As a friendly handshake and eye contact are acceptable and even expected in the white American culture, it must be acknowledged that these gestures do not have the same meaning for the Native American. Nurses may consider lack of eye contact to mean that these patients are not interested in learning, or inattentive, when in fact all along they were taking in the message of instruction being given.

The type and incidence of health problems faced by Native Americans have undergone significant change over the years. In the first half of the 20th century, acute and infectious diseases were prevalent and were the principal cause of death. Today, as a result of increased life expectancy, Native Americans are succumbing to many lifestyle diseases and chronic conditions. Chief among the causes of morbidity and mortality are heart disease, cancer, diabetes, and drug and alcohol abuse. The rates of obesity, heart disease, and diabetes for the Native American population are among the highest of all ethnic groups. All of these issues are amenable to educational intervention and need to be addressed by nurses (Gittelsohn & Rowan, 2011; Jemigan, Duran, Ahn, & Winkleby, 2010; O'Connell et al., 2010; Sequist et al., 2011; Veazie et al., 2014).

TEACHING STRATEGIES

The Indian Health Service is a government-operated health system established in 1955 to meet federal treaty obligations to provide hospitals and outpatient clinics for the delivery of healthcare services to 2 million of the country's 5.2 million Native Americans belonging to 565 tribes. With the increased focus on using health information technology and telemedicine to deliver prevention and medical management programs, important achievements have recently been made in improving diabetes control and increasing life expectancy. Nevertheless, health disparities persist in this ethnic population as compared to the overall U.S. population (Sequist et al., 2011). The Health Education program of the Indian Health Service is committed to positively influencing wellness behaviors and good lifestyle choices through health promotion and disease prevention efforts (USDHHS, 2015a).

Although all Native Americans share some of the core beliefs and practices of their culture, each tribe is unique in its customs and language. Finding the ways and means to integrate Western medicine with the traditional Native American folk medicine in caring for the varied needs of this population group presents a challenge to the nurse. It also presents a learning opportunity for the learner who is receiving these health education services. Nurses need to focus on giving information about these diseases and risk factors, emphasize the teaching of skills related to changes in diet and exercise, and help clients to build positive coping mechanisms to deal with emotional problems.

Preparing Nurses for Diversity Care

America is no longer the homogeneous melting pot society it once was. Today, numerous and varied cultures are present in the United States due to an increasing trend toward global migration of people. In addition, nurses are caring for people from many cultures due to the globalization of nursing practice. The delivery of appropriate health care now and in the future will depend on use of a culturally informed approach that goes beyond simple language translation and an understanding of the characteristics of different cultures. As primary caregivers, nurses must learn how to relate to people—including patients and their family members, fellow healthcare practitioners, and nursing students—who come from a variety of cultural backgrounds (Career Directory, 2005).

As part of former President Bill Clinton's national leadership to eliminate cultural disparities in health by the year 2010, the U.S. government introduced a series of initiatives put forth in the *Healthy People 2010* document. One goal of this 10-year plan was to eliminate racial and ethnic disparities in health (USDHHS, 2000). This initiative has been praised as being "the first explicit commitment by the government to achieve equity in health outcomes" (Jones, 2000, p. 1214). The nursing profession embraced this goal to eliminate discrepancies in health outcomes among minority populations (Carol, 2001). Since then, a follow-up *Healthy People 2020* document has been released (USDHHS, 2012). The profession continues to contribute to the expectation of eliminating these disparities by focusing on change in both academic and practice settings as well as through clinical research.

One important step to ensure culturally competent nursing care in this new century is to increase minority representation in nursing. The profession needs to recruit and retain more minority students and faculty to expand the diversity of RNs within its ranks (Carthron, 2007). Unfortunately, only 16.8% of the nursing workforce comprises people from minority groups (Figure 8–3), whereas more than 34% of the total U.S. population belongs to a variety of cultural subgroups (U.S. Census Bureau, 2011b). Another initiative to break down cultural barriers to health care calls for strengthening multicultural perspectives in the curricula of health education programs, including nursing education (Perez & Luquis, 2014; Purnell, 2013).

Nurses must be able to create an environment in which people are encouraged to express themselves and freely describe their needs. As Dreher (1996) so aptly stated many years ago, "Transcending cultural differences is more than an appreciation of cultural diversity. It is transcending one's own investment in the social and economic system as one knows it and lives it" (p. 4). Nurses must concentrate on the cultural strategies that are needed to help individuals and groups negotiate the healthcare system.

Stereotyping: Identifying the Meaning, the Risks, and the Solutions

In addressing the diversity issues of gender, socioeconomics, and culture, nurses must acknowledge the risks of stereotyping inherent in discussing these three attributes of the learner. Throughout this chapter, it has been clearly documented that differences exist in learning based on gender, socioeconomics, and culture, which in turn often require alternative approaches to teaching. It is important to realize that differences are not based on judgments as to what is good or bad, or right or wrong; rather, nurses should be acutely aware of the need to attend to these differences in a sensitive, open, and fair manner.

Nurses must relate to each person as an individual. It is important to develop an awareness that although a person can be considered a member—or may identify with members—of a certain ethnic group, the individual has his or her own abilities, experiences, preferences, and practices. Learning needs, learning styles, and readiness to learn are all factors that influence lifestyle behaviors that go beyond the culture in which someone was raised.

Nonetheless, everyone has been socialized in subtle and not-so-subtle ways according to his or her own diversity attributes, socioeconomic and political backgrounds, and other life exposures. It is important to acknowledge the prejudices, biases, and the tendency to stereotype that can come into play when dealing with others like or unlike ourselves. We must consciously attempt to recognize these possible attitudes and the effect they may have on others in our care. To address the dangers of stereotyping on more than just a superficial level, this section examines examples of what constitutes unacceptable forms of stereotyping, which pitfalls can arise in dealing with diversity, and what can be done to avoid behaviors that stereotype ourselves and others.

Stereotyping is defined by Purnell (2013) as "an oversimplified conception, opinion, or belief about some aspect of an individual or group of people" (p. 486). Exaggerated generalizations are commonly made about the characteristics, behaviors, and motives associated with any person or group of people. Actually, stereotyping can be positive or negative, depending on how, where, when, why, and about whom it is applied (Satel, 2002).

For example, stereotyping can be a useful and acceptable process to organize or classify people if based on facts and logical reasoning that helps them to identify and understand information—for example, "he's Jewish," "she's Italian," or "they're Democrats." On the other hand, stereotyping can be negative if it is used to place people in an artificial or unfair position that oversimplifies their situation and is not based on facts. Negative stereotyping leads to disrespecting, dehumanizing, and defaming an individual or group, which serves as a barrier to equality and fairness toward others.

Stereotyping deserves a bad name when it is associated with bias or clichés. There is a huge emotional component to stereotyping. The language that is used, the attitudes that are projected, the conclusions that are drawn, and the context in which stereotyping is used all determine whether it has a positive or negative quality.

Unfortunately, classification by association is often bias. Stereotyping in this sense is used to label someone. For example, Americans tend to think of themselves as the freedom fighters and liberty lovers of the world; in the same breath, they may describe members of other groups or nationalities as violators of human rights or terrorists. This threat of stereotyping is even greater today in light of the terrorist attacks occurring in the United States and worldwide in the past 2 decades. Simple appearance, such as a beard, attire, or form of speech, can be the basis of broad and deep prejudices.

People particularly tend to use an excuse to classify individuals when they do not like or respect others whose backgrounds, attitudes, abilities, values, or beliefs are different from or opposed to their own or are misunderstood or misinterpreted. Stereotyping, either conscious or subconscious, results in intolerance toward others and engenders the belief that our way is the only way or the right way. In health care, labeling, stereotyping, and stigmatizing responses by nurses and other providers marginalize patients. *Stereotype threat* is a term to describe a negative impression associated with individual's status that triggers physiological and psychological behaviors in patients as well as in providers that may be a contributor to healthcare disparities (Abdou & Fingerhut, 2014; Burgess, Warren, Phelan, Dovidio, & van Ryn, 2010; Ofri, 2011).

For example, research into gender stereotyping in the past 25 years has documented that elementary and secondary school teachers interact more actively with boys compared to girls by asking boys more questions, giving them more feedback (praise and positive encouragement), and providing them with more specific and valuable comments and guidance. In these subtle ways, stereotypical expectations are reinforced (Snowman & McCown, 2015). Attitudes toward sex-role competencies are considered a type of stereotyping. Gender bias has produced inequality in education, employment, and other social spheres.

Nurses must concentrate on treating the sexes equally when providing access to health education, delivering health and illness care, and designing health education materials that contain bias-free language. For example, they must avoid gender-specific terms, such as using *he* or *she*, unless critical to the content, and choose words that minimize ambiguity in gender identity, such as using the plural pronoun *they*. If at all possible, nurses should avoid beginning or ending words with *man* or *men*, such as *man-made*, *mankind*, or *chairmen*. Do not specify marital status unless necessary by using *Ms.* instead of *Mrs.* Suggestions for how to avoid sexist language can be found in the *Guidelines for Gender-Fair Use of Language* (2002) by the National Council of Teachers of English (www.ncte.org) and Purdue OWL's *Stereotype and Biased Language* (2010) document (https://owl.english.purdue.edu).

With respect to age, socioeconomics, culture and race, religion, or disabilities, stereotyping most definitely exists. Throughout this chapter, many cautions have been issued against stereotyping of individuals and groups. For example, just because someone belongs to a specific ethnic group does not necessarily mean that the individual adheres to all of the beliefs and practices of that particular culture.

A thorough and accurate assessment of the learner is the key to determining the particular abilities, preferences, and needs of each individual. The nurse should choose words that are accurate, clear, and free from bias whenever speaking or writing about an individual or a group of individuals. Nurses should refer to someone's ethnicity, race, religion, age, and SES only when it is essential to the content being addressed. For instance, it is more politically and socially correct to use the term *older adult* than the term *elderly* or *aged*. Do not label a member of a special population as a *disabled person*, but rather use people-first language when referring to him or her as a *person with a disability*. Also, it is more appropriate and more acceptable to refer to a *person with diabetes* rather than a *diabetic* or to a *person with AIDS* rather than an *AIDS victim*.

To avoid stereotyping, nurses should ask themselves the following questions:

- Do I use neutral language when teaching patients and families?
- Do I confront bias when evidenced by other healthcare professionals?

- Do I request information equally from patients regardless of gender, SES, age, or culture?
- Are my instructional materials free of stereotypical terminology and expressions?
- Am I an effective role model of equality for my colleagues?
- Do I treat all patients with fairness, respect, and dignity?
- Does someone's appearance influence (raise or lower) my expectations of that person's abilities or affect the quality of care I deliver?
- Do I assess the educational and experiential backgrounds, personal attributes, and economic resources of patients to ensure appropriate health teaching?
- Am I knowledgeable enough of the cultural traditions of various groups to provide sensitive care in our multicultural, pluralistic society?

It is all too easy to stereotype someone not out of malice, but rather out of ignorance. Nurses have a responsibility to keep informed of the most current beliefs and facts about various gender attributes, socioeconomic influences, and cultural traditions that could influence their teaching and learning either positively or negatively. Every day, research in nursing, social science, psychology, and medicine is yielding information that will assist in planning and revising appropriate education interventions to meet the needs of diverse patient populations.

Summary

This chapter explored the influence of gender characteristics, SES, and cultural beliefs on both the ability and the willingness of patients to learn about health and health care. The in-depth examination of these three factors serves to explain certain behaviors observed or potentially encountered in a teaching–learning situation. It also serves to assist the nurse in using strategies that sensitively address and respect the individual characteristics and particular needs of the learner.

The most important message to remember from this chapter is the care nurses must take not to stereotype or generalize common characteristics of a group to all members associated with that particular group. For example, if the nurse does not know much about an ethnic subculture, he or she should ask patients about their beliefs rather than just assuming they abide by the tenets of a certain cultural group. In that way, nurses can avoid offending learners.

In their role as teachers, nurses must be cautious to treat each learner as an individual. They must determine the extent to which patients ascribe to, exhibit beliefs in, or adhere to ways of doing things that might affect their learning. Humans live in a double environment—an outer layer of social and cultural experiences and an inner layer of innate strengths and weaknesses—which influences how they perceive and respond to their world (Griffith, 1982).

Nurses, as professionals, should constantly strive to improve the delivery of care to all people regardless of their gender orientation, socioeconomic level, or cultural origin. Nurses need to be aware of how these three factors affect the teaching–learning process before they can competently, confidently, and sensitively deliver care to satisfy the education needs of patients and their family members who come from diverse backgrounds.

Review Questions

1. What are the gender-related characteristics in cognitive functioning and personality behavior that affect learning?
2. How does the environment versus heredity influence gender-specific approaches to learning?
3. In which ways does SES negatively affect a person's health, and, conversely, how does illness impact an individual's socioeconomic well-being?
4. How does the SES of individuals influence the teaching–learning process?
5. What is meant by the term *poverty cycle*?
6. What is the definition of each of the following terms: *assimilation, acculturation, culture, ethnic group, transcultural,* and *ethnocentrism*?
7. What are the 12 cultural domains identified in Purnell's model of cultural competence that should be taken into account when conducting a nursing assessment?
8. What are the four major ethnic subcultural groups in the United States?
9. What are the prominent characteristics of each of the four major ethnic subcultural groups?
10. Which teaching strategies are most appropriate to meet the needs of individuals from each of the four major ethnic subcultural groups?
11. What can the nurse do to avoid cultural stereotyping?

Case Study

"They told us this might happen, but we were hoping this day would never come," said Kim Hoang as she and her siblings crowded into the tiny conference room—shaken to hear the news that their grandmother, Anh Hoang, a 74-year-old Vietnamese woman, was in end-stage renal failure. "My grandmother is old world. We don't know how she will cope with all of this," Kim added. The nurse and physician explained the treatment plan. Dialysis is required three times each week, and the schedule is rigid. Mrs. Hoang's diet restrictions are also significant. New medications will be added, and Mrs. Hoang needs to learn to care for her dialysis site. She will feel better once dialysis starts, but she might be fatigued and will probably require periodic blood transfusions. Kim asked to be present when her grandmother's teaching takes place. "My grandmother's English is not very good, and I can help explain things to her. She doesn't feel comfortable around strangers," Kim said.

1. How would you respond to Kim's request to serve as the interpreter for her grandmother?
2. Which areas are most important to consider when completing Mrs. Hoang's cultural assessment?
3. If during your assessment you discover conflicts between Mrs. Hoang's cultural beliefs and the treatment protocols, how will you handle them?

References

Abdou, C. M., & Fingerhut, A. W. (2014). Stereotype threat among black and white women in health care settings. *Cultural Diversity and Ethnic Minority Psychology, 20*(3), 316–323.

Adams, R. J. (2010). Improving health outcomes with better patient understanding and education. *Dove Medical Press (NZ) Ltd, 2010*(3), 61–72. doi:http://dx.doi.org/10.2147/RMPH.S7500

American Medical Student Association. (2015). *Transgender health*. Retrieved from http://www.amsa .org/advocacy/action-committees/gender-sexuality/transgender-health/

Anderson, J. M. (1987, December). The cultural context of caring. *Canadian Critical Care Nursing Journal,* 7–13.

Anderson, J. M. (1990). Health care across cultures. *Nursing Outlook, 38*(3), 136–139.

Anderson, R. M., Funnell, M. M., Arnold, M. S., Barr, P. A., Edwards, G. J., & Fitzgerald, J. T. (2000). Assessing the cultural relevance of an education program for urban African Americans with diabetes. *Diabetes Educator, 26*(2), 280–289.

Bailey, E. J., Cates, C. J., Kruske, S. G., Morris, P. S., Brown, N., & Chang, A. B. (2009, April 15). Culture-specific programs for children and adults from minority groups who have asthma. *Cochrane Database Systems Review* (2), CD006580. Retrieved from http://www.ncbi.nlm.nih.gov/pubmed/ 19370643; doi:10.1002/14651858.CD006580.pub4

Bailey, E. J., Erwin, D. O., & Belin, P. (2000). Using cultural beliefs and patterns to improve mammography utilization among African-American women: The Witness project. *Journal of the National Medical Association, 92*(3), 136–142.

Baker, D. W., Parker, R. M., Williams, M. V., Coates, W. C., & Pitkin, K. (1996). Use and effectiveness of interpreters in an emergency department. *Journal of the American Medical Association, 275*(10), 783–788.

Baron-Cohen, S. (2005). The essential difference: The male and female brain. *Phi Kappa Phi Forum, 85*(1), 23–26.

Batty, G. D., Deary, I. J., & Macintyre, S. (2006). Childhood IQ in relation to risk factors for premature mortality in middle-aged persons: The Aberdeen children of the 1950's study. *Journal of Epidemiology & Community Health, 61,* 241–247.

Begley, S. (1996, February 19). Your child's brain. *Newsweek,* 55–62.

Begley, S., Murr, A., & Rogers, A. (1995, March 27). Gray matters. *Newsweek,* 48–54.

Benjamins, M. R., & Whitman, S. (2014). Relationships between discrimination in health care and health care outcomes among 4 race/ethnic groups. *Journal of Behavioral Medicine, 37,* 402–413.

Berlin, E. A., & Fowkes, W. C. (1983). A teaching framework for cross-cultural health care: Application in family practice. *The Western Journal of Medicine, 139*(6), 934–938.

Bertakis, K. D, Azari, R., Helms, J. L., Callahan, E. J., & Robbins, J. A. (2000). Gender differences in the utilization of health care services. *Journal of Family Practice, 49*(2), 147–152. Retrieved from http://www.jfonline.com/index.php?id=22143&tx_ffnews[tt_news]=168476

Borrayo, E. (2004). Where's Maria? A video to increase awareness about breast cancer and mammography screening among low-literacy Latinas. *Preventive Medicine, 39,* 99–110.

Burgess, D. J., Warren, J., Phelan, S., Dovidio, J., & van Ryn, M. (2010, May). Stereotype threat and health disparities: What medical educators and future physicians need to know. *Journal of General Internal Medicine, 25*(Suppl. 2), 169–177. doi:10 1007/s11606-009-1221-4

Cahill, L. (2006). Why sex matters in neuroscience. *Nature Reviews/Neuroscience*. Retrieved from http://www.nature.com/nrn/index.html

Cahill, L. (2014, April 1). *Equal ≠ the same: Sex differences in the human brain*. The Dana Foundation. Retrieved from https://www.dana.org/cerebrum/2014/equal_≠_The_Same__Sex_Differences_in_ the_Human_Brain/

Campinha-Bacote, J. (2011, May 31). Delivering patient-centered care in the midst of a cultural conflict: The role of cultural competence. *OJIN: The Online Journal of Issues in Nursing, 16*(2), Manuscript 5. Retrieved from http://www.nursingworld.org/MainMenuCategories/ANAMarketplace/ANAPeriodicals/OJIN/TableofContents/Vol-16-2011/No2-May-2011/Delivering-Patient-Centered-Care-in-the-Midst-of-a-Cultural-Conflict.html

Cantore, J. A. (2001, Winter). Earth, wind, fire and water. *Minority Nurse,* 24–29.

Career Directory. (2005). Understanding transcultural nursing. *Nursing 2005,* 14–23.

Carol, R. (2001, Fall). Taking the initiative. *Minority Nurse,* 24–27.

Carpenter, C. E. (2011). Medicare, Medicaid and deficit reduction. *Journal of Financial Service Professionals, 65*(6), 27–30.

Carthron, D. (2007). A splash of color: Increasing diversity among nursing students and faculty. *Journal of Best Practices in Health Professions Diversity: Research, Education and Policy, 1*(1), 13–23.

Caudle, P. (1993). Providing culturally sensitive health care to Hispanic clients. *Nurse Practitioner, 18*(12), 40, 43–44, 46, 50–51.

Centers for Disease Control and Prevention (CDC). (2010). *Lesbian, gay, bisexual and transgender health.* Retrieved from http://www.cdc.gov/lgbthealth/

Centers for Disease Control and Prevention (CDC). (2011). *Health, United States, 2011: With special feature on socioeconomic status and health.* Retrieved from http://www.cdc.gov/nchs/data/hus/hus11.pdf

Centers for Disease Control and Prevention (CDC). (2012). *Hispanic or Latino population.* Retrieved from http://www.cdc.gov/nchs/fastats/hispanic-health.htm

Chao, R. K. (1994). Beyond parental control and authoritarian parenting style: Understanding Chinese parenting through the cultural notion of training. *Child Development, 65,* 1111–1119.

Chen, J., Bustamante , J. V., & Tom, S. E., (2015). Health care spending and utilization by race/ethnicity under the Affordable Care Act's dependent coverage expansion. *American Journal of Public Health, 105*(53), 499–507.

Christian Reformed Church in North America (CRCNA). (n.d.). *What is the cycle of poverty?* Retrieved from http://www2.crcna.org/pages/sea_cycleofpoverty.cfm

Collins, W. L. (2015). The role of African American churches in promoting health among congregations. *Social Work and Christianity, 42*(2), 193–204.

Core, L. (2008). Treatment across culture: Is there a model? *International Journal of Therapy and Rehabilitation, 15,* 519–525.

Courtenay, W. H. (2000). Constructions of masculinity and their influence on men's well-being: A theory of gender and health. *Social Science & Medicine, 50,* 1385–1401.

Crandell, T. L., Crandell, C. H., & Vander Zanden, J. W. (2012). *Human development* (11th ed.). New York, NY: McGraw-Hill.

Crimmins, E. M., & Saito, Y. (2001). Trends in healthy life expectancy in the United States, 1970–1990: Gender, race, and educational differences. *Social Science & Medicine, 52,* 1629–1641.

Darling, S. (2004). Family literacy: Meeting the needs of at-risk families. *Phi Kappa Phi Forum, 84*(2), 18–21.

Davidson, K. W., Trudeau, K. J., van Roosmalen, E., Stewart, M., & Kirkland, S. (2006). Perspective: Gender as a health determinant and implications for health education. *Health Education & Behavior, 33,* 731–743.

DeCola, P. R. (2012). *Gender effects on health and healthcare.* Retrieved from http://www.karger.com

Dignam, J. J. (2000). Differences in breast cancer prognosis among African-American and Caucasian women. *CA: A Cancer Journal for Clinicians, 50*(1), 50–64.

Dreher, M. C. (1996, 4th quarter). Nursing: A cultural phenomenon. *Reflections,* 4.

Durso, L. E., & Meyer, I. H. (2012). *Patterns and predictors of disclosure of sexual orientation to health-care providers among lesbians, gay men, and bisexuals.* Retrieved from http://williamsinstitute.law.ucla.edu/research/health-and-hiv-aids/durso-meyer-srsp-dec-2012/

Eggenberger, S. K., Grassley, J., & Restrepo, E. (2006, July 19). Culturally competent nursing care for families: Listening to the voices of Mexican-American women. *OJIN: The Online Journal of Issues in Nursing, 11*(3). Retrieved from http://www.nursingworld.org/MainMenuCategories/ANAMarketplace/ANAPeriodicals/OJIN/Tableofcontents/Volume112006/No3Sept06/ArticlePreviousTopics/CulturallyCompetentNursingCare.html

Eliot, L. (2009, September 8). Girl brain, boy brain? *Scientific American.* Retrieved from http://www.scientificamerican.com/article/girl-brain-boy-brain/

Elstad, J. I., & Krokstad, S. (2003). Social causation, health-selective mobility, and the reproduction of socioeconomic health inequalities over time: Panel study of adult men. *Social Science & Medicine, 57,* 1475–1489.

Fenway Institute. (2010a). *Ending invisibility: Better health for LGBT populations.* Retrieved from http://www.iom.edu/Activities/SelectPops/LGBTHealthIssues.aspx

Fenway Institute. (2010b). *Professional education and development for health professionals.* Retrieved from http://www.fenwayhealth.org/site/PageServer?pagename=FCHC_ins_fenway_EducProfessionals

Fernandez, R. D., & Hebert, G. J. (2000). Rituals, culture, and tradition: The Puerto Rican experience. In M. L. Kelley & V. M. Fitzsimons (Eds.), *Understanding cultural diversity: Culture, curriculum and community in nursing* (pp. 241–251). Sudbury, MA: Jones and Bartlett.

Flores, G., Abreu, M., Barone, C. P., Bachur, R., & Lin, H. (2012). Errors of medical interpretation and their potential consequences: A comparison of professional versus ad-hoc versus no interpreters. *Annals of Emergency Medicine, 60*(5), 545–553.

Forrester, D. A. (2000). Minority men's health: A review of the literature with special emphasis on African American men. In M. L. Kelley & V. M. Fitzsimons (Eds.), *Understanding cultural diversity: Culture, curriculum, and community in nursing* (pp. 283–305). Sudbury, MA: Jones and Bartlett.

Ganley, C. M., & Vasilyeva, M. (2014). The role of anxiety and working memory in gender differences in mathematics. *Journal of Educational Psychology, 16*(1), 105–120.

Gates, G. J. (2013). *Same sex and different sex couples in the American community survey: 2005–2011. Williams Institute of the UCLA School of Law.* Retrieved from http://williamsinstitute.law.ucla.edu/wp-content/uploads/ACS-2013.pdf

Giger, J. N. (2013). *Transcultural nursing: Assessment and intervention* (6th ed.). St. Louis, MO: Elsevier.

Giger, J. N., & Davidhizar, R. E. (2004). *Transcultural nursing: Assessment and intervention* (4th ed.). St. Louis, MO: Mosby–Year Book.

Giorgianni, S. S. (1998). Responding to the challenge of health literacy. *Pfizer Journal, 2*(1), 1–39.

Gittelsohn, J., & Rowan, M. (2011). Preventing diabetes and obesity in American Indian communities: The potential of environmental interventions. *American Journal of Clinical Nutrition, 93*(5), 1179S–1183S.

Gong, G., He, Y., & Evans, A. C. (2011). Brain connectivity: Gender makes a difference. *Neuroscientist, 17*(5), 575–591.

Gonzales, G. (2014). National and state-specific health insurance disparities for adults in same-sex relationships. *American Journal of Public Health, 104*(2), 96–104.

Gorman, C. (1992, January 20). Sizing up the sexes. *Time,* 42–51.

Griffith, S. (1982). Childbearing and the concept of culture. *Journal of Obstetric, Gynecologic, & Neonatal Nursing, 11*(3), 181–184.

Grønning, K., Rannestad, T., Skomsvoll, J. E., Rygg, L. O., & Steinsbekk, A. (2014). Long-term effects of a nurse-led group and individual patient education programme for patients with chronic inflammatory polyarthritis—a randomized controlled trial. *Journal of Clinical Nursing, 7–8,* 1005–1017. Retrieved from http://www.ncbi.nlm.nih.gov/pubmed/23875718; doi:10.1111/jocn.12353

Gur, R. C., Alsop, D., Glahn, D., Petty, R., Swanson, C. L., Maldjian, J. A, . . . Gur, R. E. (2000). An fMRI study of sex differences in regional activation to a verbal and a spatial task. *Brain and Language, 74,* 157–170.

Gutierrez, K. D., & Rogoff, B. (2003). Cultural ways of learning: Individual traits or repertoires of practice. *Educational Research, 32*(5), 19–25.

Hancock, L. (1996, February 19). Why do schools flunk biology? *Newsweek,* 59.

Harding, S. (1998, June). Native healers: Part 2—The circle in practice. *Alternative & Complementary Therapies,* 173–179.

Harrigan, D. O. (Ed.). (2007). The young brain: Handle with care. *SUNY Upstate Medical University Outlook, 6*(3), 3–31.

Hawthorne, K., Robles, Y., Cannings-John, R., & Edwards, A. G. (2008, July 16). Culturally appropriate health education for type 2 diabetes mellitus in ethnic minority groups. *Cochrane Database Systems Review,* (3). doi:10.1002/14651858.CD006424.pub2

Hayes, K. (2015). Black churches' capacity to respond to the mental health needs of African Americans. *Social Work and Christianity, 42*(3), 296–312.

Hebert, G. J., & Fernandez, R. D. (2000). A challenge to the Puerto Rican community: An untold story of the AIDS epidemic. In M. L. Kelley & V. M. Fitzsimons (Eds.), *Understanding cultural diversity: Culture, curriculum, and community in nursing* (pp. 253–261). Sudbury, MA: Jones and Bartlett.

Hisama, K. K. (2000, First Quarter). Japanese theory and practice: Carrying your own lamp. *Reflections on Nursing Leadership,* 30–32.

Holt, C. L., Clark, E. M., & Kreuter, M. W. (2003) Spiritual health locus of control and breast cancer beliefs among urban African American women. *Health Psychology, 22*(3), 294–299.

Holt, C. L., Kyles, A., Wiehagen, T., & Casey, C. (2003). Development of a spiritually based breast cancer educational booklet for African American women. *Cancer Control, 10*(5), 37–44.

Hosseini, H. (2015). Disparities in health care and HIV/AIDS among Hispanics/Latinos in the United States. *Journal of International Diversity, 2015*(2), 130–135.

Jantz, G. L. (2014, February 27). *Brain differences between genders: Do you ever wonder why men and women think so differently?* Retrieved from https://www.psychologytoday.com/blog/hope-relationships/201402/brain-differences-between-genders

Jemigan, V. B. B., Duran, B., Ahn, D., & Winkleby, M. (2010). Changing patterns in health behaviors and risk factors to cardiovascular disease among American Indians and Alaska Natives. *American Journal of Public Health, 100*(4), 678–683.

Jezewski, M. A. (1993). Culture brokering as a model for advocacy. *Nursing & Health Care, 14*(2), 78–85.

Joho, K. A., & Ormsby, A. (2000). A walk in beauty: Strategies for providing culturally competent nursing care to Native Americans. In M. L. Kelley & V. M. Fitzsimons (Eds.), *Understanding cultural diversity: Culture, curriculum, and community in nursing* (pp. 209–218). Sudbury, MA: Jones and Bartlett.

Jones, C. P. (2000). Levels of racism: A theoretical framework and a gardener's tale. *American Journal of Public Health, 90*(8), 1212–1214.

Juckett, G. (2013). Caring for Latino patients. *American Family Physician, 87*(1), 48–54.

Kaplan, M. A., & Inguanzo, M. M. (2011). The social implications of health reform: Reducing access barriers to health care services for uninsured Hispanic and Latino Americans in the United States. *Harvard Journal of Hispanic Policy, 23,* 83–92.

Kawamura, M., Midorikawa, A., & Kezuka, M. (2000). Cerebral localization of the center for reading and writing music. *NeuroReport, 11*(14), 3299–3303.

Kessels, R. P. C. (2003). Patients' memory for medical information. *Journal of the Royal Society of Medicine, 96,* 219–222.

Keyserling, T. C., Ammerman, A. S., Samuel-Hodge, C. D., Ingram, A. T., Skelly, A. H., Elasy, T. A., . . . Henriquez-Radan, C. F. (2000). A diabetes management program for African American women with type 2 diabetes. *Diabetes Educator, 26*(5), 796–805.

Kimura, D. (1999, Summer). The hidden mind: Sex differences in the brain. *Scientific American, 32*–37.

Krehely, J. (2009). *How to close the LGBT health disparities gap.* Center for American Progress. Retrieved from https://www.americanprogress.org/issues/lgbt/report/2009/12/21/7048/how-to-close-the-lgbt-health-disparities-gap/

Krugman, P. (2008, February 18). Poverty is poison. *New York Times.* Retrieved from http://www.ny-times.com/2008/02/18/opinion/18krugman.html

Larkin, M. (2013, July 12). *Can brain biology explain why men and women think and act differently?* Retrieved from https://www.elsevier.com/connect/can-brain-biology-explain-why-men-and-women-think-and-act-differently

Leininger, M. (1994). Transcultural nursing education: A worldwide imperative. *Nursing & Health Care, 15*(5), 254–257.

LEP patients best served with interpreter in ED. (2012). *Case Management Advisor, 23*(9), 106–108.

Lindholm, C., Burstrom, B., & Diderichsen, F. (2001). Does chronic illness cause adverse social and economic consequences among Swedes? *Scandinavian Journal of Public Health, 29,* 63–70.

Lipman, E. L., Offord, D. R., & Boyle, M. H. (1994). Relation between economic disadvantage and psychosocial morbidity in children. *Canadian Medical Association Journal, 151*(4), 431–437.

Livingston, N. A, Flentje, A., Heck, N. C., Gleason, H., Oost, K. M., & Cochran, B. N. (2015). Sexual minority stress and suicide risk: Identifying resilience through personality profile analysis. *Psychology of Sexual Orientation and Gender Identity, 2*(3), 321–328.

Lowe, J., & Struthers, R. (2001, third quarter). A conceptual framework of nursing in Native American culture. *Journal of Nursing Scholarship,* 279–283.

Mackenbach, J. P., Bos, V., Andersen, O., Cardano, M., Costa, G., Harding, S., . . . Kunst, A. E. (2003). Widening socioeconomic inequalities in mortality in six Western European countries. *International Journal of Epidemiology, 32,* 830–837.

Mackenbach, J. P., Cavelaars, A. E., Kunst, A. E., Groenhof, F., & EU Working Group on Socioeconomic Inequalities in Health. (2000). Socioeconomic inequalities in cardiovascular disease mortality: An international study. *European Heart Journal, 21*(14), 1141–1151.

Maholmes, V., & King, R. B. (Eds.). (2012). *The Oxford handbook of poverty and child development.* New York, NY: Oxford University Press.

Mail, P. D., McKay, R. B., & Katz, M. (1989). Expanding practice horizons: Learning from American Indian patients. *Patient Education and Counseling, 13,* 91–102.

Markides, K. S., & Coreil, J. (1986). The health of Hispanics in the southwestern U.S.: An epidemiological paradox. *Public Health Reports, 101*(3), 253–265.

Mattis, J. S. (2000). African American women's definitions of spirituality and religiosity. *Journal of Black Psychology, 26*(1), 101–122.

Mattis, J. S., & Jagers, R. J. (2001). A relational framework for the study of religiosity and spirituality in the lives of African Americans. *Journal of Community Psychology, 29*(5), 519–539.

Mayer, K. H., Bradford, J. B., Makadon, H. J., Stall, R., Goldhammer, H., & Landers, S. (2008). Sexual and gender minority health: What we know and what needs to be done. *American Journal of Public Health, 98*(6), 989–995.

McLeod, S. (2007). *Nature vs nurture in psychology.* Retrieved from http://www.simplypsychology.org/naturevsnurture.html

McRae, K., Ochsner, K. N., Mauss, I. B., Gabrieli, J. J. D., & Gross, J. J. (2008). Gender differences in emotion regulation: An fMRI study of cognitive reappraisal. *Group Processes & Intergroup Relations, 11,* 143–162.

Meyer, O., Castro-Schilo, L., & Agular-Gaxiola, S. (2014). Determinants of mental health and self-rated health: A model of socioeconomic status, neighborhood safety, and physical activity. *American Journal of Public Health, 104*(9), 1734–1741.

Monastersky, R. (2001, November 2). Land mines in the world of mental maps. *Chronicle of Higher Education,* A20–A21.

Monden, C. W. S., van Lenthe, F. J., & Mackenbach, J. P. (2006). A simultaneous analysis of neighborhood and childhood socioeconomic environment with self-assessed health and health-related behaviors. *Health & Place, 12,* 394–403.

Mulligan, K. (2004). Chronic illness a prescription for financial distress. *Psychiatric News, 39*(23), 17. Retrieved from http://psychnews.psychiatryonline.org/doi/full/10.1176/pn.39.23.00390017

Muronda, C. (2015, July 21). The culturally diverse nursing student: A review of the literature. *Journal of Transcultural Nursing.* Retrieved from http://www.ncbi.nlm.nih.gov/pubmed/26199289

Narayan, M. C. (2003). Cultural assessment. *Home Healthcare Nurse, 21*(9), 173–178.

Nash, J. M. (1997). Fertile minds. *Time, 149*(5), 48–56.

National Center for Education Statistics. (2006). *National Assessment of Adult Literacy (NAAL): Health literacy component.* Retrieved from http://nces.ed.gov/NAAL/index.asp

National Kids Count Program. (2011). Children in single parent families by race. Retrieved from http://datacenter.kidscount.org/data/acrossstates/Rankings.aspx?ind=107

Newlin, K., Knafl, K., & Melkus, G. D. (2002). African-American spirituality: A concept analysis. *Advances in Nursing Science, 25*(2), 57–70.

Nguyen, J., & Mills, S. (2014, May 30). Increasing racial and ethnic diversity in health psychology. *The Health Psychologist: The newsletter of the American Psychological Association.* Retrieved from http://div38healthpsychologist.com

Niedermann, K., Fransen, J., Knols, R., & Uebelhart, D. (2004). Gap between short- and long-term effects of patient education in rheumatoid arthritis patients: A systematic review. *Arthritis & Rheumatology, 51*(3), 388–398. Retrieved from http://www.ncbi.nlm.nih.gov/pubmed/15188324

Norris, T., Vines, P. L., & Hoeffel, E. M. (2011). *The American Indian and Alaska Native population: 2010.* 2010 census briefs. U.S. Department of Commerce. Retrieved from www.census.gov/prod/cen2010/briefs/c2010br-10.pdf

O'Brien, G. (2007, Fall). *Understanding ourselves: Gender differences in the brain.* Retrieved from http://www.columbiaconsult.com/pubs/v52_fall07.html

O'Connell, J., Yi, R., Wilson, C., Manson, S. M., & Acton, K. J. (2010). Racial disparities in health status: A comparison of the morbidity among American Indian and US adults with diabetes. *Diabetes Care, 33*(7), 463–470.

Ofri, D. (2011, June 21). Stereotyping patients, and their ailments. *The New York Times,* D6. Retrieved from http://www.nytimes.com/2011/06/21/health/views/21cases.html?_r=0

O'Hara, B., & Caswell, K. (2012, October). Health status, health insurance, and medical services utilization: 2010: Household economics studies. *Current Population Reports.* Retrieved from http://www.census.gov/hhes/www/hlthins.html

Pacquiao, D. F., Archeval, L., & Shelley, E. E. (2000). Hispanic client satisfaction with home health care: A study of cultural context of care. In M. L. Kelley & V. M. Fitzsimons (Eds.), *Understanding cultural diversity: Culture, curriculum, and community nursing* (pp. 229–240). Sudbury, MA: Jones and Bartlett.

Pang, K. Y. C. (2007). The importance of cultural interpretation of religion/spirituality and depression in Korean elderly immigrant women Buddhists and Christians. *Journal of Best Practices in Health Professions Diversity: Research, Education and Policy, 1*(1), 57–89.

Park, M., Chesla, C., Rehm, R., & Chun, K. M. (2011). Working with culture: Appropriate mental health care for Asian Americans. *Journal of Advanced Nursing, 67*(11), 2373–2382.

Perez, M. A., & Luquis, R. R. (2014). *Cultural competence in health education and health promotion* (2nd ed.). San Francisco, CA: Jossey-Bass.

Pew Research Center. (2010). *Hispanics, high school dropouts and the GED.* Retrieved from http://www.pewhispanic.org/files/reports/122.pdf

Portman, T., & Garrett, M. T. (2006). Native American healing traditions. *International Journal of Disability, Development and Education, 53*(4), 453–469.

Poss, J. E., & Rangel, R. (1995). Working effectively with interpreters in the primary care setting. *Nurse Practitioner, 20*(12), 43–44, 46–47.

Poverty cycle. (n.d.). *Business Dictionary*. Retrieved from http://businessdictionary.com

Powe, B. D., Daniels, E. C., Finnie, R., & Thompson, A. (2005). Perceptions about breast cancer among African American women: Do selected educational materials challenge them? *Patient Education and Counseling, 56,* 197–204.

Price, K. M., & Cortis, J. D. (2000). The way forward for transcultural nursing. *Nurse Education Today, 20,* 233–243.

Puchalski, C., & Romer, A. L. (2000). Taking a spiritual history allows clinicians to understand patients more fully. *Journal of Palliative Medicine, 3*(1), 129–137.

Purnell, L. D. (2013). *Transcultural health care: A culturally competent approach* (4th ed.). Philadelphia, PA: F. A. Davis.

Rognerud, M. A., & Zahl, P-H. (2005). Social inequalities in mortality: Changes in the relative importance of income, education, and household size over a 27-year period. *European Journal of Public Health, 16*(1), 62–68.

Ruigrok, A. N. V., Salimi-Khorshidi, G., Lai, M-C, Baron-Cohen, S., Lombardo, M. V., . . . Suckling, J. (2014). A meta-analysis of sex differences in human brain structure. *Neuroscience & Biobehavioral Reviews, 39,* 34–50. doi:10.1016/j.neubiorev.2013.12.004

Samuel-Hodge, C. D., Keyserling, T. C., France, R., Ingram, A. F., Johnston, L. F., Davis, L. P., . . . Cole, A. S. (2006). A church-based diabetes self-management education program for African Americans with type 2 diabetes. *Preventing Chronic Disease, 3*(3), 1-16.

Santrock, J. W. (2006). *Life-span development* (10th ed.). New York, NY: McGraw-Hill.

Santrock, J. W. (2013). *Life-span development* (14th ed.). New York, NY: McGraw-Hill.

Satel, S. (2002, May 26). I am a racially profiling doctor. *Post Standard,* D–6.

Scharnberg, K. (2007). Medicine men for the 21st century. *Chicago Tribune*. Retrieved from http://articles.chicagotribune.com/2007-06-04/news/0706030707_1_native-american-american-indian-21st-century

Schenker, Y., Lo, B., Ettinger, K. M., & Fernandez, A. (2008). Navigating language barriers under difficult circumstances. *Annals of Internal Medicine, 149,* 264–269.

Sequist, T. D., Cullen, T., & Acton, K. J. (2011). Indian Health Service innovations have helped reduce health disparities affecting American Indian and Alaska Native people. *Health Affairs, 30*(10), 1965–1973.

Severiens, S. E., & Ten Dam, G. T. M. (1994). Gender differences in learning styles: A narrative review and quantitative meta-analysis. *Higher Education, 27,* 487–501.

Severiens, S. E., & Ten Dam, G. T. M. (1997). Gender and gender identity differences in learning styles. *Educational Psychology, 17,* 79–93.

Shen, Z. (2015). Cultural competence models and cultural competence assessment instruments in nursing: A literature review. *Journal of Transcultural Nursing, 26*(3), 308–321.

Sincero, S. M. (2012, September 16). *Nature and nurture debate*. Retrieved from https://explorable.com/nature-vs-nurture-debate

Singh-Manoux, A., Ferrie, J. E., Lynch, J. W., & Marmot, M. (2005). The role of cognitive ability (intelligence) in explaining the association between socioeconomic position and health: Evidence from the Whitehall II prospective cohort study. *American Journal of Epidemiology, 161,* 831-839.

Smith, K. C. (2006). *Sex, gender, and health*. Johns Hopkins Bloomberg School of Public Health. Retrieved from ocw.jhsph.edu/courses/socialbehavioralaspectspublichealth/pdfs/unit2gender.pdf

Snowman, J., & McCown, R. (2015). *Psychology applied to teaching* (14th ed.). Stanford, CA: Wadsworth/ Cengage Learning.

Speck, O., Ernst, T., Braun, J., Koch, C., Miller, E., & Chang, L. (2000). Gender differences in the functional organization of the brain for working memory. *NeuroReport, 11*(11), 2581–2585.

Stanislav, L. (2006, October). When language gets in the way. *Modern Nurse,* 32–35.

Thompson, D. (2010, July 14). *Gender differences in emotional health.* Retrieved from http://www .everydayhealth.com/emotional-health/gender-differences-in-emotional-health.aspx

Titus, S. K. F. (2014). Seeking and utilizing a curandero in the United States. *Journal of Holistic Nursing, 32*(3), 189–201.

U.S. Census Bureau. (2009). *Census Bureau estimates nearly half of children under age 5 are minorities.* Retrieved from http://www.census.gov/newsroom/releases/archives/population/cb09-75.html

U.S. Census Bureau. (2010a). *The black population: 2010.* Retrieved from http://www.census.gov/prod/ cen2010/briefs/c2010br-06.pdf

U.S. Census Bureau. (2010b). *New Census Bureau report analyzes nations' linguistic diversity.* Retrieved from http://www.census.gov/newsroom/releases/archives/american_community_survey_acs/cb10- cn58.html

U.S. Census Bureau. (2010c). *Profile facts: Asian American heritage month.* Retrieved from http://www .census.gov/newsroom/releases/archives/facts_for_features_special_editions/cb11-ff06.html

U.S. Census Bureau. (2011a). *The Hispanic population: 2010.* Retrieved from http://www.census.gov/ prod/cen2010/briefs/c2010br-04.pdf

U.S. Census Bureau. (2011b). *2010 census shows America's diversity.* Retrieved from https://www .census.gov/newsroom/releases/archives/2010_census/cb11-cn125.html

U.S. Census Bureau. (2012a). *Statistical abstract of the United States.* Retrieved from https://www.census .gov/library/publications/time-series/statistical_abstracts.html

U.S. Census Bureau. (2012b). *U.S. Census Bureau projections show a slower growing, older, more diverse nation a half century from now.* Retrieved from https://www.census.gov/newsroom/releases/ archives/population/cb12-243.html

U.S. Census Bureau. (2015a). *Income and Poverty in the United States:2014.* Retrieved from http://www .census.gov/hhes/www/poverty/

U.S. Census Bureau. (2015b). *Poverty Guidelines.* Retrieved from https://aspe.hhs.gov/2015-poverty- guidelines

U.S. Department of Health and Human Services (USDHHS). (2000). *Healthy people 2010: Understanding and improving health, Volume 1.* Rockville, MD: Author.

U.S. Department of Health and Human Services (USDHHS). (2009). Death: Final data for 2006. *National Vital Statistics Reports, 57*(14).

U.S. Department of Health and Human Services (USDHHS). (2012). *Healthy people 2020.* McLean, VA: International Publishing. Retrieved from http://www.healthypeople.gov/2020/default.aspx

U.S. Department of Health and Human Services (USDHHS). (2015a). *Indian Health Service: Health Education Program.* Retrieved from http://www.ihs.gov/healthed/

U.S. Department of Health and Human Services (USDHHS). (2015b). *2015 poverty guidelines.* Retrieved from http://aspe.hhs.gov/2015-poverty-guidelines

U.S. Department of Labor. (2012). *The African American labor force in the recovery.* Retrieved from http://www.dol.gov/_sec/media/reports/blacklaborforce/

Uzundede, S. (2006, October). Respecting diversity: One patient at a time. *Modern Nurse,* 28–30.

Veazie, M., Ayala, C., Schieb, L., Dai, S., Henderson, J., & Cho, P. (2014). Trends and disparities in heart disease among American Indians/Alaska Natives 1990–2009. *American Journal of Public Health, 104*(3), 360–367.

Vidaeff, A. C., Kerrigan, A. J., & Monga, M. (2015). Cross-cultural barriers to health care. *Southern Medical Journal, 108*(1), 1–4.

Villanueva, V., & Lipat, A. S. (2000). The Filipino American culture: The need for transcultural knowledge. In M. L. Kelley & V. M. Fitzsimons (Eds.), *Understanding cultural diversity: Culture, curriculum, and community in nursing* (pp. 219–228). Sudbury, MA: Jones and Bartlett.

Ward, B. W., Clark, T. C., Freeman, C., & Schiller, J. S. (2015). *Early release of selected estimates based on data from the 2014 National Health Interview Survey.* Retrieved from http://www.cdc.gov/nchs/data/nhis/earlyrelease/earlyrelease201506.pdf

Weekes, C. (2012). African Americans and health literacy: A systematic review. *ABNF Journal, 23*(4), 1046–7041.

Wehrwein, E. A., Lujan, H. L., & DiCarlo, S. E. (2007). Gender differences in learning style preferences among undergraduate physiology students. *Advanced Physiology Education, 31*(2), 153–157.

Weiss, B. D. (2003). *Health literacy: A manual for clinicians* (pp. 1–49). Chicago, IL: American Medical Association and American Medical Association Foundation.

Whittemore, R. (2007, April 18). Culturally competent interventions for Hispanic adults with type 2 diabetes: A systematic review. *Journal of Transcultural Nursing, 2,* 157–166.

Wilson, C. J., & Auger, P. A. (2013). Gender differences in neurodevelopment and epigenetics. *European Journal of Physiology, 465*(5), 573–584.

Wilson, L. D. (2011). Cultural competency: Beyond the vital signs. Delivering holistic care to African Americans. *Nursing Clinics of North America, 46*(2), 218–232.

Winkleby, M. A., Jatulis, D. E., Frank, E., & Fortmann, S. P. (1992). Socioeconomic status and health: How education, income, and occupation contribute to risk factors for cardiovascular disease. *American Journal of Public Health, 82*(6), 816–820.

Woodiel, K. D., & Cowdery, J. E. (2014). Culture and sexual orientation. In M. A. Perez & R. R. Luquis (Eds.), *Cultural competence in health education and health promotion* (2nd ed., pp. 267–292). San Francisco, CA: Jossey-Bass.

Wright, K., & Newman-Ginger, J. (2010). California's young Hispanic children with asthma: Disparities in health care access and utilization of health care services. *Hispanic Health Care International, 8*(3), 154–164.

Yanek, L. R., Becker, D. M., Moy, T. F., Gettelsohn, J., & Koffman, D. M. (2001). Project Joy: Faith based cardiovascular health promotion for African-American women. *Public Health Reports, 116,* 68–81.

Yee, S-H., Liu, H-L., Hou, J., Pu, Y., Fox, P. T., & Gao, J-H. (2000). Detection of the brain response during a cognitive task using perfusion-based event-related functional MRI. *NeuroReport, 11*(11), 2533–2536.

Young, H. M., McCormick, W. M., & Vitaliano, P. P. (2002). Evolving values in community-based long-term care services for Japanese Americans. *Advances in Nursing Science, 25*(2), 40-56.

Educating Learners with Disabilities

Deborah L. Sopczyk

Chapter Highlights

- Scope of the Problem
- Definition of Terms
- The Language of Disabilities
- The Roles and Responsibilities of Nurses as Patient Educators
- Types of Disabilities
- Sensory Disabilities
  - *Hearing Impairments*
  - *Visual Impairments*
- Learning Disabilities
  - *Dyslexia*
  - *Auditory Processing Disorders*
  - *Dyscalculia*
- Developmental Disabilities
  - *Attention-Deficit/Hyperactivity Disorder*
  - *Intellectual Disabilities*
  - *Asperger Syndrome/Autism Spectrum Disorder*
- Mental Illness
- Physical Disabilities
  - *Traumatic Brain Injury*
  - *Memory Disorders*
- Communication Disorders
  - *Aphasia*
  - *Dysarthria*
- Chronic Illness
- The Family's Role in Chronic Illness or Disability

Key Terms

anomic aphasia
Asperger syndrome
attention-deficit/
  hyperactivity disorder
auditory processing disorder
augmentative and
  alternative communication
developmental disability
disability
dysarthria
dyscalculia
dyslexia
expressive aphasia
global aphasia
hearing impairment
intellectual disability
learning disability
people-first language
receptive aphasia
sensory disabilities
visual impairment

© wanchai/Shutterstock

Objectives

After completing this chapter, the reader will be able to

1. Recognize the scope of the disability problem from a worldwide, national, and individual patient perspective.
2. Define the term *disability*.
3. Describe the language that should be used when writing about, talking with, or talking about people with disabilities.
4. Summarize the roles and responsibilities of nurses as patient educators.
5. Name the two major types of disabilities and the six subcategories of disabilities.
6. Identify the various teaching strategies (methods and materials) that can be used when working with patients who have sensory, learning, developmental, mental, physical, and/or communication disabilities.
7. Discuss the effects of a chronic illness on people and their families in the teaching–learning process.
8. Give examples of assistive technologies and their application to enhance the lives of people with disabilities.

Teaching others about health and wellness or disease and its treatments is a challenging role for the nurse caring for individuals in any setting. The teaching–learning process is especially demanding when working with patients whose abilities to learn are challenged by disabilities that affect their capacities to see, hear, speak, move, understand, remember, or process information. In light of these challenges, education remains a critical component of care as nurses assist patients with disabilities to maintain their patterns of living or develop new ones to accommodate changes in health status or functional ability.

This chapter provides an overview of a wide range of sensory, cognitive, mental, and physical disabilities that affect the ways in which people learn. Included are the most common disabilities encountered by nurses, such as learning disabilities, mental illness, and communication disorders. Chronic illness is included because it is a situational issue that requires a change in the way the nurse approaches health education. This chapter also provides a summary of assessment, teaching, and evaluation strategies that nurses can use in designing and implementing patient education for this group of individuals and their families.

Scope of the Problem

"Disability is part of the human condition. Almost everyone will be temporarily or permanently impaired at some point in their life, and those who survive to old age will experience increasing difficulties in functioning" (World Health Organization [WHO], 2011, p. 3).

Therefore, it is not surprising that more than 1 billion people throughout the world live with a condition that is classified as a disability. This number is expected to increase as people age and the incidence of conditions such as diabetes, obesity, and cancer continues to grow (WHO, 2015b).

In the United States, nearly 60 million Americans (1 in 5) are estimated to have a disability, with almost half of these persons reporting a disability that is considered to be severe (U.S Census Bureau, 2012). Almost 1 in 12 Americans aged 18–64 report having a disability severe enough to limit their ability to work (Cornell University, 2012). If the incidence of disabilities seems high, it is important to remember that not all disabilities are readily apparent to the casual observer. For example, not all people with disabilities use a wheelchair, wear a hearing aid, or walk with the assistance of a white cane.

Individuals with disabilities are more likely than people without disabilities to have more illnesses and greater health needs and are less likely to receive health prevention services (Reichard, Stolzle, & Fox, 2011). However, it is important to avoid making assumptions about this population. This is because people with disabilities are diverse in the type and extent of health disparities they have, and the access to services that are available varies from person to person (Horner-Johnson, Dobbertin, Lee, Andresen, & the Expert Panel on Disability and Health Disparities, 2014; Wisdom et al., 2010). When health disparities arise, they do so for a number of reasons that often are directly related to a disability. Some disabilities are associated with additional chronic health problems. Other factors contributing to health disparities among people with disabilities include fear, lack of understanding, physical barriers, and cost. For example, people with Down syndrome—a common cause of intellectual disability—often have other chronic physical conditions, such as heart disease, and their intellectual disability makes it more difficult for them to access health services (Lee, Hasnain-Wynia, & Lau, 2012; Vander Ploeg Booth, 2011).

It has been said that people with disabilities represent the largest minority group in the United States, a group that comprises individuals of all ages, of all racial and ethnic backgrounds, and from all walks of life (Disability Funders Network, 2012). Health care for this group of people is often complex and costly. As patient educators, nurses can play a significant role in promoting health and wellness, ensuring proper self-care, and improving overall quality of life.

Definition of Terms

The term **disability** has been defined in a number of ways. Most definitions are broad and serve to categorize a wide variety of impairments stemming from injury, genetics, congenital anomalies, or disease. Some definitions go beyond the underlying physical or mental health issue and include different responses by societies to the individual who has a disability. For example, the World Health Organization (2015b) defines disability as "a complex phenomenon, reflecting an interaction between features of a person's body and features of the society in which he or she lives." This definition gives recognition to the environmental and social barriers faced by people who have disabilities.

In the United States, the Social Security Administration defines disability in terms of an individual's ability to work. This definition and its associated criteria are designed to be used to determine eligibility for Social Security payments for individuals with severe disabilities. The criteria used by the Social Security Administration require that the individual be classified as disabled only if he or she has a condition that interferes with basic work activities. Individuals are approved for disability benefits if they are diagnosed with a condition that is severe enough to prevent them from engaging in gainful employment for an extended period of time. The Social Security Administration (2012) does not pay benefits for partial or short-term disability.

On July 26, 1990, President George H. W. Bush signed into law the Americans with Disabilities Act (ADA). The definition of disability under the ADA is "a physical or mental impairment which substantially limits one or more of the major life activities of the individual" (U.S. Department of Justice, 2009, p. 1). A major life activity includes functions such as caring for oneself, standing, lifting, reaching, seeing, hearing, speaking, breathing, learning, and walking. This significant legislation has extended civil rights protection to millions of Americans with disabilities. The first part of the law, which became effective in January 1992, mandated accessibility to public accommodations. The second part of the law went into effect in July 1992 and required employers to make reasonable accommodations in hiring people with disabilities (Merrow & Corbett, 1994; Pelka, 2012).

ADA legislation provides the foundation on which all facets of society will be free of discrimination, including the healthcare system. Therefore, health professionals can expect to encounter people with disabilities in every setting in which they practice, such as schools, clinics, hospitals, nursing homes, workplaces, and private homes. Persons with a disability will expect nurses and other healthcare professionals to provide appropriate instruction adapted to their special needs.

The Language of Disabilities

Since the 1960s, the disability rights movement has worked to improve the quality of life of people with disabilities through political action. The disability rights movement has been successful in advocating for appropriate use of language in regard to people with disabilities—for example, use of people-first language (Haller, Dorries, & Rahn, 2006). The term **people-first language** refers to the practice of putting "the person first before the disability" in writing and speech and "describing what a person has, not what a person is" (Snow, 2012, p. 3). People-first language is based on the premise that language is powerful and that referring to an individual in terms of his or her diagnosis devalues the individual. Consider the following statements:

- Justin, a 5-year-old asthmatic, has not responded well to treatment.
- Developmentally disabled people, like Marcy, do best when provided with careful direction.

In each of these statements, the emphasis is on the disability, rather than the person. Using people-first language, these statements would be reworded as follows:

- Justin is a 5-year-old boy, recently diagnosed with asthma, who continues to have symptoms despite treatment.
- Marcy, who wants to learn how to care for herself and learns best when given careful direction, is a woman with a developmental disability.

One exception to the use of people first-language should be made for individuals who have hearing impairments because this practice is somewhat controversial in the Deaf community (Johnson & McIntosh, 2009; McLaughlin, Brown, & Young, 2004). Many Deaf people want to be recognized as deaf because it is a reflection of who they are as people. As with other cultural groups, nurses should take the steps necessary to get to know their patients and their preferences related to the use of this type of language. In regard to the word *deaf*, Strong (1996) suggests that the word *deaf* with a lowercase *d* be used when referring to the physical condition of not being able to hear, and the word *Deaf* with an uppercase *D* be used when referring to people affiliated with the Deaf community or Deaf culture.

Using people-first language is more than an exercise. It reflects a deliberate action on the part of the nurse to focus on the person with his or her unique qualities rather than to place the individual into an impersonal category based on limitations.

The words and labels nurses use to describe people have the ability to influence the way individuals think about themselves and the way individuals are perceived by society. Therefore, it is important that nurses and all health professionals be sensitive to the way in which they write about, talk about, and talk with people with disabilities. Snow (2012) offers the following suggestions for using disability-sensitive language:

- Use the phrase *congenital disability* rather than the term *birth defect*. The term *birth defect* implies that a person is defective.
- Avoid using the terms *handicapped, wheelchair bound, invalid, mentally retarded, special needs*, and other labels that have negative connotations.
- Speak of the needs of people with disabilities rather than their problems. For example, an individual does not have a hearing problem but rather needs a hearing aid.
- Avoid phrases such as *suffers from* or *victim of*, since these words encourage unnecessary and unwanted pity.
- When comparing people with disabilities to people without disabilities, avoid using phrases such as *normal* or *able-bodied*, which place the individual with a disability in a negative light.

The Roles and Responsibilities of Nurses as Patient Educators

The role of the nurse in teaching persons who have a disability continues to evolve as, more than ever before, patients expect and are expected to assume greater responsibility for self-care. The role of the nurse in working with patients who have a disability is varied and situation dependent. The nurse may encounter patients who are newly disabled or who have an illness that affects an existing disability. The nurse may also work with patients whose disability influences the way in which they learn or respond to treatment. It is the role of the nurse to teach these individuals the necessary skills required to maintain or restore health, maintain independence, and relearn or restore skills lost through illness or injury. When patients with disabilities are encountered in health and illness settings, nurses also are responsible for adapting their teaching strategies to help them learn about health, illness, treatment, and care.

When teaching patients who have a disability, the nurse must assess the degree to which families can and should be involved. Families of individuals who have a new disability are becoming increasingly involved in the individual's care and rehabilitation efforts. However, when working with a patient who has an existing disability, the appropriateness of involving family must be assessed carefully. The nurse must never assume that because a patient has a disability, he or she is incapable of self-care.

Because of the complex needs of this group, teaching often requires an interdisciplinary team effort. In developing a teaching plan, the nurse must assess the need to involve other health professionals such as physicians, social workers, physical therapists, psychologists, and occupational and speech therapists. As with other patients, the nurse has the responsibility to assess learning needs, design appropriate educational interventions, and promote an environment that will enhance learning. The teaching plan must reflect an understanding of the patient's disability and incorporate interventions and technologies that will assist the patient in overcoming barriers to learning.

Application of the teaching–learning process is intended to promote adaptive behaviors in patients that support their full participation in activities designed to promote health and, in the case of illness, optimal recovery. Emphasis on the various components of the learning process may differ depending on the disability, but it often requires changes in all three domains—cognitive, affective, and psychomotor.

Prior to teaching, assessment is always the first step in determining the nature of patients' problems or needs, the short- and long-term consequences or effects of their disability, the effectiveness of their coping mechanisms, and the type and extent of sensorimotor, cognitive, perceptual, and communication deficits they experience. When dealing with persons experiencing a new disability, the nurse must determine the extent of the patients' knowledge with respect to their disability, the amount and types of new information needed to change their behaviors, and their readiness to learn. Assessment should be based on feedback from the patient as well as on observations, testing when appropriate, and input from the healthcare team. In some cases, it may be wise to interview family members and significant others to obtain additional information.

In assessing readiness to learn, Diehl (1989) outlines the following questions to be asked, which continue to remain relevant today, when the nurse is determining if the timing of the teaching–learning process is appropriate:

1. Do the individual and family members demonstrate an interest in learning by requesting information or asking questions in an effort to determine their needs and solve problems?
2. Are there barriers to learning such as low literacy skills, vision impairments, hearing deficits, or impaired mobility?
3. If sensory or motor issues exist, is the patient willing and able to use supportive devices?
4. Which learning style best suits the patient in processing information and applying it to self-care activities?

5. Are the goals of the patient and the goals of the family similar?
6. Is the patient's environment conducive to learning?
7. Do the learners value new information and skills as a means to achieve functional improvement?

The nurse should serve as a mentor to patients and their family members in coordinating and facilitating the multidisciplinary services required to assist persons with a disability in achieving an optimal level of functioning. This role is especially important when working with a patient who has a new disability. **Appendix 9–A** provides a list of organizations that serve as resources for this population.

Types of Disabilities

Disabilities can be classified into two major categories: mental and physical. Physical disabilities typically are those that involve orthopedic, neuromuscular, cardiovascular, or pulmonary problems but may also include sensory conditions such as blindness or deafness. Mental disabilities include psychological, behavioral, emotional, or cognitive impairments.

Multiple subcategories of physical and mental disabilities exist. Seven subcategories of physical and mental disabilities have been chosen for discussion in this chapter because they represent common conditions that the nurse is likely to encounter in practice: (1) sensory disabilities, (2) learning disabilities, (3) developmental disabilities, (4) mental illness, (5) physical disabilities, and (6) communication disorders. The specific disabilities that fall under each of these subcategories are described as follows, along with the teaching strategies that should be used to meet the needs of the learners.

Sensory Disabilities

Sensory disabilities include the spectrum of disorders that affect a person's ability to use one or more of the five senses—auditory, visual, tactile, olfactory, and gustatory. The most common sensory disabilities are those that involve the ability to hear or see.

Hearing Impairments

Hearing impairment is a common disability that affects people of all ages who have either a total or partial auditory loss. It is estimated that approximately 30–48 million Americans have hearing loss in one or both ears (Lin, Niparko, & Ferrucci, 2011). Of every 1000 children born in the United States, approximately two or three are diagnosed as deaf or hard of hearing (National Institute on Deafness and Other Communication Disorders [NIDCD], (2014).

The incidence of hearing loss increases with age. Approximately 18% of all American adults aged 45–64 years have a hearing impairment. This share increases to 47% by age 75, with men being more likely to develop a hearing impairment than women (NIDCD, 2014). Although adult-onset hearing loss is often associated with exposure to loud sounds or noises, approximately 4000 new cases of sudden deafness occur in the United States every year (CDC, 2012).

People with impaired hearing—both the Deaf and the hard of hearing—have a complete loss or a reduction in their sensitivity to sounds (American Speech-Language-Hearing Association [ASHA], 2012b). Three basic types of hearing loss are as follows:

1. *Conductive hearing loss:* A type of hearing loss that occurs when the ear loses its ability to conduct sound—for example, when the ear is plugged as a result of ear wax, a foreign body, a tumor, or fluid.
2. *Sensorineural hearing loss:* A type of hearing loss that is permanent and caused by damage to the cochlea or nerve pathways that transmit sound. Although they do not cure the hearing impairment, cochlear implants and hearing aids can improve hearing in persons with this type of disability.
3. *Mixed hearing loss:* A type of hearing loss that is a combination of conductive and sensorineural losses.

People with hearing loss may have a problem with one or both ears. The degree of hearing loss experienced by people with a hearing impairment is classified on a scale ranging from slight to profound. Although health professionals may use the scale to differentiate people who are classified as being deaf or hard of hearing, patients themselves do not always agree with this classification. Therefore, the nurse must determine if the patient prefers to be referred to as deaf or hard of hearing (National Association of the Deaf, 2010).

Regardless of the degree of hearing loss, any person with a hearing impairment faces communication barriers that interfere with efforts at patient teaching (Stock, 2002). Some individuals who are deaf or hearing impaired also may be unable to speak or have limited verbal abilities and vocabularies (Lederberg, Schick, & Spenser, 2012). This is especially true for adults who are prelingually deaf—that is, they have been deaf since birth or early childhood. Problems with understanding health- and illness-related vocabulary also may occur with patients who are deaf (Pollard & Barnett, 2009).

It is clear that individuals who are deaf will have different skills and needs depending on the type of deafness and the amount of time they have been without a sense of hearing. Those who have been deaf since birth did not have the benefit of acquiring language skills. As a result, they may not possess understandable speech and may have limited reading and vocabulary skills. Most likely, their primary modes of communication will be sign language and lipreading (Alliance for Students with Disabilities in Science, Technology, Engineering, and Mathematics, 2010; Vicars, 2003).

If deafness has occurred after language has been acquired, Deaf people may speak quite understandably and have facility with reading and writing and some lipreading abilities. If deafness has occurred in later life, affected individuals will probably have poor lipreading ability, but their reading and writing skills should be within average range, depending on their educational and experiential background. In older adults, visual impairments may be a compounding factor. The combination of these deficits poses major communication problems when teaching older patients.

People with hearing impairments, like other individuals, require health care and health education information at various periods during their lives. Because of the diversity of this population, assessment is a critical first step in patient education. It is important to determine the extent of the patient's hearing loss and the use of hearing aids, cochlear implants, or other types of assistive equipment.

Individuals with hearing loss often experience social isolation and feelings of inadequacy (Fusick, 2008). These feelings may contribute to a lack of confidence when faced with health challenges. Nurses should assess the patient's prior knowledge of the issue being addressed, recognizing that people with hearing impairments may not have been exposed to the same kinds of health information as people who can hear (Pollard, Dean, O'Hearn, & Haynes, 2009).

Finally, it is important to remember that individuals who are deaf will always rely on their other senses for information input, especially their sense of sight. For patient education to be effective, then, communication must be visible. Because there are several different ways to communicate with a person who is deaf, one of the first things nurses need to do is ask patients to identify their communication preferences. Sign language, written information, lipreading, and visual aids are some of the common choices. Although one of the simplest ways to transfer information is through visible communication signals such as hand gestures and facial expressions, this method will not be adequate for any lengthy teaching sessions.

The following modes of communication are suggested as ways to decrease the barriers of communication and facilitate teaching and learning for patients with hearing impairments in any setting.

SIGN LANGUAGE

Many people who are deaf consider American Sign Language (ASL) to be their primary language and preferred mode of communication. ASL differs from simple finger spelling, which is a method of using different hand positions to represent letters of the alphabet. In contrast, ASL is a complex language made up of signs as well as finger spelling combined with facial expressions and body position. Eye gaze and head and body shift are also incorporated into the language (NIDCD, 2015).

The nurse who does not know ASL is advised to obtain the services of a professional interpreter. Sometimes a family member or friend of the patient skilled in signing is willing and available to act as an interpreter during teaching sessions. However, family members and friends may have difficulty translating medical words and phrases and may be hesitant to convey information that may be upsetting to the patient. Therefore, it is usually preferable to use a professional interpreter, especially if the teaching session will involve sensitive or confidential information (Scheier, 2009). Prior to enlisting the assistance of an interpreter, whether family member or professional, the nurse should always be certain to obtain the patient's permission to do so. Information communicated regarding health issues may be considered personal and private.

Federal law (Section 504 of the Rehabilitation Act of 1973, PL 93-112) requires that health facilities receiving federal funds secure the services of a professional interpreter upon request of a patient. If the patient cannot provide the names of interpreters, the nurse can contact the state registry of interpreters of the deaf. This registry can provide an up-to-date list of qualified sign language interpreters.

During a teaching session, the nurse should stand or sit next to the interpreter. He or she should talk at a normal pace and look and talk directly to the Deaf person when speaking. The interpreter will convey information to the patient as well as share patient responses with the nurse. It is important to remember that ASL does not provide a word-for-word translation of the spoken or written word and that misunderstandings can occur. Patient education involves the exchange of what is often detailed and important information. To determine if the information given is understood, the nurse should ask questions of the patient, request teach-back or demonstrations, allow the patient to ask questions, and use other appropriate assessment strategies (Scheier, 2009).

LIPREADING

Lipreading is the process of interpreting speech by observing movements of the face, mouth, and tongue (Feld & Sommers, 2009). One common misconception is that all people who are deaf can read lips. However, even among those who do, lipreading may not be appropriate for health education or other forms of patient communication. Among Deaf persons in general, word comprehension while lipreading is only about 35%. Therefore, only a skilled lipreader will obtain any real benefit from this form of communication (Rouger et al., 2007).

When working with a patient who is lipreading, it is not necessary to exaggerate lip movements, because this action will distort the movements of the lips and interfere with interpretation of the words. If the patient prefers to lipread, speakers must be sure to provide sufficient lighting on their faces and remove all barriers from around the face, such as gum, pencils, hands, and surgical masks. Beards, mustaches, and protruding teeth also present a challenge to the lipreader. Because less than half of the English language is visible on the lips, one should supplement this form of communication with signing or written materials.

WRITTEN MATERIALS

Written information is probably the most reliable way to communicate, especially when understanding is critical. In fact, nurses should always write down the important information in addition to using the spoken word even when the Deaf person is versed in lipreading or an interpreter is involved. Written communication is always the safest approach.

Printed education materials must always match the reading level of the learner. When preparing written materials for patients who are deaf, it is important to keep the message simple. Although recent studies suggest that students who are deaf are making strides in their reading performance, many people with deafness struggle with the written word (Easterbrook & Beal-Alvarez, 2012).

When providing handwritten or typewritten instructions or using commercially prepared printed education materials, remember that a person with limited reading ability often interprets words literally (the actual meaning of them). Therefore, instructions should be clear, with minimum use of words or phrases that could be misinterpreted.

For example, instead of writing, "When running a fever, take two aspirin," write "For a fever of 100.5°F or higher, take two aspirin." The second message is clearer in that it avoids misinterpretation of the word *running* and also provides clarification of the word *fever*. In addition, visual aids such as simple pictures, drawings, diagrams, and models are also very useful to increase understanding of written materials.

VERBALIZATION BY THE CLIENT

Sometimes patients who are deaf will choose to communicate through speaking, especially if they have established a trusting relationship with the nurse. The tone and loudness of the voice of a patient who is deaf may differ from the average speaker, so nurses must listen carefully, remembering that time may be needed to become accustomed to the patient's particular voice sounds (pitch) and speech rhythms. A quiet, private place should be selected for teaching so that the patient's words can be heard. If the patient's words are difficult to understand, it may help to write down what is heard, which may help those listening to get the gist of the message.

SOUND AUGMENTATION

For those patients who have a hearing loss but are not completely deaf, hearing aids are often a useful device. A patient who has already been fitted for a hearing aid should be encouraged to use it, and it should be readily accessible, fitted properly, turned on, and with the batteries in working order. With permission of the patient and family, the nurse should make a referral to an auditory specialist for any patient who needs to be evaluated for use of a hearing aid.

Only one out of five people who could benefit from a hearing aid actually wear one (NIDCD, 2014). Cost contributes to this problem. Although Medicare policies vary from state to state, as a rule, Medicare does not pay for routine hearing examinations or hearing aids. Under some circumstances, Medicare will pay for diagnostic hearing tests when hearing loss is suspected as a result of illness or treatment (Medicare, 2012).

Another means by which sounds can be strengthened or increased is by cupping one's hands around the client's ear or using a stethoscope in reverse. That is, the patient puts the stethoscope in his or her ears, and the nurse talks into the bell of the instrument (Babcock & Miller, 1994).

When working with a client who is deaf, nurses should always stand or sit nearer to the patient's good ear, use slow speech, and provide adequate time for the patient to respond. Shouting, which distorts sounds, should be avoided.

TELECOMMUNICATIONS

Technology can be used effectively to teach a person who is deaf. The Deaf also can be taught to use technology to enhance life skills. Some examples of telecommunication devices that accomplish both of these goals include television decoders for closed captioned programs, captioned telephones that transcribe everything a person says into writing on a screen, and alerting devices that warn of a crying baby, ringing doorbell, or ringing phone.

Caption films for patient education are available free of charge through Modern Talking Pictures and Services. Text telephones (TTY or Teletype), sometimes referred to as TDD (telecommunication devices for the deaf), are typewriter-like devices that allow for text messages between two parties. These devices use a relay station to translate messages if only one party has the TTY device.

Under federal law, these technology-based devices are considered to be reasonable accommodations for persons with deafness and hearing impairments. However, nurses should note that translation of the spoken word on health-related videos created for the hearing population, without the tone of voice, voice level, and other strategies speakers use to emphasize a point, may alter the message that is conveyed to patients who are deaf (Pollard et al., 2009; Wallhagen, Pettengill, & Whiteside, 2006).

In summary, nurses as patient educators can apply the following guidelines when using any of the already mentioned modes of communication (McConnell, 2002; Navarro & Lacour, 1980).

- Nurses should:
  - Be natural, not rigid or stiff, or not attempt to overexaggerate speech.
  - Use short, simple sentences.
  - Speak at a moderate pace, pausing occasionally to allow for questions.
  - Be sure to get the Deaf person's attention by a light touch on the arm before beginning to talk.
  - Face the patient and stand no more than 6 feet away when trying to communicate.
  - Ask the patient's permission to eliminate environmental noise by lowering the television, closing the door, and so forth.
  - Make sure the patient's hearing aid is turned on, the batteries are working, and his or her glasses are clean and in place.
- Nurses must avoid the following:
  - Talking and walking at the same time.
  - Moving their head excessively.
  - Speaking while in another room or turning away from the person with hearing loss while communicating.
  - Standing directly in front of a bright light, which may cast a shadow or glare.
  - Joking, using slang, or using vocabulary the patient might misinterpret or not understand.
  - Placing an intravenous line in the hand of the patient who uses sign language.

No matter which methods and materials of communication for teaching are chosen, it is important to confirm that health messages have been received and correctly understood. It is essential to check patient comprehension in a nonthreatening manner, such as using the teach-back approach. However, in attempts to avoid embarrassing or offending one another, patients as well as healthcare providers will often acknowledge with a smile or a nod in response to what either party is trying to communicate when, in fact, the message is not well understood. To be sure that the health education requirements of patients who are deaf and hearing impaired are being met, the nurse must find effective strategies to communicate the intended message clearly (Harrison, 1990). Patients who have lived with a hearing impairment for a while usually can indicate which modes of communication work best for them.

Visual Impairments

A **visual impairment** is defined as some form and degree of difficulty seeing and includes a spectrum range of deficits, ranging from total blindness to partial loss of sight, which may include visual field limitations (e.g., tunnel vision), alternating areas of total blindness and vision, and color blindness. Approximately 285 million people worldwide are visually impaired. Of this total, 39 million are blind, and 246 million have low vision (WHO, 2015a). The American Foundation for the Blind (AFB) estimates that more than 20 million people in the United States are blind or visually impaired. Although almost 5 million of these people are older than the age of 65, visual impairment is not a problem that is restricted to older adults. Approximately 1.3 million Americans have vision problems severe enough to classify them as legally blind, and about 60,000 of these individuals are children (AFB, 2012; National Federation for the Blind, 2015).

Blindness and visual impairment are caused by many factors (**Figure 9–1**). Disease is the major cause of loss of vision in adults, with cataracts, age-related macular degeneration, glaucoma, and diabetic retinopathy accounting for the greatest number of disease-related impairments (Braille Institute, 2012; National Institutes of Health, 2015). Although vitamin A deficiency is the leading cause of blindness in children worldwide, amblyopia and strabismus, optic nerve neuropathy, prematurity, low birth weight, and congenital conditions such as congenital cataracts are the most common factors leading to blindness in children in the United States (Lighthouse International, 2015).

In the United States, a person is determined to be legally blind if vision is 20/200 or less in the better eye with correction or if visual field limits in both eyes are within 20 degrees in diameter. Approximately 90% of people who are legally blind have some degree of vision. Typically, a person who is legally blind is unable to read the largest letter on the eye chart with corrective lenses (Braille Institute, 2012). In comparison, total blindness is defined as an inability to perceive any light or movement (Braille Institute, 2012).

Patients who seem to be legally blind but have not been evaluated by a low-vision specialist should be put in contact with local sources, such as the Blind Association and the Commission for the Blind and Visually Handicapped. Patients may require assistance in obtaining help from these services.

The following are some tips nurses might find helpful when teaching patients with visual impairments:

- As a first step, assess patients to avoid making assumptions about their needs because a person who is blind may be very different from one who has low vision.
- Make sure to speak directly to patients rather than to their sighted companions.
- Contact a low-vision specialist who can prescribe optical devices, such as a magnifying lens (with or without a light), a telescope, a closed-circuit TV, or a pair of sun shields, that will help nurses to adapt their teaching materials to the specific needs of patients.

Major diseases causing serious vision impairment that cannot be corrected with conventional spectacles or lenses are cataract, macular degeneration, glaucoma, and diabetic retinopathy. People who have advanced stages of these diseases have difficulty performing ordinary visual tasks, like reading.

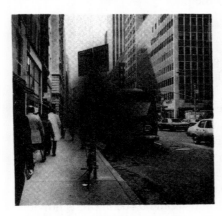

MACULAR DEGENERATION—The deterioration of the macula, the central area of the retina, results in an area of decreased central vision. Peripheral, or side, vision remains unaffected. This is the most prevalent eye disease.

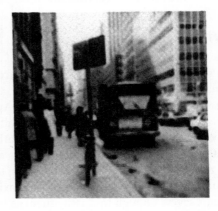

CATARACT—An opacity of the lens results in diminished acuity but does not affect the field of vision. There are no blind spots, but the person's vision is hazy overall, particularly in glaring light.

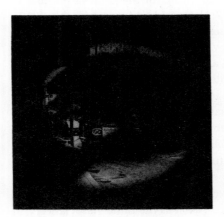

GLAUCOMA—Chronic elevated eye pressure in susceptible individuals may cause atrophy of the optic nerve and loss of peripheral vision. Early detection and close medical monitoring can help reduce complications.

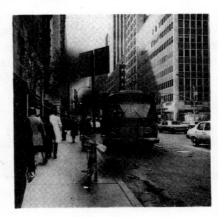

DIABETIC RETINOPATHY—Leaking of retinal blood vessels in advanced or long-term diabetes can affect the macula or the entire retina and vitreous, producing blinding areas.

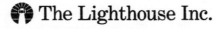

The Lighthouse Inc.

Figure 9–1 Photo essay on partial sight (low vision)

© 2016 Lighthouse Guild.

- Rely on patients' other senses of hearing, taste, touch, and smell when conveying messages as a means to help them take in information from their environment. Usually their listening skills are particularly acute; it is not necessary to shout. When teaching, the nurse should speak in a normal tone of voice.

- Always approach patients by announcing your presence, identifying yourself or others, and explaining clearly why you are there and what you are doing, because people who are blind cannot take advantage of nonverbal cues such as hand gestures, facial expressions, and other body language and instead use their talents of memory and recall to maximize learning (Babcock & Miller, 1994).

- When teaching psychomotor skills, describe as clearly as possible the steps of a procedure, explain any noises associated with treatments or the use of equipment, and allow patients to touch, handle, and manipulate equipment so that they can perform return demonstrations. Use the tactile learning technique when teaching them the characteristics and the placement of objects. For example, allow patients to identify their medications by feeling the shape, size, and texture of tablets and capsules; to locate their various medicines, glue pills and tablets to the tops of bottle caps or put them in different-sized or different-shaped containers (Boyd, Gleit, Graham, & Whitman, 1998); keep items in the same place at all times so they can independently locate their belongings; and arrange things in front of them in a regular clockwise fashion to facilitate learning to perform a task that must be accomplished in an orderly, step-by-step manner (McConnell, 1996).

- Enlarge the font size of letters in printed and handwritten materials as a typical important first step in using these types of instructional tools.

- Use bold colors to provide contrast, which is a key factor in helping a person with limited sight distinguish objects. Assess whether black ink on white paper or white ink on black paper is better, if using a dark placemat with white dishes or serving black coffee in a white cup helps them to see items more clearly, and if placing pills, equipment, or other materials on a contrasting background helps them locate objects they are working with.

- Use proper lighting, which is of utmost importance in assisting patients to read or locate objects. Regardless of the print size, the color of the type, or the paper used, if the light is not sufficient, patients will have a great deal of difficulty distinguishing printed words or manipulating objects.

- Provide large-print watches and clocks with either black or white backgrounds that are available through a local chapter for the visually handicapped.

- Make use of audiotapes and cassette recorders as useful instructional tools to convey patient education information, some of which are available as talking books and can be obtained through the National Library Service or through the state library for the blind and visually handicapped. Also, audiotape oral instructions that can be listened to as necessary at another time and place and can be played over again as many times as necessary to reinforce learning.

- Make use of standard computer features such as screen magnifiers (which can change the text to be 2 to 16 times larger than the normal view), high contrast (which can invert typical black-on-white to other color options), and screen-resolution adjustments to make information on the patient's computer screen easier to see. Advanced assistive technology comes equipped with text-to-speech converters, synthetic speech, screen readers, and Braille keyboards, displays, and printers (University of Washington, 2012).

- Access appropriate resources for information, such as a Braille library, the National Braille Press, or local blind associations for printed education materials.
- When teaching ambulation, always use the sighted guide technique by allowing the patient to grasp your forearm while walking about one half-step ahead, or seek the referral of a mobility specialist available through the local associations for the blind.
- Hold teaching sessions in quiet, private spaces, whenever possible, to minimize distractions and to allow adequate time to deliver instruction in an unhurried manner.

Diabetes education consumes a great deal of a nurse's teaching time and presents unique challenges. Because of the high incidence of this disease in the American population, diabetic retinopathy is a major cause of blindness. Patients who have lost their sight as a result of this disease probably have already mastered some of the necessary skills to care for themselves but will need continued assistance. Of course, it is also possible for persons with visual impairments to be diagnosed at a later time with diabetes. In either case, at some point in the course of their lives, these persons will need to learn how to use appropriate adaptive equipment.

Fortunately, there also has been continuous improvement in the equipment used for self-monitoring of blood glucose levels and for self-injection of insulin. Easy-to-use monitors with large display screens or voice instructions are available now, as are new nonvisual adaptive devices for measuring insulin, and insulin pens that contain prefilled dosages; in addition, built-in magnifiers have made insulin administration much easier for patients who have difficulty reading a syringe (Cohen & Ayello, 2005).

Learning Disabilities

Learning disabilities have emerged as a major issue in the United States (CDC, 2015a). Although often associated with school-aged children, these neurologically based disorders begin in childhood and persist through adulthood (Taymans et al., 2009). Learning disorders are complex conditions that are frequently hidden and vary from individual to individual. As a result, they are often misunderstood and underestimated (Child Development Institute, 2012; LDOnline, 2012; National Joint Committee on Learning Disabilities, 2011; Practitioners' Task Force on Adults With Learning Disabilities, 2007; Santrock, 2013; Snowman & McCown, 2015).

A number of definitions of learning disabilities can be found in the literature. The Individuals with Disabilities Education Act (IDEA) in 2004 retained the original definition of specific learning disability as first defined in 1975. IDEA defines **learning disability** as a "disorder in one or more of the basic psychological processes involved in understanding or in using language, spoken or written, that may manifest itself in an imperfect ability to listen, think, speak, read, write, spell or do mathematical calculations" (ASHA, 2004). This definition stands as the accepted working definition to assess, diagnose, and categorize an array of learning disabilities.

Learning disabilities is an umbrella term that includes such conditions as dyslexia, dyscalculia, and auditory processing disorders. The statistics on learning disabilities are sobering. Almost 2.4 million school-aged children have some form of a learning problem (National Center for Learning Disabilities, 2014), and overall, as many as one out of every five people in the United States has a learning disability (U.S. Department of Education, 2006).

About three to four times as many boys as girls are identified as having a learning disability, but this gender difference is thought to be due to referral bias—more boys are referred for treatment because of their behavior (Crandell, Crandell, & Vander Zanden, 2011; Santrock, 2013). Children with learning disabilities represent the largest segment of children in special education classes, accounting for nearly 40% of the group (Aron & Loprest, 2012).

In the past, a learning disability was thought to be a problem involving only children. Now, however, evidence supports the belief that most individuals do not outgrow the problem (Crandell et al., 2011; Gerber, 2012). Indeed, the rate of learning disabilities in adults is probably similar to the rate in children.

The causes of learning disabilities are varied and often unclear. Genetics plays a role in approximately 50% of cases. It is also suspected that a number of factors that affect the brain, especially during gestation, delivery, and the early years of life, can result in a learning disability. For example, the use of alcohol during pregnancy, difficulties during delivery, and exposure to toxins such as lead paint can all result in learning disabilities (Learning Disabilities Association of America, 2015).

Despite the statistics that reveal the lifelong challenges of individuals with learning disabilities, many of these individuals have been found to have at least average, if not superior (gifted), intelligence. In fact, learning disabilities are often labeled "the invisible handicap" because they do not necessarily result in low achievement. Some very famous and successful people in world history are thought to have had some type of learning disability—ranging from artists (Leonardo da Vinci), to political leaders (Woodrow Wilson, Winston Churchill, and Nelson Rockefeller), to military figures (George Patton), to scientists (Albert Einstein and Thomas Edison) (Crandell et al., 2011). **Table 9–1** lists common myths and corresponding facts about learning disabilities.

The most common learning disorders are discussed in the following subsections.

Dyslexia

Dyslexia is "a neuro-developmental learning disorder that is characterized by slow and inaccurate word recognition" despite traditional and regular instruction, adequate intelligence, and intact sensory abilities (Peterson & Pennington, 2012, p. 1997). Dyslexia accounts for the largest percentage of people with learning disabilities, affecting approximately 10% to 15% of this population (Crandell et al., 2011; Dyslexia Research

Table 9–1 Myths and Facts About Learning Disabilities

Myth:	Children are labeled "learning disabled" because they can't learn.
Fact:	They can learn, but their preferred learning modality must be identified.
Myth:	Children who have a learning disability must be spoken to more slowly.
Fact:	Those who learn in an auditory manner may become impatient with slower speech and stop listening; those who learn visually would benefit more from seeing the information.
Myth:	Children who are learning disabled just have to try harder.
Fact:	Telling these children to try harder is a turnoff. They already do try hard.
Myth:	Children outgrow their disabilities.
Fact:	Children do not outgrow their disabilities. They develop strategies to compensate for and minimize their disabilities.
Myth:	Children with learning disabilities should be treated like everyone else.
Fact:	That treatment would be unfair; they would not get what they need.
Myth:	Nearly all children with learning disabilities are boys.
Fact:	Boys are more often referred for proper identification of learning disabilities because they are more overt in acting out their frustrations.

Reproduced from Greenberg, L. A. (1991, September/October). Teaching children who are learning disabled about illness and hospitalization. *MCN: American Journal of Maternal/Child Nursing, 16*(5), 260–263. Used with permission.

Institute, 2015). Often associated with reading difficulty, dyslexia is actually a language disorder that results in a wide array of symptoms, including reading difficulty, problems with writing and spelling, and delays in speech (Dyslexia Research Institute, 2015; International Dyslexia Association, 2015). Individuals with dyslexia often have other learning disabilities, including attention-deficit/hyperactivity disorder, language impairment disorder, and speech sound disorder (Dyslexia Research Institute, 2015; Peterson & Pennington, 2012).

It is a common misconception that people with dyslexia simply see letters in reverse order. In reality, the problem of dyslexia is much more complex. Recent research indicates several subtypes of dyslexia exist, each characterized by a different neurologic deficit (Heim et al., 2008; Menghini et al., 2010; Wajuhian & Naidoo, 2012). These subtypes are made up of a combination of problems, including the inability to break down words into individual sounds, difficulty distinguishing letters visually, and an inability to associate sounds with letters (Heim et al., 2008; Hultquist, 2006; PBS, 2010). Furthermore, people with dyslexia have been shown to have a deficit in working or short-term memory, making it difficult for them to process complex sentences (Crandell et al., 2011; Wiseheart, Altmann, Park, & Lombardino, 2008).

Levine (2002) has created a website, Misunderstood Minds, that includes exercises that simulate the reading difficulties of someone with dyslexia; Dr. Levine's site can be accessed at http://www.pbs.org/wgbh/misunderstoodminds. Although people with dyslexia can learn to read, the challenges they face can result in self-esteem issues. Young children often experience problems at school because of their disability (Ingesson,

2007), and older adults who were never diagnosed or who did not receive reading help are at greatest risk. The nurse must be sensitive to these issues when teaching.

People with visual perception problems such as dyslexia face a number of other challenges. For example, they may experience a figure–ground problem such that the person is unable to attend to a specific object within a group of objects, such as finding a cup of juice on a food tray. Furthermore, judging distances or positions in space or dealing with spatial relationships may prove difficult, resulting in the person's bumping into things, being confused about left and right or up and down, or being unable to throw a ball or do a puzzle.

Nurses face a number of issues when teaching patients with dyslexia and other types of perceptual deficits. Assessment is a critical first step. A discussion with the patient is advisable to determine the extent of the individual's abilities and disabilities and the manner in which he or she learns best. For example, many people with visual perceptual deficits tend to be auditory learners. Those who learn best by hearing need to have visual stimulation kept to a minimum.

Visual materials such as pamphlets and books are ineffective unless the content is explained orally or the information is read aloud. If visual items are used, nurses should give only one item at a time, with a sufficient period in between times to allow for the patient to focus on and master the information. It may also be helpful to add pictures to written material wherever possible to help convey information. CDs and audiotapes (with or without earphones) and verbal instruction may be beneficial as well.

Some patients with dyslexia have difficulty with the spoken word and may struggle to express themselves or understand what is being said to them (International Dyslexia Association, 2015). For these patients, it is important to proceed in an unhurried manner, presenting small amounts of information over a period of time with frequent assessment of learning. If a patient has difficulty with spoken as well as written words, a combined approach using both oral instruction and visual information may be effective. Nurses can assess recall and retention of information by oral questioning, allowing learners to express orally what they understand and remember about the content that has been presented.

Finally, when teaching motor skills, it is important that nurses remember that people with dyslexia may have impaired left–right discrimination. They may become confused during instruction and coaching if the nurse makes reference to a left hand or right foot. To help overcome this problem, nurses can tape an *X* on the appropriate hand or reference the "arm with the watch."

Auditory Processing Disorders

Auditory processing disorder (APD), also known as central auditory processing disorder (CAPD), is a broad term used to describe a condition that results in an inability of the central nervous system to efficiently process or interpret sound impulses (Kids Health, 2011). Under usual conditions, sound vibrations are converted to electrical impulses in the ear and then transmitted by the auditory nerves to the brain, where they are interpreted. Auditory processing disorders occur when the brain fails to process or interpret these sound impulses effectively. This type of disability affects approximately 5% of children (Kids Health, 2011). Although its cause is usually unknown, this condition can be developmental or acquired and is associated with ear infections and head trauma in both adults and children (Musiek, Barran, & Shinn, 2004).

Auditory processing disorders are characterized by the inability to distinguish subtle differences in sounds—for example, *blue* and *blow* or *ball* and *bell*. There also may be a problem distinguishing speech when others are speaking in the same room. Auditory lags may occur, whereby sound input cannot be processed at a normal rate. Parts of conversations may be missed unless one speaks at a speed that allows the individual enough time to process the information.

During instruction, it is important to limit the noise level and eliminate background distractions. Using as few words as possible and repeating them when necessary (using the same words to avoid confusion) are useful strategies. Nurses should work with the patient to determine the volume and rate of speech that are best understood. For example, some patients find that speech delivered a little slower and a little louder works well (Musiek et al., 2004). Direct eye contact helps keep the learner focused on the task at hand.

Visual teaching methods such as demonstration and return demonstration, gaming (e.g., puppetry), role modeling, and role play, as well as providing written materials, pictures, charts, films, books, puzzles, printed handouts, and using the computer, are the best ways to communicate information. Hand signs for key words when giving verbal instructions and allowing the learner to have hands-on experiences and opportunities for observation are useful techniques. Individuals with auditory processing problems often rely on tactile learning as well. They enjoy doing things with their hands, want to touch everything, prefer writing and drawing, engage in physical exploration, and enjoy physical movement through sports activities.

Individuals with auditory processing disorders may rely on vision to help them learn. The visual learner may closely watch the instructor's face for the formation of words, expressions, eye movements, and hand gestures. If the learner does not understand something being taught, he or she may exhibit frustration in the form of becoming irritable and inattentive. Patients may want instruction to be audiotaped so that they can replay the information as needed.

Dyscalculia

Dyscalculia is a severe learning disability that impairs those parts of the brain involved in mathematical processing (Shalev & Gross, 2001), resulting in an inability to understand sets of numbers. Therefore, the problem for individuals with dyscalculia is not related to difficulty learning mathematical functions but rather to an inability to comprehend the relationship between a numerical symbol and the objects it represents (Spinney, 2009).

Dyscalculia can be either developmental (i.e., acquired at birth) or the result of injury to the brain. The developmental form of this condition is present in 5% to 6% of school-aged children and persists for some individuals into adulthood (Wilson, 2012). Acquired dyscalculia can occur at any time. Individuals with dyscalculia often have other learning or developmental disabilities such as attention-deficit/hyperactivity disorder (ADHD) or dyslexia (Lindsay, Tomazic, Levine, & Accardo, 2001).

It is important for nurses to recognize that the impact of dyscalculia on a patient extends beyond his or her ability to calculate an insulin dose or count the correct number of pills. Such individuals may also have some other issues as follows (British Dyslexia Association, 2015):

- Difficulty grasping the abstract concept of time. As a result, these clients may be unable to read a clock, follow a schedule, or understand the sequence of past and future events.
- Inability to differentiate between right and left.
- Problems with learning specific activities that require sequential processing—that is, any activity in which steps must be followed.
- Problems with reading numbers, such as on a prescription bottle.
- Confusion when schedules or routines change.

The approach to working with a patient with dyscalculia varies depending on the age of the individual and his or her experience with this disorder. A teenager or adult who has lived with dyscalculia for a number of years may have developed strategies for addressing issues such as time, schedules, and numbers. It is important that assessment be done prior to teaching to determine the extent of the disability and the coping strategies that have been successful for the patient. As with any patient who has a learning disability, teaching should be done in an environment that is free from distraction as much as possible and conducted in an unhurried manner. Nurses may find it helpful to begin with the concrete when teaching and then move to the abstract slowly and carefully. Pictures and diagrams may help the patient grasp more abstract concepts. Assessment is vital to determine that the patient has learned the content or skills presented, and reinforcement of learning is critical.

Developmental Disabilities

Child development is a "progressive process that follows along a course of expected outcomes" (Quinn, 2000, p. 17) or milestones in areas such as language, cognition, gross and fine motor control, and social and emotional behavior. Children who do not meet developmental milestones are considered to have a developmental delay. Approximately 13% of preschool children demonstrate developmental delays severe enough to make them eligible for early intervention services (Rosenberg, Zhang, & Robinson, 2008). Many of these children are simply developing at a slower than normal rate and, with intervention, will eventually achieve developmental milestones (Quinn, 2000).

A developmental delay is a temporary or short-term challenge whereas a **developmental disability** represents a lifelong condition resulting from a change in the pattern or nature of a child's development. "Children with developmental disabilities are not traveling at a slower pace; they are traveling a different route altogether" (Quinn, 2000, p. 22). Although children with developmental disorders may find alternative paths to meeting developmental milestones, many are left with deficits that persist into adulthood. Examples of developmental disorders include ADHD and Down syndrome as well as pervasive developmental disorders, or those that involve impairment in the development of socialization and communication skills (National Institute of Neuro-logical Disorders and Stroke, 2012b). Examples of pervasive developmental disorders include autism and Rett syndrome.

Public policy has been enacted to protect the 3 to 4 million people in the United States with developmental disabilities. The Developmental Disabilities Assistance and Bill of Rights Act of 2000 (U.S. Department of Health and Human Services [USDHHS], 2000) establishes state councils on developmental disabilities; university centers for ex-cellence in disability education, research, and service; and national initiatives to collect data and provide assistance as needed.

The Individuals With Disabilities Education Act, originally passed in 1975 as the Education of All Handicapped Children Act, addresses the educational needs of chil-dren with developmental disabilities. Amended several times since its inception in 1975, IDEA assures that children with disabilities receive a free and appropriate public education as well as early intervention services starting in infancy (Crandell et al., 2011; Snowman & McCown, 2015).

When working with a child with a developmental disability, it is important for the nurse to recognize the important role of parents, who are the individuals who know the child best. It is a wise nurse who invites these parents to participate and assist the staff dur-ing their child's hospitalization and works with them in the home. Likewise, when caring for an adult with a developmental disability, caregivers are often the people who know the patient best. However, the nurse needs to be sensitive to the arduous schedule involved in caring for a child or adult with a severe developmental disability and recognize that dur-ing times of illness, parents and family members are often stressed and fatigued.

Managing the treatment of persons with developmental disabilities accounts for an increasing portion of healthcare practice today. Because developmental disabilities usu-ally are diagnosed during infancy and are likely to last a lifetime, nurses must acquire sensitivity to family issues and learn to be flexible in their approaches to meet the intel-lectual, emotional, and medical concerns of patients with special needs (Webb, Tittle, & VanCott, 2000). Several of the common developmental disabilities are described in de-tail in the following subsections.

Attention-Deficit/Hyperactivity Disorder

The many controversies surrounding the diagnosis and treatment of attention-deficit/hyperactivity disorder have made this developmental disability a household word. How-ever, despite the debate about diagnosis, treatment, and unnecessary labeling of children, it is recognized as a legitimate medical condition by the American Medical Association, the American Psychiatric Association, and multiple other major professional and health organizations. **Attention-deficit/hyperactivity disorder** (ADHD) is a disorder of both children and adults that is characterized by difficulty focusing on everyday tasks, as demonstrated by inappropriate behavior such as lack of attention and being impulsive. Although many individuals display some symptoms of ADHD from time to time, an actual diagnosis of ADHD is dependent upon the individual displaying symptoms most of the time and across settings, for example, at home, in school, and on the playground. Furthermore, a child must display six or more symptoms for 6 months or more, and an adult must display five or more symptoms before the diagnosis is confirmed (Block, Macdonald, & Piotrowski, 2015; CDC, 2015a).

ADHD is a developmental condition that manifests in three forms according to the National Institute of Mental Health (NIMH, 2012a):

- ADHD, predominantly inattentive type—a form of ADHD that is characterized by inability to attend to tasks, forgetfulness, and distraction.
- ADHD, predominantly hyperactive impulsive type—a type of ADHD that results in restlessness and a lack of control. Individuals with this form of ADHD are hyperactive and exhibit impulsive behavior.
- ADHD, combined type—a combination of the first two types.

Although all three types are referred to as ADHD, hyperactivity is not present in all cases.

Heredity plays a role in ADHD, making individuals susceptible to certain environmental factors that are associated with the condition. These environmental risk factors include, but are not limited to, low birth weight, traumatic brain injury (TBI), and maternal smoking (Kessler et al., 2006).

ADHD is a common and growing problem. Approximately 2 million children between the ages of 6 and 11 years are diagnosed with this disorder (Crandell et al., 2011). Although boys outnumber girls by at least three to one in terms of the incidence of this disorder, recent research suggests that gender bias might have a role in overdiagnosing boys (Bruchmuller, Margraf, & Schneider, 2012; M. Miller, Ho, & Hinshaw, 2012; Snowman & McCown, 2015). Some children outgrow symptoms of ADHD, but many do not.

Research on the incidence of ADHD in the adult population is inconclusive; however, estimates range from 4% to 5% (Davidson, 2008). ADHD in the adult population is estimated to be underdiagnosed and undertreated and often exists with comorbid mental health and substance abuse disorders (Antshel et al., 2011; Chen, 2015; Kessler et al., 2006). Adults with ADHD may be unaware that they have the condition or be reluctant to disclose this diagnosis because of the stigma associated with it (Sherman, 2012; CDC, 2015a).

ADHD affects individuals at all levels of intelligence and is often compounded with other learning disabilities (Davidson, 2008). The classic symptoms of ADHD include inattention, hyperactivity, and impulsivity. These symptoms present numerous challenges for adults and children; as a result, people with ADHD often struggle in school, at work, and in society. Often, medication therapy, in combination with psychological interventions, is the treatment of choice for both children and adults with ADHD.

Careful assessment is critical before working with any patient with ADHD. Nurses should have an open discussion with the patient and the parents, if the patient is a child, to determine how he or she learns best. If the patient is unable to identify the strategies that have worked well in school or work, the nurse must assess the patient's response to various techniques and make accommodations as necessary. The nurse can then develop an individualized education plan to promote learning through use of patient education strategies that compensate for or minimize the effect of the disability (Crandell et al., 2011; Greenberg, 1991). It is also important to remember, especially when working with adults or children who have symptoms of ADHD, that they may be undiagnosed or may choose to hide this diagnosis.

Nurses should consider the following strategies when working with adults and children with ADHD:

- Provide encouragement during teaching because both adults and children with ADHD are likely to have experienced failure in school and in work settings and may lack confidence in their abilities to manage their health care.
- Focus on the positives rather than on the deficits. Research has shown that individuals with ADHD have many of the same cognitive strengths as those without ADHD (Climie & Mastoras, 2015).
- Consider the learning style of the individual. For visual learners, use colorful handouts and slides; for kinesthetic learners, incorporate movement and activity; and for auditory learners, have them read out loud and consider the use of a recorder so that teaching sessions can be replayed.
- Because patients with ADHD have difficulty maintaining appropriate attention levels, use strategies to attract and hold their attention, such as breaking content to be taught into small, focused sessions whenever possible and, if patients have multiple care-related tasks to accomplish on their own, teaching them to break their care into smaller tasks.
- Structure the environment to eliminate unnecessary distractions.
- Consider using stress reduction techniques prior to teaching to help patients who may be anxious about teaching to relax, which may result in better learning.

Intellectual Disabilities

Intellectual disabilities are among the most common developmental disabilities, affecting approximately 6.5 million people in the United States alone (Center for Parent Information and Resources [CPIR], 2015). An **intellectual disability** is a condition that originates before the age of 18 and results in impaired reasoning, learning, problem solving, and adaptive behavior (American Association on Intellectual and Developmental Disabilities, 2012). A score of less than 75 on an IQ test is one of the major indicators of intellectual disability; use of such an instrument for diagnosis is typically supplemented with tests to assess limitations in conceptual, practical, and social skills (CPIR, 2015).

Intellectual disabilities have multiple causes. First, intellectual disability is a major characteristic of several syndromes such as Down syndrome, fragile X syndrome, and fetal alcohol syndrome. Second, any factor that affects the developing neurologic system of the fetus can result in intellectual disability—for example, drugs, disease, and trauma. Third, birth trauma, low birth weight, disease, and other factors that negatively affect the newborn or young child can cause intellectual disability (Harris, 2005). Finally, intellectual disability can occur as a result of social factors such as lack of education and lack of stimulation as a result of adults not responding to infants and young children (CPIR, 2015).

When planning a teaching intervention with an individual who has an intellectual disability, the nurse must keep in mind the patient's developmental stage, not his or her chronological age. If the patient does not communicate verbally, the nurse should note whether certain nonverbal cues, such as gestures, signing, or other symbols, are used for communication purposes. Most patients with intellectual disabilities are incapable of abstract thinking. Although the majority can understand simple explanations, examples must be given in concrete terms. For example, instead of saying, "Lunch will be here in a few minutes," the nurse could show a clock and point to the time. For children scheduled to have surgery, giving them a surgical mask to play with will help dispel fears they may have when entering the operating room. Likewise, adults with intellectual disabilities benefit from clear explanations and simple demonstrations prior to treatments. Lack of explanation can result in misunderstandings and unnecessary anxieties.

When communicating with patients, nurses must always remember that facial expression and voice tone are more important than words spoken. They should talk with family members or other caregivers to learn about any unique ways in which the patient communicates, including words they may use for body parts or any nonverbal gestures or cues for "yes" or "no" responses. Nurses should lavish any positive behavior with great praise. They should keep the information simple, concrete, and repetitive, and they should be consistent, but firm, setting appropriate limits. Nurses should be careful not to dominate any teaching session, but rather let patients actively participate and gain a sense of accomplishment. Nurses must assign simple tasks with simple directions and show what is to be done, rather than relying on verbal commands. They should give only one direction at a time. A reward system often works very well as, for example, giving children stickers with familiar childhood characters to place on their bed or pajamas that will remind the child of a job well done. For adults, rewards that are important to that individual will work as well.

Asperger Syndrome/Autism Spectrum Disorder

Asperger syndrome is a pervasive developmental disability that falls at the high end of the autism spectrum (Atwood, 2006). It is estimated that 2 out of every 10,000 children in the United States are diagnosed with Asperger syndrome every year (National Institute of Neurological Disorders and Stroke, 2012a). Asperger syndrome is caused by a brain dysfunction that is typically genetic in origin (Atwood, 2006).

Although Asperger syndrome was officially classified as a distinct diagnosis in the early 1990s, the American Psychiatric Association voted to eliminate it as a separate diagnosis in the 2013 edition of *Diagnostic and Statistical Manual of Mental Disorders*. Instead, now this syndrome falls under the umbrella term "autism spectrum disorder" (Autism Research Institute, 2013). This decision is somewhat controversial, particularly among the Asperger syndrome community. Therefore, although the actual diagnostic label has changed, it is likely that the term *Asperger syndrome* will continue to be used for some time.

Children with Asperger syndrome may exhibit a variety of symptoms, including impaired social interaction, repetitive rituals, clumsiness, and limited areas of interest (National Institute of Neurological Disorders and Stroke, 2012a). Although they have good language and cognitive skills, with average or above average vocabularies, they have difficulty modulating the pitch of their voice and typically speak in a flat, monotone manner (Medical News Today, 2015). Asperger syndrome cannot be cured, but with treatment, children with this condition can learn to grow into functioning adults. However, adults with Asperger syndrome may continue to display subtle symptoms of the disorder, particularly in relation to social interactions (Bauer, 2008).

Teaching the child with Asperger syndrome presents many challenges. Although intellectual disability is usually not present, the communication and social problems associated with the disorder make it difficult both for the child to attend to instruction and for the nurse as educator to assess the child's response. For example, children with Asperger syndrome have significantly more difficulty following verbal instructions than do other children (Saalasti et al., 2008). The nurse should provide multiple cues and a lot of repetition when teaching.

Also, children with Asperger syndrome have limitations in telling a story, and their stories tend to be shorter and less coherent than stories told by other children. Therefore, when assessing a child with Asperger syndrome, the nurse may choose to ask direct questions rather than open-ended questions requiring a lengthy response (Rumpf & Becker, 2012).

Like other individuals with autism, "Asperger patients do not use the human face as a source of important clues in social interactions and avoid eye contact" (Topel & Lachmann, 2008, p. 603). Thus, when shown a human face, they have difficulty interpreting emotions conveyed by facial expressions (Falkmer, Bjallmark, Larsson, & Falkmer, 2012). Therefore, the nurse must recognize that patients with this syndrome may need verbal cues rather than facial cues during teaching sessions.

Creative strategies are often helpful in teaching the patient with Asperger syndrome. Because these individuals often have difficulty generalizing to other situations what they have been taught, it may be helpful to teach the child skills in context with something familiar. For example, Hayhurst (2008) suggests that if working on motor skills, patients might practice climbing the steps on the bus or using equipment in the playground.

Mental Illness

In the United States, mental disorders are classified according to the categories outlined in *Diagnostic and Statistical Manual of Mental Disorders,* fifth edition. Mental disorders affect an estimated 20% of Americans (1 in 5) ages 18 and older (Substance Abuse and Mental Health Services Administration, 2014). Mental disorders are the leading cause of disability in the United States and Canada for people aged 15–44, and only a fraction of those affected receive treatment (NIMH, 2012b). These statistics reveal the relative prevalence of mental illness in our society and indicate that nurses will often care for patients with a psychiatric problem as a primary or secondary diagnosis.

Although educating patients with mental disorders requires the same basic principles of patient teaching, some specific teaching strategies should be considered. As with any other nursing intervention, the first step is to begin with a comprehensive assessment. In this case, it is wise to determine whether the patient has any cognitive impairment or inappropriate behavior as well as to assess the patient's level of anxiety.

The emotional threat that a person perceives as a result of a psychiatric disorder may result in an increased anxiety level and subsequently trigger a chain of physiological reactions that then decrease his or her readiness to learn (Haber, Krainovich-Miller, McMahon, & Price-Hoskins, 1997).

High anxiety can make learning nearly impossible (Kessels, 2003; Stephenson, 2006). Despite the nurse's best efforts, patients with a mental disorder may not be able to identify their need to learn and may not be sufficiently ready to learn. The nurse, however, may not be able to wait for readiness to happen. Therein lies the challenge.

Although persons with mental disorders are able to learn given the right circumstances and strategies, it is important to remember that people with mental illness can experience difficulty in processing information and verbally communicating information. In addition, they may experience decreased concentration and become easily distracted, which can limit their ability to stay on task. These symptoms of their disease can be compounded by the medications used to treat mental illness, which can cause drowsiness, difficulty concentrating, blurred vision, or agitation.

It is very important that care, including education, of the patient with mental illness build upon the individual's strengths and skills (Jackson, 2009). The nurse must enter into a partnership with the patient and, when appropriate, with his or her family or caregiver. Also, because the patient's behavior can be unpredictable, it is very important that the family or significant other participate in the patient education sessions (Haber et al., 1997).

Three essential strategies have proved especially successful when teaching people with mental illness (Haber et al., 1997):

1. Teach by using simple and brief words, repeating information over and over to help patients remember important messages, writing down important information by placing it on index cards, and using simple drawings or symbols to assist with improving memory. Be creative.
2. Keep sessions short and frequent. For instance, instead of a half-hour session, break the learning period into two 15-minute sessions or three 10-minute sessions.
3. Involve all possible resources, including the patient and his or her family, by actively engaging them in helping to determine the patient's preferred learning styles as well as by using computer-assisted instruction, videotapes, and role modeling to reinforce content.

As with any teaching program, it is important to set goals and determine outcomes with the patient. The specific behavioral objectives depend on individual learning needs as well as overall learning outcomes. These would include empowering patients to take as much control over their health as possible.

Motivating the patient with a chronic mental illness can be challenging. A certificate of recognition may be given to each patient when he or she completes a program, which can be a powerful motivator. Independence and self-management remain goals that, if achieved, can have a positive effect on the quality of life of the chronically mentally ill.

Physical Disabilities

Traumatic Brain Injury

A fall, car accident, gunshot wound, and a blow to the head are just a few potential causes of traumatic brain injury (TBI). Falls are the leading cause of TBI, particularly for children from birth to the age of 4 and adults older than 65 years of age. Approximately 2.5 million people sustain a TBI each year in the United States. Of these cases, approximately 75% involve concussions or other mild forms of head injury (CDC, 2014). Males are more likely than females to sustain a TBI, as are individuals with preexisting developmental disabilities, such as ADHD (Schachar, Park, & Dennis, 2015). The two age groups at highest risk for the injury are infants to 4-year-olds and 15- to 19-year-olds. Of course, military duty increases the risk of sustaining a TBI (Marchione, 2007). The CDC (2014) estimates that at least 5.3 million Americans currently have a long-term or lifelong need for help to perform activities of daily living as a result of a TBI.

The cognitive deficits that occur depend on the severity and location of the injury but may include poor attention span, slowness in thinking, confusion, difficulty with short-term and long-term memory, being easily distracted, impulsive and socially inappropriate behaviors, poor judgment, mental fatigue, and difficulty with organization, problem solving, reading, and writing (ASHA, 2015). As might be expected, communication skills will more than likely be an issue. Cognitive deficits may persist for an extended period of time.

The treatment of people with severe brain injury is most often divided into three stages:

1. Acute care (in an intensive care unit)
2. Acute rehabilitation (in an inpatient brain-injury rehabilitation unit)
3. Long-term rehabilitation after discharge (at home or in a long-term care facility)

At every stage of treatment, there are many hurdles to conquer. Throughout the rehabilitation process, family teaching must be consistent and thoughtful, because most of the residual impairments are not visible, with the exception of the sensorimotor deficits. The communication, cognitive-perceptual, and behavioral changes associated with TBI may be dramatic. However, the most difficult problem for the family is often the recognition that their relative will probably never be the same person again. In fact, personality changes present the biggest burden for the family. Studies have shown that the level of the family's stress is directly related to the extent of the individual's personality changes and the relative's own perception of the symptoms arising from the head injury (Grinspun, 1987).

Although most of the literature deals with the importance of including the family during the rehabilitation period, it is clear that persons with brain injury will always need the involvement of their family. Again, the benefits of participation in family groups are immeasurable. Considerable strength is gained from group participation, and learning is accomplished through a friendly, informal approach. Of particular importance for persons with brain injury is the need for unconditional acceptance from their friends and family.

Patients recovering from TBI face many challenges. Just as the family needs to adjust to the changes in their injured family member, so patients themselves must cope with loss of identity. The significant physical and cognitive changes caused by the brain injury often alter how the individual interacts with the world (Fraas & Calvert, 2009). Patients face not only recovery from physical injury, but often an uncertain future.

Learning needs for this population center on the issues of patient safety and family coping. Safety issues are related to cognitive and behavioral capabilities. Families are faced with a life-changing event and will require ongoing support and encouragement to take care of themselves. Recovery may require several years, and most often the person is left with some form of impairment.

According to the CDC (2014), 40% of all persons hospitalized with a TBI have at least one unmet need for services 1 year after the injury. The most frequently noted needs relate to managing stress and emotional upsets, controlling one's temper, improving one's job skills, and regaining memory and problem-solving ability. **Table 9–2** lists guidelines for teaching persons with a TBI.

Memory Disorders

Memory is a complex process that allows people to retrieve information that has been stored in the brain (Cherry, 2012). Short-term memory refers to information that is remembered as long as one is paying attention to it—for example, being able to complete the steps of a procedure in a return demonstration. Individuals with short-term memory deficits may be unable to recall what they learned an hour before, but they may be able to recall the information at a later point in time. Long-term memory consists of information that has been repeated and stored and becomes available whenever the individual thinks about it, such as being able to remember a telephone number over a long period of time. Brain injury, a wide range of diseases, and medical disorders can all result in mild to severe memory disorder.

Table 9–2 Guidelines for Effective Teaching of the Brain-Injured Patient

Do	Don't
Use simple rather than complex statements.	Stop talking or give up trying to communicate.
Use gestures to enhance what you are saying.	Speak too fast.
Give step-by-step directions.	Talk down to the person.
Allow time for responses.	Talk to the family member or significant other as if the patient is not there.
Recognize and praise all efforts to communicate.	
Use listening devices.	
Keep written instructions simple, with as small an amount of information as possible.	
Seek the assistance of a speech-language pathologist.	

Brain injury often results in a memory disorder referred to as amnesia. Individuals with anterograde amnesia have memory up until the brain injury but are unable to form memories in the present. Individuals with retrograde amnesia have memory loss for a period of time prior to the brain injury. Most people with brain injury have a combination of both types of amnesia (Mastin, 2010).

Alzheimer's disease, multiple sclerosis, Parkinson's disease, brain tumors, and depression are just a few of the conditions that can result in some degree of memory disorder. The following strategies may be helpful when working with patients who have memory loss for whatever reason and to whatever extent.

- To relearn the memory process, emphasize memory techniques that focus on the need for attention, the benefit of repeating information, and the importance of practicing recall to grasp the information being taught (Thomas, 2009).
- If the patient has intact communication skills, encourage him or her to take notes during teaching sessions, or the session can be audiotaped to provide the patient and his or her family with a resource for referral.
- If a patient has minor memory problems, assist him or her to create a system of reminders—for example, use of a personal digital assistant (PDA), calendar, or sticky notes.
- Use vivid pictures to help them visualize concepts (Wadsley, 2010).
- Teach patients to "chunk information." For example, rather than remembering the seven numbers in a phone number, they can think about a phone number in double digits—for example, 7-45-86-42 (Wadsley, 2010). The same principle can be applied to any procedure that has multiple steps.
- Structure teaching sessions to allow for brief, frequent repetitive sessions that provide constant reinforcement of learning.

Communication Disorders

Communication disorders can affect an individual's ability to both send and receive messages. A cerebrovascular accident (stroke) is the most common cause of impaired communication. This section covers some useful strategies that are appropriate for working with an individual with an impaired communication disorder such as aphasia, a common occurrence following stroke.

Stroke is the leading cause of long-term disability in the United States. A stroke occurs about every 40 seconds, and death from a stroke happens on average every 4 minutes. African Americans and Native Americans are at greatest risk of having a stroke (American Heart Association, 2015). More than 7 million Americans are living with the long-term effects of stroke, with about one third having mild impairments, another third becoming moderately impaired, and the remainder being severely impaired (National Stroke Association, 2015).

Aphasia

One of the most common effects of a stroke is aphasia. "Aphasia is an acquired communication disorder that impairs a person's ability to process language but does not affect intelligence" (National Aphasia Association, 2015). Aphasia results from damage to the language center of the brain. Primary signs of this disorder include some combination of deficits in the ability to express oneself, to understand speech, to read, and to write. Although seen commonly in adults who have suffered a stroke, aphasia can also result from a brain tumor, infection, head injury, or dementia.

An estimated 1 million people in the United States today suffer from aphasia (National Aphasia Association, 2015). Many forms of aphasia are possible, and newly diagnosed clients usually work with a speech therapist. Some of the more common types of aphasia include global aphasia, expressive aphasia, receptive aphasia, and anomic aphasia (National Aphasia Association, 2015). Determining the type of aphasia involved will assist the nurse in developing an appropriate teaching plan for the patient.

Global aphasia is the most severe form and produces deficits in both the ability to speak and the ability to understand language. **Expressive aphasia** affects the dominant cerebral hemisphere and results in patients having difficulty conveying their thoughts, speaking haltingly, and using sentences consisting of a few disjointed words, but understanding what is being said to them. When this is caused by a stroke, the stroke often leaves the person with right-sided paralysis as well. **Receptive aphasia** is a result of damage to the temporal lobe and affects auditory and reading comprehension. Although the patient's hearing is not impaired, she is nevertheless unable to understand the significance of the spoken or written word. Individuals with **anomic aphasia** understand what is being said to them and are able to speak in full sentences, but they have difficulty finding the right noun or verb to convey their thoughts, so they often talk around an issue or switch thoughts when they cannot remember a word.

The inability to communicate normally is a devastating consequence of a brain injury and requires the full support of the healthcare team. Aphasia has the potential to be a highly frustrating experience for both the patient and his or her caregivers. Speech therapy should be one of the earliest interventions, and the nurse will need to incorporate those strategies identified as effective by the speech therapist into the teaching–learning plan. Every effort must be made to establish communication at some level. Remember, regardless of how severe the communication deficit is, it is almost always possible to assist patients who have had a stroke to communicate in some manner and to some extent.

First and foremost, when working with a patient who has expressive aphasia, it is important to remember that communication will take time. Patients who struggle to find the right word may need time to express themselves, so communication cannot be hurried. As these patients struggle to speak, nurses must resist the temptation to finish sentences or fill in gaps for them without asking permission to do so. Patients with receptive aphasia may suddenly find that their native language sounds foreign. These individuals may need extra time to process and understand what is being said. They may find it especially difficult to follow very fast speech, like that heard on the radio or television news, and can easily misinterpret the subtleties of language (e.g., taking the literal meaning of sarcasm or a figure of speech such as "He kicked the bucket"). In either type of aphasia, the nurse should focus on what the patient can do rather than on the speech deficits (National Aphasia Association, 2015; Sander, 2014).

Environmental control is critical for all teaching sessions with patients who have aphasia. The nurse must make sure that he or she has the patient's full attention before attempting to communicate and that a quiet, disruption-free area is created. Because patients are often frustrated or embarrassed by their disability, a private area is also preferred. Moreover, the nurse must always remember that the patient's difficulty with communication is not reflective of an inability to think or understand. Therefore, neither the nurse nor members of the family should talk down to the patient. Ample praise and positive reinforcement for attempts to speak or efforts to understand are also important. It is unnecessary and demoralizing to correct every misunderstanding or error in word selection and pronunciation—the goal is communication rather than perfection. Finally, it is important that the nurse, as well the family, avoid the tendency to protect the patient by shielding him or her from group conversations, especially those conversations that are important to the patient (National Aphasia Association, 2015).

The term **augmentative and alternative communication** describes the strategies and technologies that can be used to aid communication with a patient who has aphasia following a brain injury, such as a stroke (Wallace & Bradshaw, 2011). Additional strategies and technologies that can be used by the nurse include the following (McKelvey, Hux, Dietz, & Beukelman, 2010; Wallace & Bradshaw, 2011):

- For patients who have difficulty with expression, establish a consistent system for everyone to use that allows the patient to respond to yes/no questions—for example, moving the head up and down for "yes" or side to side for "no." The nurse should use this system not only to get information from the patient but also to verify that the patient is grasping the material being presented in a teaching session.
- Teach the patient to point to certain objects to quickly express common needs. For example, the nurse might explain to the patient, "When you point to your water pitcher, I will know that you want a drink of water."
- Use simple sentence structure, speak slowly, and emphasize important words. Repeat important points using different words or phrases. Ask only one question at a time. Break questions down into parts so that simple answers are acceptable.
- Avoid jumping from topic to topic. Keep like topics together, and announce when you are changing topics—for example, "We just finished talking about *when* to take your medication; now I will talk about *how* to take your pills."
- Teach the patient to use exaggerated facial expressions, hand movements, or tone of voice to improve speech comprehension. For example, a patient who grimaces when attempting to ask for pain medication is more easily understood. It is important that the patient, the family, and the nurse be open to using different ways to enhance communication. The nurse also can model messages using exaggerated facial expressions to assist the patient who has difficulty with comprehension.
- Make use of available communication boards. A communication board is a platform that uses pictures, letters, or other symbols that can be pointed or gestured to so as to convey a message. Communication boards range in style and level of technological enhancement, but all provide a simplified way of assisting patients to communicate. Many communication boards allow for digitized messages to

be used. For example, a question mark on a communication board might be programmed to elicit a voice that says, "I don't understand; please repeat." If a communication board with pictures or letters is not available, the nurse can create one. When using pictures with patients who have severe aphasia, the nurse should present personally relevant, context-related photographs whenever possible. In addition, the nurse might create a picture board that is specific to the learning that needs to take place. For example, when teaching the patient about medications, the nurse might develop a picture board illustrating the medications ordered, the purpose of each, and how it should be taken. When assessing the patient's understanding of the information, the nurse could then say, "Point to the pill you will take for pain" or "Show me whether you are supposed to take this medicine with food or with water."

- Support patients' speech therapy programs by having them recall word images and by naming first commonly used objects (e.g., spoons, knives, forks) and then those objects in the immediate environment (e.g., bed, table). Another strategy is to have the person repeat the words spoken by the nurse. It is wise to begin with simple terms and work progressively toward more complex phrases.

The act of communicating may be exhausting for the patient with expressive aphasia, so it is important to keep teaching sessions short and focused. Most people become tired when sessions are longer than 30 minutes. Often patients' speech will become slurred at this point, and they will experience mental fatigue. Whenever possible and if the patient agrees, it may be helpful to have a family member or significant other present during teaching sessions so that he or she can reinforce learning as needed.

As nurses attempt to work with and engage patients with aphasia in a teaching–learning intervention, they must be aware of their own attitudes. The effort to communicate with someone without using his or her usual speech and language can be a frustrating experience. Nurses should be sure to take time out and reflect on the rewards of assisting the client and family in overcoming this barrier.

Dysarthria

Many people with degenerative disorders, such as Parkinson's disease, multiple sclerosis, and myasthenia gravis, also have dysarthria. **Dysarthria** is a neuro-motor disorder that is caused by damage to the nerves or muscles associated with eating and speaking, including the mouth, tongue, larynx, or vocal cords. The result may range from mild changes to totally unintelligible speech. The type and severity of dysarthria depend on which area of the nervous system is affected (ASHA, 2012a). Individuals with dysarthria have problems making their speech intelligible, audible, natural, and efficient (Mackenzie, 2011; Sander, 2014).

The intervention of a speech-language pathologist may help improve the function of various muscles used for speech in patients with dysarthria. In some cases, for example, Parkinson's disease medication may help to improve speech. Some mechanical devices have been developed as well, such as a prosthetic palate, which is used to control hypernasality.

Sign language may be used if the person's arm and hand muscles are not significantly affected. The nurse should work with the speech-language pathologist to determine whether any of the other nonverbal aids would be appropriate, such as communication boards or a portable electronic voice synthesizer. With the advent of adaptive technologies, the possibilities are limitless.

To improve communication with people with dysarthria, Yorkston et al. (2001) make the following suggestions:

- Control the communication environment by reducing distractions.
- The person with dysarthria should pay attention to the speaker and watch him or her as he or she talks.
- When the patient has difficulty understanding a speaker, the patient should be honest and let the speaker know.
- When asking a patient to repeat something, be specific. Convey the part of the message that was misunderstood so that the patient does not have to repeat the entire message.
- If the patient's message cannot be understood, ask questions that require a yes or no answer or have the patient write his or her message.

Chronic Illness

Chronic illness is the leading cause of death in the United States. It is a major cause of disability resulting in blindness, amputations, stroke, and other cognitive, sensory, and physical impairments and accounts for 86% of the nation's healthcare costs (CDC, 2015b). Every aspect of an individual's life is touched by the illness—physical, psychological, social, economic, and spiritual. Because successful management of a chronic illness is a lifelong process, the development of good learning skills is a matter of survival. It is impossible within this chapter to cover specific teaching strategies for each chronic illness; instead, some general teaching and learning principles are suggested in the following pages.

Life with a chronic illness is characterized by unpredictability and uncertainty. Most illnesses have several phases that affect the educational needs of both the individual and his or her family. No single approach will fit each teaching–learning situation.

It is important to be aware of the timing, acuity, and severity of the disease progression. The family's reaction and perception of the chronic illness are also important influences on the teaching–learning process (E. T. Miller, 2011). Families need information and education to deal with the limitations and changes in their loved one's lifestyle.

Strauss et al. (1984) identified eight key problem areas experienced by chronically ill patients and their families that are still relevant today:

1. Prevention of medical crises and the management of problems once they occur
2. Control of symptoms
3. Carrying out prescribed regimens and dealing with problems associated with continuous self-care management

4. Prevention of, or living with, social isolation that decreases contact with others
5. Adjustment to changes in the course of the disease through periods of exacerbation or remission
6. Keeping interactions normal with others as well as maintaining one's lifestyle as consistent as possible
7. Funding (finding the necessary money to pay for treatments or to survive with partial or complete loss of employment)
8. Confronting psychological, marital, and family problems that often arise in dealing with long-term illness

Patients who are chronically ill often manage complex therapeutic regimens. Braden's self-help model (learned response to chronic illness experience) is a nursing theory that provides a framework with which to describe factors that enhance learning and moderate responses in chronic illness (Lubkin & Larsen, 2016). This model proposes a teaching approach that the nurse can use to encourage independence in patients versus them feeling helpless or responding passively to interventions.

The Family's Role in Chronic Illness or Disability

Families are often the care providers and the support system for the person with a chronic illness or disability, and they need to be included in all the teaching–learning interactions. Their reactions and perceptions of the impact of chronic illness or disability, rather than the illness or disability itself, influence all aspects of adjustment. Family participation does have a profound influence on the success of a patient's rehabilitation program (Lubkin & Larsen, 2016; Turner et al., 2007).

When assessing the patient and family, it is important to note what the family considers high-priority learning needs. Most often, such needs will be related to the caregiver's perceived lifestyle change. A caregiver might ask, "Can I continue working outside the home?" or "Will I be able to maintain my relationships with friends?" It is important that the nurse assist the patient and family to identify problems and develop mutually agreed-upon goals. Adaptation is key. Communication between and among family members is crucial. If a family has open communication, the nurse is in a good position to help the family mobilize their resources to obtain needed educational and emotional support.

The education process also needs to take into consideration the family's strategies for coping with their relative's illness or disability. Without a doubt, the overwhelming nature of chronic illness or disability affects the quality of life not only for the person who is ill or disabled but also for all the family members (Lubkin & Larsen, 2016). In their role as caregivers, family members have their own anxieties and fears.

A chronic illness or disability can either destroy or strengthen family unity. Siblings and children of the person who is ill or disabled may be at different stages of acceptance. Denial may be present during the initial diagnosis of an illness or disability. Later, as the patient and his or her family realize that the situation is permanent and has many consequences, the nurse may witness them pass through periods of

Table 9–3 Relieving External Tensions in Client and Family Education

Problem	Response
Family Dynamics	
Patient or family member feeling overwhelmed	Goal setting: Help family refocus on tasks at hand. Review goals that have been attained to boost morale.
Anxiety and fear of performing complex procedures	Establish an atmosphere of acceptance. Don't be in a hurry. Offer opportunities for discussion and questions and answers. Reassure patient and family that they have made the right treatment choice.
Emotions associated with chronic or terminal conditions	Provide opportunities to express feelings. Offer referrals to community resources.
Caregiver burnout and illness	Simplify patient management where possible (e.g., scheduling drug doses to reduce nighttime treatment). Remain accessible. Remember: When caregiver needs are not being met, resentments increase. Provide information on respite care.
Patient fatigue, especially with chronic illness	Help the patient identify individual ability for as much active participation in the family life as possible.
Young patients overwhelmed by complex emotions about their situation and therapy	Encourage both children and adolescents to use artwork to express their feelings. Suggest support groups. Offer support to parents and siblings who must alter their family lifestyle.
Geriatric Considerations	
An increase in the number of drugs taken daily (on average four or more per day) leading to increase in the potential for adverse reactions	Use only one pharmacy so that one source keeps track of medications. Continually evaluate all drugs taken for need, safety, compatibility, potential adverse reactions, and expiration dates.
Decreased visual acuity	Use teaching materials with large, bold type. Encourage the use of corrective lenses or a magnifying glass.

Modified by permission from LaRocca, J. C. (1994). *Mosby's home health nursing pocket consultant.* St. Louis, MO: Mosby–Year Book.

anger, guilt, depression, fear, and hostility. As these feelings gradually become less intense, teaching lessons will need to be readjusted to fit the new circumstances. Flexibility is vital to achieving successful outcomes. Be sure to treat each family member as unique and recognize that some family members may never fully adjust to the altered circumstances. **Table 9–3** lists some of the most common sources of tension in patient and family education.

Nurses need to value their teaching role when they work with the family of a person with a chronic illness or disability. Unlike families dealing with an acutely ill member, families with a member who is permanently ill or disabled will have contact with the healthcare system off and on throughout their lives. Therefore, whenever teaching sessions are required, the availability of families to be present should be a primary consideration. Given adequate support and resources, families with a member who is chronically ill or disabled can adapt, make adjustments, and live healthy, happy, full lives.

Summary

This chapter covered some of the most common disabilities experienced by millions of Americans as a result of disease, injury, heredity, aging, and congenital defects. These conditions affect physical, cognitive, or sensory capacities and require behavioral change in one or more of these domains of learning. The nurse as patient educator must be creative, innovative, flexible, and persistent when applying the principles of teaching and learning to meet the needs of these special populations of individuals, their families, and their significant others.

The shock of any disability, whether it occurs at the beginning of life or toward the end, has a tremendous impact on individuals and their families. At the onset of the condition and throughout the transition and recovery or rehabilitation process, the patient and family face the prospect of having to learn new information or relearn previous skills to adapt to their situation. Inner strength and courage are attributes needed to face each new day, as the effort for most patients to live a normal life never ends. The physical, social, emotional, and vocational implications of living with a disability or the permanence of a chronic illness require the nurse as patient educator to be well prepared to meet all members of these special populations right where they are in their struggle to live a life of quality and independence.

Review Questions

1. How widespread is the disability issue in the United States and worldwide?
2. What is meant by the term *disability*?
3. What is people-first language, and why should nurses use it in their writing and speaking?
4. Which questions should the nurse ask when assessing readiness to learn in a person with a disability?
5. How can the nurse enhance communication with a patient who has a hearing impairment?
6. Which techniques can the nurse use when teaching a patient who has a visual impairment?
7. How can the nurse adapt teaching strategies to meet the needs of a patient with dyslexia?
8. What are the characteristic behaviors of persons with ADHD, and which patient education interventions should be used with this population for effective teaching and learning?
9. How is the term *developmental disability* defined, and what approaches can be used by the nurse when teaching children with mental or physical impairments?
10. What are the key problem areas experienced by patients who are chronically ill and by their family members or significant others?
11. How can assistive technology devices improve the quality of life for a person with a disability?

Case Study

It is early morning on the pediatric unit, and the staff are conducting morning rounds. They are discussing 10-year-old Matthew Yoakum, who was transferred to the unit yesterday evening from the ICU. Matt had a below-the-elbow amputation of his right arm following an accident on his family farm. The following conversation takes place.

Jose Garcia, MSW: Matt and his family are having a very hard time. Apparently Matt was helping his father when he started fooling around, slipped, and fell into the hay elevator. His lower arm was so badly mangled that the surgeon couldn't save it.

Kristen Stryker, PT: I've met with the family. They are feeling very guilty. Matt has ADHD and has had a lot of behavior problems at school. His dad told me that he should have been watching Matt more carefully because he knows that his son has a hard time concentrating on what he is doing.

Usha Gupta, RN: We have seen some behavior problems here as well. Last night one of the staff went into his room to ask him to lower his radio and he refused. When she turned the radio off, Matt began spitting and swearing at her.

Carly Thomas, OTR: I think he and his family are very frightened. This has all happened so quickly and the consequences of his injury are significant.

Usha Gupta RN: We need to develop a teaching plan. Maybe if they have a better sense of what is going to happen, they will begin to feel more in control.

Develop a teaching plan for the Yoakum family by responding to the following questions.

1. Which information should be collected as part of the assessment of this family?
2. Which factors in this situation might interfere with the patient's and family members' readiness to learn?
3. Which teaching strategies would you use to facilitate learning?

References

Alliance for Students with Disabilities in Science, Technology, Engineering, and Mathematics (AccessSTEM). (2010). *How can I work with a student who is deaf and speaks ASL but struggles with written English?* Retrieved from http://www.washington.edu/doit/Stem/articles?77

American Association on Intellectual and Developmental Disabilities. (2012). *FAQ on intellectual disability.* Retrieved from http://www.aaidd.org/intellectual-disability/definition/faqs-on-intellectual-disability

American Foundation for the Blind (AFB). (2012). *Statistical snapshots from the American Foundation for the Blind.* Retrieved from http://www.afb.org/section.aspx?FolderID=2&SectionID=15

American Heart Association. (2015). *Heart disease and stroke statistics: 2015 update.* Retrieved from http://circ.ahajournals.org/

American Speech-Language-Hearing Association (ASHA). (2004). *Specific learning disability.* Retrieved from http://www.asha.org/advocacy/federal/idea/04-law-specific-ld/

American Speech-Language-Hearing Association (ASHA). (2012a). *Dysarthria.* Retrieved from http://www.asha.org/public/speech/disorders/dysarthria.htm

American Speech-Language-Hearing Association (ASHA). (2012b). *Type, degree, and configuration of hearing loss.* Retrieved from http://www.asha.org/public/hearing/disorders/types.htm

American Speech-Language-Hearing Association (ASHA). (2015). *Traumatic brain injury.* Retrieved from http://www.asha.org

Antshel, K., Hargrave, T. M., Simonescu, M., Kaul, P., Hendricks, K., & Faraone, S. V. (2011). Advances in understanding and treating ADHD. *BMC Medicine, 9*(72). Retrieved from http://www.biomedcentral.com/1741-7015/9/72

Aron, L., & Loprest, P. (2012). Disability and the education system. *The Future of Children, 22*(1), 97–122.

Atwood, T. (2006). *The complete guide to Asperger's syndrome.* London, England: Jessica Kingsley.

Autism Research Institute. (2013). *DSM-V: What changes may mean.* Retrieved from http://www.autism.com/index.php/news_dsmV

Babcock, D. E., & Miller, M. A. (1994). *Client education: Theory and practice.* St. Louis, MO: Mosby.

Bauer, S. (2008). *Asperger's syndrome: General information across the lifespan.* Retrieved from http://www.education.com/reference/article/Ref_Asperger_Long/

Block, R. W., Macdonald, N. E., & Piotrowski, N. A. (2015). Attention deficit hyperactivity disorder (ADHD). In B. C. Auday (Ed.), *Magill's medical guide* (online edition).

Boyd, M. D., Gleit, C. J., Graham, B. A., & Whitman, N. I. (1998). *Health teaching in nursing practice* (3rd ed.). Stamford, CT: Appleton & Lange.

Braille Institute. (2012). *Facts about sight loss and definitions of blindness.* Retrieved from http://www.brailleinstitute.org/resources/sight-loss-news.html?start=4

British Dyslexia Association. (2015, January). *Dyscalculia.* Retrieved from http://www.bdadyslexia.org.uk/dyslexic/dyscalculia

Bruchmuller, K., Margraf, J., & Schneider, S. (2012). Is ADHD diagnosed in accord with diagnostic criteria? Overdiagnosis and influence of client gender on diagnosis. *Journal of Consulting Psychology, 80*(1), 128–138.

Center for Parent Information and Resources (CPIR). (2015, July). *Intellectual disability.* Retrieved from http://www.parentcenterhub.org

Centers for Disease Control and Prevention (CDC). (2012). *Hearing loss in children.* Retrieved from http://www.cdc.gov/ncbddd/hearingloss/data.html

Centers for Disease Control and Prevention (CDC). (2014). *Injury, prevention and control: Traumatic brain injury.* Retrieved from http://www.cdc.gov/TraumaticBrainInjury/

Centers for Disease Control and Prevention (CDC). (2015a, October 9). *Attention-Deficit/Hyperactivity Disorder (ADHD): Data and statistics.* Retrieved from http://www.cdc.gov/ncbddd/adhd/data.html

Centers for Disease Control and Prevention (CDC). (2015b, October 6). *Chronic disease prevention and health promotion.* Retrieved from http://www.cdc.gov/chronicdisease

Chen, G. (2015). The secret signs of undiagnosed adult attention deficit disorder. *Community College Review.* Retrieved from http://www.communitycollegereview.com/blog/the-secret-signs-of-undiagnosed-adult-attention-deficit-disorder

Cherry, K. (2012). *What is memory? An overview of memory and how it works.* Retrieved from http://psychology.about.com/od/cognitivepsychology/a/memory.htm

Child Development Institute. (2012). *About learning disabilities.* Retrieved from http://www.childdevelopmentinfo.com/learning/learning_disabilities.shtml

Climie, E.A., & Mastoras, S. M. (2015). ADHD in schools: Adopting a strengths-based perspective. *Canadian Psychology, 56*(3), 293–300.

Cohen, A. S., & Ayello, E. (2005). Diabetes has taken a toll on your patients. *Nursing, 35*(5), 44–47.

Cornell University. (2012). *Disability statistics.* Retrieved from http://disabilitystatistics.org

Crandell, T. L., Crandell, C. H., & Vander Zanden, J. W. (2011). *Human development* (10th ed.). New York: NY: McGraw-Hill.

Davidson, M. A. (2008). ADHD in adults: A review of the literature. *Journal of Attention Disorders, 11,* 628–641.

Diehl, I. N. (1989). Client and family learning in the rehabilitation setting. *Nursing Clinics of North America, 24*(1), 257–264.

Disability Funders Network. (2012). *Disability stats and facts.* Retrieved from http://www.disabilityfunders.org/disability-stats-and-facts

Dyslexia Research Institute. (2015). *Dyslexia.* Retrieved from http://www.dyslexia-add.org/issues.html

Easterbrook, S. R., & Beal-Alvarez, J. S. (2012). States' reading outcomes of students who are deaf and hard of hearing. *American Annals of the Deaf, 157*(1), 27–40.

Falkmer, M., Bjallmark, A., Larsson, M., & Falkmer, T. (2012). Recognition of facially expressed emotions and visual searches in adults with Asperger syndrome. *Research in Autism Spectrum Disorders, 5*(1), 210–217.

Feld, J. E., & Sommers, M. S. (2009). Lipreading, processing speed, and working memory in younger and older adults. *Journal of Speech, Language and Hearing Research, 52,* 155–156.

Fraas, M., & Calvert, M. (2009). The use of narratives to identify characteristics leading to a productive life following acquired brain injury. *American Journal of Speech-Language Pathology, 18,* 315–328.

Fusick, L. (2008). Serving clients with hearing loss: Best practices in mental health counseling. *Journal of Counseling & Development, 86*(1), 102–111.

Gerber, P. (2012). The impact of learning disabilities on adulthood: A review of the evidenced-based literature for research and practice in adult education. *Journal of Learning Disabilities, 45*(1), 31–46.

Greenberg, L. A. (1991). Teaching children who are learning disabled about illness and hospitalization. *MCN: The American Journal of Maternal/Child Nursing, 16*(5), 260–263.

Grinspun, D. (1987). Teaching families of traumatic-brain-injured adults. *Critical Care Nursing Quarterly, 10*(3), 61–72.

Haber, J., Krainovich-Miller, B., McMahon, A. L., & Price-Hoskins, P. (1997). *Comprehensive psychiatric nursing* (5th ed.). St. Louis, MO: Mosby.

Haller, B., Dorries, B., & Rahn, J. (2006). Media labeling versus the U.S. disability community identity: A study of shifting cultural language. *Disability & Society, 21*(1), 61–75.

Harris, J. (2005). *Intellectual disability: Understanding its development, causes, classification, evaluation and treatment.* New York, NY: Oxford University Press.

Harrison, L. L. (1990). Minimizing barriers when teaching hearing-impaired clients. *MCN: The American Journal of Maternal/Child Nursing, 15*(2), 113.

Hayhurst, C. (2008). Treating kids with autism. *PT: The Magazine of Physical Therapy, 16,* 20–27.

Heim, S., Tschierse, J., Amunts, K., Wilms, M., Vossel, S., Willmes, K., . . . Haber, W. (2008). Cognitive subtypes of dyslexia. *Acta Neurobiologiae Experimentalis, 68*(1), 73–82.

Horner-Johnson, W., Dobbertin, K., Lee, J., Andresen, E. M., & the Expert Panel on Disability and Health Disparities. (2014). Disparities in health care access and receipt of preventive services by disability type: Analysis of the medical expenditure panel survey. *Health Research and Educational Trust, 49*(6), 1980–1999.

Hultquist, A. (2006). *Introduction to dyslexia for parents and professionals.* London, England: Jessica Kingsley.

Ingesson, S. G. (2007). Growing up with dyslexia: Interviews with teenagers and young adults. *School Psychology International, 28,* 574–590.

International Dyslexia Association. (2015). *IDA fact sheets on dyslexia and related language-based learning differences.* Retrieved from http://www.interdys.org/FactSheets.htm

Jackson, C. (2009). Keys to unlocking better care. *Mental Health Practice, 12*(9), 6–7.

Johnson, J. R., & McIntosh, A. (2009). Toward a cultural perspective and understanding of the disability and deaf experience in special and multicultural education. *Remedial and Special Education, 30*(2), 67–83.

Kessels, R. P. C. (2003). Patients' memory for medical information. *Journal of the Royal Society of Medicine, 96,* 212–222.

Kessler, R. C., Adler, L., Barkley, R., Biederman, J., Conners, C. K., Demler, O., . . . Zaslavsky, A. M. (2006). The prevalence and correlates of ADHD in the United States: Results for the national comorbidity survey replication. *The American Journal of Psychiatry, 163,* 716–723.

Kids Health. (2011). *Auditory processing disorder.* Retrieved from http://www.kidshealth.org

LDOnline. (2012). *What is a learning disability?* Retrieved from http://www.ldonline.org/ldbasics/whatisld

Learning Disabilities Association of America. (2015). *Adults with learning disabilities: An overview.* Retrieved from http://www.ldaamerica.org/adults-with-learning-disabilities-an-overview/

Lederberg, A. R., Schick, B., & Spenser, P. E. (2012). Language and literacy development of deaf and hard of hearing children: Successes and challenges. *Developmental Psychology, 12,* 1–16.

Lee, J. C., Hasnain-Wynia, R., & Lau, D. T. (2012). Delay in seeing a doctor due to cost: Disparity between older adults with and without disabilities in the United States. *Health Services Research, 47*(2), 698–720.

Levine, M. (2002). *Misunderstood minds.* Retrieved from http://www.pbs.org/wgbh/misunderstoodminds

Lighthouse International. (2015). *Statistics on vision impairment.* Retrieved from http://li129-107 .members.linode.com/research/statistics-on-vision-impairment/

Lin, F. R., Niparko, J. K., & Ferrucci, L. (2011). Hearing loss prevalence in the United States. *Archives of Internal Medicine, 17*(20), 1851–1852.

Lindsay, R. L., Tomazic, T., Levine, M., & Accardo, P. (2001). Attention function as measured by a continuous performance task in children with dyscalculia. *Journal of Developmental & Behavioral Pediatrics, 22,* 287–292.

Lubkin, I. M., & Larsen, P. (2016). *Chronic illness: Impact and intervention* (9th ed.). Burlington, MA: Jones & Bartlett Learning.

Mackenzie, C. (2011). Dysarthria in stroke: A narrative review of its description and the outcome in intervention. *International Journal of Speech-Language Pathology, 13*(2), 125–136.

Marchione, M. (2007, September 10). *Thousands of GIs cope with brain damage.* Retrieved from http://www.washingtonpost.com/wp-dyn/content/article/2007/09/10/AR2007091000248.html

Mastin, L. (2010). *The human memory.* Retrieved from http://www.human-memory.net/disorders.html

McConnell, E. A. (1996). Clinical do's and don'ts: Caring for a patient with a vision impairment. *Nursing, 26*(5), 28.

McConnell, E. A. (2002). How to converse with a hearing-impaired patient. *Nursing, 32*(8), 20.

McKelvey, M., Hux, K., Dietz, A., & Beukelman, D. (2010). Impact of personal relevance and contextualization on word–picture matching by people with aphasia. *American Journal of Speech-Language Pathology, 19,* 22–33.

McLaughlin, H., Brown, D., & Young, A. M. (2004). Consultation, community and empowerment: Lessons from the deaf community. *Journal of Social Work, 4*(2), 153–166.

Medicare. (2012). *Medicare.gov.* http://www.medicare.gov/

Menghini, D., Finzi, A., Benassi, R., Botzani, R., Facoetti, A., Giovagnoli, S., . . . Vicari, S. (2010). Different underlying neurocognitive deficits in developmental dyslexia: A comparative study. *Neuropsychologia, 48*(i4), 863–873.

Merrow, S. L., & Corbett, C. (1994). Adaptive computing for people with disabilities. *Computers in Nursing, 12*(4), 201–209.

Miller, E. T. (2011). Client and family education. In I. M. Lubkin & P. Larsen (Eds.), *Chronic illness: Impact and interventions* (8th ed., pp. 319–343). Sudbury, MA: Jones & Bartlett Learning.

Miller, M., Ho, K., & Hinshaw, J. (2012). Executive functions in girls with ADHD followed prospectively into young adulthood. *Neuropsychology, 26*(3), 278–287.

Medical News Today. (2015). *What is Asperger's syndrome?* Retrieved from http://www.medicalnewstoday .com

Musiek, F., Barran, J., & Shinn, J. (2004). Assessment and remediation of an auditory processing disorder associated with head trauma. *Journal of the American Academy of Audiology, 15,* 117–132.

National Aphasia Association. (2015). *What is aphasia?* Retrieved from http://www.aphasia.org/

National Association of the Deaf. (2010). *Community and culture.* Retrieved from http://www.nad.org /issues/american-sign-language/community-and-culture-faq

National Center for Learning Disabilities. (2014). *The state of learning disabilities: Facts, trends, and emerging issues.* Retrieved from http://www.ncld.org/wp-content/uploads/2014/11/2014-State-of -LD.pdf

National Federation for the Blind. (2015, September). *Blindness statistics.* Retrieved from http://nfb.org /blindness-statistics

National Institute of Mental Health (NIMH). (2012a). *Attention deficit hyperactivity disorder.* Retrieved from http://www.nimh.nih.gov/health/publications/attention-deficit-hyperactivity-disorder/complete -index.shtml

National Institute of Mental Health (NIMH). (2012b). *Statistics.* Retrieved from http://www.nimh.nih .gov/statistics/index.shtml

National Institute of Neurological Disorders and Stroke. (2012a). *Asperger syndrome fact sheet.* Retrieved from http://www.ninds.nih.gov/disorders/asperger/detail_asperger.htm

National Institute of Neurological Disorders and Stroke. (2012b). *NINDS pervasive developmental disorders information page.* Retrieved from http://www.ninds.nih.gov/disorders/pdd/pdd.htm

National Institute on Deafness and Other Communication Disorders (NIDCD). (2014). *Quick statistics.* Retrieved from http://www.nidcd.nih.gov/health/statistics/Pages/quick.aspx

National Institute on Deafness and Other Communication Disorders (NIDCD). (2015, June 24). *American sign language.* Retrieved from http://www.nidcd.nih.gov/health/hearing/pages/asl.aspx

National Institutes of Health. (2015). *Eyes and vision.* Retrieved from http://health.nih.gov/category /EyesandVision

National Joint Committee on Learning Disabilities. (2011, March). Learning disabilities: Implications of policy regarding research and practice: A report by the National Joint Committee on Learning Disabilities. *Learning Disability Quarterly, 34*(4), 237–241.

National Stroke Association. (2015). *National Stroke Association's complete guide to stroke.* Retrieved from http://www.academia.edu/6010090/National_Stroke_Associations_Complete_Guide_to_Stroke

Navarro, M. R., & Lacour, G. (1980). Helping hints for use with deaf patients. *Journal of Emergency Nursing, 6*(6), 26–28.

PBS. (2010). *A primer on dyslexia.* Retrieved from http://www.pbs.org/parents/readinglanguage /articles/dyslexia/main.html

Pelka, F. (2012). *What we have done: An oral history of the disability rights movement.* Amherst, MA: University of Massachusetts Press.

Peterson, R., & Pennington, B. (2012). Developmental dyslexia. *Lancet, 379,* 1997–2007.

Pollard, R. Q., & Barnett, S. (2009). Health-related vocabulary knowledge among deaf adults. *Rehabilitation Psychology, 54*(2), 182–185.

Pollard, R. Q., Dean, R. K., O'Hearn, A., & Haynes, S. L. (2009). Adapting health education materials for deaf audiences. *Rehabilitation Psychology, 54,* 232–238.

Practitioners' Task Force on Adults with Learning Disabilities. (2007). *Screening for learning disabilities in adult education programs.* Retrieved from http://www.aceofflorida.org/userfiles/file/TAP%20 B%20Screening-Learning%20Disabilitie%20FINALs.pdf

Quinn, B. (2000). *Pervasive developmental disorder.* London, England: Jessica Kingsley.

Rehabilitation Act of 1973, PL 93-112, Section 504. Retrieved from http://www.dol.gov/oasam/regs/statutes/sec504.htm

Reichard, A., Stolzle, H., & Fox, M. (2011). Research paper: Health disparities among adults with physical disabilities or cognitive limitations compared to individuals with no disabilities in the United States. *Disability and Health Journal, 4*(2), 59–67.

Rosenberg, S. A., Zhang, D., & Robinson, C. (2008). Prevalence of developmental delays and participation in early intervention services for young children. *Pediatrics, 121*(6), 1503–1509.

Rouger, J., Lagleyre, S., Fraysse, B., Deneve, S., Deguine, O., & Barone, P. (2007). Evidence that cochlear-implanted deaf patients are better multisensory integrators. *Proceedings of the National Academy of Science of the United States of America, 104*(17), 7295–7300.

Rumpf, A., & Becker, I. K. (2012). Narrative competence and internal state language of children with Asperger syndrome and ADHD. *Research in Developmental Disabilities, 33*(5), 1395–1407.

Saalasti, S., Lepisto, T., Toppila, E., Kujala, T., Laakso, M., Niemeien von Mendt, T., & Jansson-Verkassalo, E. (2008). Language abilities of children with Asperger's syndrome. *Journal of Autism and Developmental Disorders, 38*, 1574–1580.

Sander, D. J., (2014). An overview of communication, movement and perception difficulties after stroke. *Nursing Older People, 26*(5), 32–37.

Santrock, J. W. (2013). *Lifespan development* (14th ed.). New York, NY: McGraw-Hill.

Schachar, R. J., Park L. S., & Dennis, M. (2015). Mental health implications of traumatic brain injury (TBI) in children and youth. *Journal of the Canadian Academy of Child and Adolescent Psychiatry, 24*(2), 100–108.

Scheier, D. B. (2009, Spring/Summer). Barriers to health care for people with hearing loss: A review of the literature. *Journal of the New York State Nurses' Association*, 4–10.

Shalev, R., & Gross, T. (2001). Developmental dyscalculia. *Pediatric Neurology, 24*, 337–342.

Sherman, C. (2012). *Overcoming the ADHD stigma.* Retrieved from http://www.additudemag.com/adhd/article/2003.html

Snow, K. (2012). *People first language.* Retrieved from http://www.disabilityisnatural.com.

Snowman, J., & McCown, R. (2015). *Psychology of applied teaching* (14th ed.). Stanford, CA: Wadsworth/Cengage Learning.

Social Security Administration. (2012). *What we mean by disability.* Retrieved from http://www.ssa.gov/dibplan/dqualify4.htm

Spinney, L. (2009). How dyscalculia adds up. *New Scientist, 201*(2692), 40–43.

Stephenson, P. L. (2006). Before teaching begins: Managing patient anxiety prior to providing education. *Clinical Journal of Oncology Nursing, 10*(2), 241–245.

Stock, S. (2002, January 21). When science isn't golden. *Advance for Nurses*, 28–29.

Strauss, A. L., Corbin, J., Fagerhaugh, S., Glaser, B., Mames, D., & Weiner, C. (1984). *Chronic illness and quality of life* (2nd ed.). St. Louis, MO: Mosby.

Strong, M. (1996). *Language learning and deafness.* New York, NY: Cambridge University Press.

Substance Abuse and Mental Health Services Administration. (2014, November 20). *Nearly one in five adult Americans experienced mental illness in 2013.* Retrieved from http://www.samhsa.gov/newsroom/press-announcements/201411200115

Taymans, J. M., Swanson, H. L., Schwarz, R. L., Gregg, N., Hock, M., & Gerber, P. J. (2009, June). *Learning to achieve: A review of the research literature on serving adults with learning disabilities.* National Institute for Literacy. Retrieved from https://lincs.ed.gov/publications/pdf/L2ALiteratureReview09.pdf

Thomas, D. (2009). The journey back to effective cognitive function after brain injury: A patient perspective. *International Journal of Therapy and Rehabilitation, 16*, 497–501.

Topel, E., & Lachmann, F. M. (2008). Life begins on an ant farm for two patients with Asperger's syndrome. *Psychoanalytic Psychology, 25*, 602–617.

Turner, B., Fleming, J., Cornwell, L., Haines, T., Kendell, M., & Chenoweth, L. (2007). A qualitative study of the transition from hospital to home for individuals with acquired brain injury and their family caregivers. *Brain Injury, 21*, 1119–1130.

University of Washington. (2012). *Working together: Computers and people with sensory impairments.* DO-IT. Retrieved from http://www.uw.edu/doit/

U.S. Census Bureau. (2012). *Nearly 1 in 5 people have a disability in the U.S., Census Bureau reports.* Retrieved from http://www.census.gov/newsroom/releases/archives/miscellaneous/cb12-134.html

U.S. Department of Education. (2006). *Twenty-sixth annual report to Congress on the implementation of the Individuals with Disabilities Education Act.* Retrieved from http://www2.ed.gov/about/reports/annual/osep/2004/index.html

U.S. Department of Health and Human Services (USDHHS). (2000). *The Developmental Disabilities Assistance and Bill of Rights Act of 2000.* Retrieved from http://www.acl.gov/Programs/AIDD/Index.aspx

U.S. Department of Justice. (2009). *A guide to disabilities rights laws.* Retrieved from http://www.ada.gov/cguide.htm

Vander Ploeg Booth, K. (2011). Health disparities and intellectual disabilities: Lessons from individuals with Down syndrome. *Developmental Disabilities Research Reviews, 17*, 32–35.

Vicars, M. (2003). *The relationship between literacy and ASL.* Retrieved from http://www.lifeprint.com/asl101/pages-layout/literacy1.htm

Wadsley, P. (2010, Spring). Healthy living: Memory loss. *Momentum*, 38–41.

Wajuhian, S. O., & Naidoo, K. S. (2012). Dyslexia: An overview. *Optometry & Vision Development, 43*(1), 24–33.

Wallace, T., & Bradshaw, A. (2011). Technologies and strategies for people with communication problems following brain injury or stroke. *NeuroRehabilitation, 28*(211), 199–209.

Wallhagen, M. I., Pettengill, E., & Whiteside, M. (2006). Sensory hearing impairment in older adults. *American Journal of Nursing, 106*(10), 40–48.

Webb, M., Tittle, M., & VanCott, M. (2000). Increasing students' sensitivity to families of children with disabilities. *Nurse Educator, 25*(1), 43–47.

Wilson, A. J. (2012). *Dyscalculia primer and resource guide.* Retrieved from http://www.oecd.org/fr/sites/educeri/dyscalculiaprimerandresourceguide.htm

Wisdom, J., McGee, M. G., Horner Johnson, W., Michael, Y., Adams, E., & Berlin, M. (2010). Health disparities between women with and without disabilities: A review of the research. *Social Work in Public Health, 25*(3/4), 368–386.

Wiseheart, R., Altmann, L. J. P., Park, H., & Lombardino, L. J. (2008). Sentence comprehension in young adults with developmental dyslexia. *Annals of Dyslexia, 59*, 151–167.

World Health Organization (WHO). (2011). *World report on disability.* Geneva, Switzerland: WHO Press. Retrieved from http://www.disabled-world.com/disability/statistics/who-disability.php

World Health Organization (WHO). (2015a). *Visual impairment and blindness.* Retrieved from http://www.who.int/mediacentre/factsheets/fs282/en/

World Health Organization (WHO). (2015b). *World report on disability.* Geneva, Switzerland: WHO Press.

Yorkston, K. M., Spencer, K. A., Duffy, J. R., Beukelman, D. R., Golper, L. A., Miller, R. M., . . . Sullivan, M. (2001). Evidence-based practice guidelines for dysarthria: Management of pharyngeal function. *Journal of Medical Speech-Language Pathology, 9*(4), 257–273.

APPENDIX 9–A

Resources and Organizations for People with Disabilities

Assistive Technology

AbleData
103 W. Broad Street, Suite 400
Falls Church, VA 22046
800-227-0216
E-mail: abledata@neweditions.net
www.abledata.com

The International Center for Disability Resources on the Internet (ICDRI)
4312 Birchlake Court
Alexandria, VA 22309
919-349-6661
www.icdri.org

Augmentative and Alternative Communication

American Speech-Language-Hearing Association (ASHA)
2200 Research Boulevard
Rockville, MD 20810-3289
888-498-6699 or 800-638-8255
www.asha.org

International Society for Augmentative and Alternative
    Communication (ISAAC)
312 Dolomite Drive, Suite 216
Toronto, ON M3J 2N2, Canada
905-850-6848
www.isaac-online.org

Blindness

American Diabetes Association
1701 N. Beauregard Street
Alexandria, VA 22311
800-342-2383
www.diabetes.org

American Foundation for the Blind
2 Penn Plaza, Suite 1102
New York, NY 10121
800-232-5463 (800-AFB-LINE) or 212-502-7600
www.afb.org

Library of Congress
101 Independence Avenue S.E.
Washington, DC 20540
202-707-5000
www.loc.gov
Administers a free program of Braille and audio materials.

National Braille Press
88 St. Stephen Street
Boston, MA 02115
617-266-6160 or 888-965-8965
E-mail: orders@nbp.org
www.nbp.org

National Library Service for the Blind and Physically Handicapped
1291 Taylor Street N.W.
Washington, DC 20542
202-707-5100
www.loc.gov/nls/contact.html

Deafness

Gallaudet College National Academy
800 Florida Avenue N.E.
Washington, DC 20002-3695
www.gallaudet.edu

Helen Keller National Center
141 Middle Neck Road
Sands Point, NY 11050
516-944-8900
www.hknc.org

National Institutes of Health
National Institute on Deafness and Other Communication
   Disorders (NIDCD)
31 Center Drive, MSC 2320
Bethesda, MD 20892-2320
800-241-1044 or 301-496-4000
E-mail: nidcdinfo@nidcd.nih.gov
www.nidcd.nih.gov

Registry of Interpreters for the Deaf, Inc.
333 Commerce Street
Alexandria, VA 22314
703-838-0030
www.rid.org

Provides information on interpreting and interpreters; referral to local agencies and state chapters of the Registry of Interpreters for the Deaf for assistance in locating interpreters.

Developmental Disabilities

National Institute of Child Health and Human Development (NICHD)
P.O. Box 3006
Rockville, MD 20847
800-370-2943
TTY: 1-888-320-6942
E-mail: NICHDInformationResourceCenter@mail.nih.gov
www.nichd.nih.gov

Disability Services

Americans with Disabilities Act (ADA)
U.S. Department of Justice
Civil Rights Division, Disabilities Rights Section—NYA
900 Pennsylvania Ave. N.W.
Washington, DC 20530
800-514-0301 (voice) or 800-514-0383 (TTY) or Section
    phone 202-307-0063
www.ada.gov

Autism Speaks
1 East 33rd Street, 4th Floor
New York, NY 10016
646-843-5240
www.autismspeaks.org

Disability Resources, Inc.
3602 Clack Street
Abilene, TX 79604
325-677-6815
www.disabilityresources.org

National Council on Disability
1331 F. Street N.W., Suite 850
Washington, DC 20004
202-272-2004 (voice) or 206-272-2074 (TTY)
www.ncd.gov

Head Injury

Brain Injury Association of America
1608 Spring Hill Road, Suite 110
Vienna, VA 22182
800-444-6443 or 703-761-0750
www.biausa.org

Healthcare-Related Federal Agencies

Centers for Disease Control and Prevention
1600 Clifton Road
Atlanta, GA 30333
404-639-3311 or 800-232-4636 (800-CDC-INFO) or 888-232-6348 (TTY)
www.cdc.gov

National Institute on Disability and Rehabilitation Research (NIDRR)
U.S. Department of Education
400 Maryland Avenue S.W., Room 3060
Washington, DC 20202
202-245-7640
www.ed.gov/about/offices/list/osers/nidrr

National Institutes of Health
National Center for Medical Rehabilitation Research, NIHD, NIH
800-370-2943
www.nichd.nih.gov

Learning Disabilities

A.D.D. Warehouse
300 N.W. 70th Avenue, #102
Fort Lauderdale, FL 33317
954-792-8944
www.addwarehouse.com/shopsite_sc/store/html/index.html

Attention Deficit Disorder Association
P.O. Box 7557
Wilmington, DE 19083-9997
800-939-1019
info@add.org
www.add.org

Learning Disabilities Association of America
4156 Library Road
Pittsburgh, PA 15234-1349
412-341-1515
www.ldaamerica.org

Mental Health

Mental Health America
2000 N. Beauregard Street, 6th Floor
Alexandria, VA 22311
703-684-7722 or 800-969-6642
TTY: 800-433-5959
www.mentalhealthamerica.net

National Institute of Mental Health (NIMH)
Public Information and Communications Branch
6001 Executive Boulevard
Rockville, MD 20852
301-443-4513 or 866-615-6464
TTY: 301-443-8431 or TTY toll-free: 866-415-8051
E-mail: nimhinfo@nih.gov
www.nimh.nih.gov

Neuromuscular Disorders

ALS Association National Headquarters
1275 K Street N.W., Suite 250
Washington, DC 20005
800-782-4747 or 202-407-8580
www.alsa.org

Epilepsy Foundation of America
8301 Professional Place East, Suite 200
Landover, MD 20785-2353
301-459-1569 (online store) or 800-332-1000
www.epilepsy.com

Multiple Sclerosis Foundation
6520 North Andrews Avenue
Fort Lauderdale, FL 33309-2132
800-225-6495 or 954-776-6805 or 888-MSFOCUS
E-mail: admin@msfocus.org or support@msfocus.org
www.msfocus.org

Muscular Dystrophy Association—USA
National Office
222 S. Riverside Plaza, Suite 1500
Chicago, IL 60606
800-572-1717
E-mail: mda@mdausa.org
www.mda.org

Myasthenia Gravis Foundation of America, Inc.
355 Lexington Avenue, 15th Floor
New York, NY 10017
800-541-5454
E-mail: mgfa@myasthenia.org
www.myasthenia.org

Parkinson's Disease Foundation, Inc.
1359 Broadway, Suite 1509
New York, NY 10018
800-457-6676 or 212-923-4700 or 800-4PD-INFO (help line)
E-mail: info@pdf.org
www.pdf.org or www.parkinson.org

Program Services Assistance, MS Helpline
888-MSFOCUS
954-776-6805
E-mail: support@msfocus.org
www.msfocus.org

Stroke

National Aphasia Association
P.O. Box 87
Scarsdale, NY 10581
800-922-4622
E-mail: naa@aphasia.org
www.aphasia.org

National Institute of Neurological Disorders and Stroke (NINDS)
P.O. Box 5801
Bethesda, MD 20824
800-352-9424 or 301-496-5751
www.ninds.nih.gov

National Stroke Association
9707 E. Easter Lane, Suite B
Centennial, CO 80112-3747
800-STROKES (787-6537) or 303-649-9299
E-mail: info@stroke.org
www.stroke.org

PART III

Techniques and Strategies for Teaching and Learning

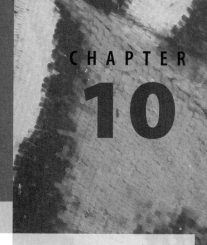

Behavioral Objectives and Teaching Plans

Susan B. Bastable | Eleanor Price McLees

Chapter Highlights

- Characteristics of Goals and Objectives
- The Importance of Using Behavioral Objectives
- Writing Behavioral Objectives and Goals
  - *Performance Words With Many or Few Interpretations*
- Common Mistakes When Writing Objectives
- Taxonomy of Objectives According to Learning Domains
  - *The Cognitive Domain*
  - *The Affective Domain*
  - *The Psychomotor Domain*
- Development of Teaching Plans
- Use of Learning Contracts
- The Concept of Learning Curve

Key Terms

affective domain
augmented feedback
behavioral (learning) objectives
cognitive domain
distributed practice
goal
intrinsic feedback
learning contract
learning curve
massed practice
mental imaging
   (mental practice)
objective
psychomotor domain
subobjectives
taxonomy
teaching plan
transfer of learning

Objectives

After completing this chapter, the reader will be able to

1. Identify the differences between goals and objectives.
2. Recognize the value of using behavioral objectives for teaching and learning.
3. Write behavioral objectives accurately and concisely using the four components of condition, performance, criterion, and who will do the performing.
4. List the common errors made in writing objectives.
5. Define the three domains of learning: affective, cognitive, and psychomotor.
6. Identify the instructional methods appropriate for teaching in each domain.
7. Develop teaching plans that reflect internal consistency between elements.
8. Recognize the role of the nurse in developing objectives for the planning, implementation, and evaluation of teaching and learning.
9. Identify the potential application of the learning curve concept to the development of psychomotor skills.

Previous chapters have looked at the unique aspects of the learner. These characteristics and attributes relate to learning needs, readiness to learn, and learning styles. The assessment of the learner is the first step in the teaching and learning process and cannot be underestimated. As in the clinical setting, an incomplete nursing assessment may lead to an incorrect nursing diagnosis and plan. So, too, a thorough assessment of learners is essential to determine what they need to know, when and under which conditions they are most receptive to learning, and how they actually learn best or prefer to learn.

Before deciding on the content to be taught, the nurse must first identify the learning need(s) of each patient and then decide what the learner is expected to learn. The needs of patients and their families are determined by identifying gaps in their knowledge, attitudes, or skills. Learning needs may be identified by the patient, by their family members, by the nurse, or even by the facility, such as providing required education on patients' rights. Identifying these learning needs is necessary before writing behavioral objectives. These objectives guide the planning, teaching, and evaluation of the educational process (Nothwehr, Dennis, & Wu, 2007).

Educators and educational psychologists have designed ways of writing and classifying behavioral objectives. This helps teachers organize content for the learner. Writing and classifying behavioral objectives also looks at learners with various levels of ability. For example, the discharge teaching for a 20-year-old with a learning disability will have different objectives than those for the discharge teaching of a 75-year-old with corrective lenses, even if both patients have the same diagnosis.

The classic research by Bloom, Englehart, Furst, Hill, and Krathwohl (1956) added an understanding of learning objectives by creating categories and levels of behaviors. This is the concept of **taxonomy**, which is the ordering of behaviors according to their type and complexity.

Knowing how to write and categorize **behavioral (learning) objectives** is important if goals are to be consistent with the objectives, be measurable, and be attainable. In today's economically driven healthcare environment, these skills are necessary for measuring and justifying the need to teach others in the most cost-efficient manner.

This chapter examines the importance of behavioral objectives for effective teaching; describes how to write clear and precise behavioral objectives; provides an overview of the taxonomy levels of cognitive, affective, and psychomotor domains; and outlines the development of teaching plans and learning contracts. Lastly, the concepts of the learning curve as they apply to mastering psychomotor skills also are discussed. Each element provides a framework for successful teaching.

Characteristics of Goals and Objectives

The terms goal and objective are often used as if they are one and the same. However, a real difference exists between the two terms. This distinction must be clearly understood because it is common to find confusion on the meaning of these terms among nurses and educators alike (Krau, 2011; Wittman-Price & Fasolka, 2010).

Two factors differentiate goals from objectives: their relationship to time and their level of specificity (Haggard, 1989). A **goal** is the outcome that is to be achieved at the end of the teaching and learning process. Goals are global and broad and are a long-term target for both the learner and the teacher. Goals are the desired outcomes of learning that realistically can be achieved, usually in weeks or months. For a goal to be reached, at least several objectives will need to be met first.

In contrast to a goal, an **objective** is a specific, single, one-dimensional behavior. Objectives are short term and should be achieved at the end of one teaching session, or shortly after several teaching sessions. Objectives are statements of specific, short-term behaviors. They lead step-by-step to the more general, overall goal. While there are several types of objectives, a behavioral (learning) objective is the planned outcome of the teaching and learning process that is action oriented and learner centered (Bastable, 2014).

Also, **subobjectives** that reflect aspects of a main objective may be written. They, too, are specific statements of short-term behaviors that lead to the achievement of the primary objective. Objectives and subobjectives specify what the learner will be able to do as a result of being taught.

Objectives must be achieved before the goal can be reached. They must be observable and measurable for the nurse as teacher to decide if they have been met by the learner. Objectives are related to the goal. As an analogy, a goal can be thought of as an entire pie, the objectives as individual slices of the pie that make up the goal, and the smaller subobjectives as bite-sized pieces of a single slice of the pie.

Together, objectives and goals form a map that provides directions (objectives) as to how to arrive at a particular destination (goal). For example, a goal might be that a patient with heart failure will learn to manage his or her disease. To reach this goal, which the nurse and the patient have agreed on, specific objectives must be outlined to address changes in behavior. These changes would be related to diet, medications, exercise, and fluid monitoring (Buck, McAndrew, Dionne-Odom, Wion, & Riegel, 2015). The objectives to accomplish the goal become the blueprint for attaining the desired outcomes of learning.

Both the teacher and learner need to be part of setting goals and objectives if the teaching and learning process is to be truly successful. It is absolutely crucial that the learner be involved with creating goals and objectives right from start. Otherwise, both the teacher and the learner have wasted their time because the learner may know the content already or view it as unimportant, irrelevant, impractical, and/or unrealistic. The learner may then choose not to take an active role in the educational process in spite of the teacher's efforts.

Objectives and goals must be clearly written, realistic, and learner centered. If the objectives and goals do not specifically identify what the learner is expected to do or understand, then the learning process may not be clear for reaching an obvious end. Also, goals and objectives are often unrealistic. Thus, the learner can easily become discouraged. This affects motivation and certainly impacts the learner's compliance. For example, a goal that a patient with hypertension will maintain a totally salt-free diet is unrealistic. Rather, a more realistic goal would be maintaining a low-salt diet with the objectives of learning to avoid eating and preparing foods high in sodium. Also, goals and objectives must be directed to what the learner is expected to be able to do, not what the teacher is expected to teach. This keeps teachers focused on results, not on the act of teaching. Anderson et al. (2001) emphasize that not all learners will take away the same thing from the same instruction, unless objectives are specific and clear.

The Importance of Using Behavioral Objectives

Using behavioral objectives for teaching far outweighs the arguments against using them. The following key points justify the need for writing behavioral objectives (Ferguson, 1998; Krau, 2011; Morrison, Ross, & Kemp, 2004; Phillips & Phillips, 2010). The careful construction of well-written objectives:

- Helps to keep the teachers' thinking on target and learner centered.
- Communicates to learners and healthcare team members what is planned for teaching and learning.
- Helps learners understand what is expected of them so they can keep track of their progress.
- Forces teachers to organize educational materials so they do not get lost in the content and forget the learner's role in the process.
- Encourages nurses as teachers to evaluate their own motives for teaching.
- Tailors teaching to the learner's unique needs.
- Creates guideposts for teacher evaluation and documentation of success or failure.
- Focuses attention on what the learner will come away with once the teaching–learning process is completed, not on what is taught.
- Orients teacher and learner to the end results of the educational process.
- Makes it easier for the learner to visualize performing the required skills.

Robert Mager (1997) points out three other major advantages in writing clear objectives:

1. They provide the solid foundation for the selection or design of instructional content, methods, and materials.
2. They provide learners with ways to organize their efforts to reach their goals.
3. They help determine whether an objective has, in fact, been met.

As Mager (1997) asks, "If you don't know where you're going, how will you know which road to take to get there?" (p. 14). For example, mechanics do not select specific tools until they know what has to be repaired; nurses would not choose their sterile supplies until they know what type of wound needs to be dressed; and builders do not buy construction materials before drafting a blueprint. Likewise, after the teacher has identified a learning need, it is important that she clearly states the intended results of instruction even before she proceeds with any other part of the educational process.

Haggard (1989) summarizes the following questions that arise if objectives are not consistently written:

- How will anyone else know which objectives have been set?
- How will the teacher evaluate and document success or failure?
- How will learners keep track of their progress?

Developing behavioral objectives not only helps nurses explore their own knowledge, values, and beliefs about teaching and learning, but also encourages them to examine the experiences, values, motivations, and knowledge of patients and their families. Establishing objectives and goals is considered by many nurses to be the initial, most important consideration in the teaching and learning process (Haggard, 1989; Mager, 1997).

Writing Behavioral Objectives and Goals

Well-written behavioral objectives give learners very clear statements about what is expected of them. They also assist teachers in being able to measure learner progress toward achieving the objectives. Over the years, Robert Mager's (1997) approach to writing behavioral objectives has become widely accepted among teachers. His message to them is that for objectives to be meaningful, they must precisely, clearly, and very specifically communicate the teacher's instructional intent (Arends, 2011).

According to Mager (1997), the format for writing concise and useful behavioral objectives includes the following three important characteristics:

1. *Performance:* Describes what the learner is expected to be able to do to demonstrate the kinds of behaviors the teacher will accept as evidence that objectives have been achieved. Activities performed by the learner may be observable and quite visible, such as being able to write or list something, whereas other activities may not be as visible, such as being able to identify or recall something.
2. *Condition:* Describes the situations under which the behavior will be observed or the performance will be expected to occur.
3. *Criterion:* Describes how well, with what accuracy, or within what time frame the learner must be able to perform the behavior in order to be considered competent.

These three characteristics translate into the following key questions: (1) What should the learner be able to do? (2) Under which conditions should the learner be able to do it? (3) How well must the learner be able to do it? A fourth component must also be included; it should describe the who to guarantee that the behavioral objective is indeed learner centered. Behavioral objectives are statements that communicate *who* will do *what* under *which conditions* and *how well* (Cummings, 1994).

An easy way to remember the four elements that should be in a behavioral objective is to follow the ABCD rule proposed by Smaldino, Lowther, and Russell (2012):

A—audience (who)
B—behavior (what)
C—condition (under which circumstance)
D—degree (how well; to what extent; within what time frame)

For example, the following behavioral objective includes these four elements: "After a 20-minute teaching session on relaxation techniques (C—condition), Mrs. Smith (A—audience/learner) will be able to identify (B—behavior or performance) three distinct techniques for lowering her stress level (D—degree or criterion)."

Table 10–1 outlines the four-part method of objective writing. **Table 10–2** gives examples of well-written and poorly written objectives.

Performance Words With Many or Few Interpretations

When writing behavioral objectives using the format suggested by Mager (1997), the recommendation is to use precise action words or verbs as labels that are open to few interpretations when describing learner performance. An objective is considered most useful when it clearly states what a learner must demonstrate for mastery in a knowledge, attitude,

Table 10–1 The Four-Part Method of Objective Writing

Condition (Testing Situation)	Who (Identify Learner)	Performance (Learner Behavior)	Criterion (Quality or Quantity of Mastery)
Without using a calculator	the student	will solve	5 out of 6 math problems
Using a model	the staff nurse	will demonstrate	the correct procedure for changing sterile dressings
Following group discussion	the patient	will list	at least two reasons for losing weight
After watching a video	the caregiver	will select	high-protein foods with 100% accuracy

Table 10–2 Samples of Written Objectives

Well-Written Objectives
Following a class on hypertension, the patient will be able to state three out of four causes of high blood pressure.
On completing the reading materials provided on the care of a newborn, the mother will be able to express any concerns she has about caring for her baby after discharge.
After a 20-minute teaching session, the patient will verbalize at least two feelings or concerns associated with wearing a colostomy bag.
After reading handouts, the patient will be able to state three examples of foods that are sources of protein.

Poorly Written Objectives
The patient will be able to prepare a menu using low-salt foods. [Condition and criterion missing]
Given a list of exercises to relieve low back pain, the patient will understand how to control low back pain. [Performance not stated in measurable terms; criterion missing]
The nurse will demonstrate crutch walking postoperatively to the patient. [Teacher-centered]
During discharge teaching, the patient will be more comfortable with insulin injections. [Performance not stated in measurable terms; condition missing; criterion missing]
The patient will verbalize and demonstrate the proper steps to performing self-catheterization. [Contains two expected behaviors; criterion missing; time frame missing]
After a 20-minute teaching session, the patient will appreciate knowing the steps required to complete a fingerstick. [Performance not stated in measurable terms; criterion missing; condition missing]

or skill area. A performance verb describes what the learner is expected to do. A performance may be visible or audible. For example, the learner is able *to list, to write, to state,* or *to walk.* These performances are directly observable. A performance also may be invisible. For example, the learner is able *to identify, to solve, to recall,* or *to recognize.* Any performance, whether it is visible/audible or invisible, described by a "doing" word is measurable.

Verbs that describe an internal state of thinking, feeling, or believing should be avoided because they are difficult to measure or observe. Words that are used to describe something a learner can *be,* rather than can *do,* are known as *being words.* Examples of being words, which also are called abstractions, include *to understand, to know, to enjoy,*

Table 10–3 Verbals With Many or Few Interpretations

Terms With Many Interpretations (Not Recommended)	Terms With Few Interpretations (Recommended)	
to know	to apply	to explain
to understand	to choose	to identify
to appreciate	to classify	to list
to realize	to compare	to order
to be familiar with	to construct	to predict
to enjoy	to contrast	to recall
to value	to define	to recognize
to be interested in	to describe	to select
to feel	to demonstrate	to state
to think	to differentiate	to verbalize
to learn	to distinguish	to write

Data from Gronlund, N. E. (1985). *Stating objectives for classroom instruction* (3rd ed.). New York: Macmillan; Gronlund, N. E. (2004). *Writing instructional objectives for teaching and assessment* (7th ed.). Upper Saddle River, NJ: Pearson Merrill Prentice Hall.

and *to appreciate* (Mager, 1997). Understanding, knowing, enjoying, and appreciating are considered abstract states of being that cannot be directly measured but merely implied.

It is impossible to identify all behavioral terms that might potentially be used in objective writing. The important thing to remember in selecting verbs to describe performance is that they must be specific, observable or measurable, and action oriented. As stated by Anderson et al. (2001), if the teacher is able to describe the behavior to be attained, it will be easily recognized when learning has occurred. **Table 10–3** gives examples in two columns of terms: one column listing verbs that are not recommended for use because they are too broad, ambiguous, and imprecise to evaluate, and the other column listing verbs that are recommended because they are specific and relatively easy to measure (Gronlund, 1985, 2004; Gronlund & Brookhart, 2008).

Common Mistakes When Writing Objectives

In creating behavioral objectives, a number of common mistakes can be easily made by novice and seasoned teachers alike. The most frequent errors made in writing objectives are as follows:

- Describing what the teacher does rather than what the learner is expected to do
- Including more than one expected behavior in a single objective (avoid using *and* to connect two verbs—e.g., the learner will select *and* prepare)
- Forgetting to identify all four components of condition, performance, criterion, and who the learner is
- Using terms for performance that are open to many interpretations, are not action oriented, and are difficult to measure

Table 10–4 Writing SMART Objectives

Specific	Be specific about what is to be achieved (i.e., use strong action verbs, be concrete).
Measurable	Quantify or qualify objectives by including numeric, cost, or percentage amounts or the degree/level of mastery expected.
Achievable	Write attainable objectives.
Realistic	Resources (i.e., personnel, facilities, equipment) must be available to achieve objectives.
Timely	State when the objectives will be achieved (e.g., within a week, a month, by the day of patient discharge).

Data from Glenn M. Parker Associates, Inc. (2000). *Team workout*. Amherst, MA: HRD Products.

- Writing objectives that are unattainable and unrealistic given the ability level of the learner
- Writing objectives that do not relate to the stated goal
- Cluttering objectives by including unnecessary information
- Being too general so as not to specify clearly the expected behavior to be achieved

If you use the SMART rule, it is easy to create effective objectives for different audiences in diverse settings. This objective-setting process is shown in **Table 10–4**.

Taxonomy of Objectives According to Learning Domains

A taxonomy is a way to categorize things according to how they are related to one another. In science, biologists use taxonomies to classify plants and animals based on their natural characteristics. In the late 1940s, psychologists and educators became concerned about the need to develop a system for defining and ordering levels of behavior according to their type and complexity (Reilly & Oermann, 1990). Bloom et al. (1956) and Krathwohl, Bloom, and Masia (1964) developed a very useful taxonomy, known as the taxonomy of educational objectives, as a tool for classifying behavioral objectives. This taxonomy is divided into three broad categories or domains: cognitive (thinking domain), affective (feeling domain), and psychomotor (doing or skills domain).

Although these three domains of cognitive, affective, and psychomotor learning are described as existing as separate entities, they are interdependent and can be experienced simultaneously. Humans do not possess thoughts, feelings, and actions in isolation from one another. For example, the affective domain influences the cognitive domain and vice versa; the processes of thinking (cognitive) and feeling (affective) influence psychomotor performance, and vice versa (Menix, 1996).

In addition to each objective being classified by a domain, each domain is ordered in a taxonomic form of hierarchy. Behavioral objectives are classified into low, medium, and high levels, with simple behaviors listed first (at the lower end), followed by behaviors of moderate difficulty, and with the more complex behaviors listed last (at the higher end). This concept of hierarchy realizes that learners must successfully achieve behaviors at lower levels of the domains before they are able to adequately learn behaviors at higher levels of the domains. Thus, to use an analogy of climbing a ladder, you cannot get to the top unless you go up one step at a time. See **Figure 10–1** for a diagram of the level of complexity of the behaviors in each domain.

A. COGNITIVE DOMAIN

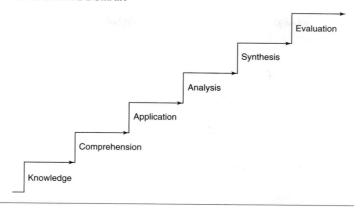

B. AFFECTIVE DOMAIN

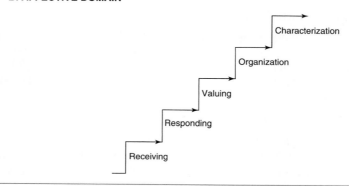

C. PSYCHOMOTOR DOMAIN

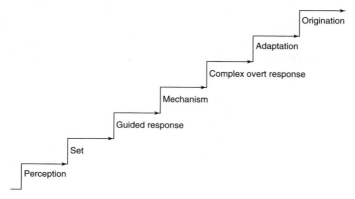

Figure 10–1 Domain hierarchies

A. Data from Gronlund, N. E., & Brookhart, S. M. (2008). *Gronlund's writing instructional objectives* (8th ed.). Upper Saddle River, NJ: Pearson Merrill Prentice Hall.
B. Data from Krathwohl, D. R., Bloom, B. J., & Masia, B. B. (1964). *Taxonomy of educational objectives: The classification of educational goals. Handbook II: The affective domain.* New York, NY: David McKay.
C. Data from Simpson, E. J. (1972). The classification of educational objectives in the psychomotor domain. In M. T. Rainer (Ed.), *Contributions of behavioral science to instructional technology: The psychomotor domain* (3rd ed.). Englewood Cliffs, NJ: Gryphon Press, Prentice Hall.

The Cognitive Domain

The **cognitive domain** is known as the "thinking" domain. Learning in this domain involves acquiring information and addressing the development of the learner's intellectual abilities, mental capacities, understanding, and thinking processes (Eggen & Kauchak, 2012). Objectives in this domain are divided into six levels (Bloom et al., 1956), each specifying cognitive processes ranging from the simple (knowledge) to the more complex (evaluation) as seen in Figure 10–1.

Levels of Behavioral Objectives and Examples in the Cognitive Domain

Knowledge level: Ability of the learner to memorize, recall, define, recognize, or identify specific information, such as facts, rules, principles, conditions, and terms, presented during instruction. For example: After a 20-minute teaching session, the patient will be able to state with accuracy the definition of chronic obstructive pulmonary disease (COPD).

Comprehension level: Ability of the learner to demonstrate an understanding of what is being communicated by recognizing it in a translated form, such as grasping an idea by defining it or summarizing it in his or her own words (knowledge is a prerequisite behavior). Example: After watching a 10-minute video on nutrition following gastric bypass surgery, the patient will be able to give at least three examples of food choices that will be included in his diet.

Application level: Ability of the learner to use ideas, principles, abstractions, or theories in particular situations, such as figuring, writing, reading, or handling equipment (knowledge and comprehension are prerequisite behaviors). Example: On completion of a cardiac rehabilitation program, the patient will modify three exercise regimes that can fit into her lifestyle at home.

Analysis level: Ability of the learner to recognize and structure information by breaking it down into its separate parts and specifying the relationship between the parts (knowledge, comprehension, and application are prerequisite behaviors). Example: After reading handouts provided by the nurse, the family member will calculate the correct number of total grams of protein included on average per day in the family diet.

Synthesis level: Ability of the learner to put together parts into a unified whole by creating a unique product that is written, oral, or in picture form (knowledge, comprehension, application, and analysis are prerequisite behaviors). Example: Given a sample list of foods, the patient will create a menu to include foods from the four food groups (dairy, meat, vegetables and fruits, and grains) in the recommended amounts for daily intake.

Evaluation level: Ability of the learner to judge the value of something by applying appropriate criteria (knowledge, comprehension, application, analysis, and synthesis are prerequisite behaviors). Example: After three teaching sessions, the patient will judge her readiness to function independently in the home setting.

Table 10–5 lists verbs commonly used in writing cognitive-level behavioral objectives.

Table 10–5 Commonly Used Verbs According to Domain Classification

Cognitive Domain
Knowledge: choose, circle, define, identify, label, list, match, name, outline, recall, report, select, state
Comprehension: describe, discuss, distinguish, estimate, explain, generalize, give example, locate, recognize, summarize
Application: apply, demonstrate, illustrate, implement, interpret, modify, order, revise, solve, use
Analysis: analyze, arrange, calculate, classify, compare, conclude, contrast, determine, differentiate, discriminate
Synthesis: categorize, combine, compile, correlate, design, devise, generate, integrate, reorganize, revise, summarize
Evaluation: appraise, assess, conclude, criticize, debate, defend, judge, justify
Affective Domain
Receiving: accept, admit, ask, attend, focus, listen, observe, pay attention
Responding: agree, answer, conform, discuss, express, participate, recall, relate, report, state willingness, try, verbalize
Valuing: assert, assist, attempt, choose, complete, disagree, follow, help, initiate, join, propose, volunteer
Organization: adhere, alter, arrange, combine, defend, explain, express, generalize, integrate, resolve
Characterization: assert, commit, discriminate, display, influence, propose, qualify, solve, verify
Psychomotor Domain
Perception: attend, choose, describe, detect, differentiate, distinguish, identify, isolate, perceive, relate, select, separate
Set: attempt, begin, develop, display, position, prepare, proceed, reach, respond, show, start, try
Guided response, mechanism, and complex overt response: align, arrange, assemble, attach, build, change, choose, clean, compile, complete, construct, demonstrate, discriminate, dismantle, dissect, examine, find, grasp, hold, insert, lift, locate, maintain, manipulate, measure, mix, open, operate, organize, perform, pour, practice, reassemble, remove, repair, replace, separate, shake, suction, turn, transfer, walk, wash, wipe
Adaptation: adapt, alter, change, convert, correct, rearrange, reorganize, replace, revise, shift, substitute, switch
Origination: arrange, combine, compose, construct, create, design, exchange, reformulate

Data from Gronlund, N. E. (1985). *Stating objectives for classroom instruction* (3rd ed.). New York: Macmillan; Gronlund, N. E. (2004). *Writing instructional objectives for teaching and assessment* (7th ed.). Upper Saddle River, NJ: Pearson Merrill Prentice Hall.

TEACHING IN THE COGNITIVE DOMAIN

Several teaching methods and tools exist for the purpose of developing cognitive abilities. The methods most often used to stimulate learning in the cognitive domain include lecture, group discussion, one-to-one instruction, and self-instruction activities, such as computer-assisted instruction. Verbal, written, and visual tools are all particularly successful in enhancing the teaching methods to help learners master cognitive content. For example, research has shown computer-assisted instruction to be effective in teaching clients about HIV prevention (Evans, Edmunson-Drane, & Harris, 2000). However, cognitive skills can be gained by exposure to all types of educational experiences, including the instructional methods used primarily for affective and psychomotor learning. For example, the concept of group discussion for prenatal care has been shown to improve perinatal outcomes (Rotundo, 2012).

Cognitive domain learning is the traditional focus of most teaching. In education of patients, as well as nursing staff and students, emphasis remains on the sharing of facts, theories, and concepts. Perhaps this emphasis has evolved because teachers typically feel more confident and more skilled in being the giver of information than in being the facilitator and coordinator of learning. Lecture and one-to-one instruction are the most frequently used methods of teaching in the cognitive domain.

With respect to cognitive learning, how much time for practice is necessary to influence the short-term and long-term retention of factual information? Generally, research findings indicate that learning distributed over several sessions leads to better memory than information learned in a single session. This phenomenon has been described by Willingham (2002) as the "spacing effect." That is, learning information all at once on one day, an approach known as **massed practice**, is much less effective for remembering facts than learning information over successive periods of time, an approach known as **distributed practice**. Massed practice, similar to what is commonly identified as "cramming," might allow the recall of information for a short time, but evidence strongly supports that distributed practice is very important in forging memories that last for years.

The effect of spreading out learning over time is very clear. The average person exposed to distributed practice remembers 67% better than people who receive massed training. That is, spacing the time allocated for learning significantly increases memory. Such scientific findings explain, for example, why teaching a patient only on the day of discharge from the hospital is ineffective.

The Affective Domain

The **affective domain** is known as the "feeling" domain. Learning in this domain involves influencing feelings expressed as emotions, interests, beliefs, attitudes, values, and appreciations. The affective domain is divided into categories that specify the degree of a person's depth of emotional responses to tasks. The affective domain includes emotional and social development goals. As stated by Eggen and Kauchak (2012), educators use the affective domain to help learners realize their own attitudes and values.

Although nurses recognize the need for individuals to learn in the affective domain, a person's attitudes, beliefs, and values cannot be directly observed but can only be inferred from words and actions (Maier-Lorentz, 1999). Nurses tend to be less confident and more challenged in writing behavioral objectives for the affective domain because it is difficult to develop easily measurable objectives and evaluation of learning outcomes based on inferences of someone's observed behavior (Goulet & Owen-Smith, 2005; Morrison et al., 2004).

Reilly and Oermann (1990) differentiate among the terms *beliefs, attitudes,* and *values*. Beliefs are what an individual perceives as reality; attitudes represent feelings about an object, person, or event; and values are operational beliefs that guide actions and ways of living. Objectives in the affective domain are divided into five categories (Krathwohl et al., 1964), each specifying the associated level of affective responses as seen in Figure 10–1.

Levels of Behavioral Objectives and Examples in the Affective Domain

Receiving level: Ability of the learner to show awareness of an idea or fact or a consciousness of a situation or event in the environment. This level represents a willingness to selectively attend to or focus on data or to receive a stimulus. Example: During a group discussion session, the patient will admit to any fears he may have about needing to undergo a repeat angioplasty.

Responding level: Ability of the learner to respond to an experience, at first obediently and later willingly and with satisfaction. This level indicates a movement beyond denial and toward voluntary acceptance, which can lead to feelings of pleasure or enjoyment as a result of some new experience (receiving is a prerequisite behavior). Example: At the end of one-to-one instruction, the child will verbalize feelings of confidence in managing her asthma using the peak-flow tracking chart.

Valuing level: Ability of the learner to regard or accept the worth of a theory, idea, or event, demonstrating sufficient commitment or preference to an experience that is seen as having value. At this level, there is a definite willingness and desire to act to further that value (receiving and responding are prerequisite behaviors). Example: After attending a grief support group meeting, the patient will complete a journal entry reflecting her feelings about the experience.

Organization level: Ability of the learner to organize, classify, and prioritize values by integrating a new value into a general set of values, to determine interrelationships of values, and to establish some values as dominant and pervasive (receiving, responding, and valuing are prerequisite behaviors). Example: After a 45-minute group discussion session, the patient will be able to explain the reasons for her anxiety and fears about her self-care management responsibilities.

Characterization level: Ability of the learner to display adherence to a total philosophy or worldview, showing firm commitment to the values by generalizing certain experiences into a value system (receiving, responding, valuing, and organization are prerequisite behaviors). Example: Following a series of teaching sessions, the patient will display consistent interest in maintaining good hand-washing technique to control the spread of infection to family members and friends.

Table 10–5 lists verbs commonly used in writing affective-level behavioral objectives.

TEACHING IN THE AFFECTIVE DOMAIN

Several teaching methods are reliable in helping the learner acquire affective behaviors. Role modeling, role play, simulation, gaming, questioning, case studies, and group discussion sessions are examples of methods of instruction that can be used to help patients and their families develop values and explore attitudes, interests, and feelings.

The affective domain encompasses three levels (Menix, 1996) that govern attitudes and feelings:

- The *intrapersonal level* includes personal perceptions of one's own self, such as self-concept, self-awareness, and self-acceptance.
- The *interpersonal level* includes the perspective of self in relation to other individuals.
- The *extrapersonal level* involves the perception of others as established groups.

All three levels are important in affective skill development and can be taught through a variety of methods specifically geared to affective domain learning.

Focusing on behaviors in the affective domain is critically important but is often underestimated. Unfortunately, priority is rarely given to teaching in the affective domain. The nurse's focus more often emphasizes cognitive and psychomotor learning, with little time being set aside for exploration and clarification of the learner's feelings, emotions, and attitudes (Morrison et al., 2004; Zimmerman & Phillips, 2000).

Nurses must address the needs of the whole person by recognizing that learning is subjective and value driven (Schoenly, 1994). For nurses practicing in any setting, affective learning is especially important because they constantly face ethical issues and value conflicts (Tong, 2007). The diversity of our society requires nurses to respect the racial and ethnic diversity in the population groups they serve (Marks, 2009). Additionally, advancing technology also places nurses in advocacy positions when patients, families, and other healthcare professionals struggle with treatment decisions. In turn, patients and family members face the prospects of making moral and ethical choices as well as learning to internalize the value of complying with prescribed treatment regimens and incorporating health promotion and disease prevention practices into their daily lives.

The teaching and learning setting is key in meeting affective behavioral outcomes. An open, empathetic, and accepting attitude by nurses sets the foundations for engaging patients and their families in learning. Staff nurses' beliefs, attitudes, and values significantly influence their affective behavior as they integrate cultural competency into their practice.

A nurse who is teaching patients and their families must have a personal value system that coincides with the values of the profession. Three American Nurses Association documents—*Code of Ethics for Nurses With Interpretive Statements* (2015), *Nursing's Social Policy Statement* (2010a), and *Standards of Clinical Nursing Practice* (2010b)—provide nurses with ethical guidelines for professional practice.

The Psychomotor Domain

The **psychomotor domain** is known as the "skills" domain. Learning in this domain involves acquiring fine and gross motor abilities, such as walking, handwriting, manipulating equipment, or performing a procedure. Psychomotor skill learning, according to Reilly and Oermann (1990), "is a complex process demanding far more knowledge than suggested by the simple mechanistic behavioral approach" (p. 81). To develop psychomotor skills, integration of both cognitive and affective learning is required as well. The affective component recognizes the value of the skill being learned. The cognitive component relates to knowing the principles, relationships, and processes involved in the skill. Although all three domains are involved in demonstrating a psychomotor competency, the psychomotor domain can be examined separately and requires different teaching approaches and evaluation strategies (Reilly & Oermann, 1990). Psychomotor skills are easy to identify and measure because they include primarily movement-oriented activities that are relatively easy to observe.

Psychomotor learning can be classified in a variety of ways (Dave, 1970; Harrow, 1972; Moore, 1970; Simpson, 1972). Simpson's system seems to be the most widely recognized as relevant to patient teaching. Objectives in this domain, according to Simpson (1972), are divided into seven levels, from simple to complex, as seen in Figure 10–1.

Levels of Behavioral Objectives and Examples in the Psychomotor Domain

Perception level: Ability of the learner to show sensory awareness of objects or cues associated with some task to be performed. This level involves reading directions or observing a process with attention to steps or techniques in developing a skill. Example: After a 10-minute teaching session on aspiration precautions, the family caregiver will describe the best position to place the patient in during mealtimes to prevent choking.

Set level: Ability of the learner to exhibit readiness to take a particular kind of action as evidenced by expressions of willingness, sensory attending, or body language favorable to performing a motor act (perception is a prerequisite behavior). Example: Following a demonstration of how to do proper wound care, the patient will express a willingness to practice changing the dressing on his leg using the correct procedural steps.

Guided response level: Ability of the learner to exert effort via overt actions under the guidance of an instructor to imitate an observed behavior with conscious awareness of effort. Imitating may be performed hesitantly but with compliance to directions and coaching (perception and set are prerequisite behaviors). Example: After watching a 15-minute video on the procedure for self-examination of the breast, the patient will perform the exam on a model with 100% accuracy.

Mechanism level: Ability of the learner to repeatedly perform steps of a desired skill with a certain degree of confidence, indicating mastery to the extent that some or all aspects of the process become habitual. The steps are blended into a meaningful whole and are performed smoothly with little conscious effort (perception, set, and guided response are prerequisite behaviors). Example: After a 20-minute teaching session, the patient will demonstrate the proper use of crutches while repeatedly applying the correct three-point gait technique.

Complex overt response level: Ability of the learner to automatically perform a complex motor act with independence and a high degree of skill, without hesitation and with minimum expenditure of time and energy; performance of an entire sequence of a complex behavior without the need to attend to details (perception, set, guided response, and mechanism are prerequisite behaviors). Example: After three 20-minute teaching sessions, the patient will demonstrate the correct use of crutches while accurately performing a number of tasks, such as going up stairs, getting in and out of the car, and using the toilet.

Adaptation level: Ability of the learner to modify or adapt a motor process to suit the individual or various situations, indicating mastery of highly developed movements that can be suited to a variety of conditions (perception, set, guided response, mechanism, and complex overt response are prerequisite behaviors). Example: After reading handouts on healthy food choices, the patient will be able to replace unhealthy food items she normally chooses to eat at home with healthy alternatives.

Origination level: Ability of the learner to create new motor acts, such as novel ways of manipulating objects or materials, as a result of an understanding of a skill and developed ability to perform skills (perception, set, guided response, mechanism, complex overt response, and adaptation are prerequisite behaviors). Example: After simulation training, the parents will respond correctly to a series of scenarios that demonstrate skill in recognizing respiratory distress in their child with asthma.

Table 10–5 lists verbs commonly used in writing psychomotor-level behavioral objectives.

Another taxonomic system for psychomotor learning proposed by Dave (1970) is based on behaviors that include muscular action and neuromuscular coordination. Dave's system recognizes that levels of skill attainment can be achieved and refined over a period of months depending on the frequency with which the learner uses certain skills in practice. Objectives in this domain, according to Dave (1970), are divided into five levels, as shown in **Table 10–6**.

These taxonomic criteria for the development of psychomotor skill competency suggest that accuracy should be stressed rather than the speed at which a skill is acquired (Reilly & Oermann, 1990). Dave's levels will apply when considering aspects of the learning curve, discussed later in this chapter. Nevertheless, the levels of psychomotor behavior, no matter which taxonomic system is used, require the general and orderly steps of observing, imitating, practicing, and adapting.

TEACHING OF PSYCHOMOTOR SKILLS

A number of different teaching methods, such as demonstration, return demonstration, simulation, and self-instruction, are useful for the development of motor skills. Also, instructional materials, such as videos (DVDs), audiotapes (CDs), models, diagrams, and posters, are effective approaches for teaching and learning in the psychomotor domain.

When teaching psychomotor skills, it is important for the nurse to remember to keep skill instruction separate from a discussion of principles underlying the skill (cognitive component) or a discussion of how the learner feels about carrying out the skill (affective component). Psychomotor skill development is very egocentric and usually requires a great deal of concentration as the learner works toward mastery of a skill.

Table 10–6 Dave's Levels of Psychomotor Learning

Imitation. At this level, observed actions are followed. The learner's movements are gross, coordination lacks smoothness, and errors occur. Time and speed required to perform are based on learner needs.
Manipulation. At this level, written instructions are followed. The learner's coordinated movements are variable, and accuracy is measured based on the skill of using written procedures as a guide. Time and speed required to perform vary.
Precision. At this level, a logical sequence of actions is carried out. The learner's movements are coordinated at a higher level, and errors are minimal and relatively minor. Time and speed required to perform remain variable.
Articulation. At this level, a logical sequence of actions is carried out. The learner's movements are coordinated at a high level, and errors are limited. Time and speed required to perform are within reasonable expectations.
Naturalization. At this level, the sequence of actions is automatic. The learner's movements are coordinated at a consistently high level, and errors are almost nonexistent. Time and speed required to perform are within realistic limits, and performance reflects professional competence.

It is easy to interfere with psychomotor learning if the teacher asks a knowledge (cognitive) question while the learner is trying to focus on the performance (psychomotor response) of a skill. For example, while the patient is learning to self-administer parenteral medication, the nurse might simultaneously ask the patient to respond cognitively to the question, "What are the actions or side effects of this medicine?" or "How do you feel about injecting yourself?" These questions demand cognitive and affective responses during psychomotor performance.

What the nurse is doing in this situation is asking the learner to demonstrate at least two different behaviors at the same time. This approach can result in frustration and confusion, and ultimately it may result in failure to achieve either of the behaviors successfully. It is essential for the teacher to keep in mind that questions related to the cognitive or affective domain should be posed only *before* or *after* the learner practices a new psychomotor skill (Oermann, 1990).

In psychomotor skill development, the ability to perform a skill is not equivalent to having learned or mastered a skill. Performance is a transitory action, whereas learning is a more permanent behavior that follows from repeated practice and experience (Oermann, 1990). The actual mastery of a skill requires practice to allow the individual to repeat the performance time and again with accuracy, coordination, confidence, and out of habit. Practice does make perfect, so repetition leads to perfection and reinforcement of the behavior.

Riding a bicycle is a perfect example of the difference between being able to perform a skill and having mastered that skill. When one first attempts to ride a bicycle, movements tend to be very jerky, and a great deal of concentration is required. Falling off the bicycle is not unexpected in the learning process. Once the skill is learned, however, bicycle riding becomes a smooth, automatic operation that requires minimal concentration.

Some behaviors that are learned do not require much reinforcement, even over a long period of disuse. Yet, other behaviors, once mastered, need to be rehearsed or relearned to perform them at the level of skill once achieved. The amount of practice required to learn a new skill varies with the individual, depending on many factors. Oermann (1990) and Bell (1991) have addressed some of the more important variables:

Readiness to learn: The motivation to learn affects the degree of effort exhibited by the learner in working toward mastery of a skill.

Past experience: If the learner is familiar with equipment or techniques similar to those needed to learn a new skill, then mastery of the new skill may be achieved at a faster rate. The effects of learning one skill on the subsequent performance of another related skill are collectively known as **transfer of learning** (Gomez & Gomez, 1984). For example, if a family member already has experience with aseptic technique in changing a dressing, then learning to suction a tracheostomy tube using sterile technique should not require as much time to master.

Health status: An illness state or other physical or emotional impairments in the learner may affect the time it takes to acquire or successfully master a skill.

Environmental stimuli: Depending on the type and level of stimuli as well as the learning style (degree of tolerance for certain stimuli), distractions in the immediate surroundings may interfere with the ability to acquire a skill.

Anxiety level: The ability to concentrate can be dramatically affected by how anxious someone feels. Nervousness about performing in front of another person is a particularly important factor in psychomotor skill development. High anxiety levels interfere with coordination, steadiness, fine muscle movements, and concentration levels when performing complex psychomotor skills. It is important to reassure learners that they are not necessarily being tested during psychomotor skill performance. Reassurance and support reduce anxiety levels related to the fear of not meeting expectations of themselves or of the teacher.

Developmental stage: Physical, cognitive, and psychosocial stages of development all influence an individual's ability to master a movement-oriented task. Certainly, a young child's fine and gross motor skills as well as cognitive abilities are at a different level from those of an adult. The older adult, too, likely exhibits slower cognitive processing and increased response time (needing more time to perform an activity) compared to younger clients.

Practice session length: During the beginning stages of learning a motor skill, short and carefully planned practice sessions and frequent rest periods are valuable techniques to help increase the rate and success of learning. These techniques are thought to be effective because they help prevent physical fatigue and restore the learner's attention to the task at hand.

Mental imaging (also known as **mental practice**) has surfaced as a helpful alternative for teaching motor skills, particularly for patients who have suffered a stroke (Page, Levine, Sisto, & Johnson, 2001). Research indicates that learning psychomotor skills can be enhanced through use of such imagery. Mental practice, which involves imagining or visualizing a skill without body movement prior to performing the skill, can enhance motor skill acquisition (Page, Levine, & Khourey, 2009).

Another hallmark of psychomotor learning is the type and timing of the feedback given to learners. Psychomotor skill development allows for spontaneous feedback so that learners have an immediate idea of how well they performed. During skill practice, learners receive **intrinsic feedback**. This is feedback that is generated from within the learners, giving them a sense of or a feel for how they have performed. They may sense that they either did quite well or that they felt awkward and need more practice. The teacher also has the opportunity to provide **augmented feedback**. In this case, the teacher shares information or an opinion with the learners or conveys a message through body language about how well they performed (Oermann, 1990). The immediacy of the feedback, along with intrinsic and augmented feedback, makes it a unique feature of psychomotor learning. In addition, performance checklists can serve as guides for teaching and learning and are another effective tool for evaluating the level of skill performance.

An important point to remember is that making mistakes is an expected part in the process of teaching or learning a psychomotor skill. If the teacher makes an error when demonstrating a skill or the learner makes an error during return demonstration, this occasion is the perfect teaching opportunity to offer anticipatory guidance: "Oops, I made a mistake. Now what do I do?" Unlike in cognitive skill development, where errorless learning is the objective, in psychomotor skill development, a mistake made represents an opportunity to demonstrate how to correct an error and to learn from the not-so-perfect initial attempts at performance. The old saying "You learn by your mistakes" is most applicable to psychomotor skill mastery.

The spacing of practice time improves the likelihood that learners will remember new facts, as described by Willingham (2002) earlier in this chapter. The spacing effect seems to apply to the learning of simple and complex motor skills. Willingham (2004) also addressed the necessity for practice to be repeated beyond the point of perfection if skill learning is to be long lasting, automatic, and achieved with a high level of competence.

In summary, learning is a very complex phenomenon. It can occur in all three domains simultaneously, can happen formally or informally, and can occur in a variety of settings. Evaluation of learning is equally challenging, especially in the affective domain because affective behaviors are not as obvious and clearly observable as the skills acquired in the cognitive and psychomotor domains.

It is clear that the cognitive, affective, and psychomotor domains represent separate behaviors, yet these domains are interrelated. For example, the performance of a psychomotor skill requires cognitive knowledge or understanding of information. Knowledge might be about the scientific principles underlying a practice or the rationale explaining why a skill is important to carry out. Also, an affective component to performing the skill must be acknowledged. Understanding the feelings and attitudes of learners is essential if the psychomotor behavior is to become integrated into their overall experience. Mastering behavioral objectives in all domains is necessary for the learner to attain the ultimate goal of competence and independence in self-care.

Development of Teaching Plans

After mutually agreed-upon goals and objectives have been written, it should be clear what the learner is to learn and what the teacher is to teach. A predetermined goal and related objectives serve as a basis for developing a teaching plan.

A **teaching plan** is a blueprint to achieve the goal and the objectives that have been developed. Along with listing the goal and objectives, this plan should indicate the purpose, content, methods, tools, timing, and evaluation of instruction. The teaching plan should clearly and concisely identify the order of these various parts of the education process. Teaching plans are created for three major reasons:

1. To direct the teacher to look at the relationship between each of the steps of the teaching process to make sure that there is a logical approach to teaching.
2. To communicate in writing exactly what is being taught, how it is being taught and evaluated, and the time allotted to meet each of the behavioral objectives. This is essential for the involvement of the patient and each member of the healthcare team.
3. To legally document that an individual plan for each learner is in place and is being properly implemented.

Many healthcare agencies require evidence of teaching plans to meet internal policies, validate evidenced-based practices, and adhere to guidelines for accreditation.

Agencies may look to standardized documented teaching plans through the electronic medical record as a way to measure improved outcomes (Zynx Health, 2015). Teaching plans can be presented in a number of different formats to meet institutional requirements or the preference of the user. However, all eight components must be included for the teaching plan to be considered comprehensive and complete.

A teaching plan should incorporate the following eight basic elements (Bastable, 2014; Ryan & Marinelli, 1990):

1. The purpose (the *why* of the educational session)
2. A statement of the overall goal
3. A list of objectives
4. An outline of the content to be covered in the teaching session
5. The instructional method(s) used for teaching the related content
6. The time allotted for the teaching of each objective
7. The instructional resources (materials/tools and equipment) needed
8. The method(s) used to evaluate learning

A sample teaching plan template is shown in **Figure 10–2**. This format is highly recommended because the columns allow the teacher, as well as anyone else who is using it, to see all parts of the teaching plan at one time. Also, this format provides the best structure for determining whether all the elements of a plan fit together cohesively.

When creating a teaching plan, the educator must be certain that, above all else, *internal consistency* exists within the plan (Ryan & Marinelli, 1990). A teaching plan is said to be internally consistent when all of its eight parts are related to one another. This concept of internal consistency requires that the domain of learning for each objective be reflected across each of the elements of the teaching plan, from the purpose all the way through to the end process of evaluation. All parts of the teaching plan need to relate to each other, with the overall intention of meeting the goal.

Internal consistency is the major criterion for judging the integrity of a teaching plan. For example, if the nurse has decided to teach a skill with an objective in the psychomotor domain, then the purpose, goal, objectives, content, methods of instruction, instructional materials, amount of time allocated for teaching, and evaluation methods should be reflective of that particular psychomotor domain. Nurses need to know how to organize and present information in an internally consistent teaching plan.

The following is an example of consistency among the first three elements of a teaching plan (Bastable, 2014, p. 661):

Purpose: To provide mothers of male newborns with the information necessary to perform postcircumcision care.

Goal: The mother will independently manage postcircumcision care for her baby boy.

Objective: Following a 20-minute teaching session, the mother will be able to demonstrate the procedure for postcircumcision care with each diaper change (psychomotor).

In this example, the purpose, goal, and objective reflect the psychomotor domain. The other elements of content, methods of instruction, instructional resources, time allotment, and evaluation methods also must be appropriate to the psychomotor domain

PURPOSE:					
GOAL:					
Objectives and Subobjectives	Content Outline	Method of Instruction	Time Allotted (in min.)	Resources (instructional materials)	Method of Evaluation

Figure 10–2 Sample teaching plan template

as well to ensure internal consistency of the plan. See **Figure 10–3** for a complete teaching plan on postcircumcision care.

Several considerations must be taken into account when developing a teaching plan and organizing each of the eight components. Even before the teaching plan is developed, a decision needs to be made about what domains should be included. If the purpose and goal are written to accomplish a skill that may include more than one domain,

Figure 10–3 Post-Circumcision Care

Purpose: To provide mothers of male newborns with the information necessary to perform postcircumcision care.
Goal: The mother will independently manage postcircumcision care for her baby boy.

Objectives	Content Outline	Method of Instruction	Time Allotted	Resources	Method of Evaluation
Following a 20-minute teaching session, the mother will be able to:					

1. Demonstrate procedure for postcircumcision care with each diaper change (psychomotor)	A. Definition of circumcision
	B. Circumcision care
	  1. Washing penis
	  2. Applying petroleum jelly and gauze
	  3. Diapering baby
		Demonstration
		–
		–
		Return demonstration
			10 minutes	Written/pictorial flip chart
				Infant doll
				Washcloth
				Warm water
				Petroleum jelly
				Gauze
				Diaper
					Observation of return demonstration

2. Identify three reasons to call the doctor or nurse (cognitive)	Post-circumcision complications 1. Bleeding 2. Weak or absent stream of urine 3. Drainage 4. Swollen penis 5. Baby acts sick or more fussy than expected	1:1 instruction	5 minutes	Written/pictorial flip chart	Posttest
3. Express any concerns about circumcision care (affective)	A. Summarize common concerns B. Explore feelings	Discussion	5 minutes	White board	Question and answer

Developed as part of teaching project assignment by Eleanor P. McLees, BSN, RN, CNM, and Julie-Lynn Corsoniti, BS, RN, in NSG 561 course during spring 2007 semester at Le Moyne College, Syracuse, NY.

then the teaching plan should reflect one or more objectives for each domain. In addition, the content, methods of teaching, time allocation, resources, and methods of evaluation should flow across the plan in parallel with each objective and be appropriate for accomplishing the domain of learning related to each objective.

Also, the teacher needs to be conscious and realistic about developing certain elements of a teaching plan. For example, selecting self-instruction in an online format as a method of teaching may not be available to some learners who do not know how to use or who cannot afford to have computers, smartphones, certain types of software, and access to the Internet. While the nurse may find one-on-one teaching the most effective with patients, the expense may be prohibitive. Selecting group discussion may be more cost effective and more appropriate in meeting the goals and objectives of a teaching plan that is the same for more than one patient with a similar diagnosis.

The *content outline* for each objective depends on the complexity of that objective and how it relates to the goal. The detail of the content to be taught, that is, the amount and depth of information required, depends on the assessment of the learner's needs, readiness to learn, and learning style.

The *method of instruction* chosen also should be appropriate for the information being taught, the learners, and the setting. If, for example, the purpose is to teach a client to self-administer medication from an asthma inhaler (psychomotor domain), then the primary method of teaching should be demonstration and return demonstration. However, if the purpose is to provide knowledge of what is in a low-fat diet to a group of individuals with high cholesterol (cognitive domain), then lecture, programmed instruction, or group discussion would be more appropriate teaching methods.

The amount of *time* for teaching each objective also must be specified. A teaching session should be no more than 15 to 20 minutes in length and certainly no more than 30 minutes (Bastable, 2014). Additional teaching sessions may be required for the learner to achieve each objective and eventually reach the learning goal.

The *resources* to be used should match the content and support the teaching methods. For example, to teach breast self-examination, an anatomic model of the breast plus written and audiovisual materials would be useful instructional tools. Using a variety of resources is ideal to keep the learner's attention, address various learning styles, and serve to reinforce information. Incorporating many different types of resources is especially helpful to the learner with low literacy skills.

Finally, the *method of evaluation* should match the domains of each objective and validate that the goal has been met or not met. Evaluation methods must measure the desired learning outcomes to determine if and to what extent the learner achieved the goal. For example, a learner recently diagnosed with coronary artery disease may have a learning objective to be able to *state*, *list*, or *circle* the three most important symptoms of a heart attack. In this teaching situation, the evaluation method to test that knowledge could be a written posttest or the oral question-and-answer approach.

In summary, nurses need to be able to develop teaching plans as part of their professional practice. Developing teaching plans is a challenging skill that should not be underestimated. Just as with any nursing care plan, all elements of a teaching plan need to relate to each other to be truly effective. Figure 10–3 is an example of a teaching plan that meets all the rules of construction and has internal consistency. The goal is reflective of the purpose, the objectives are derived from the goal, the content meets the objectives, and the teaching and evaluation methods as well as the resources and timing relate to the content. If any aspect in a teaching plan is not related to the overall goal, then these components must be revised. Keep in mind that the economics of the teaching plan are a realistic consideration in today's cost-driven healthcare system.

Use of Learning Contracts

The concept of learning contracts is an increasingly popular approach to patient and family education. A contract can be implemented with any individual learner or group of learners. Learning contracts are based on the principle that learners are active partners, rather than passive recipients, in the teaching–learning process (Atherton, 2005).

A **learning contract** is defined as a written (formal) or verbal (informal) agreement between the teacher and the learner, which specifies the teaching and learning activities that are to occur within a certain time frame. A learning contract is a mutually negotiated agreement, usually in the form of a written document, drawn up together by the teacher and the learner, that outlines what the learner will learn, what resources will be needed, how learning will be achieved and within what time period, and which criteria will be used for measuring the success of the experience (Jones-Boggs, 2008; Keyzer, 1986; Knowles, Holton, & Swanson, 1998; Matheson, 2003). Inherent in the learning contract is the existence of some type of reward for upholding the contract agreement (Wallace & Mundie, 1987). For patients and families, this reward may be recognition of their success in mastering a task that helps them move closer to independence in self-care and a high quality of life.

Learning contracts are considered to be an effective teaching strategy for empowering the learner because they emphasize self-direction, mutual negotiation, and mutual evaluation of established competency levels (Jones-Boggs, 2008). A number of terms have been used to describe this approach, such as independent learning, self-directed learning, and learner-centered or project-oriented learning (Chan & Chien, 2000; Lowry, 1997; Waddell & Stephens, 2000).

Learning contracts stress shared accountability for learning between the teacher and the learner. The method of contract learning actively involves the learner at all stages of the teaching-learning process, from assessment of learning needs and identification of learning resources to the planning, implementation, and evaluation of learning activities (Jones-Boggs, 2008; Knowles et al., 1998). Translating the concept of learning contracts to the healthcare environment, they are a unique way of presenting information to patients. They are the essence of an equal and cooperative partnership, which challenges the traditional nurse–patient relationship through a redistribution of power and control. Allowing patients to negotiate a contract for learning shifts the control and emphasis of the learning experience from a traditionally teacher-centered focus to a learner-centered focus.

Learning contracts can be especially useful in facilitating the discharge of patients to their home from the hospital or rehabilitation settings. In situations involving the care of a complex patient by multidisciplinary team members, a contract provides a patient-centered, cohesive communication tool between the patient, family caretakers, and the healthcare team (Cady & Yoshioka, 1991; Yetzer, Goetsch, & St. Paul, 2011).

The Concept of Learning Curve

The **learning curve** is a common phrase used to describe how long it takes a learner to learn anything new. This phrase, however, often is used incorrectly when referring to learners who have acquired new knowledge (cognitive domain) or have developed new attitudes, beliefs, or values (affective domain). Research, to date, only supports the correct use of the term *learning curve* in relation to psychomotor domain learning.

McCray and Blakemore (1985) note that the learning curve "is basically nothing more than a graphic depiction of changes in performance or output during a specified time period" (p. 5). A learning curve shows the relationship between practice and performance of a skill. It provides a concrete measure of the rate at which someone learns a task. In many situations, evidence of learning (improvement) follows a very productive and predictable pattern. Understanding the key concepts surrounding the learning curve is essential for any teacher who is approaching the teaching and learning process when it involves skill development.

Although the learning curve concept has been used for decades in business and industry to measure employee productivity, a thorough search of the nursing literature reveals little documentation that this concept has been applied to skill practice. Only in the last few years has reference been found in the medical literature to describe the application of this concept to the learning of surgical and other invasive techniques (Gawande, 2002). Medicine is just beginning to realize the usefulness of the learning curve concept in determining how long it takes for physicians to become competent in performing procedures using new technologies, such as simulators, laparoscopes, or robotic instruments (Eversbusch & Grantcharov, 2004; Flamme, Stukenborg-Colsman, & Wirth, 2006; Hernandez et al., 2004; Savoldi et al., 2009).

Lee Cronbach (1963) was an educational psychologist whose classic work provides the foundation to understanding the concept of the learning curve. Cronbach defines the learning curve, specifically related to psychomotor skill development, as "a record of an individual's improvement made by measuring his ability at different stages of practice and plotting his scores" (p. 297).

According to Cronbach (1963), the learning curve is divided into the following six stages (**Figure 10–4**):

1. *Negligible progress:* Initially very little improvement is detected during this stage. This prereadiness period is when the learner is not ready to perform the entire task, but relevant learning is taking place. This period can be relatively long in young children who are developing physical and cognitive abilities, such as

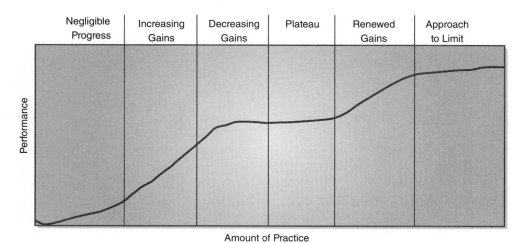

Figure 10–4   A schematic learning curve

Modified from Cronbach, L. J. (1963). *Educational psychology* (2nd ed., p. 299). New York, NY: Harcourt, Brace & World.

focused attention and gross and fine motor skills, and in older adults who may have difficulty in perceiving key discriminations.

2. *Increasing gains:* Rapid gains in learning occur during this stage as the learner grasps the essentials of the task. Motivation may account for increased gains when the learner has interest in the task, receives approval from others, or experiences a sense of pride in discovering the ability to perform.

3. *Decreasing gains:* During this stage the rate of improvement slows, and additional practice does not produce substantial gains. Learning occurs in smaller increments as the learner incorporates changes by using cues to smooth out performance.

4. *Plateau:* During this stage there are no substantial gains. This leveling-off period is characterized by a minimal rate of progress in performance. Instead, the learner is making other adjustments in mastering the skill. The belief that there is a period of no progress is considered false because gains in skills can occur even though overall performance scores remain stable.

5. *Renewed gains:* During this stage the rate of performance rises again and the plateau period has ended. These gains usually are from growth in physical development, renewed interest in the task, a response to challenge, or the drive for perfection.

6. *Approach to limit:* During this stage progress becomes negligible. The ability to perform a task has reached its potential, and no matter how much more the learner practices a skill, he or she is not able to improve. However, this is a hypothetical stage because individuals never truly stop learning.

Individual learning curves are irregular (**Figure 10–5**) and often do not follow a smooth theoretical curve, as seen in Figure 10–4. Such factors as attention, interest,

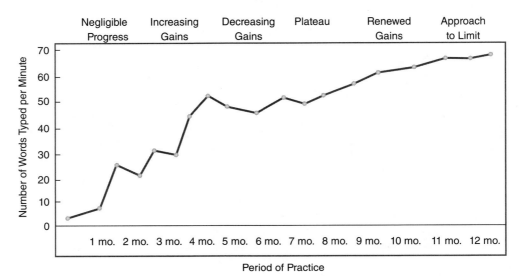

Figure 10–5 Learning curve during one year of typing practice

Data from Cronbach, L. J. (1963). *Educational psychology* (2nd ed., p. 303). New York, NY: Harcourt, Brace & World.

energy, ability, situational circumstances, and favorable or unfavorable conditions for learning provide the ups and downs that are expected in performance (Barker, 1994; Cronbach, 1963; Gage & Berliner, 1998; Woolfolk, 2010). It is important to note that the learning curve can be skewed by the reliability of the performance. As stated by Atherton (2005), "Any novice can get it right occasionally (beginner's luck), but it is consistency which counts and the progress of learning is often assessed on this basis" (p. 1). As Atherton further elaborates, it is incorrect to use the cliché "steep learning curve" to imply that something is difficult to learn. In fact, the opposite is true. As a learner practices a difficult skill, in almost all cases the line rises slowly, not quickly, over time. In other words, a steep, short learning curve indicates that the learner was able to master a skill rapidly and easily.

More nursing research needs to be conducted on applying the learning curve concept to the teaching and learning of psychomotor skills. Such studies would help nurses to improve their understanding of various dimensions of the teaching and learning process related to mastering skills. In relation to patient teaching, research might answer such questions as the following:

- Can a learning curve be shortened given the characteristics of the learner, the situation, or the task at hand?
- Why is the learning curve steeper, more drawn out, or more irregular for some learners than for others?
- Can we predict the learning curves of our patients depending on their educational or experiential backgrounds?
- How many times, on average, does a particular skill need to be practiced to improve competency and ensure consistency of performance?
- What can we do from an educational standpoint to influence the pace and pattern of learning that may result in earlier or more complete achievement of expected outcomes?
- How can the learning curve concept be applied to improve staff performance, thereby increasing work satisfaction and productivity, decreasing costs of care, and improving the quality and safety of care?

Answers to these questions might provide new approaches for evidence-based practice changes for nurses involved in the teaching and learning process.

Many advantages can result by applying concepts of the learning curve to patient teaching. Perhaps the most important understanding of this concept is the realization that the pattern and pace of learning are typically irregular. The learning of any task is initially slow, then more rapid, inevitably decreases, reaches a plateau, and then increases again. After this point a limit is reached when likely no more significant improvement is likely to be achieved. Understanding this phenomenon can help teachers adjust their expectations (or deal with their frustrations) when different paces and patterns of learning occur in patients and their family members as they attempt to master any psychomotor skill.

When the teacher shares with patients that the amount of practice needed to improve performance is very individualized, they may find their frustrations are reduced and their expectations become more realistic. For example, a patient who is undergoing rehabilitation to learn how to walk again following an injury may easily become discouraged with the lack of progress he is making. This happens as the pace of learning varies over time. Also, the patient may experience a time at the beginning or in the middle of the curve when he or she seems not to be learning at all. Teachers can realistically support the learner if they understand that the pace and pattern of skill development are based on the concept of the learning curve.

Summary

The major portion of this chapter focused on differentiating goals from objectives; preparing accurate and concise objectives; classifying objectives according to the three domains of learning; and teaching cognitive, affective, and psychomotor skills using appropriate instructional methods and materials. The writing of effective behavioral objectives is fundamental to the education process. Goals and objectives serve as a guide to the teacher in the planning, implementation, and evaluation of teaching and learning. The communication of desired behavioral outcomes and the mechanisms for accomplishing behavioral changes in the learner are essential elements in the decision-making process with respect to both teaching and learning.

Assessment of the learner is a prerequisite to formulating objectives. The teacher must have a clear understanding of what the learner is expected to be able to do well before selecting the content to be taught and the methods and materials to be used for instruction. Objectives setting must be a partnership effort engaged in by both the learner and the teacher for any learning experience to be successful and rewarding in the achievement of expected outcomes.

Also, this chapter outlined the development of teaching plans and briefly discussed learning contracts and the concept of the learning curve. Teaching plans provide the blueprint for organizing and presenting information in a coherent manner. Nurses need to develop skills in writing teaching plans that reflect internal consistency of all the components. Learning contracts are an innovative, unique, patient-centered alternative to structuring an adult learning experience, especially in the home and rehabilitation settings. They are designed to encourage learners to be self-directed, which increases their level of active involvement and accountability. For the nurse, understanding the concept of the learning curve is essential to teaching psychomotor skills. More nursing research needs to be done to yield findings from evidence-based practice in applying the learning curve concept to patient care.

Review Questions

1. What are the definitions of the terms *goal* and *objective*?
2. Which two major factors distinguish goals and objectives from each other?
3. What reasons justify the importance of using behavioral objectives in teaching?
4. What are the four components that should be included in every written behavioral objective?
5. Which types of mistakes are commonly made when writing behavioral objectives?
6. What are the three domains of learning?

7. What levels of behavior are considered the most simple and the most complex in the cognitive, affective, and psychomotor domains?
8. Why is it important for the nurse to keep psychomotor skill instruction for the novice learner separate from the cognitive and affective components of skill development?
9. Which factors influence the amount of practice required to learn any new skill?
10. What are the eight basic components of a teaching plan?
11. Why is the concept of the learning curve important in the development of psychomotor skills?

Case Study

Suppose you are a new nurse working the day shift on a busy postpartum unit. You have an assignment of five mother–baby units and expect at least one more mother–baby admission later in the morning. Two nurses have called in sick.

Three of your patients are Anna B. and her twin boys born at 37 weeks. Anna B. is a 21-year old first-time mother who delivered yesterday morning by cesarean section under spinal anesthesia. Because Anna has as a history of asthma and pneumonia as well as being a half-pack-per-day smoker, she needs to start using an incentive spirometer every 2 hours while awake.

Anna was last medicated 4 hours ago with oral pain medication and states her pain is currently 5 out of 10. Her vital signs are stable, her incision is clean and dry, she has moderate lochia, and her lungs are clear on auscultation. She has been out of bed to ambulate and her Foley catheter was removed by the night shift nurses. She has not yet voided on her own.

Anna takes an oral antihistamine daily and occasionally uses a bronchodilator via an inhaler. Her asthma was well controlled during her pregnancy. She has not smoked while she has been in the hospital.

Anna is bottle feeding her twins. Anna is married and works as a library aide at an area middle school and states that she graduated from a local high school. She speaks English, although Ukrainian is her primary language.

You are responsible for doing the teaching with Anna on using the incentive spirometer.

1. List two factors or variables that might impact the practice time needed by Anna to learn this new skill.
2. List the goal and purpose for learning in Anna's teaching plan.
3. List one cognitive, one affective, and one psychomotor objective to achieve the goal for learning.
4. List the teaching methods and instructional materials you will use to teach Anna, including the reason why they were selected.
5. What evaluation methods will you use to identify that Anna has met the goal?

References

American Nurses Association. (2010a). *Nursing's social policy statement*. Washington, DC: Author.

American Nurses Association. (2010b). *Standards of clinical nursing practice*. Washington, DC: Author.

American Nurses Association. (2015). *Code of ethics for nurses with interpretive statements*. Washington, DC: American Nurses Publishing. Retrieved from http://www.nursingworld.org/MainMenuCategories /EthicsStandards/CodeofEthicsforNurses.aspx

Anderson, L. W., Krathwohl, D. R., Airasian, P. W., Cruikshank, K. A., Mayer, R. E., Pintrich, P. R., . . . Wittrock, M. C. (2001). *A taxonomy for learning, teaching, and assessing* (Rev. ed.). New York, NY: Longman.

Arends, R. I. (2011). *Learning to teach* (9th ed.). New York, NY: McGraw-Hill.

Atherton, J. S. (2005). *Learning contracts*. Retrieved from http://www.learningandteaching.info/teaching /learningcontracts.htm

Barker, L. M. (1994). *Learning and behavior: A psychobiological perspective*. New York, NY: Macmillan College Publishing.

Bastable, S. (2014). *Nurse as educator: Principles of teaching and learning for nursing practice* (4th ed.). Burlington, MA: Jones & Bartlett Learning.

Bell, M. L. (1991). Learning a complex nursing skill: Student anxiety and the effect of preclinical skill evaluation. *Journal of Nursing Education*, *30*(5), 222–226.

Bloom, B. J., Englehart, M. S., Furst, E. J., Hill, W. H., & Krathwohl, D. R. (1956). *Taxonomy of educational objectives: The classification of educational goals. Handbook 1: Cognitive domain*. New York, NY: David McKay.

Buck, H., McAndrew, L., Dionne-Odom, J., Wion, R., & Riegel, B. (2015). What were they thinking? Patients' cognitive representation of heart failure self-care. *Journal of Hospice & Palliative Nursing*, *17*(3), 249–256.

Cady, C., & Yoshioka, R. S. (1991). Using a learning contract to successfully discharge an infant on home total parenteral nutrition. *Pediatric Nursing*, *17*(1), 67–70, 74.

Chan, S. W., & Chien, W. T. (2000). Implementing contract learning in a clinical context: Report on a study. *Journal of Advanced Nursing*, *31*(2), 298–305.

Cronbach, L. J. (1963). *Educational psychology* (2nd ed.). New York, NY: Harcourt, Brace & World.

Cummings, C. (1994). Tips for writing behavioral objectives. *Nursing Staff Development Insider*, *3*(4), 6, 8.

Dave, R. (1970). *Psychomotor levels in developing and writing objectives*. Tucson, AZ: Educational Innovators Press.

Eggen, P. D., & Kauchak, D. P. (2012). *Strategies for teachers teaching content and thinking skills* (6th ed.). Boston, MA: Allyn & Bacon.

Evans, A. E., Edmunson-Drane, E. W., & Harris, K. K. (2000). Computer-assisted instruction: An effective instructional method for HIV prevention? *Journal of Adolescent Health*, *26*, 244–251.

Eversbusch, A., & Grantcharov, T. P. (2004). Learning curves and impact of psychomotor training on performance in simulated colonoscopy: A randomized trial using virtual reality endoscopy trainer. *Surgical Endoscopy*, *18*(10), 1514–1518.

Ferguson, L. M. (1998). Writing learning objectives. *Journal of Nursing Staff Development*, *14*(2), 87–94.

Flamme, C. H., Stukenborg-Colsman, C., & Wirth, C. J. (2006). Evaluation of the learning curves associated with uncemented primary total hip arthroplasty depending on the experience of the surgeon. *Hip International*, *16*(3), 191–197.

Gage, N. L., & Berliner, D. C. (1998). *Educational psychology* (6th ed.). Boston, MA: Houghton Mifflin.

Gawande, A. (2002, January 28). The learning curve: Annals of medicine. *The New Yorker*, 52–61.

Gomez, G. E., & Gomez, E. A. (1984). The teaching of psychomotor skills in nursing. *Nurse Educator*, *9*(4), 35–39.

Goulet, C., & Owen-Smith, P. (2005). Cognitive-affective learning in physical therapy education: From implicit to explicit. *Journal of Physical Therapy Education*, *19*(3), 67–72.

Gronlund, N. E. (1985). *Stating objectives for classroom instruction* (3rd ed.). New York, NY: Macmillan.

Gronlund, N. E. (2004). *Writing instructional objectives for teaching and assessment* (7th ed.). Upper Saddle River, NJ: Pearson Merrill Prentice Hall.

Gronlund, N. E., & Brookhart, S. M. (2008). *Gronlund's writing instructional objectives* (8th ed.). Upper Saddle River, NJ: Pearson Merrill Prentice Hall.

Haggard, A. (1989). *Handbook of patient education*. Rockville, MD: Aspen.

Harrow, A. J. (1972). *A taxonomy of the psychomotor domain: A guide for developing behavioral objectives*. New York, NY: David McKay.

Hernandez, J. D., Bann, S. D., Munz, Y., Moorthy, K., Datta, V., Martin, S., . . . Rockall, T. (2004). Qualitative and quantitative analysis of the learning curve of a simulated surgical task on the da Vinci system. *Surgical Endoscopy*, *18*(3), 372–378.

Jones-Boggs, K. (2008). Perceived benefits of the use of learning contracts to guide clinical education in respiratory care students. *Respiratory Care*, *53*, 1475–1481.

Keyzer, D. (1986). Using learning contracts to support change in nursing organizations. *Nurse Education Today*, *6*(8), 103–108.

Knowles, M. S., Holton, E. F., & Swanson, R. A. (1998). *The definitive classic in adult education and human resource development* (3rd ed.). Houston, TX: Gulf.

Krathwohl, D. R., Bloom, B. J., & Masia, B. B. (1964). *Taxonomy of educational objectives: The classification of educational goals. Handbook II: The affective domain*. New York, NY: David McKay.

Krau, S. D. (2011). Creating educational objectives for patient education using the new Bloom's taxonomy. *Nursing Clinics of North America*, *46*(3), 299–312.

Lowry, M. (1997). Using learning contracts in clinical practice. *Professional Nurse*, *12*(4), 280–283.

Mager, R. F. (1997). *Preparing instructional objectives* (3rd ed.). Atlanta, GA: Center for Effective Performance.

Maier-Lorentz, M. M. (1999). Writing objectives and evaluating learning in the affective domain. *Journal for Nurses in Staff Development*, *15*(4), 167–171.

Marks, R. (2009). Ethics and patient education: Health literacy and cultural dilemmas. *Health Promotion Practice*, *10*, 328–332.

Matheson, R. (2003). Promoting the integration of theory and practice by the use of a learning contract. *International Journal of Therapy and Rehabilitation*, *10*(6), 264–270.

McCray, P., & Blakemore, T. (1985). *A guide to learning curve technology to enhance performance prediction in vocational evaluation*. Menomonie, WI: Research and Training Center, Stout Vocational and Rehabilitation Institute, School of Education and Human Services, University of Wisconsin–Stout.

Menix, K. D. (1996). Domains of learning: Interdependent components of achievable learning outcomes. *Journal of Continuing Education in Nursing*, *27*(5), 200–208.

Moore, M. R. (1970). The perceptual–motor domain and a proposed taxonomy of perception. *Audio Communications Review*, *18*, 379–413.

Morrison, G. R., Ross, S. M., & Kemp, J. E. (2004). *Designing effective instruction* (4th ed.). Hoboken, NJ: Wiley.

Nothwehr, F., Dennis, L., & Wu, H. (2007). Measurement of behavioral objectives for weight management. *Health Education & Behavior*, *34*, 793–807.

Oermann, M. H. (1990). Psychomotor skill development. *Journal of Continuing Education in Nursing*, *21*(5), 202–204.

Page, S. J., Levine, P., & Khourey, J. (2009). Modified constraint-induced therapy combined with mental practice: Think through better motor outcomes. *Stroke, 40*(2), 551–554.

Page, S. J., Levine, P., Sisto, S. A., & Johnston, M. V. (2001). Mental practice with physical practice for upper-limb motor deficit in subacute stroke. *Physical Therapy, 81*, 1455–1462.

Phillips, J. J., & Phillips, P.P. (2010). The power of objectives: Moving beyond learning objectives. *Performance Improvement, 49*(6), 17–24.

Reilly, D. E., & Oermann, M. H. (1990). *Behavioral objectives: Evaluation in nursing* (3rd ed.). Pub. No. 15–2367. New York, NY: National League for Nursing.

Rotundo, G. (2012). Centering pregnancy: The benefits of group prenatal care. *Nursing for Women's Health, 15*(6), 510–518.

Ryan, M., & Marinelli, T. (1990). *Developing a teaching plan.* Unpublished self-study module, College of Nursing, State University of New York Health Science Center at Syracuse.

Savoldi, G. L., Schiffer, E., Abegg, C., Baeriswyl, V., Clerique, F., & Weber, J. (2009). Learning curves of the Glidescope, the McGrath, and the Airtraq laryngoscopes: A manekin study. *European Journal of Anaesthesiology, 26*, 554–558.

Schoenly, L. (1994). Teaching in the affective domain. *Journal of Continuing Education in Nursing, 25*(5), 209–212.

Simpson, E. J. (1972). The classification of educational objectives in the psychomotor domain. In M. T. Rainier (Ed.), *Contributions of behavioral science to instructional technology: The psychomotor domain* (3rd ed.). Englewood Cliffs, NJ: Gryphon Press, Prentice Hall.

Smaldino, S. E., Lowther, D. L., & Russell, J. D. (2012). *Instructional technology and media for learning* (10th ed.). Boston, MA: Pearson.

Tong, R. (2007). *New perspectives in health care ethics: An interdisciplinary and cross-cultural approach.* Upper Saddle River, NJ: Pearson Education.

Waddell, D. L., & Stephens, S. (2000). Use of learning contracts in a RN-to-BSN leadership course. *Journal of Continuing Education in Nursing, 31*(4), 179–184.

Wallace, P. L., & Mundie, G. E. (1987). Contract learning in orientation. *Journal of Nursing Staff Development, 3*(4), 143–149.

Willingham, D. T. (2002, Summer). Allocating student study time: "Massed" versus "distributed" practice. *American Educator*, 37–39, 47.

Willingham, D. T. (2004, Spring). Practice makes perfect—but only if you practice beyond the point of perfection. *American Educator*, 31–33, 38.

Wittmann-Price, R. A., & Fasolka, B. J. (2010). Objectives and outcomes: The fundamental difference. *Nursing Education Perspectives, 31*(4), 233–236.

Woolfolk, A. (2010). *Educational psychology* (11th ed.). Upper Saddle River, NJ: Merrill.

Yetzer, E. A., Goetsch, N., & St. Paul, M. (2011). Teaching adults SAFE medication management. *Rehabilitation Nursing, 36*(6), 255–260.

Zimmerman, B. S., & Phillips, C. Y. (2000). Affective learning: Stimulus to critical thinking and caring practices. *Journal of Nursing Education, 39*(9), 422–425.

Zynx Health. (2015). *Interdisciplinary evidence-based plans of care that support clinical excellence.* Retrieved from http://www.zynxhealth.com

Teaching Methods and Settings

Kathleen Fitzgerald | Kara Keyes

Chapter Highlights

- Teaching Methods
  - *Lecture*
  - *Group Discussion*
  - *One-to-One Instruction*
  - *Demonstration and Return Demonstration*
  - *Gaming*
  - *Simulation*
  - *Role Play*
  - *Role Modeling*
  - *Self-Instruction*
- Selection of Teaching Methods
- Evaluation of Teaching Methods
- General Principles for Teaching Across Methodologies
- Settings for Teaching

Key Terms

demonstration
gaming
group discussion
healthcare-related setting
healthcare setting
lecture
nonhealthcare setting
one-to-one instruction
pacing
return demonstration
role modeling
role play
scaffolding
self-instruction
settings for teaching
simulation
skill inoculation
teaching method

Objectives

After completing this chapter, the reader will be able to

1. Define the term *teaching method*.
2. Explain the various types of teaching methods.
3. Describe how to use each method effectively.
4. Identify the advantages and limitations of each method.
5. Discuss the variables that influence the selection of the various methods.
6. Recognize techniques to enhance teaching effectiveness.
7. Explain how to evaluate teaching methods.
8. Classify settings for teaching according to the primary purpose of the organization or agency in which the nurse functions as teacher.

© wanchai/Shutterstock

After an excellent learning experience, a patient might comment, "Now, there is a born teacher!" This statement would seem to indicate that effective teaching by nurses comes naturally. In reality, being able to teach well is a learned skill. Developing this skill requires the nurse to understand the educational process, including which teaching methods to use under what circumstances. Determining the most appropriate teaching methods to instruct patients and their family members depends on a variety of differences: the age and developmental level of the learners; what the learners already know and what they need to know to succeed; the subject-matter content; the objectives for learning; the available time, space, and material resources; and the physical setting. Stimulating and effective teaching–learning experiences are designed, not accidental or automatic, and involve the use of one or several methods of instruction to achieve the desired learning outcomes (Rothwell & Kazanas, 2008).

A **teaching method** is the way information is taught that brings the learner into contact with what is to be learned. Examples of such methods include lecture, group discussion, one-to-one instruction, demonstration and return demonstration, gaming, simulation, role play, role modeling, and self-instruction modules. As the use of technology evolves, these methods also are being offered over the Internet as online learning opportunities (Cook et al., 2008).

Instructional materials are the objects or vehicles, such as printed handouts, videos, podcasts, and posters, used to communicate information that supplements the teaching method. It is important at this point to draw a distinction between the terms *teaching methods* and *instructional materials*. Although they often are treated as being one and the same thing, they are very distinct and separate features. See Chapter 12 for more information.

This chapter focuses on the types of teaching methods available and considers how to choose and use them most efficiently and effectively. In doing so, the advantages and limitations of each method, the variables influencing the selection of various methods, and the approaches for evaluating the methods are identified to improve the delivery of instruction. In all types of situations and settings, nurses are expected to teach a variety of patients and their family members. Therefore, throughout this chapter, examples are provided about how to apply the various methods to enhance teaching and learning experiences.

Teaching Methods

There is no one perfect method for teaching all learners in all settings. Also, no one method is necessarily more effective for changing behavior in any of the three learning domains (cognitive, affective, and psychomotor). Whatever the method chosen, people learn best when it is used in conjunction with another method or with one or more of the instructional materials available to accompany the teaching approach (Friedman, Cosby, Boyko, Hatton-Bauer, & Turnbull, 2011).

The importance of selecting appropriate methods to meet the needs of learners should not be underestimated. The popular Chinese proverb "Tell me; I forget. Show me; I remember. Involve me; I understand" (author unknown) clearly implies that information retention rates vary with different teaching methods. Using methods of instruction that actively involve the learner improves the amount of information they retain and, thus, positively affects their learning outcomes (Ridley, 2007).

The nurse functions in the vital role of teacher by facilitating, guiding, and supporting the learner in acquiring new knowledge, attitudes, and skills. Even though a nurse may tend to rely on one teaching method, he or she rarely adheres to that single method in a pure fashion. Instead, various methods are often used in combination with one another. For example, a nurse may choose lecture as the primary teaching approach but also allow the opportunity for question-and-answer periods and short group discussions during the teaching session.

Deciding which method(s) to select must be based on a consideration of such major factors as the following:

- Audience characteristics (size, diversity, learning style preferences)
- Nurse's expertise as a teacher
- Objectives of learning
- Potential for achieving learning outcomes
- Cost-effectiveness
- Instructional setting
- Evolving technology

These and many other variables are addressed in the following review of the methods of instruction available for teaching and learning.

Lecture

Lecture can be defined as a highly structured method by which the nurse verbally transmits information directly to a group of learners for the purpose of instruction. It is one of the oldest and most often used approaches to teaching. The word *lecture* comes from the Latin term *lectura*, which means "to read."

The lecture method has been highly criticized in recent years because, in its purest form, the nurse does all of the talking and the learner remains in a passive role (DeYoung, 2014). However, as Brookfield (2006) points out, "An abused method calls into question the expertise of those abusing it, not the validity of the method itself" (p. 99). Therefore, if a lecture is well organized and delivered effectively, it can be a very useful method of instruction (Bain, 2004; Bartlett, 2003; Brookfield, 2006; Woodring & Woodring, 2014).

The lecture format is useful in demonstrating patterns, highlighting main ideas, and presenting unique ways of viewing information, such as explaining diabetes mellitus to a group of patients. The lecture should not be employed, however, to give people the same information that they could read independently at another time and place. It is the teacher's expertise, both in theory and experience, that contributes significantly to the learner's understanding of a topic.

The lecture is an ideal way to provide foundational background information as a basis for follow-up group discussions. Also, it is a means to summarize data and current research findings not available elsewhere (Boyd, Gleit, Graham, & Whitman, 1998; Brookfield, 2006). In addition, the lecture can easily be supplemented with instructional materials, such as printed handouts and audiovisual tools.

Lecturing is an acquired skill that is learned and perfected over time, and it is a more complex task than commonly thought (Young & Diekelmann, 2002). Specific strategies exist to strengthen the effectiveness of a lecture (Cantillon, 2003). According to Silberman (2006), five approaches to the effective transfer of knowledge during a lecture are the following:

- *Use opening and summary statements.* At the beginning of the lecture, present major points to help learners become oriented to the subject and at the end provide conclusions to remind learners about the main points made.
- *Present key terms.* Reduce the major points in the lecture to some key words that act as verbal cues or memory jogs.
- *Offer examples.* When possible, provide real-life illustrations of the ideas in the lecture.
- *Use analogies.* If possible, compare the content that is being presented to the knowledge that learners may already have.
- *Use visual backups.* Use a variety of media to help learners see as well as hear what is being said.

Each lecture should include three main parts: introduction, body, and conclusion. These three parts are described in the following subsections (Miller & Stoeckel, 2016; Woodring & Woodring, 2014).

INTRODUCTION

During the introduction phase of a lecture, the nurse should present learners with an overview of the behavioral objectives related to the lecture topic, along with an explanation as to why these objectives are significant. The use of set (the opening to a presentation) engages learners' attention and focuses the group on the teacher, which creates the stage for learners to be ready to listen (Kowalski, 2004). This technique of set captures attention, clarifies goals and objectives, motivates the learner, and demonstrates the relevance of the content in a way that can stimulate the interest of learners in the subject. Nurses also might engage learners' attention by conducting an informal survey of the group or stating the behavioral objectives as questions that will be answered during the body of the lecture.

If the lecture is one of a series, the nurse needs to make a connection with the overall subject and the topic being presented as well as explain its relationship to previous topics covered in prior lectures and those that will follow. Last, the nurse should establish a rapport with the audience by letting his or her personality shine through and by using humor, if appropriate.

BODY

The next portion of the lecture involves the actual delivery of the content related to the topic being addressed. Reading a printed copy of the entire presentation word for word is extremely boring and is a sure way to turn off the audience. Careful preparation is needed so that the important aspects are covered in an organized, accurate, logical, and interesting manner. Examples should be used throughout to enhance the important points, but additional facts and repetition of information should be avoided so as not to reduce the impact of the message. Because the lecture format tends to be a passive approach to learning, the nurse can enhance the effectiveness of the presentation by combining it with other instructional methods, such as discussion or question-and-answer sessions, to engage learners to actively participate.

CONCLUSION

The nurse as teacher should include a wrap-up with every lecture. This final section of the lecture format summarizes the information provided in the presentation. At this point, the nurse can review the major concepts presented. Try to leave some time for questions and answers. During this time, questions asked should be repeated so that the rest of the audience can hear them and understand the response. If time runs short, the nurse can limit the question-and-answer session, but then welcome immediate follow-up by meeting with interested individuals alone or in a smaller group or by suggesting relevant readings.

The nurse's speaking skills also are important to the delivery of a lecture. According to Jacobs (2009), the following variables of speech need to be considered:

- Volume
- Rate
- Pitch/tone
- Pronunciation
- Enunciation
- Proper grammar
- Avoiding annoying habits such as the use of "ums"

Not only are speaking skills important, but body language should also be considered and includes the following:

- Demonstrate enthusiasm.
- Make frequent eye contact with audience.
- Use posture and movement.
  - Convey self-confidence.
  - Demonstrate professionalism.
- Use gestures.
  - Avoid repetitive movement.
  - Rely on head and hands to emphasize points and to keep the audience's attention.

Using audiovisual materials, such as a video, a podcast, or PowerPoint slides, can also add variety to a lecture. The widespread availability of technology makes it easy to enhance a presentation—but only if the technology is used wisely. When developing PowerPoint slides, for example, nurses should adhere to the following general guidelines (Evans, 2000):

- Do not put all content on slides, but include only the key concepts to supplement the presentation.
- Use the largest font possible.

- Do not exceed 25 words per slide.
- Choose colors that provide a high level of contrast between background and text if presenting in a large room with bright lights.
- Use graphics (figures and tables) to summarize important points, to succinctly present information, or to share large amounts of numerical data.
- Do not overdo the use of animation (moving figures), which can be very distracting to the audience.

Overall, it is important to keep the following points in mind: Make sure that the visual aids are large enough and positioned well enough for all to see, and keep them simple and easy to understand (Jacobs, 2009).

Thanks to new technologies, lectures are now being delivered to an even wider variety of learners in locations remote from one another. Distance learning is an ideal way to maximize resources and to transmit current information to people separated by space and time. Through this strategy, the cost, time, and inconvenience of travel no longer can keep an audience from meeting face-to-face with an expert (Cook et al., 2008). **Table 11–1** highlights the major advantages and limitations of lecture as a method of instruction.

Group Discussion

Group discussion is defined as a method of teaching whereby a small number of patients and/or their family members get together to actively exchange information, feelings, and opinions with one another and with the nurse. The nurse's role is to act as a facilitator to keep the discussion focused and to tie important points together. The nurse must be well versed in the subject matter to field questions, to move the discussion along in the direction intended, and to give appropriate feedback (Miller & Stoeckel, 2016).

Table 11–1 Major Advantages and Limitations of Lecture

Advantages
• An efficient, cost-effective means for transmitting large amounts of information to a large number of people at the same time and within a relatively reasonable time frame.
• Useful to demonstrate patterns, highlight main ideas, summarize data, and present unique ways of viewing information.
• An effective approach for cognitive learning, especially at lower levels of the cognitive domain.
• Useful in providing foundational background information as a basis for subsequent learning, such as group discussion.
• Easily supplemented with printed handouts and audiovisual materials to enhance learning.

Limitations
• Largely ineffective in influencing behaviors in the affective and psychomotor domains.
• Does not provide for much stimulation or involvement of learners.
• Very instructor centered, and thus the most active participant—the nurse—is frequently the most knowledgeable one.
• Does not account for individual differences in background, attention span, or learning style.
• All learners are exposed to the same information regardless of their cognitive abilities, learning needs, or stages of coping.
• The diversity within groups makes it challenging, if not impossible, for the nurse to reach all learners equally.

In general, the benefits of group discussions are that they lead to deeper understanding and longer retention of information, increased social support, greater transfer of learning from one situation to another, more positive interpersonal relationships, more favorable attitudes toward learning, and more active learner participation (Brookfield, 2006; Johnson, Johnson, & Smith, 2007; Oakley & Brent, 2004; Springer, Stanne, & Donovan, 1999). As a commonly used instructional technique, this method is learner centered as well as subject centered. Group discussion is an effective method for teaching in both the affective and cognitive domains (Springer et al., 1999).

Group size is a major consideration and should be determined by the purpose or task to be accomplished. Group size can vary somewhat, but discussion is most effective with relatively small groups (ideally between 4 to 8 people). This allows learners to have the opportunity to ask questions and to be more interactive with one another (DeYoung, 2014).

Nurse involvement and control of the process will vary with the needs of the group members. Group discussion requires the nurse to be able to tolerate less structure and organization than other teaching methods, such as lecture or one-to-one instruction. In addition, the group itself must have some knowledge of the content before this method can be effective (Billings & Halstead, 2012); otherwise, the discussion will be based on pooled ignorance. For example, an experienced support group of patients or their significant others may need little input while they work out a complex self-care problem. In contrast, a new group of patients or family members with little understanding of a topic will need to access information directly from the nurse or another source before they can meaningfully participate in problem solving as part of the discussion process.

The nurse's responsibility is to make sure that every member of the group has interpreted information correctly, because failure to do so will lead to conclusions based on faulty data. Although diversity within a group is beneficial, a wide range of literacy skills, states of anxiety, and experiences with acute and chronic conditions within the group may lead to difficulty in meeting any one member's needs. For this reason, patient groups need to be prescreened.

It is important for the nurse to sustain trust within the group. Everyone must feel safe and comfortable enough to express his or her point of view, otherwise the relationship between the nurse and the learners as well as relationships among learners will break down, which creates an environment unsuitable for learning. One helpful approach is for the nurse to tell the group at the beginning of the session that the goal is to hear from all members by asking for their input and points of view during the discussion period. Learners who tend to dominate the discussion should be requested to hold questions that can be handled privately at the end of the session, because these inquiries are important but unique to their circumstances.

Respectful attention and tolerance toward others should be modeled by the nurse and required of all group members. Of course, this consideration does not eliminate the need to correct errors or disagreements. A clear message must be given that while personal opinions may be debatable, the inherent value of what each member has to say and the member's right to participate is guaranteed (Ridley, 2007).

Teaching people in groups rather than individually allows the nurse to reach a number of learners at the same time. The group discussion method is economically beneficial from a time-efficiency perspective when compared with educating each learner individually. With healthcare costs rising, this method should be considered as an efficient and effective method to teach simultaneously a number of patients and family members who have similar learning needs, such as information to prepare for childbirth or cardiac bypass surgery. In a study on the effects of educational interventions on patient satisfaction, Oermann (2003) reported that a group of patients in a waiting room of an ambulatory care center were educated via a videotape about glaucoma, which was then followed by group interaction with a nurse to discuss key points and answer questions. This approach led to higher satisfaction with the education received during their visit.

Discussion is effective in assisting learners to identify resources and to internalize the topic being discussed by helping them to reflect on its personal meaning (Brookfield & Preskill, 2005). Through group work, members share common concerns and receive reinforcement from one another. The ideas that everyone is in the same boat or if one person can do it, so can the others serve to stimulate motivation for learning as a result of peer support.

Group discussion has proved particularly helpful to patients and families dealing with chronic illness. This instructional method is most effective during the accommodation stage of psychological adjustment to chronic illness, because the interactions reduce isolation and foster identification with others who are in similar circumstances (Fredette, 1990). Discussion in a group offers members a forum in which to share information for cognitive growth as well as an opportunity to learn self-efficacy. The resulting increase in the confidence levels of patients and families enhances their ability to handle an illness (Cooper, Booth, Fear, & Gill, 2001; Deakin, McShane, Cade, & Williams, 2005; Lorig & Gonzalez, 1993).

The group process informs people about how to respond to situations, improves their coping mechanisms, and explores ways to incorporate needed changes into their lives. Group self-management education for people with diabetes, for example, has been found in some instances not only to be more cost-effective but also to result in greater treatment satisfaction and to be slightly better in supporting lifestyle changes (Tang, Funnell, & Anderson, 2006). **Table 11–2** highlights the main advantages and limitations of group discussion as a method of instruction.

One-to-One Instruction

One-to-one instruction, which may be given either formally or informally, involves face-to-face delivery of information specifically designed to meet the needs of an individual learner. This type of patient education strategy has been found to have a positive effect on learning and on compliance (Vermeire, Hearnshaw, Van Royen, & Denekens, 2001). Formal one-to-one instruction is a planned activity, whereas informal one-to-one instruction is an unplanned interaction, such as capitalizing on a teachable moment that occurs unexpectedly when the patient demonstrates a readiness to learn (Miller & Stoeckel, 2016). Such instruction offers an opportunity for both the nurse and the learner to communicate knowledge, ideas, and feelings primarily through oral exchange,

Table 11–2 Major Advantages and Limitations of Group Discussion

Advantages
• Enhances learning in both the affective and cognitive domains.
• Is both learner centered and subject centered.
• Stimulates learners to think about issues and problems.
• Encourages members to exchange their own experiences, thereby making learning more active and less isolating.
• Provides opportunities for sharing of ideas and concerns.
• Fosters positive peer support and feelings of belonging.
• Reinforces previous learning.

Limitations
• One or more members may dominate the discussion.
• Easy to stray from the topic, which interferes with achievement of the objectives.
• Shy learners may refuse to become involved or may need a great deal of encouragement to participate.
• Requires skill to tactfully redirect learners who go off on tangents or who dominate without losing their trust and that of other group members.
• Particularly challenging for the novice teacher when members do not easily interact.
• More time consuming to transmit information than other methods such as lecture.
• Requires teacher's presence at all sessions to act as facilitator and resource person.

although nonverbal messages can be conveyed as well. Thus this method of teaching is a process of mutual interchange between the patient and the health professional. It requires interpersonal skill and sensitivity on the part of the nurse and the ability to establish rapport with the learner (Falvo, 2010; Gleasman-DeSimone, 2012).

One-to-one instruction should never be a lecture delivered to an audience of one to meet the nurse's goals. Instead, the experience should actively involve the learner and be based on his or her unique learning needs. Ideally, a one-to-one teaching session should be 15 to 20 minutes in length, and the nurse should offer information in small, bite-sized portions to allow time for processing (Haggard, 1989). Research shows that the more information that is given at any one time, the less it is remembered and correctly recalled. Thus, effective communication depends more on the quality of the information presented than on the quantity to increase adherence to, and patient participation in, a recommended plan of care (Kessels, 2003).

One-to-one instruction can be tailored to meet objectives in all three domains of learning. It begins with an assessment of the learner and the mutual setting of objectives to be accomplished (Burkhart, 2008). As part of the assessment process, it is very important to determine whether any problem behaviors exist, such as smoking, and at which stage of change the person is with respect to dealing with such behaviors. Once this information is determined, the nurse can tailor educational interventions to that stage (Prochaska, DiClemente, Velicer, & Rossi, 1993).

The stages of change model can be generalized across a broad range of behaviors, including but not limited to smoking cessation, weight control, avoidance of high-fat diets, safer sex, and exercise initiation (Prochaska et al., 1994; Saarmann, Daugherty, & Riegel, 2000). For example, the patient with a chronic problem such as obesity must consider the options available for weight control; only then can the patient and the nurse mutually design an action plan that the patient thinks can be accomplished. This patient's confidence level can be assessed by asking on a scale of 0–10 how certain he is of achieving this goal. A score of 7 or higher makes it more likely he will be successful (Lorig, 2003). See Chapter 6 for the stages of change model that explains motivation and compliance for behavioral change.

Whenever teaching is done on a one-to-one basis, instructions should be specific and time should be given for an immediate response from the learner, followed by direct feedback from the nurse. Allowing patients and their family members the opportunity to state their understanding of information gives the nurse an opportunity to evaluate the extent of learning. The teach-back or tell-back strategy that asks learners to restate in their own words what they understood should always be used by the nurse to be sure patients heard and interpreted the information correctly and completely (Fidyk, Ventura, & Green, 2014; Hyde & Kautz, 2014; Jager & Wynia, 2012; Kemp, Floyd, McCord-Duncan, & Lang, 2008). So often nurses ask learners "Do you understand what I just taught you?" A question that is closed ended and only requires a "yes" or "no" response does not provide information for the nurse to confirm that the message was, in fact, received as intended. This type of question should almost always be avoided. This is because, more likely than not, learners will say "yes," indicating they understood something even when research shows that on average only about half of the information taught the first time is remembered, and only about 20% of it is recalled accurately (Ley, 1972; Kessels, 2003). Also, communicating to learners what further information is forthcoming allows them to connect what they have just learned with what they will be learning in the future (Falvo, 2010). For example, the nurse teaching a patient about hypoglycemia might say, "Now that you understand what causes low blood sugar, we will talk about how to tell when you have it and what to do if you experience it after discharge."

The process of one-to-one instruction involves moving learners from repeating the information that was shared to applying what they have just learned. In the previous example regarding hypoglycemia, the nurse might offer the learner a hypothetical situation similar to what the patient might experience given his lifestyle and have him work through how to respond to it. In this type of one-to-one exchange, a potentially threatening situation can be presented in a nonthreatening manner (Boyd et al., 1998). For instance, the nurse might ask a busy executive who has diabetes how he would respond to feeling shaky and sweaty at 2:00 p.m. on a day when a meeting runs late and he misses lunch. The nurse must clearly state that these types of scenarios are not meant to be a test but rather a dress rehearsal for real-world situations. They can change the scenarios with further questioning to help learners plan how they could prevent such occurrences in the future. This technique gives learners a chance to use the information at a higher cognitive level and provides an opportunity for the nurse to evaluate the patient's learning in a safe environment.

With the one-to-one method of instruction, questioning is an excellent technique. It encourages learners to be active participants in the learning process and gives nurses important feedback on their progress (Falvo, 2010). Questions can be matched with the behavioral objectives to be achieved. For example, to determine a patient's knowledge level in the cognitive domain, the nurse might ask, "What is the next step that you should take?"

Questioning should not be interpreted by learners as a test of their knowledge but rather as a way to exchange information and stimulate thinking. However, two problems can occur with questioning: (1) Questions can be so unclear that the learner does not know what the question is, or (2) they can contain too many facts to process effectively (House, Chassie, & Spohn, 1990). The nurse should watch the learner's nonverbal reactions and rephrase the question if he or she detects either of these problems. If the learner seems confused, it is helpful to state that perhaps the question was not clear. This technique guards against the learner feeling guilty or becoming discouraged if the answer to a question was incorrect (Falvo, 2010).

Also, it is important to give patients and their family members time to process information and respond to your questions. Sometimes nurses are uncomfortable waiting in silence for an answer or are impatient and attempt to correct an answer before learners complete their responses. Questioning is ineffective as a technique when nurses do not give learners enough time to process information. Preliminary interruption may further interfere with a learner's thinking abilities and create a tense atmosphere.

One-to-one instruction has much strength as a teaching method. However, it also has its drawbacks. **Table 11–3** summarizes the major advantages and limitations of this method.

From an economic standpoint, one-to-one instruction is a very labor-intensive method and should be thoughtfully tailored to make the expense worthwhile in terms of achieving learner outcomes. One-to-one teaching of patients and families is often considered an inefficient approach to learning because the nurse is reaching only one person at a time.

Table 11–3 Major Advantages and Limitations of One-to-One Instruction

Advantages
• The pace and content of teaching can be tailored to meet individual needs.
• Ideal as an intervention for initial assessment and ongoing evaluation of the learner.
• Good for teaching behaviors in all three domains of learning.
• Especially suitable for teaching those who are learning disabled, low literate, or educationally disadvantaged.
• Provides opportunity for immediate feedback to be shared between the nurse and the learner.

Limitations
• The learner is isolated from others who have similar needs or concerns.
• Deprives learners of the opportunity to identify with others and share information, ideas, and feelings with those in like circumstances.
• Can put learners on the spot because they are the sole focus of the nurse's attention.
• Questioning may be interpreted by learners as a technique to test their knowledge and skills.
• The learner may feel overwhelmed and anxious if the nurse makes the mistake of cramming too much information into each session.

Demonstration and Return Demonstration

It is important to begin this discussion by making a clear distinction between demonstration and return demonstration. **Demonstration** by the nurse is done to show the learner how to perform a particular skill. **Return demonstration** by the learner is carried out in an attempt to establish competence by performing a task with cues from the nurse as needed. These two methods require different abilities by both the nurse and the learner. In particular, they are effective in teaching psychomotor domain skills. However, demonstration and return demonstration may also be used to enhance cognitive and affective learning.

Prior to giving a demonstration, learners should be informed of the purpose of the procedure, the sequential steps involved, the equipment needed, and the actions expected of them. It is important to stress why the demonstration is important or useful to the participants. Equipment should be tested prior to the demonstration to ensure that it is complete and in good working order. For the demonstration method to be employed effectively, learners must be able to clearly see and hear the steps being taught. Therefore, the demonstration method is best suited to teaching individuals or small groups. A large screen or multiple screens for video presentations of demonstrations can allow larger groups to participate.

Demonstrations can be a passive activity for learners, whose role is to observe the nurse presenting an exact performance of a required skill. Demonstrations are more effective when instructions are explained verbally either prior to or during the demonstration. This method of instruction can be enhanced if the nurse slows down the pace of performance, exaggerates some of the steps (Radhakrishna, John, & Edgar, 2011), or breaks lengthy procedures into a series of shorter steps. This incremental approach to sequencing discrete steps of a procedure is known as **scaffolding** and provides the learner with a clear and exacting image of each stage of skill development (Brookfield, 2006).

In the process of demonstrating a skill to patients and their significant others, it is important to explain why each step needs to be carried out in a certain manner to prevent bad habits from being acquired prior to the learner performing a new skill set (Brookfield, 2006; DeYoung, 2014; Lorig, 2003). Demonstration as a teaching method provides nurses with the opportunity to model their commitment to a learning activity, builds credibility, and inspires learners to achieve a level of excellence (Brookfield, 2006).

The key to performing the demonstration is practice, practice, and practice. If the demonstration is difficult for the nurse, how can you expect your learner to perform the skill? Determine whether the skill is appropriate for the experience level of your learner (Radhakrishna et al., 2011). The nurse's performance should be flawless, but it is important that the nurse take advantage of a mistake to show how errors can be handled. If an error does occur, it may serve to increase rapport with the learners and allow them to relax and not feel intimidated, knowing mistakes do happen and can be corrected (Brookfield, 2006). However, too many mistakes disrupt the mental image that the learners are forming.

When demonstrating a psychomotor skill, if possible, the nurse should work with the exact equipment that the learner is expected to use. This consideration is particularly important for novice learners. For instance, the patient or family member who is learning to carry out an activity of daily living at home will be anxious and frustrated if taught in the hospital or community-based agency with one type of assistive device, such as a wheelchair or shower seat, when another type is used after discharge. Often the learner is too inexperienced to follow the skill pattern and, instead, may become confused when using a different device.

Return demonstration should be planned to occur as close as possible to when the demonstration was given. Learners may need reassurance to reduce their anxiety prior to beginning the performance because the opportunity for return demonstration by them may be viewed as a test. Such a perception may lead them to believe they are expected to carry out a perfect performance the very first time around. Once a learner recognizes that the nurse is a coach and not an evaluator, the climate will be less tense and the learner will be more comfortable in attempting to practice a new skill. Nurses can stress the fact that the initial performance is not expected to be perfect.

In addition, allowing the learner to manipulate the equipment before being expected to use it may help to reduce anxiety levels. Some patients, however, may experience an increased sense of unease when faced with learning a new skill because they identify the need to learn a skill with their illness. For example, a young woman learning to care for a venous access device may be very anxious because her diagnosis of cancer has necessitated the need for this device.

It is important to note that when the learner is giving a return demonstration, the nurse should remain silent except for offering cues when necessary or briefly answering questions. Learners may be prompted by a series of pictures or coached by a partner with a checklist. The first time patients perform a return demonstration, they may need a significant amount of coaching. Nurses should limit their help to coaching—they should *not* do the task for the patients. The next time the patient practices the skill, the nurse should observe and coach only if needed (Lorig, 2003). Also, the nurse should avoid casual conversations or asking questions because they merely serve to interrupt the learner's thought processes and interfere with efforts to focus on mentally imprinting the procedure while performing the task.

Breaking the steps of the procedure into small increments will give the learner the opportunity to master one sequence before attempting the next one. Praising the learner along the way for each step correctly performed reinforces behavior and gives the learner confidence in being able to successfully accomplish the task in its entirety. Emphasis should be on what to do, rather than on what not to do. Practice should be supervised until the learner is competent enough to perform steps accurately.

Different learners will need different amounts of practice to become competent, but once they have acquired the skill, they can then practice on their own to increase speed and proficiency. The value of practice should not be underestimated. For a new skill to become automatic and long lasting, repeated practice beyond the point of mastery is essential (Willingham, 2004). However, if a task is similar to one performed before, less time will be required to master the new skill. For example, a mother who has already learned to use sterile technique at home to change the dressing on her son's abdominal wound will likely learn more quickly and with much more ease how to properly use aseptic measures if she also has to learn how to manage home intravenous therapy.

Table 11–4 Major Advantages and Limitations of Demonstration and Return Demonstration

Advantages
• Especially effective for learning in the psychomotor domain.
• Actively engages the learner through stimulation of visual, auditory, and tactile senses.
• Repetition of movement and constant reinforcement increases confidence, competence, and skill retention.
• Provides opportunity for overlearning to achieve the goal.
Limitations
• Requires plenty of time to be set aside for teaching as well as learning.
• Size of audience must be kept small to ensure opportunity for practice and close supervision.
• Equipment can be expensive to purchase and replace.
• Extra space and equipment is needed for practicing certain skills.
• Competency evaluation requires 1:1 teacher:learner ratio.

Return demonstration sessions should be planned to occur close enough together that the learner does not lose the benefit of the most recent practice session. As with demonstration, the equipment for return demonstration needs to exactly match that used by the nurse and expected to be used by the learner. Learners also will require help in compensating for individual differences. For instance, if you are right-handed and the learner is left-handed, sitting across from each other during instruction would be more helpful than sitting next to one another. The person with difficulty seeing the increments on a syringe may need a magnifying device to accurately perform the skill.

Table 11–4 summarizes the advantages and limitations of demonstration and return demonstration. Perhaps the biggest drawbacks to demonstration and return demonstration are the expenses associated with these methods. Group size must be kept small to ensure that each learner is able to visualize the procedures being performed and to have the opportunity for practice. Individual supervision is required during follow-up practices. Furthermore, the cost of obtaining, maintaining, and replacing equipment can be significant and must be factored into the process.

Gaming

Gaming is a method of instruction requiring the learner to participate in a competitive activity with preset rules (Allery, 2004). The goal is for the learners to win a game by applying knowledge and rehearsing skills previously learned. Games can be simple, or they can be more complex to challenge the learner's ability to use higher-order thinking and problem-solving strategies (Jaffe, 2014).

Gaming activities do not have to reflect reality, but they are designed to accomplish educational objectives. Gaming is primarily effective for improving cognitive functioning but also can be used to enhance skills in the psychomotor domain and to influence affective behavior through increased social interaction (Berbiglia, Goddard, & Littlefield, 1997; Beylefeld & Struwig, 2007; Henry, 1997; Robinson, Lewis, & Robinson, 1990).

In comparison with other teaching methods, gaming is an interactive strategy that creates a dynamic environment for learning. As an experiential approach to learning, the use of games has been found to stimulate enjoyment of learning, increase active participation and engagement of learners, provide variety from a teaching/learning perspective, enhance skill acquisition, and improve problem-solving abilities (Jaffe, 2014; Raines, 2010). Also, evidence suggests that gaming may improve recall and long-term retention of information (Allery, 2004; Beylefeld & Struwig, 2007; Blakely, Skirton, Cooper, Allum, & Nelmes, 2008; O'Leary, Diepenhorst, Churley-Strom, & Magrane, 2005).

Games can be placed anywhere in the sequence of a learning activity (Joos, 1984). For example, they can be used as a device to introduce a topic, check learner progress, or summarize information. However, some games may require prerequisite knowledge for the learner to participate effectively. Therefore, a prior session of teaching may be required before the game can be played (Henry, 1997).

Games can be designed for a single individual, such as puzzles, or for a group of players, such as bingo or Jeopardy! For gaming activities that involve multiple participants, the nurse's role is that of a facilitator. At the beginning of a game, the nurse tells learners the objectives and the rules, distributes any materials required to play the game, and assigns the various teams. Once the game starts, the nurse needs to keep the flow going and interpret the rules. The game should be interrupted as seldom or as briefly as possible so as not to disturb the pace (Joos, 1984).

When the game is completed, winners should be rewarded. Prizes do not have to be expensive because their main purpose is to acknowledge achievement of learners in a public manner (Robinson et al., 1990). At the end of the game, the nurse should conduct a debriefing session to evaluate the gaming experience. Learners should be given a chance to discuss what they learned, ask questions, receive feedback regarding the outcome of the game, and offer suggestions for improving the process.

Games may be either purchased or designed. Well-known commercial games such as Trivial Pursuit, bingo, Monopoly, and Jeopardy! have the advantage in that their formats can be modified, the equipment is reusable for different topics, and many players already have familiarity with the rules of the games (Bender & Randall, 2006). Word searches, crossword puzzles, treasure hunts, and card and board games also are flexible in format and can be developed inexpensively and with relative ease. Nurses should be sure to test any games prior to widespread use. An example of a game used for patient education is a word search puzzle for foods (**Figure 11–1**) known to elevate serum potassium, which is appropriate for use by patients with end-stage renal disease (Robinson et al., 1990).

Computer games, although much more expensive, are becoming increasingly available and are a popular option for many learners (Begg, 2008). Such games, which are also referred to as edutainment (meaning educational software disguised in a game format), introduce content or involve the process of competition to attain a learning goal. They are an enjoyable and effective way to teach specific cognitive, psychomotor, and affective skills. The Game Show Presenter—software that is now available to nurses to create many types of games—can be accessed at http://www.gameshowpresenter.com.

Gaming is an instructional method that is particularly attractive to children, who enjoy the challenge of learning through playlike activity. Lieberman (2001) described an interactive video game designed for patients aged 8–16 years with type 1 diabetes. This

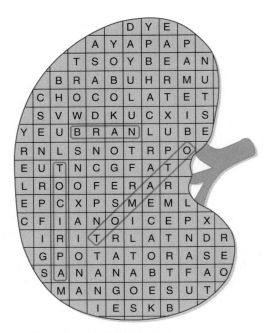

Figure 11–1 Sample word search game for patients

Reprinted with permission of the American Nephrology Nurses Association, publisher, *ANNA Journal*, 17(4), (August 1990), p. 307.

game modeled the daily challenges of self-care, and participants were told to play the game as much or as little as they wished. By the end of the 6-month trial, there was a 77% drop in diabetes-related urgent care as well as an increase in self-efficacy in communication with parents about diabetes and in self-care related to diabetes.

It is particularly important to remember that games, whether purchased or self-developed, must serve the purpose of helping the learner accomplish the predetermined behavioral objectives. Are people learning while they are having fun? Lieberman (2001) also reported that children and adolescents improved their self-care after engaging in interactive games related to smoking prevention, asthma, and diabetes. Other research indicates that electronic games as a tool for patient education have the potential to improve health outcomes ("Editorial," 2009).

Table 11–5 outlines the advantages and limitations of gaming as an instructional method. Economic considerations include either the cost of purchasing a game or the time taken by the nurse to design, test, and update the gaming material. Also, some types of games require the nurse to be present as facilitator each time that they are played.

Simulation

Simulation is a trial-and-error method of teaching whereby an artificial experience is created that engages the learner in an activity that reflects real-life conditions but without the risk-taking consequences of an actual situation. As Gaba (2004) explains, "Simulation is a technique, not a technology, to replace or amplify real experiences with guided

Table 11–5 Major Advantages and Limitations of Gaming

Advantages
• Fun with a purpose.
• Retention of information promoted by stimulating learner enthusiasm and increasing learner involvement.
• Easy to devise or modify for individual or group learning.
• Adds variety to the learning experience.
• Excellent for dull or repetitious content that must be periodically reviewed.

Limitations
• Creates a competitive environment that may be threatening to some learners.
• Requires group size to be kept small for participation by all learners.
• Requires more flexible space for teamwork than a traditional conference or patient education room.
• Potentially higher noise level; special space accommodations are needed as a result.
• May be more physically demanding than many other methods.
• Not possible for learners with some disabilities to participate.

experiences that . . . replicate substantial aspects of the real world in a fully interactive manner" (p. i2). No longer seen as a technological toy for learning basic skills, simulation is now used to help patients learn psychomotor and cognitive skills.

To some extent, overlap exists between the methods of gaming, simulation, and role play, in that all three instructional approaches require learners to engage in experiential learning (Allery, 2004). Simulation allows participants to make decisions in a safe and controlled environment, witness the consequences, and evaluate the effectiveness of their actions (Corbridge et al., 2008; DeYoung, 2014).

A follow-up discussion with learners after use of these experiential methods is important to facilitate their analysis of the experience. Simulation should always be followed by a debriefing session that includes a discussion of events that happened during the experience, the decisions made, the actions taken, the consequences of the choices, the possible alternatives, and suggestions for improvement in skill performance. Simulations provide the opportunity for anticipatory learning (Allery, 2004; Childs & Sepples, 2006; Jeffries, 2005).

When planning a simulation, it is most effective if the nurses make the learning experience resemble real life as much as possible but in a nonthreatening way. The activity should challenge the decision-making ability of the patient and family members by imposing time constraints, providing realistic levels of tension, and using actual equipment or other important features of the environment in which the specific skill will be performed. For example, a scenario could be developed to help parents prevent sudden infant death syndrome by working through a situation in which a monitor signals respiratory difficulty in their baby. As another example, provide the patient in a diabetic self-management education program the opportunity to select foods from a restaurant menu and set his or her insulin pump for the correct bolus of insulin to learn how to master these skills. Such simulations are created for the purpose of determining whether the learner has the necessary skills to perform the activity correctly.

Table 11–6 Major Advantages and Limitations of Simulation

Advantages
• Excellent for psychomotor skill development.
• Enhances higher level problem-solving and interactive abilities in the cognitive and affective domains.
• Provides for active learner involvement in a lifelike situation with consequences determined by variables inherent in the situation.
• Guarantees a safe, nonthreatening environment for learning.

Limitations
• Can be expensive.
• Very labor intensive in many cases.
• Not readily available to all learners yet.

The learning laboratory recently has become a teaching environment for patients and family members to use models, computers, videotapes, and actual equipment, with the nurse in the role of the facilitator, to practice various skills such as sterile techniques and care-giving activities. Simulated experiences for the learner should be followed with actual experiences as soon as possible. Simulation is never exactly the same as the real thing to prepare the learner. Therefore, the learner will need help with the transfer of skills acquired in a simulated experience to the actual situation. Virtual reality technology, which remains in its infancy in healthcare settings, has the potential to narrow the distance even more between simulation and real life for the education of patients and family members (Gaba, 2009; Kaphingst et al., 2009).

Table 11–6 summarizes the main strengths and drawbacks of the simulation method of instruction.

Role Play

Role play is a method of instruction by which patients and family members actively participate in an unrehearsed dramatization. Participants are asked to play an assigned character as they think the character would act in reality. This technique is intended to arouse feelings and elicit emotional responses in the learners. It is used primarily to achieve behavioral objectives in the affective domain. Unlike high-fidelity simulation, which teaches learners to master skills for application to their own real-life situations, role play—a form of simulation—places learners in real-life situations to help them develop understanding of other people and why they behave the way they do (Comer, 2005; Lowenstein & Harris, 2014; Redman, 2007). For example, children may use role play with puppets to explore their responses to such illnesses as asthma (Ramsey & Siroky, 1988).

As a teaching method, role play is a very useful technique because it serves multiple functions: It helps learners to explore their own and others' feelings; gain insight into their values, attitudes, and beliefs; develop problem-solving and decision-making skills; explore a topic in more depth; and develop a better understanding of interpersonal relationships (Billings & Halstead, 2012; Lowenstein & Harris, 2014).

The responsibility of the nurse is to design a situation with enough information for learners to be able to assume the role of someone else without actually giving a script to them to follow. Occasionally, people are assigned to play themselves to rehearse desired behavior, or the nurse takes a part in the role-playing session to act as a positive role model for the learners. Most often, however, the nurse acts as the facilitator and designates members in a group to play particular characters. They then pretend to be these people for the duration of the exercise. Participants do and say things that they perceive actual persons would do, say, and feel.

For role play to be employed effectively, the nurse must be sure that the group has attained a comfort level that allows each member to feel secure enough to participate in a dramatization. This method should never be used with learners at the beginning of a group session encounter. Members need time to establish a rapport with one another as well as with the nurse, or else learners may feel embarrassed or self-conscious about playing a part. All members of the group should be given an assignment to ensure that they are actively involved in the teaching–learning experience (Haggard, 1989). Those who are actual participants need to be informed about the roles they are to portray so that they can effectively develop the appropriate actions. Those who are designated as observers require specific instructions about what to attend to during the role-play session.

The actual length of a role-play session can be as short as 5 minutes, but it should not exceed 15 to 20 minutes (Lowenstein & Harris, 2014). Role play is best done in small groups so that all learners can serve as either players or observers. Active participation by learners is particularly important during a postactivity discussion or debriefing session. Because this instructional method is most effective for learning in the affective domain, all participants need to discuss how they felt and share what they observed to gain insight into their understanding of interpersonal relationships and their reactions to role expectations or conflicts (Comer, 2005).

Table 11–7 summarizes the main advantages and limitations of role play.

Role Modeling

The use of self as a role model is often overlooked as a teaching method. Learning from **role modeling** is called identification and emanates from learning and developmental theories such as Bandura's social learning theory and Erickson's psychosocial stages of development, which explain how people acquire new behaviors and social roles (Crandell,

Table 11–7 Major Advantages and Limitations of Role Play

Advantages
• Opportunity to explore feelings and attitudes.
• Potential for bridging the gap between understanding and feeling.
• Narrows the role distance between and among patients and professionals.

Limitations
• Limited to small groups.
• Tendency by some participants to overly exaggerate their assigned roles.
• A role part loses its realism and credibility if played too dramatically.
• Discomfort felt by some participants in their roles or inability to develop them sufficiently.

Table 11–8 Major Advantages and Limitations of Role Modeling

Advantages
• Influences attitudes to achieve behavior change in the affective domain.
• Potential of positive role models to instill socially desired behaviors.
Limitations
• Requires rapport between the role model and the learner.
• Potential of negative role models to instill unacceptable behaviors.

Crandell, & Vander Zanden, 2012; Snowman & McCown, 2015). This instructional method primarily achieves behavior change in the affective domain.

Nurses have many opportunities to demonstrate behaviors they would like to instill in learners, whether they are patients or family members. The competency with which the nurse as teacher performs a skill, the way he or she interacts with others, the personal example he or she sets, and the enthusiasm and interest he or she conveys about a subject or problem all can influence learners' motivation levels and the extent to which they successfully perform a desired behavior.

Table 11–8 summarizes the advantages and limitations of this method of instruction.

Self-Instruction

Self-instruction is a teaching method used by the nurse to provide or design instructional activities that guide the learner in independently achieving the objectives of learning. Each self-study module usually focuses on one topic, and the hallmark of this format is independent study. The self-instruction method is effective for learning in the cognitive and psychomotor domains, where the goal is to master information and apply it to practice. Self-study also can be an effective adjunct for introducing principles and step-by-step guidelines prior to demonstration of a psychomotor skill.

This teaching method is sometimes difficult to identify as a singular entity because of the variety of terms used to describe it, such as *minicourse, self-instructional package, individualized learning activities,* and *programmed instruction.* For the purposes of this discussion, the term *self-instruction* is used. It is defined as a self-contained instructional activity that allows learners to progress by themselves at their own pace (Abruzzese, 1996).

Self-instruction modules come in a variety of forms, including, but not limited to, workbooks, study guides, workstations, videotapes, Internet modules, and computer programs. They are specifically designed to be used independently. With this instructional technique, the nurse serves as a facilitator/resource person to provide motivation and reinforcement for learning. This method requires less nurse time to give information, and each session with the learner is intended to meet individual needs. For example, patients might learn breast self-examination or CPR techniques by using specifically prepared self-study materials.

Some learners resist the self-instruction method because it appears to depersonalize the teaching–learning process. That perception is not necessarily valid. Communication can still occur between the nurse and the learner, but the focus of instruction is different. The amount of time for direct interaction is more limited than with other methods of teaching such as lecture, group discussion, and one-to-one instruction. This method adheres to the principles of adult education whereby the learner assumes responsibility for learning and is self-directed (Knowles, Holton, & Swanson, 2011).

A self-instruction module is carefully designed to achieve preset objectives by bringing learners from diverse knowledge and skill backgrounds to a similar level of achievement. Modules can be made readily accessible to learners along with any resources that are needed to complete the self-study program. Each self-instruction module needs to contain the following elements:

- An introduction with statement of purpose and directions for how to use the module.
- A list of prerequisite skills that the learner needs to have to use the module.
- A list of behavioral objectives, which are clear and measurable statements describing which skills the learner is expected to acquire.
- A pretest to determine whether the learner needs to proceed with the module based on his or her areas of strength or weakness.
- An identification of resources and learning activities, such as videos, slides, or written materials.
- An outline of the actual learning activities that will be presented in small units of discrete information called frames.
- An estimated total length of time to complete the module. A well-designed module is kept relatively short so as not to dampen the motivation to learn.
- Different presentations for the material based on the objectives and the resources available. For example, information may be given via programmed instruction or through a series of readings.
- Periodic self-assessments to provide feedback to the learner throughout the module to decide whether the previous information has been processed sufficiently enough to move on to the next unit.
- A posttest to evaluate the learner's level of mastery in achieving the objectives. If learners are aware that a posttest needs to be completed, this requirement encourages them to pay attention to the information. Keeping a record of final outcomes is helpful in patient education as documentation of competency.

Self-instruction modules have been found to be cost effective because they are designed for use by large numbers of individuals with minimal and infrequent revisions. It may be less time consuming and more efficient to purchase, rather than produce, a self-instruction module if the information presented in a commercial product is appropriate for the target audience.

The Internet offers a variety of patient education self-instruction modules. The information explosion, coupled with the rapidly advancing technology of computers, has made web-based teaching and learning available to patients and their family members. Also, computer-assisted instruction (CAI) is an individualized method of self-study using technology to deliver an educational activity. CAI allows learners to proceed at their

Table 11–9 **Major Advantages and Limitations of Self-Instruction**

Advantages
• Allows for self-pacing.
• Stimulates active learning.
• Provides opportunity to review and reflect on information.
• Built-in, frequent feedback.
• Indicates mastery of material accomplished in a particular time frame.

Limitations
• Limited with learners who have low literacy skills.
• Not appropriate for learners with visual and hearing impairments.
• Requires high levels of motivation.
• Not good for learners who tend to procrastinate.
• May induce boredom if this method is overused with a population with no variation in the activity design.

own pace with immediate and continuous feedback on their progress as they respond to a software program. Most computer programs assist the learner in primarily achieving cognitive domain skills. CAI offers consistent presentation of material and around-the-clock accessibility. This instructional method not only saves time but also accommodates different types of learners. It allows slow learners to repeat lessons as many times as necessary, while learners who are already familiar with material can skip ahead to more advanced material (DeYoung, 2014).

Some concern has been voiced that computer instruction might depersonalize the learning process (DeYoung, 2014). However, the use of CAI does not preclude the nurse's availability for guidance in learning. While this technology delivers content, it allows more time for the nurse to concentrate on the personal aspects of individual reinforcement and ongoing assessments of learning. For example, CAI has been used with good patient acceptance for precolposcopy education (Martin, Hoffman, & Kaminski, 2005). Recently, computer programs, known as interactive health communication applications (IHCAs), have been used by people with chronic disease. Research findings indicate that IHCAs can improve user knowledge, have a positive effect on social support, lead to better clinical outcomes, and increase self-efficacy (a person's belief in his or her capacity to take specific action) when compared to nonusers of IHCAs (Murray, Burns, Tai, Lai, & Nazareth, 2005).

Table 11–9 lists major advantages and limitations of this method of instruction.

Selection of Teaching Methods

The process of selecting a teaching method requires a prior determination of the behavioral objectives to be accomplished and an assessment of the learners who will be involved in achieving the objectives. Also, consideration must be given to available resources such as time, money, space, and materials to support learning activities as

Table 11–10 General Characteristics of Teaching Methods

Methods	Domain	Learner Role	Nurse Role	Advantages	Limitations
Lecture	Cognitive	Passive	Presents information	Cost effective Targets large groups	Not individualized
Group discussion	Affective Cognitive	Active—if learner participates	Guides and focuses discussion	Stimulates sharing ideas and emotions	Shy or dominant member High levels of diversity
One-to-one instruction	Cognitive Affective Psychomotor	Active	Presents information and facilitates individualized learning	Tailored to individual's needs and goals	Labor intensive Isolates learner
Demonstration	Psychomotor Cognitive	Passive	Models skill or behavior	Preview of exact skill/behavior	Small groups needed to facilitate visualization
Return demonstration	Psychomotor	Active	Individualizes feedback to refine performance	Immediate individual guidance	Labor intensive to view individual performance
Gaming	Cognitive Affective	Active—if learner participates	Oversees pacing Referees Debriefs	Captures learner enthusiasm	Environment too competitive for some learners
Simulation	Cognitive Psychomotor	Active	Designs environment Facilitates process Debriefs	Practice reality in safe setting	Labor intensive Equipment costs
Role playing	Affective	Active	Designs format Debriefs	Develops understanding of others	Exaggeration or underdevelopment of role
Role modeling	Affective Cognitive	Passive	Models skill or behavior	Helps with socialization to role	Requires rapport
Self-instruction	Cognitive Psychomotor	Active	Designs package Gives individual feedback	Self-paced Cost effective Consistent	Procrastination Requires literacy

well as the comfort level of the nurse using particular teaching methods. **Table 11–10** summarizes the general characteristics of teaching methods.

Nurses are at different levels of teaching on the novice-to-expert continuum, which influences their choices of teaching methods. For example, an expert skilled at facilitating small-group discussion may be a novice in the design and selection of games. Also, nurses tend to focus on a particular teaching method because it is the one they feel most comfortable using without considering all the criteria for selection. There is no one right method, because the best approach depends on many variables, such as the audience, the content to be taught, the setting in which teaching and learning are to take place, and the resources available.

A novice should begin instruction with very familiar content so that he or she can focus on the teaching process itself and feel more confident in trying out different techniques and strategies for instruction. He or she should ask questions of patients and family members in the evaluation process to determine whether the teaching method chosen was appropriate for accomplishing the behavioral objectives and for meeting the expectations of different learners in terms of their learning needs and styles, and readiness to learn.

Evaluation of Teaching Methods

An important aspect of evaluating any instructional program is to assess the effectiveness of the method (Friedman et al., 2011). Was the option selected as effective, efficient, and appropriately used as possible? Nurses should ask four major questions to help decide which teaching method to choose or whether the method of instruction selected should be revised or rejected:

1. *Does the teaching method help the learners to achieve the stated objectives?* This question is the most important criterion for evaluation—if the method does not help to accomplish the objectives, then all the other criteria are unimportant.
2. *Is the learning activity accessible and acceptable to the learners who have been targeted?* Patients and their family members need programs to be offered at suitable times and accessible locations. For example, childbirth preparation classes scheduled during the daytime hours likely would not be convenient for expectant couples who are working. Also, does the teaching method appeal to the learner(s) in terms of their learning needs, learning style(s), and readiness to learn characteristics?
3. *Is the teaching method efficient given the time, energy, and resources available in relation to the number of learners the nurse is trying to reach?* To teach large numbers of learners, nurses must choose a method that can accommodate groups, such as lecture, discussion sessions, or role play, or a method that can reach many individuals at one time, such as the use of various self-instructional formats. Sufficient resources and equipment are needed to adequately deliver the message intended. In this era of cost containment, employers and insurers want their money invested in patient education methods that yield the best possible outcomes at the lowest price—as measured in terms of preventing illness and injury, minimizing the severity and extent of illness, and reducing lengths of stay and readmissions—and that lead to consumer satisfaction.
4. *To what extent does the teaching method allow for active participation to accommodate the needs, abilities, and style of the learner?* Active participation has been well documented as a way to increase interest in learning and the retention of

information. Evaluate how active learners want to be or are able to be in the process of gaining knowledge and skills. No one method can satisfy all learners, but adhering to one method exclusively addresses the preferred style of only a segment of the audience.

General Principles for Teaching Across Methodologies

No matter which teaching method is chosen to reach the intended learner(s) and to accomplish the behavioral objectives set forth, it is important to consider some basic rules that will enhance the teaching–learning experience. The following, in no order of priority, are some of the key principles nurses should adhere to when teaching patients and their significant others (Bradshaw & Lowenstein, 2014; Crandell et al., 2012; Falvo, 2010; Miller & Stoeckel, 2016; Phillips, 1999; Snowman & McCown, 2015).

Give Positive Reinforcement

Educational research clearly indicates the effects of positive reinforcement on learning. Acknowledging ideas, actions, and opinions of others by using words of praise or approval, such as "That's a good answer," "I agree with you," and "You have a very good point," or using nonverbal expressions of acceptance, such as smiling, nodding, or a reassuring pat on the back, encourages learners to participate more readily or try harder to improve their performance. Rewarding even a small success can instill satisfaction in the learner. Positive reinforcers, in the form of recognition, tangible rewards, or opportunities, should closely follow the desired behavior. The clearer the correlation between the desired behavior and the reward, the more meaningful the reinforcement. Criticism, on the other hand, dampens motivation and causes learners to withdraw.

What constitutes positive reinforcement for one individual may not suffice for another, because rewards are closely tied to value systems. Also, the quantity of reinforcement varies in its effectiveness from one individual to another. A small amount of praise can have a strong effect on the learner who is not used to succeeding, whereas significant praise may be relatively ineffective for a consistently high achiever. In addition, an incentive that works for a learner at one time may not work well at another time depending on the circumstances.

Project an Attitude of Acceptance and Sensitivity

The ease with which nurses conduct themselves, the willingness to receive and answer questions, the simple courtesies extended, and the responsiveness demonstrated toward an audience are all actions that set the tone for a friendly, warm, and receptive atmosphere for learning. If the nurse exhibits self-confidence and self-respect, the learner will feel comfortable, confident, and secure in the learning environment. If the nurse comes across as believable, trustworthy, considerate and competent, he or she helps to put the patients and family members at ease, which serves as an invitation for them to learn. When the nurse exercises patience and sensitivity with respect to age, race, culture, and gender, this attitude projects an acceptance of others, which serves to establish a rapport and opens up avenues of communication for the sharing of ideas and concerns.

People learn better in a comfortable and supportive environment. Not only is it important that the physical environment be conducive to learning, but the psychological climate also should be respectful of learners and focused on their need for an atmosphere of support and acceptance. Nurses must have a clear view of their role as facilitators and expert coaches and avoid acting as controlling givers of information.

Be Organized and Give Direction

Instruction should be logically organized, objectives clearly defined and presented up front, and directions given in a straightforward, specific, and easily understood manner. Audiovisual materials selected to supplement various methods of teaching should clarify or enhance a message.

Instructional sessions should be relatively brief, so as not to overload the learner with too much detail and extraneous content. Regardless of the method of instruction used, the attention span of the learner waxes and wanes over time, and what is learned first and last is retained the most (Ley, 1972). Need-to-know information should take precedence over nice-to-know information, thereby ensuring that enough time is allotted to cover the essentials. As Kessels (2003) has clearly documented, "40–80% of medical information provided by healthcare practitioners is forgotten immediately. The greater the amount of information presented, the lower the proportion correctly recalled; furthermore, almost half of the information that is remembered is incorrect" (p. 219).

Advance organizers—that is, topic headings that clue the learner into what will be presented and help focus the learner's attention on the message—should be used to structure information. These headers assist the learner in identifying the subject to be addressed and anticipating in which order the information will be presented.

Elicit and Give Feedback

Feedback should be a two-way process. It is a strategy to give information to the learner as well as to receive information from the learner. Both the nurse and the learner need to seek information about the quality of their performance. Feedback should be encouraged during and at the end of each teaching–learning encounter as well as at the completion of an educational program. It can take the form of either verbal or nonverbal responses to a situation.

Feedback that learners receive can be subjective or objective. Subjective data, whether physiological or psychological, come from within the learners themselves. People sense how they are reacting to a situation. Internally, they usually know how well they performed or how they feel by their own responses, such as fatigue, anxiety, disinterest, or satisfaction. Learners are able to compare their own performance to what they expect of themselves or what they think others expect of them.

Objective data come to learners from the nurse, who measures their behavior based on a set of standards or criteria and who gives them an opinion on the progress they have made. To get feedback, the learner might ask, "How well did I do?" "Am I on track?" "Did I do all right?" or "What do you think?"

Feedback to the nurse is equally important, because the effectiveness of teaching depends to a great extent on the learners' reactions. Whether positive or negative, verbal or nonverbal, feedback enables the nurse to determine whether he or she should maintain or modify his or her approach to teaching. Feedback indicates whether to proceed, take time to review or explain, or cease instruction altogether for the moment.

The nurse should be direct in requesting feedback from the learners by asking questions such as "What questions do you have?" "How clear is this to you?" "What needs to be explained further?" or "What more can I help you with?" In addition, the nurse should be sensitive to nonverbal expressions such as a nod, a smile, a look of bewilderment, or a frown indicating an understanding or lack thereof.

Feedback is neutral unless it is compared with established norms, preset criteria, or past behavior. How much someone learned, for example, is meaningless unless compared to what the person knew previously or how the person stacks up against other learners under similar conditions.

Feedback, either positive or negative, is needed by both the learner and the teacher. Praise reinforces behavior and increases the likelihood that the behavior will continue. Constructive criticism tends to redirect behavior to conform with expected norms. Labeling someone's personality as cooperative, smart, stubborn, unmotivated, or uncaring is harmful, but it is helpful to label someone's performance as excellent or in need of further practice to give that person specific information for improving, correcting, or continuing the behavior.

Use Questions

Questioning is a means by which both the nurse and the learner can elicit feedback about performance. If the nurse is skillful in the use of questioning, it serves multiple purposes in the teaching–learning process. Questions may help to clarify concepts, assess what the learner already knows about the topic, stimulate interest in a new subject, or evaluate the learner's mastery of the predetermined behavioral objectives.

Babcock and Miller (1994) identified three types of questions that can be used to elicit different types of answers:

1. Factual or descriptive questions begin with words such as *who, what, which, where, how,* or *when* and ask for recall-type responses from the learner. Factual questions such as "Which foods are high in fat?" "Who should you call if you run out of medication?" or "How often on average do you use your inhaler?" elicit straightforward facts. Descriptive questions take a more open-ended approach, such as "Which kinds of exercise do you get daily?" "What problems do you have with activities of daily living?" or "What are the signs and symptoms of infection?" These questions require a more detailed and organized response from the learner.

2. Clarifying questions ask for more information and help the learner to convey thoughts and feelings. Such questions might include "What do you mean when you say . . .?" or "When do you feel most anxious?"
3. Higher order questions require more than memory or perception to answer. They ask the learner to draw conclusions, establish cause and effect, or make comparisons. Examples include "Why does a low-salt diet help to control blood pressure?" "What do you think will happen if you don't take your medication?" and "What do you see as the advantages and disadvantages in following the treatment plan?"

After asking questions, a period of silence may occur. This gap can be uncomfortable for both the nurse and the learner. Nurses can reduce anxiety over silence by encouraging the learner to think about the answer before responding. In a group, this strategy also allows all participants to have a chance to think through their responses to the questions, which gives them the opportunity to make more thoughtful and deliberate responses. How long a nurse should wait for a response depends on many variables, such as how complex the question is, who the learners are, and what they are expected to know. Wait time is a matter of judgment on the part of the nurse.

Questioning helps the nurse appropriately pace the material being presented. Also, answers to questions allow the nurse to arrive at an evaluative judgment as to the progress the learner is making in the achievement of the behavioral objectives.

Use the Teach-Back or Tell-Back Strategy

Many patients who have been taught about their health problem, how to prevent disease, or how to follow recommended treatment regimens to promote or maintain their health do not always fully and accurately understand the information that has been given to them. When patients are asked to explain what they have been told by their nurse or other healthcare provider, it becomes evident that for various reasons there are many gaps and errors in the information they interpreted and remembered (Floyd, Lang, McCord, & Keener, 2004; Ley, 1972, 1979; Kessels, 2003).

Thus, nurses who teach patients using various teaching methods and instructional materials must assess how well and how much patients understood the information given to them before they are expected to independently care for themselves. It is important that nurses ask patients to restate in their own words what they learned to confirm their retention of information and the effectiveness of the patient education interventions. A key strategy to determine the extent of patients' understanding following each patient education encounter is known as the teach-back, tell-back, or show me approach to evaluate learning.

This specific educational technique is patient and family centered and results in improved nurse–patient communication, increased patient satisfaction with care, improved quality of care, and the opportunity to assess patient health literacy (Fidyk et al., 2014; Jager & Wynia, 2012; Kandula, Malli, Zei, Larson, & Baker, 2011; Nigolian & Miller, 2011). It also has been shown to decrease hospital average lengths of stay and readmission rates (Fidyk et al., 2014). Multiple studies have demonstrated that patients prefer and perceive the teach-back, tell-back, or show me strategy because they find it most effective for learning (Hyde & Kautz, 2014; Kemp et al., 2008).

Know the Audience

The effectiveness of teaching can be severely limited when the choice of instructional method is based on the interest and comfort level of the nurse and not on the assessed needs of the learner. Nurses must use methods that match the topic rather than their own personality (Glenn, 2009).

Most nurses have a preferred style of teaching and tend to rely on that approach regardless of the content to be taught. Nurses skilled at teaching, however, adapt themselves to a teaching style appropriate to the subject matter, setting, and various styles of the learners. Flexibility is their hallmark in tailoring the instructional design to the unique needs of each population of learners. All nurses should be willing to use a variety of teaching methods to provide the best possible experience for achievement of objectives.

Use Repetition and Pacing

Repetition, if used in the right amount, is a technique that strengthens and reinforces learning by aiding in the retention of information (Willingham, 2004). If overused, however, repetition can lead to boredom and frustration because the nurse is repeating what is already understood and remembered. If used carefully, it can assist the learner in focusing on important points and can help keep the learner on track.

Repetition is especially important when presenting new or difficult material. The opportunity for repeated practice of behavioral tasks is called **skill inoculation**. Repetition can take the form of a simple reminder, a review of previously learned material, or the continued practice of a skill. Assessing the learner's understanding helps nurses use repetition effectively.

Pacing refers to the speed at which information is presented. Some self-instruction methods of teaching, such as programmed instruction, allow for individualized pacing so that learners can move along at their own speed, depending on their abilities and style of learning. Other methods, such as group learning, require the nurse to take command of the rate at which information is presented and processed.

Many factors determine the optimal rate of teaching, such as the following:

- Previous history with learning
- Attention span
- The domain in which learning is to take place
- The learner's eagerness and determination to obtain a reward or attain a goal
- The degree of progress in learning
- The learner's ability to cope with frustration and discomfort

Keeping in touch with the learner(s) helps nurses pace their teaching. It should be slow enough to allow learners to absorb the information presented, yet fast enough to maintain their interest and enthusiasm.

Summarize Important Points

Summarizing information at the completion of the teaching–learning session gives a perspective on what has been covered, how it relates to the objectives, and what the nurse expects the learner to have achieved. Summarizing also reviews key ideas to instill information in the mind and helps the learner to see the parts of a whole. Closure should be achieved at the end of one lesson before proceeding to a new topic. Summary reinforces retention of information. It also provides feedback as to the progress made, thereby leaving the learner with a feeling of satisfaction with what has been accomplished.

Settings for Teaching

Traditionally, the primary focus of nursing practice has been on the delivery of acute care in hospital settings. In recent years, however, the practice of nursing in community-based settings has experienced tremendous growth. The reasons for the shift in orientation of nursing practice from inpatient to outpatient care sites relate to the trends affecting the nation's healthcare system as a whole. These trends include public and private reimbursement policies, changing population demographics, advances in healthcare technology, an emphasis on wellness care, and increased consumer interest in health. In response to these trends, nursing practice has broadened to include a greater emphasis on the delivery of care in community settings such as homes, clinics, health maintenance organizations, physicians' offices, public schools, and the workplace.

With the increased focus on prevention, promotion, and independence in self-care activities, today's newly emerging healthcare system mandates the education of consumers to a greater extent than ever before. Opportunities for patient teaching have become increasingly more varied in terms of the types of patients encountered, their particular learning needs, and the settings in which healthcare teaching occurs. Because health education has become an increasingly important responsibility of nurses in all practice environments, it is important to acknowledge the various settings where clients, well or ill, may be consumers of health care.

Settings for teaching are classified according to the relationship health education has to the primary purpose of the organization or agency that provides health instruction. An *instructional setting* is defined as any place where nurses engage in teaching for disease prevention, health promotion, and health maintenance and rehabilitation. It comprises any environment in which health education takes place to provide individuals with learning experiences for the purpose of improving their health or reducing their risk for illness and injury. O'Halloran (2003) identified three types of settings for the education of patients:

1. A **healthcare setting** is one in which the delivery of health care is the primary or sole function of the institution, organization, or agency. Hospitals, visiting nurse home care associations, public health departments, outpatient clinics,

extended-care facilities, health maintenance organizations, physicians' offices, and therapist-owned and -managed centers are some examples of organizations whose primary purpose is to deliver health care. Health education is a part of the overall care delivered within these settings. Nurses function to provide direct patient care in this setting, and their role encompasses the teaching of patients as part of that care.

2. A **healthcare-related setting** is one in which healthcare-related services are offered as a complementary function of the agency. Examples of this type of setting include the American Heart Association, the American Cancer Society, the American Arthritis Association, and the Muscular Dystrophy Association. These organizations provide patient advocacy, conduct health screenings and self-help groups, distribute health education information and materials, and support research on disease and lifestyle issues for the benefit of consumers within the community. Education on health promotion, disease prevention, and improving the quality of life for those who live with a particular illness or disability is the key function of nurses within these agencies.

3. A **nonhealthcare setting** is one in which health care is an incidental or supportive function of an organization. Examples of this type of setting include businesses, industries, schools, and military and penal institutions. The primary purpose of these organizations is to produce a manufactured product or offer a non-health-related service to the public. Industries, for example, are involved in health care only to the extent of providing health screenings and nonemergency health coverage to their employees through a health office within their place of employment, making available instruction in job-related health and safety issues to meet Occupational Safety and Health Administration (OSHA) regulations, or providing opportunities for health education through wellness programs to reduce absenteeism or improve employee health status and morale.

Nurses must recognize the numerous opportunities available for the teaching of those individuals who are currently or potentially consumers of health care. Given that teaching is an important aspect of healthcare delivery and that nurses function as teachers in a multitude of settings, they will inevitably encounter patients of differing ages and at various stages along the wellness-to-illness continuum. Wherever and whenever teaching takes place, nurses need to recognize the importance of consciously applying the principles of teaching and learning to these encounters for maximum effectiveness in helping patients to attain and maintain optimal health.

Professional nurses involved in patient health education should use available opportunities to share resources among the three identified settings (**Figure 11–2**). Many already perform this service, as printed or audiovisual materials are borrowed, rented, or purchased for small fees from area institutions, organizations, or agencies; nurses from one setting are contracted for or voluntarily provide health education programs to small and large groups in another setting; and nurses from each category of setting collaborate on individual patient situations or on major community health projects.

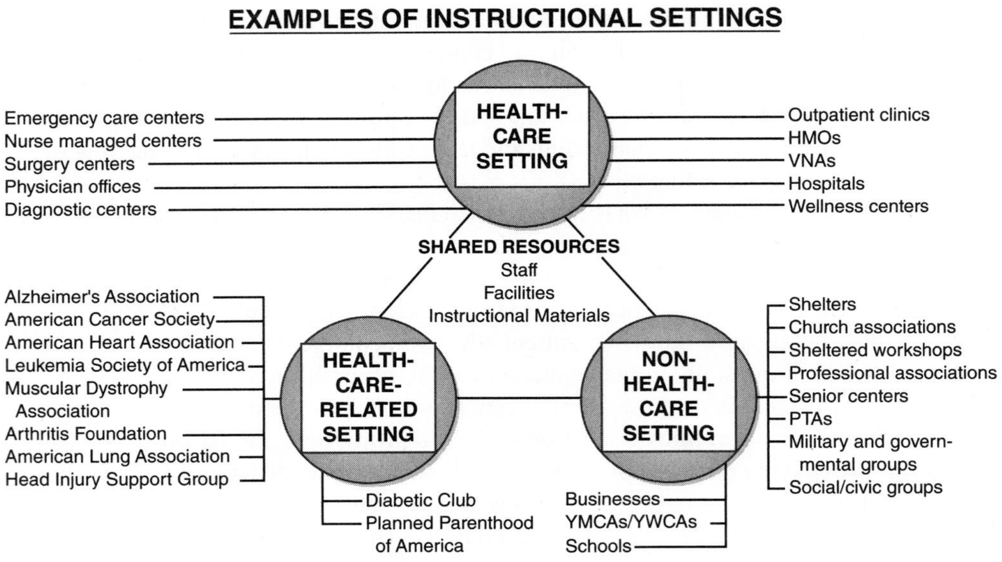

EXAMPLES OF INSTRUCTIONAL SETTINGS

Figure 11–2   Types of settings for health teaching

Summary

This chapter presented an in-depth review of the various teaching methods and compared the advantages and limitations of each approach. Also, it briefly addressed the settings in which teaching takes place. Emphasis was given to the importance of taking into account the patients' and family members' characteristics, the behavioral objectives, the nurse's characteristics, and available resources prior to selecting and using any of the vast array of methods at the nurse's disposal.

In many instances, guidelines were put forth to assist nurses in planning and developing their own instructional activities. In addition, the major questions to be considered when evaluating the effectiveness of teaching methods were assessed in detail. Finally, some general principles to increase the effectiveness of all methods of instruction were discussed.

What must be stressed are the qualities specific to each method and the fact that no one method is better than another. The effectiveness of any method depends on the purpose for and the circumstances under which it is used. Nurses in the role of teachers are urged to take different approaches to teaching rather than rely on any one particular method. Varying the teaching methods or using methods in combination with one another can assist nurses in accomplishing the objectives for learning while meeting the different needs and styles of each and every learner.

Review Questions

1. How is the term *teaching method* defined?
2. What are the advantages and limitations of each teaching method?

3. Which methods used for instruction are most effective in encouraging active participation by the learner?
4. Which teaching methods are best for learning cognitive skills? Psychomotor skills? Affective skills?
5. Which variables influence the selection of any method of instruction?
6. Which major questions should nurses ask themselves when evaluating the effectiveness of a teaching method? Which question is the most important criterion for evaluation?
7. What are the general principles that can be applied to teaching no matter what method is chosen?
8. Are teachers born or made? Explain.
9. What are the three classifications of settings for teaching?

Case Study

Mary Beech, a 67-year-old white female, is newly diagnosed with type 2 diabetes. She has a history of hypertension, obesity, and peripheral vascular disease. At her doctor's appointment today, the nurse, Karen, plans to provide patient teaching on how to manage diabetes at home. She has gathered teaching materials, including the brochures *Facts about Diabetes* and *How to Manage Diabetes at Home*. Karen also plans to show a video that covers basic information about diabetes management, such as how to use the blood glucose meter.

After Mrs. Beech is provided with the brochures to read and she is shown the video, Karen asks, "What questions do you have about diabetes management?" Mrs. Beech replies, "I don't know. I'm overwhelmed with all this information and don't have any idea where to begin!"

1. If the nurse wants to encourage Mrs. Beech to take an active role in managing her diabetes at home, what teaching methods can she select that complement the instructional materials she has provided? Why?
2. What are the advantages of the teach-back approach after information has been given to the patient? Are there any limitations to using this approach?
3. An evaluation of any educational session is vitally important to determine the effectiveness of the teaching method(s) used. What four major questions should be asked to determine if a teaching method was appropriate?

References

Abruzzese, R. S. (1996). *Nursing staff development: Strategies for success* (2nd ed.). St. Louis, MO: Mosby-Year Book.

Allery, L. A. (2004). Educational games and structured experiences. *Medical Teacher, 26*(6), 504–505.

Babcock, D. E., & Miller, M. A. (1994). *Patient education: Theory and practice*. St. Louis, MO: Mosby-Year Book.

Bain, K. (2004, April 9). What makes great teachers great? *Chronicle of Higher Education*, B7–B9.

Bartlett, T. (2003, May 9). Big, but not bad. *Chronicle of Higher Education*, 35–38.

Begg, M. (2008). Leveraging game-informed healthcare education. *Medical Teacher, 30*, 155–158.

Bender, D., & Randall, K. E. (2006). Description and evaluation of an interactive Jeopardy game designed to foster self-assessment. *Internet Journal of Allied Health Sciences and Practice, 3*(4), 1–7.

Berbiglia, V. A., Goddard, L., & Littlefield, J. H. (1997). Gaming: A strategy for honors programs. *Journal of Nursing Education, 36*(6), 289–291.

Beylefeld, A. A., & Struwig, M. C. (2007). A gaming approach to learning medical microbiology: Students' experiences of flow. *Medical Teacher, 29*, 933–940.

Billings, D. M., & Halstead, J. A. (2012). *Teaching in nursing: A guide for faculty* (4th ed.). St. Louis, MO: Saunders Elsevier.

Blakely, G., Skirton, H., Cooper, S., Allum, P., & Nelmes, P. (2008, August 13). Educational gaming in the health sciences: Systematic review. *Journal of Advanced Nursing*, 259–269.

Boyd, M. D., Gleit, C. J., Graham, B. A., & Whitman, N. I. (1998). *Health teaching in nursing practice: A professional model* (3rd ed.). Stamford, CT: Appleton & Lange.

Bradshaw, M. J., & Lowenstein, A. J. (2014). *Innovative teaching strategies in nursing and related health professions* (6th ed.). Burlington, MA: Jones & Bartlett Learning.

Brookfield, S. D. (2006). *The skillful teacher: On technique, trust, and responsiveness in the classroom.* San Francisco, CA: Jossey-Bass.

Brookfield, S. D., & Preskill, S. (2005). *Discussion as a way of teaching: Tools and techniques for democratic classrooms* (2nd ed.). San Francisco, CA: Jossey-Bass.

Burkhart, J. A. (2008). Training nurses to be teachers. *Journal of Continuing Education in Nursing, 39*(11), 503–510.

Cantillon, P. (2003, February 22). ABC of learning and teaching in medicine: Teaching large groups. *British Medical Journal, 326*, 437–440.

Childs, J. C., & Sepples, S. (2006). Clinical teaching by simulation: Lessons learned from a complex patient care scenario. *Nursing Education Perspectives, 27*(3), 154–158.

Comer, S. K. (2005). Patient care simulations: Role playing to enhance clinical understanding. *Nursing Education Perspectives, 26*(6), 357–361.

Cook, D., Levinson, A., Garside, S., Dupras, D., Erwin, P., & Montori, V. (2008). Internet-based learning in the health professions: A meta-analysis. *Journal of the American Medical Association, 300*(10), 1181–1196.

Cooper, H., Booth, K., Fear, S., & Gill, G. (2001). Chronic disease patient education: Lessons from meta-analyses. *Patient Education and Counseling, 44*, 107–117.

Corbridge, S., McLaughlin, R., Tiffen, J., Wade, L., Templin, R., & Corbridge, T. C. (2008). Using simulation to enhance knowledge and confidence. *Nurse Practitioner, 33*(6), 12–13.

Crandell, T. L., Crandell, C. H., & Vander Zanden, J. W. (2012). *Human development* (11th ed.). New York, NY: McGraw-Hill.

Deakin, T., McShane, C. E., Cade, J. E., & Williams, R. D. (2005). Group-based training for self-management strategies in people with type 2 diabetes mellitus. *Cochrane Database of Systematic Reviews, 2*, CD003417. doi:10.1002/14651858. CD1858.CD003417.pub2

DeYoung, S. (2014). *Teaching strategies for nurse educators* (3rd ed.). Upper Saddle River, NJ: Prentice Hall.

Editorial: Games people play could be good for their health, sense of empowerment. (2009). *Patient Education Management, 16*(12), 133–135.

Evans, M. (2000). Polished, professional presentation: Unlocking the design elements. *Journal of Continuing Education in Nursing, 31*(5), 213–218.

Falvo, D. R. (2010). *Effective patient education: A guide to increased adherence* (4th ed.). Sudbury, MA: Jones & Bartlett Learning.

Fidyk, L., Ventura, K., & Green, K. (2014). Teaching nurses how to teach. *Journal of Nurses in Professional Development, 30*(5), 248–253.

Floyd, M. R., Lang, F., McCord, R. S., & Keener, M. (2004). Patients with worry: Presentations of concerns and expectations for response. *Patient Education and Counseling, 57,* 211–216.

Fredette, S. L. (1990). A model for improving cancer patient education. *Cancer Nursing, 13,* 207–215.

Friedman, A. J., Cosby, R., Boyko, S., Hatton-Bauer, J., & Turnbull, G. (2011). Effective teaching strategies and methods of delivery for patient education: A systematic review and practice guideline recommendations. *Journal of Cancer Education, 26,* 12–21.

Gaba, D. M. (2004). The future vision of simulation in health care. *Quality and Safety in Health Care, 13,* i2–i10.

Gaba, D. M. (2009). Do as we say, not as you do: Using simulation to investigate clinical behavior in action. *Simulation in Healthcare, 4*(2), 67–69.

Gleasman-DeSimone, S. (2012). *How nurse practitioners educate their adult patients about healthy behaviors: A mixed method study* (Unpublished dissertation in partial fulfillment for the degree of Doctor of Philosophy). Capella University.

Glenn, D. (2009, December 15). Matching teaching style to learning style may not help students. *Chronicle of Higher Education.* Retrieved from http://chronicle.com/article/Matching-Teaching-Style-to /49497/

Haggard, A. (1989). *Handbook of patient education.* Rockville, MD: Aspen.

Henry, J. M. (1997). Gaming: A teaching strategy to enhance adult learning. *Journal of Continuing Education in Nursing, 28,* 231–234.

House, B. M., Chassie, M. B., & Spohn, B. B. (1990). Questioning: An essential ingredient in effective teaching. *Journal of Continuing Education in Nursing, 21,* 196–201.

Hyde, Y. M., & Kautz, D. D. (2014). Enhancing health promotion during rehabilitation through information-giving, partnership-building, and teach-back. *Rehabilitation Nursing, 39,* 178–182.

Jacobs, K. (2009). Professional presentations and publications. In E. Creapeau, E. Cohn, & B. Boyt Schell (Eds.), *Willard and Spackman's occupational therapy* (11th ed., pp. 411–417). Philadelphia, PA: Wolters Kluwer/Lippincott Williams & Wilkins.

Jaffe, L. (2014). Games are multidimensional in educational situations. In M. J. Bradshaw & A. J. Lowenstein (Eds.), *Innovative teaching strategies in nursing and related health professions* (6th ed., pp. 183–202). Burlington, MA: Jones & Bartlett Learning.

Jager, A. J., & Wynia, M. K. (2012). Who gets a teach-back? Patient-reported incidence of experiencing a teach-back. *Journal of Health Communications, 17,* 294–302.

Jeffries, P. R. (2005). A framework for designing, implementing, and evaluating simulations used as teaching strategies in nursing. *Nursing Education Perspectives, 26*(2), 96–103.

Johnson, D. W., Johnson, R. T., & Smith, K. (2007). The state of cooperative learning in post-secondary and professional settings. *Educational Psychology Review, 19,* 15–29.

Joos, I. R. M. (1984). A teacher's guide for using games and simulation. *Nurse Educator, 9*(3), 25–29.

Kandula, N. R., Malli, T., Zei, C. P., Larson, E., & Baker, D. W. (2011). Literacy and retention of information after a multimedia diabetes educational program and teach-back. *Journal of Health Communications, 16,* 89–102.

Kaphingst, K. A., Persky, S., McCall, C., Lachance, C., Lowenstein, J., Beall, A. C., & Blascovich, J. (2009). Testing the effects of educational strategies on comprehension of a genomic concept using virtual reality technology. *Patient Education and Counseling, 77,* 224–230.

Kemp, E. C., Floyd, M. R., McCord-Duncan, E., & Lang, F. (2008). Patients prefer the method of "Tell-Back Collaborative Inquiry" to assess understanding of medical information. *Journal of the American Board of Family Medicine, 21*(1), 24–30.

Kessels, R. P. (2003). Patients' memory for medical information. *Journal of the Royal Society of Medicine, 96,* 219–222.

Knowles, M. S., Holton, E. F., & Swanson, R. A. (2011). *The adult learner: The defensive classic in adult education and human resource development* (7th ed.). Houston, TX: Gulf Publishing.

Kowalski, K. (2004). The use of set. *Journal of Continuing Education in Nursing, 35*(2), 56–57.

Ley, P. (1972). Primacy, rated importance, and recall of medical statements. *Journal of Health and Social Behavior, 13*, 311–317.

Ley, P. (1979). Memory for medical information. *British Journal of Social Clinical Psychology, 18*, 245–266.

Lieberman, D. (2001). Management of chronic pediatric diseases with interactive health games: Theory and research findings. *Journal of Ambulatory Care Management, 24*(1), 26–38.

Lorig, K. R. (2003). Taking patient ed to the next level: Patients with chronic illnesses need more than traditional patient education. They need you to help them develop the self-management skills that they'll use for the rest of their lives. *RN, 66*(12), 35–44.

Lorig, K., & Gonzalez, V. M. (1993). Using self-efficacy theory in patient education. In B. Gilroth (Ed.), *Managing hospital-based patient education* (pp. 327–337). Chicago, IL: American Hospital Publishing.

Lowenstein, A. J., & Harris, M. (2014). Role play. In M. J. Bradshaw & A. J. Lowenstein, *Innovative teaching strategies in nursing and related health professions* (6th ed., pp. 183–202). Burlington, MA: Jones & Bartlett Learning.

Martin, J. T., Hoffman, M. K., & Kaminski, P. F. (2005). NPs vs. IT for effective colposcopy patient education. *Nurse Practitioner, 30*(4), 52–57.

Miller, M. A., & Stoeckel, P. R. (2016). *Patient education: Theory and practice* (2nd ed.). Burlington, MA: Jones & Bartlett Learning.

Murray, E., Burns, J., Tai, S. S., Lai, R., & Nazareth, I. (2005). Interactive health communication applications for people with chronic disease (review). *Cochrane Database of Systematic Reviews, 4*, 70.

Nigolian, C. J., & Miller, K. L. (2011). Teaching essential skills to family caregivers: Nurses can use "teachable moments" to help the transition from hospital to home care. *The American Journal of Nursing, 111*(11), 52–57.

Oakley, B., & Brent, R. (2004). Turning student groups into effective teams. *Journal of Student Centered Learning, 2*(1), 9–34.

Oermann, M. H. (2003). Effects of educational intervention in waiting room on patient satisfaction. *Journal of Ambulatory Care Management, 26*(2), 150–158.

O'Halloran, V. E. (2003). Instructional settings. In S. B. Bastable (Ed.), *Nurse as educator: Principles of teaching and learning for nursing practice* (2nd ed., pp. 465–492). Sudbury, MA: Jones and Bartlett.

O'Leary, S., Diepenhorst, L., Churley-Strom, R., & Magrane, D. (2005). Educational games in an obstetrics and gynecology core curriculum. *American Journal of Obstetrics & Gynecology, 193*, 1848–1851.

Phillips, L. D. (1999). Patient education: Understanding the process to maximize time and outcomes. *Journal of Intravenous Nursing, 22*(1), 19–35.

Prochaska, J., DiClemente, C., Velicer, W., & Rossi, J. (1993). Standardized, individualized, interactive, and personalized self-help programs for smoking cessation. *Health Psychology, 12*(5), 399–405.

Prochaska, J., Velicer, W., Rossi, J., Goldstein, M., Marcus, B., Rakowski, W., Rossi, S. R. (1994). Stages of change and decisional balance for 12 problem behaviors. *Health Psychology, 13*(1), 39–46.

Radhakrishna, R., John, C. E., & Edgar, P. Y. (2011). Teaching tips/notes. *NACTA Journal, 55*(2), 92–95.

Raines, D. A. (2010). An innovation to facilitate student engagement and learning: Crossword puzzles in the classroom. *Teaching and Learning in Nursing, 5*(2), 85–90.

Ramsey, A. M., & Siroky, A. S. (1988). The use of puppets to teach school-aged children with asthma. *Pediatric Nursing, 14*, 187–190.

Redman, B. K. (2007). *The practice of patient education: A case study approach* (10th ed.). St. Louis, MO: Mosby Elsevier.

Ridley, R. T. (2007). Interactive teaching: A concept analysis. *Journal of Nursing Education, 46*(5), 203–209.

Robinson, K. J., Lewis, D. J., & Robinson, J. A. (1990). Games: A way to give laboratory values meaning. *American Nephrology Nurses Association Journal, 17*(4), 306–308.

Rothwell, W. J., & Kazanas, H. C. (2008). *Mastering the instructional design process: A systematic approach* (4th ed.). San Francisco, CA: Pfeiffer.

Saarmann, L., Daugherty, J., & Riegel, B. (2000). Patient teaching to promote behavior change. *Nursing Outlook, 48*(6), 281–287.

Silberman, M. (2006). *Active training: A handbook of techniques, designs, case examples and tips.* San Francisco, CA: Pfeiffer, John Wiley & Sons.

Snowman, J., & McCown, R. (2015). *Psychology applied to teaching* (14th ed.). Stamford, CA: Wadsworth/ Cengage Learning.

Springer, L., Stanne, M. E., & Donovan, S. S. (1999). Effects of small-group learning on undergraduates in science, mathematics, engineering, and technology: A meta-analysis. *Review of Educational Research, 69*(1), 21–51.

Tang, T. S., Funnell, M. M., & Anderson, R. M. (2006). Group education strategies for diabetes self-management. *Diabetes Spectrum, 19*(2), 99–105.

Vermeire, E., Hearnshaw, H., Van Royen, P., & Denekens, J. (2001). Patient adherence to treatment: Three decades of research. A comprehensive review. *Journal of Clinical Pharmacy and Therapeutics, 26,* 331–342. doi:10.1046/j.1365-2710.2001.00363.x

Willingham, D. T. (2004, Spring). Practice makes perfect: But only if you practice beyond the point of perfection. *American Educator*, 31–33, 38.

Woodring, B. C., & Woodring, R. C. (2014). The lecture: Long-lasting, logical, and legitimate. In M. S. Bradshaw & A. J. Lowenstein (Eds.), *Innovative teaching strategies in nursing and related health professions* (pp. 127–148). Burlington, MA: Jones & Bartlett Learning.

Young, P., & Diekelmann, N. (2002). Learning to lecture: Exploring the skills, strategies, and practices of new teachers in nursing education. *Journal of Nursing Education, 41*(9), 405–412.

Instructional Materials

Diane Hainsworth | Susan Bastable | Kara Keyes

Chapter Highlights

- General Principles
- Choosing Instructional Materials
- The Three Major Components of Instructional Materials
  - *Delivery System*
  - *Content*
  - *Presentation*
- Types of Instructional Materials
  - *Written Materials*
  - *Demonstration Materials*
  - *Audiovisual Materials*
- Evaluating Instructional Materials

Key Terms

analogue
audiovisual materials
blended learning
characteristics of the learner
characteristics of the medium
characteristics of the task
delivery system
illusionary representations
instructional materials
multimedia learning
realia
replica
symbol
symbolic representations
tailored instruction

Objectives

After completing this chapter, the reader will be able to

1. Differentiate between instructional materials and teaching methods.

2. Discuss general principles that apply to all types of instructional materials.

3. Identify the three major variables (learner, task, and medium characteristics) to be considered when selecting, developing, and evaluating instructional materials.

4. Cite the three components of instructional materials required to effectively communicate patient education messages.

5. Identify the many types of instructional materials—printed, demonstration, and audiovisual media—available for teaching patients and their family members.

6. Describe the general guidelines for development of printed materials.

7. Analyze the advantages and disadvantages specific to each type of instructional material.
8. Evaluate the type of materials suitable for instruction depending on such variables as the size of the audience, the resources available, and the characteristics of the learner.
9. Identify where instructional materials can be found.
10. Critique instructional materials for value and appropriateness.
11. Recognize the supplemental nature of instructional materials in patient education.

Whereas teaching methods are the approaches the nurse uses to deliver patient education, **instructional materials** are the objects or vehicles by which information is communicated. Often these terms are used interchangeably and are frequently referred to in combination with one another as teaching strategies and techniques. Nevertheless, teaching methods and instructional materials are not one and the same, and a clear distinction can and should be made between them. Teaching methods are the way information is taught. Instructional materials, which include printed, demonstration, and audiovisual media, are the tools used to enhance teaching and learning. How effective these multimedia approaches are must be based on theory about the way people learn, on studies that examine the effects of each tool on the learner, and on evidence from practice (R. E. Mayer, 2014).

Instructional materials are the tools and aids used to transmit information that supplement, rather than replace, the act of teaching and the role of the nurse as teacher. These materials by which information is shared with the learner must be examined closely because they represent an important aspect of the education process. Given the numerous factors affecting both the teacher and the learner, such as the increase in nursing staff workloads, the decrease in length of inpatient stays or outpatient visits, the increase in patient acuity, the alternative settings in which education is now delivered, the varied learner characteristics and preferences, and the shrinking resources for patient education, it is imperative that nurses understand the various types of printed, demonstration, and audiovisual materials available to help nurses teach efficiently and effectively.

Instructional materials provide the nurse with tools to deliver information creatively, clearly, accurately, and in a timely manner. They help nurses reinforce information, clarify abstract concepts, and simplify complex messages. Multimedia resources serve to stimulate a learner's senses as well as add variety, realism, and enjoyment to the teaching–learning experience. They have the potential to assist patients and their family members not only in acquiring knowledge and skills but also in retaining more effectively what they learn. Research indicates that a variety of printed, demonstration, and audiovisual materials do, indeed, enhance teaching and learning (Friedman, Cosby, Boyko, Hatton-Bauer, & Turnbull, 2011).

This chapter provides an overview of how to select, develop, implement, and evaluate instructional materials. The advantages and disadvantages of the various types of instructional materials are discussed. The choice of one or more of them often depends on availability and cost. This chapter is intended to assist nurses to make informed decisions about choosing and using appropriate instructional materials that fit the learner, that affect the motivation of the learner, and that accomplish the expected learning outcomes.

General Principles

Before selecting or developing instructional materials from the many available options, nurses should be aware of the following general principles regarding the effectiveness of these tools:

- The teacher must be familiar with the content and mechanics of a tool before using it.
- Printed, demonstration, and audiovisual materials can change learner behavior by influencing cognitive, affective, and psychomotor development.
- No one tool is better than another to enhance learning because the suitability of any particular instructional material depends on many variables.
- Instructional materials should complement, reinforce, and supplement—not substitute for—the nurse's teaching efforts.
- The choice of material should match the content and the tasks to be learned.
- The instructional material(s) selected should match available financial resources.
- Instructional aids must be appropriate for the physical conditions of the learning environment, such as the number of learners, the space, the lighting, the sound projection, and the hardware (delivery mechanisms) used to display information.
- Instructional materials should match the sensory abilities, developmental stages, and educational level of the learners.
- The messages conveyed by instructional materials must be accurate, up to date, appropriate, unbiased, and free of any unintended content.
- The tools used should contribute in a meaningful way to the learning situation by adding or clarifying information.

Choosing Instructional Materials

Nurses must consider many important variables when selecting instructional materials. The role of the nurse goes beyond the giving of information only; it also involves skill in designing and planning for instruction. Learning can be made more enjoyable for both the learner and the teacher if the nurse knows which instructional materials are available, as well as how to choose and use them so as to best enhance the teaching–learning experience.

Knowledge of the different instructional materials available and their appropriate use helps nurses make patient education more interesting, challenging, and effective for all types of learners. With current trends in healthcare reform, instructional materials for patient education need to include content on health promotion, illness prevention, health maintenance, and rehabilitation.

Making appropriate choices of instructional materials depends on a broad understanding of three major variables: (1) **characteristics of the learner**, (2) **characteristics of the medium**, and (3) **characteristics of the task** to be achieved (Frantz, 1980). A useful mnemonic for remembering these variables is LMAT—standing for learner, medium, and task.

1. *Characteristics of the learner.* Many variables are known to influence learning. Nurses, therefore, must know their audience so that they can choose those tools best suited to the needs and abilities of various learners. They must consider sensory and motor abilities, reading skills, motivational levels (locus of control), developmental stages, learning styles, gender, socioeconomic characteristics, and cultural backgrounds.

2. *Characteristics of the medium.* A wide variety of mediums—printed, demonstration, and audiovisual—are available to enhance teaching methods. Print materials are the most common form through which information is communicated, but demonstration tools and nonprint media, which include a large range of audio and visual possibilities, are popular and useful choices. Because no single medium is more effective than all other options, the nurse should be flexible in considering a multimedia approach to complement methods of instruction.

3. *Characteristics of the task.* Identifying the type of learning domain (cognitive, affective, and/or psychomotor), as well as the complexity of behaviors to be achieved to meet identified objectives, defines the task(s) that must be accomplished.

The Three Major Components of Instructional Materials

Depending on the teaching methods chosen to communicate information, nurses must decide which instructional materials are potentially best suited to assist with the process of teaching and learning. The delivery system (Weston & Cranston, 1986), content, and presentation (Frantz, 1980) are the three major components that nurses should keep in mind when selecting print and nonprint materials for instruction.

Delivery System

The **delivery system** includes both the software and the hardware used in presenting information. For instance, the nurse giving a lecture might choose to enhance the information being presented by using PowerPoint slides (software) delivered via a computer (hardware). The content on DVDs (software), in conjunction with a DVD player (hardware), and CD-ROM programs (software), in conjunction with computers (hardware), are other examples of delivery systems.

The choice of the delivery system is influenced by the number of learners to be taught at any one time, the size of the intended audience, the pacing and flexibility needed for the effective delivery of information, and the sensory aspects most suitable to an individual patient or group of patients and family members.

Content

The content (intended message) is independent of the delivery system and is the actual information being communicated to the learner. When selecting instructional material(s), the nurse must consider several factors:

- The accuracy of the information being conveyed. Is it up to date and accurate?
- The appropriateness of the medium to convey particular information. Pamphlets, posters, and podcasts, for example, can be very useful tools for sharing information to change behavior in the cognitive or affective domain but are not ideal for skill development in the psychomotor domain. Videos as well as real equipment or models with which to perform demonstrations and return demonstrations are much more effective tools for learning psychomotor behaviors.
- The appropriateness of the readability level of materials for the learner(s). Is the content written at a literacy level suitable for the patient's reading and comprehension abilities? The more complex the task, the more important it is to write clear, simple, succinct instructions enhanced with illustrations so that patients can understand the content.

Presentation

The form of the message is a very important component for selecting or developing instructional materials. However, a consideration of this aspect of any tool is frequently ignored. Weston and Cranston (1986) describe the form of the message as occurring along a continuum from concrete (real objects) to abstract (symbols).

REALIA

Realia (the condition of being real) refers to the most concrete form of stimuli that can be used to deliver information. For instance, a woman demonstrating breast self-examination is the closest example to reality. Because this form of presentation might be less acceptable for a wide range of teaching situations, the next best choice would be a manikin. Such a model, which is similar to a human figure, has many characteristics that simulate reality, including size and three dimensionality (width, breadth, and depth), but without being the true figure that may very well cause embarrassment for the learner. The message is less concrete, yet using an imitation of a person as an instructional tool allows for an accurate presentation of information to stimulate the learners' perceptual abilities. Further along the continuum of realia is a video presentation of a woman performing breast self-examination. The learner could still visualize a breast self-examination done accurately, but the aspect of three dimensionality is absent in a video format. In turn, the message becomes less concrete and more abstract.

ILLUSIONARY REPRESENTATIONS

The term **illusionary representations** applies to a less concrete, more abstract form of stimuli through which to deliver a message, such as moving or still photographs, audiotapes projecting true sounds, and real-life drawings. Although many realistic cues, such as dimensionality, are missing, this category of instructional materials has the advantage of offering learners a variety of real-life visual and auditory experiences to which they might otherwise not have access or exposure because of such factors as location, availability, or expense.

SYMBOLIC REPRESENTATIONS

The term **symbolic representations** refers to the most abstract types of messages, though they are the most common form of instructional materials to communicate information. These types of representations include numbers and letters of the alphabet, symbols that are written and spoken as words that convey ideas or represent objects. Audiotapes of someone speaking, graphs, written texts, handouts, posters, flip charts, and whiteboards on which to display words and images are vehicles to deliver messages in symbolic form. The chief disadvantage of symbolic representations is that they lack being concrete. The more abstract and sophisticated the message, the more difficult it is to comprehend. Consequently, symbolic representations may be inappropriate as instructional materials for patients who are very young, from different cultures, with significant literacy problems, or with cognitive and sensory impairments.

When making decisions about which tools to select to best accomplish teaching and learning objectives, the nurse should carefully consider these three media components. When choosing from a wide range of print, demonstration, and audiovisual options, key issues to be taken into account include the various delivery systems available, the content or message to be conveyed, and the form in which information will be presented. Nurses must remember that no single medium is suitable for all learners to acquire and retain information. Most important, the function of instructional materials must be understood—that is, to supplement, complement, and support the nurse's teaching efforts for the successful achievement of learner outcomes.

Types of Instructional Materials

Written Materials

Handouts, such as leaflets, books, pamphlets, brochures, and instruction sheets (all symbolic representations), are the most widely used and most accessible type of tools for teaching. Printed materials have been described as "frozen language" (Redman, 2007, p. 34) and are the most common form of teaching aid because of the distinct advantages they provide to enhance teaching and learning.

The greatest strengths of written materials are as follows:

- Available as a reference to reinforce information for learners when the nurse is not immediately present to answer questions or clarify information.
- Widely used at all levels of society, so this medium is acceptable and familiar to the public.
- Easily obtained through commercial sources, usually at relatively low cost and on a wide variety of subjects, for distribution by nurses.

- Provided in convenient forms, such as pamphlets, which are portable, reusable, and do not require software or hardware resources for access.
- Becoming more widely available in languages other than English as a result of the recognition of significant cultural and ethnic shifts in the general population.
- Suitable to a large number of learners who prefer reading as opposed to receiving messages in other formats.
- Flexible in that the information is absorbed at a speed controlled by the reader.

The disadvantages of printed materials include the following facts:

- Written words are the most abstract form through which to convey information.
- Immediate feedback on the information presented may be limited.
- A large percentage of materials are written at too high levels for reading and comprehension by the majority of patients (Doak, Doak, Friedell, & Meade, 1998; G. Mayer & Villaire, 2009).
- Written materials are inappropriate for persons with visual or cognitive impairment.

COMMERCIALLY PREPARED MATERIALS

A variety of brochures, posters, pamphlets, and patient-focused instructional sheets are available from commercial vendors. Whether such materials enhance the quality of learning is an important question for nurses to consider when evaluating these products for content, readability, and presentation. Commercial products may or may not be produced in collaboration with health professionals, which raises the question of how factual and understandable the information may be. For example, materials prepared by pharmaceutical companies or medical supply companies might not be free of bias and may contain complex language. Nurses must ask several questions when reviewing printed materials that have been prepared commercially, including the following:

- Who produced the item?
- Can the item be previewed?
- Is the price of the instructional tool consistent with its educational value?
- Can the tool be used with large numbers of learners?
- How quickly will the information become outdated?

The main advantage of using commercial materials is that they are readily available and can be obtained in bulk for free or at a relatively low cost (Fraze, Griffith, Green, & McElroy, 2010). A nurse might need to spend hours researching, writing, and copying materials to create informational resources of equal quality and value, so commercially produced materials can save valuable time. Also, some commercial materials that can be customized to the needs of individual patients are accessible online.

The disadvantages of using commercial materials include issues of cost, accuracy and adequacy of content, and readability of the materials. Some educational booklets are expensive to purchase and impractical to give away in large quantities. Fraze and associates (2010) have developed a checklist to help healthcare providers determine the appropriateness of printed education materials for use by their patients to improve health outcomes in various clinical settings.

SELF-COMPOSED MATERIALS

Nurses may choose to write their own instructional materials to save costs or to tailor content to specific audiences. Composing materials offers many advantages (Brownson, 1998; Doak et al., 1998). For example, by writing their own materials, nurses can tailor the information to accomplish the following points:

- Fit the institution's policies, procedures, and equipment
- Build in answers to those questions asked most frequently by patients
- Highlight points considered especially important by the team of physicians, nurses, and other health professionals at their institution or agency
- Reinforce specific oral instructions that clarify difficult concepts and address specific patient needs

Doak and colleagues (1998) outline specific suggestions for tailoring information to help patients read and remember the message and to act on it. These authors define **tailored instruction** as personalizing the message so that the content, structure, and image fit an individual patient's learning needs. To accomplish this goal, they suggest techniques such as writing the patient's name on the cover of a pamphlet and opening a pamphlet with a patient and highlighting the most important information as it is verbally reviewed. In another example, Feldman (2004) describes successful use of childcare checklists that had simple line drawings (no more than two to a page) along with brief written descriptions that led parents with cognitive disabilities through specific care tasks, such as bathing a baby, in a step-by-step fashion. Audiotapes also accompanied these pictures and simple instructions. Additional studies support the effectiveness of tailored instruction over nontailored messages in achieving reading, recall, and follow-through in health teaching (Campbell et al., 1994; Skinner, Strecher, & Hospers, 1994).

Of course, composing materials also has disadvantages. Nurses need to be extra careful to be sure that materials are well written, attractive, and well laid out, which can be a time-consuming task. Although nurses are expected to enhance their methods of teaching with instructional materials, few have ever had formal training in the development and application of written materials. Many tools produced by nurses are too long, too detailed, and written at too high a level for the target audience. See Chapter 7 for the 27 guidelines on how to simplify printed education materials (PEMs) so that they are more readable.

Also, Doak, Doak, and Root (1996) and Brownson (1998) suggest the following important tips to be sure self-composed PEMs are clear and appropriate:

- Make certain the content is accurate and up to date.
- Organize the content in a logical, step-by-step, simple fashion so that learners are being informed adequately but are not overwhelmed with large amounts of information. Avoid giving details because they may unnecessarily lengthen the written information and make it more complex than it should be. Prioritize the content to address only what learners need to know. Content that is nice to know can be addressed verbally on an individual basis.
- Make sure the information clearly and concisely discusses the *what*, *how*, and *when*. Follow the KISS rule: Keep it simple and smart. This can best be accomplished by putting the information into a question-and-answer format or by dividing the content into subheadings according to key topics to be addressed.

- Avoid medical jargon whenever possible, and define any technical terms using simple, everyday language. If it is important to expose patients to technical terms because these are what they will hear when dealing with their medical situation and with the medical team, define the terms carefully and simply and be consistent with the words used.
- Find out the average grade in school completed by the targeted patient population, and write the education materials two to four grade levels below the average calculated. For patients and their family members who are not literate, pictures can increase recall of spoken medical instruction (Houts et al., 1998; Houts, Doak, Doak, & Loscalzo, 2006; Kessels, 2003).

Always state things in positive, not negative, terms. Never illustrate incorrect messages. For example, showing a hand holding a metered-dose inhaler in the mouth not only incorrectly illustrates a drug delivery technique (Weixler, 1994) but also reinforces that message through the image's visual impact alone. **Figure 12–1** illustrates the correct way to use an inhaler and reinforces a positive message.

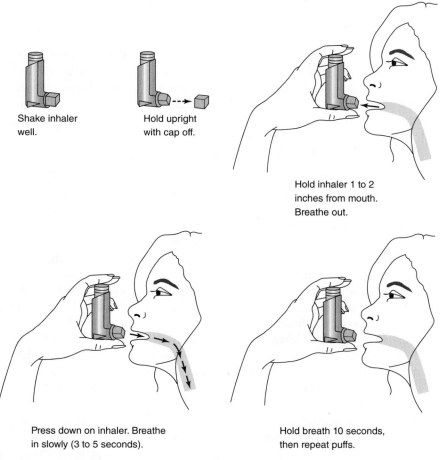

Shake inhaler
well.

Hold upright
with cap off.

Hold inhaler 1 to 2
inches from mouth.
Breathe out.

Press down on inhaler. Breathe
in slowly (3 to 5 seconds).

Hold breath 10 seconds,
then repeat puffs.

Figure 12–1 Diagram illustrating proper technique for inhaler use

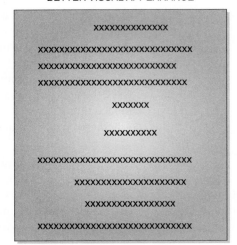

CLUTTERED APPEARANCE   BETTER VISUAL APPEARANCE

Figure 12–2   Inadequate versus adequate appearance and formatting

In addition to the guidelines for clarity in constructing written materials, format and appearance are equally important in motivating learners to read the printed word. If the format and appearance are too detailed, learners will feel overwhelmed; in such a case, instead of attracting the learners, you will discourage and turn them off. **Figure 12–2** illustrates how a simple rather than lengthy format is much more appealing to any reader.

EVALUATING PRINTED MATERIALS

When evaluating PEMs, nurses should keep in mind the following considerations.

1. *Nature of the audience.* What is the average age of the audience? For instance, adults who are literate tend to prefer printed materials that they can read at their leisure. Children or adult patients who have low literacy skills, however, like short and simple printed materials with many illustrations.

    Also, what is the preferred learning style of the particular audience? Printed materials with few illustrations are poorly suited to patients who not only have difficulty reading but also do not like to read. Information in the form of simple pictures, graphs, and charts can be included with the content of printed materials for the benefit of those individuals who have low literacy skills or who are visual and conceptual learners (Houts et al., 2006).

    In addition, does the audience have any sensory deficits? Vision problems are common among older adult patients, and deficits in short-term memory may pose a problem for comprehension. Having materials that can be reread at the learner's own convenience and pace can reinforce earlier learning and reduce confusion over treatment instructions. For those individuals with vision impairments, use a large typeface and lots of white space, separate one section from another with plenty of spacing, highlight important points, and use black print on white paper.

2. *Literacy level required.* PEMs for helping patients accomplish behavioral objectives will not be effective if the materials are written at a level beyond the ability of the learner to understand (G. Mayer & Villaire, 2009). The Joint Commission mandates that health information be presented in a manner that can be understood by patients and family members. Therefore, it is important to screen potential educational tools that will be used with various teaching methods. A number of formulas (e.g., Fog, SMOG, Fry) are available to determine the reading difficulty level as outlined in Chapter 7 and **Appendix 7–A**.

3. *Linguistic variety available.* This refers to choices of printed materials in different languages that may be accessed. However, these options often are limited because duplicate materials in more than one language are costly to publish and not likely to always be produced unless the publisher anticipates a large demand. The growth of minority populations in the United States has promoted increasing attention to the need for non-English teaching materials. Regional differences exist, such that there may be greater availability of Asian language materials on the West Coast and more Spanish-language materials in the Southwest and Northeast than in other parts of the United States.

4. *Clarity and brevity.* Simpler is better. Shorter also is better. Remind yourself of the KISS rule: Keep it simple and smart. Address the important facts only. What does the patient need to know? Choose words that explain *how*; the *why* can be filled in later during, for example, one-to-one instruction or group discussion. Include uncomplicated pictures and basic illustrations that show step by step the written instructions. **Figure 12–3** provides a good example of a clear, brief, easy-to-follow instructional tool that is used to teach a patient with asthma how to determine when a metered-dose inhaler is empty. By using simple, clear graphics and few words, the learner is guided through the procedure with very little room for misunderstanding, and this tool is suitable for a wide range of audiences.

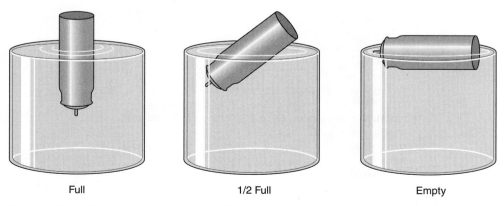

Full   1/2 Full   Empty

Figure 12–3 Example of a clear, easy-to-follow instructional tool for an asthma patient

5. *Layout and appearance.* How written materials look is crucial in attracting the attention of patients and getting them to read the information. If a tool has too much wording, with few spaces between sentences and paragraphs, small margins, and many pages of content, the patient may find it much too difficult and too time consuming to read (see Figure 12–2).

   Allowing plenty of white space is the most important step that nurses can take to improve the appearance of written materials. This means creating a lot of blank space between and around the words by double spacing, leaving wide margins, indenting important points, using bold lettering, and separating key statements with extra space. Putting a graphic in the middle of the text can break up the print and provide a way to reinforce the written information. Redman (2007) states that pictures rather than spoken words are better for learning because they increase recognition and recall. An example used earlier in this chapter is teaching the psychomotor task of using a metered-dose inhaler (see Figure 12–1). **Figure 12–4** includes simple step-by-step instructions written in the active voice on how to carry out this technique correctly.

6. *Opportunity for repetition.* Written materials can be read later and again and again by the learner to reinforce the teaching when the nurse is not there to answer questions. Thus it is an advantage if materials are laid out in a simple question-and-answer format. Questions demand answers, and this format allows patients to find information easily for repeated reinforcement of important messages. If nurses write their own materials, they also must be mindful of the need to keep information current and to update it for changing protocols and varied patient populations.

7. *Concreteness and familiarity.* Using the active voice (present tense) is more immediate, directive, and concrete. For example, "Shake the inhaler very well three times" is more effective than "The inhaler should be shaken thoroughly" (see Figure 12–4). Also, the importance of using plain language instead of medical jargon cannot be stressed enough. Inadequate patient understanding of common

---

STEPS FOR CORRECT INHALER TECHNIQUE

1. Shake the inhaler very well three times.
2. Remove cap and hold inhaler upright.
3. Hold the inhaler 1 to 2 inches from your mouth.
4. Tilt your head back slightly and breathe out fully.
5. Press down on the inhaler and start to breathe in slowly.
6. Breathe in slowly and deeply (3 to 5 seconds) to pull the medicine down into your lungs.
7. Hold your breath for 10 seconds to keep the medicine in your lungs.
8. Take a few normal breaths.
9. Repeat puffs by following steps 1–8 again.

Figure 12–4 Example of instructions written in an active voice

medical terms used by healthcare providers is a significant factor in noncompliance with medical regimens. A number of studies indicate that patients understand medical terms at a much lower rate than nurses expect (D'Alessandro, Kingsley, & Johnson-West, 2001; Estey, Musseau, & Keehn, 1994; Friedman et al, 2011; Lerner, Jehle, Janicke, & Moscati, 2000; G. Mayer & Villaire, 2009).

In summary, nurse-designed or commercially produced PEMs are widely used for a broad range of audiences. They vary in literacy demand levels and may be found written in several languages. Studies on the effectiveness of PEMs on patient health outcomes have reported varied results. If PEMs are used alone, the effect has been small (Giguere et al., 2012). If used in combination with written and verbal information, they improved patients' knowledge and satisfaction with care (Johnson & Sandford, 2005). The literacy level of written communication materials is a major factor in the usefulness of print materials (D'Allessandro et al., 2001; G. Mayer & Villaire, 2009). **Table 12–1** summarizes their basic advantages and disadvantages.

Demonstration Materials

Demonstration materials include many types of visual, hands-on mediums. Models and real equipment are one type, and a combination of printed words and visual illustrations (diagrams, graphs, charts, photographs, and drawings) in the form of displays are another type. Displays include such instructional tools as posters, bulletin boards, flannel boards, flip charts, chalkboards, and whiteboards. These types of mediums represent unique ways of communicating messages to the learner. Demonstration materials primarily stimulate the visual senses but can combine the sense of sight with touch and sometimes even smell and taste. From these various forms of demonstration materials, the nurse can choose one or more to complement teaching efforts that will help patients achieve the objectives for learning. Just as with written materials, these tools must be accurate and appropriate for the intended audience. Ideally, they will bring the learner closer to reality and actively engage him or her in a visual and active manner. As such, demonstration tools are useful for cognitive, affective, and psychomotor skill development. The major forms of demonstration materials—models and displays—are discussed in detail here.

Table 12–1 Basic Advantages and Disadvantages of Printed Materials

Advantages	Disadvantages
Materials are easily accessible and available on many topics.	They are impersonal.
The rate of reading is controlled by the reader.	There is limited feedback; the absence of an instructor lessens opportunity to clear up misinterpretation.
Complex concepts can be explained both fully and adequately.	
Procedural steps can be outlined.	Printed materials are passive tools.
Verbal instruction can be reinforced.	Highly complex materials may be overwhelming to the learner.
The learner is always able to refer back to instructions given in print.	Literacy skill of the learner may limit effectiveness.
	Materials may not be available in different languages.

MODELS

Models are three-dimensional objects that allow the learner to immediately apply knowledge and psychomotor skills by observing, examining, manipulating, handling, assembling, and disassembling them while the teacher provides feedback (Rankin & Stallings, 2005). In addition, these demonstration aids encourage learners to think abstractly and to use many of their senses (Boyd, Gleit, Graham, & Whitman, 1998). Whenever possible, the use of real objects and actual equipment is preferred—but a model is the next best thing when the real object is not available, accessible, or feasible, or is too complex to use. Because approximately 30% to 40% of people are visual learners and 20% to 25% are kinesthetic (hands-on) learners, using models not only capitalizes on their learning styles (preference for learning) but also enhances their retention and understanding of new information (Aldridge, 2009).

Three specific types of models are used for teaching and learning, as differentiated by Babcock and Miller (1994):

- Replicas, associated with the word *resemble*
- Analogues, associated with the words *act like*
- Symbols, associated with the words *stands for*

A **replica** is an exact copy constructed to scale that resembles the features or substance of the original object. The dimensions of the reproduction may be decreased or enlarged in size to make demonstration easier and more understandable. A replica of the DNA helix is an excellent example of a model used to teach the complex concept of genetics. Replicas can be examined and manipulated by the learner to get an idea of how something looks and works. They are excellent choices for teaching psychomotor skills because they give the learner an opportunity for active participation through hands-on experience. Not only can the learner assemble and disassemble parts to see how they fit and operate, but the learner can also control the pace of learning.

Replicas are used frequently by the nurse when teaching the anatomy and physiology of different parts of the body. Models of the brain, limbs, heart, kidney, ear, eye, joints, and pelvic organs, for example, allow the learner to visualize parts of the body not readily viewed or impossible to see without these teaching aids. Resuscitation dolls are a popular type of replica used to teach the skills of cardiopulmonary resuscitation. Learners who regularly refresh their skills using demonstration models as instructional tools are more likely to maintain their knowledge of and ability to use techniques as compared with those learners who do not (Pinto, 1993).

Using a replica first to learn a technique can desensitize patients and their family members before they are taught to do an invasive procedure on themselves or on a loved one. Instructional models have been found to be effective in reducing fear and enhancing acceptance of certain procedures (Cobussen-Boekhorst, Van Der Weide, Feitz, & DeGier, 2000). For example, teaching a patient with diabetes how to draw up and inject insulin can best be accomplished by using a combination of real equipment and replicas. Patients first draw up sterile saline in real syringes, practice injecting oranges, and then progress to a model of a person before actually injecting themselves. Sometimes showing a video before directly handling equipment may be helpful if learners are very anxious about performing various procedures. For lessons aimed at psychomotor learning, nurses can use skills checklists as a way to evaluate the accuracy of return demonstrations. Simulation laboratories, for example, often use this evaluation method (Jeffries, 2005; Siwe, Bertero, Pugh, & Wijma, 2009).

The second type of model is known as an **analogue** because it has the same properties and performs like the real object. Unlike replicas, analogue models are effective in explaining and representing dynamic systems. Although costly, a sophisticated human patient simulator is an analogue. The patient simulator is a manikin that physiologically responds to treatment in a manner similar to what would occur in live human beings. Clinical simulators for patient education have been an untapped resource for teaching and learning that shows promise in changing knowledge and attitudes (Siwe et al., 2009).

The third type of model is a **symbol**, which is used frequently in teaching situations. Written words, mathematical signs and formulas, diagrams, cartoons, printed handouts, and traffic signs are all examples of symbolic models that convey a message to the receiver through a visual image or association. International signs, for example, communicate familiar messages that individuals with different language abilities or from multicultural backgrounds can understand. However, abbreviations common to healthcare personnel, such as NPO, PRN, and QD, should be avoided when interacting with patients and their families because they are likely to be unfamiliar with these abbreviations.

The advantage of models is that they can adequately take the place of a real object, which may be too small, too large, too expensive, too complex, unavailable, or inappropriate for use in a teaching–learning situation. A variety of models can be purchased from commercial vendors at varying prices (some for free) or can be made by the teacher. Models do not need to be expensive or elaborate to get concepts and ideas across (Aldridge, 2009; Rankin & Stallings, 2005). In particular, models enhance learning in the following ways:

- Allow learners to practice acquiring new skills without being afraid of hurting themselves or others
- Stimulate active learner involvement
- Provide the opportunity for immediate testing of psychomotor and cognitive behaviors
- Allow learners to receive instant feedback
- Appeal to the kinesthetic (movement oriented) learner who prefers the hands-on approach to learning

In terms of their disadvantages, some models may not be suitable for learners with poor abstract thinking skills or visual impairments unless each individual is given the chance to learn about the object using other senses. Also, some models can be fragile, very expensive, bulky to store, and difficult to transport. Unless models are very large, they cannot be observed and manipulated by more than a few learners at any one time. However, this drawback can be overcome by using team teaching and by creating different stations at which to arrange replicas for demonstration purposes (Babcock & Miller, 1994).

DISPLAYS

Whiteboards, posters, storyboards, flip charts, and bulletin boards are examples of displays that can be used for patient education. Displays are two-dimensional objects that serve as useful tools for a variety of teaching purposes. They can be used to convey simple or short messages and to clarify, reinforce, or summarize information on important topics and themes. Although they have been referred to as static instructional tools given that they are often stationary (Haggard, 1989), some displays can be transported, and some can be altered to change the message when necessary. Demonstration tools can effectively achieve behavioral objectives by vividly representing relationships between subjects or objects. Whiteboards and flip charts are particularly versatile means of delivering information. Storyboards—visual tools that use pictures and written text to explain a sequence of events—are effective in providing consistent messages to patients in a simple, easy-to-understand format (Lowenstein, Foord, & Romano, 2009).

Information on displays can be added, corrected, or deleted quickly and easily while the learners are actively following what the teacher is doing or saying. Such tools are excellent means of encouraging active participation, keeping the learners' attention on the topic at hand, and reinforcing the contributions of others. Flexible and handy, they provide opportunities for the teacher, in an immediate and direct fashion, to organize data, capture ideas, perform on-the-spot problem solving, and compare various points of view. Also, unlike some other types of visuals, these display tools can allow learners to see parts of a whole picture while assisting the teacher in filling in the gaps.

The following are important guidelines suggested by Babcock and Miller (1994) for nurses using chalkboards and whiteboards to teach:

- Be sure writing is legible and large enough to be seen.
- Step aside and face the learner(s) after putting notes on the board to maintain contact with the audience.
- Allow learners time to copy or think about the message.
- Ask a note taker to capture a creative design or record an idea before the contents on the board are erased or changed.

The following are some specific advantages of displays as teaching tools:

- They are a quick way to attract attention and get an idea across.
- Most are flexible, easily modified, and reusable.
- Many are portable and easily assembled or disassembled.
- They stimulate interest or ideas in the observer.
- They are effective ways of influencing cognitive and affective behaviors.

In contrast, some of the disadvantages of displays include the following:

- They may take up a lot of space.
- The more static types, such as posters, can be time consuming to have prepared and for that reason tend to be used as displays for a long time, which increases the risk of them becoming outdated.
- Some displays (e.g., posters and bulletin boards) are not suitable for large audiences if information needs to be viewed at the same time.

- Only limited amounts of information can be included at one time.
- Displays are not effective for teaching psychomotor skills.
- They may become too cluttered when a lot of information is placed on them.
- If permanently mounted, they cannot be transported.
- The symbolic nature of the message may not be well understood by some learners.

POSTERS

Although they are a type of display material, posters are addressed separately here because they have become an increasingly popular and important instructional tool (www .cdc.gov; www.uptodate.org; www.accenthealth.com). Essentially hybrids of print and visual media, posters use the written word along with graphic illustrations. Posters are an effective and reasonable option for conveying information (Daley, 1997; Duchin & Sherwood, 1990; Flournoy, Turner, & Combs, 2000; Moneyham, Ura, Ellwood, & Bruno, 1996; Pulley, Brace, Bernard, & Masys, 2007). They serve as a visual supplement to oral instruction of patients and families in various healthcare settings, and they are a common format for communicating health information to patients. However, a recent review of multiple studies on the effectiveness of posters in promoting knowledge determined that further evidence is needed to determine how effective they are in comparison to other teaching and learning approaches (Ilic & Rowe, 2013).

Posters can serve as an independent source of information or can be used along with other instructional methods and materials. Some critics view the poster as a passive instructional medium, but if designed and used properly, the message conveyed by a well-constructed poster is brief, constant, and interactive for teaching and learning (Daley, 1997; Duchin & Sherwood, 1990; Ilic & Rowe, 2013). Because the primary purpose of a poster is visual stimulation, it is meant to attract attention (Flournoy et al., 2000). Effective posters instill a mental image that may be remembered long after they are seen. This mental image serves as a cue to the viewer to remember the message being delivered. Much like a bumper sticker on a car, effective poster displays can potentially leave lasting impressions that are easily recalled at some future date. **Figure 12–5** is an excellent example.

The advantages of posters are that they can be used as a way to reinforce and condense information, and they can be used multiple times for different teaching–learning encounters. For example, when nurses in clinic and office settings are teaching a patient and significant other about osteoarthritis (degenerative arthritis), a poster with a series of pictures can show how joints can be affected over time, why pain occurs, and the actions certain treatments have on reducing inflammation. The value of posters is that the messages being conveyed are repeated every time they are viewed (Bach, McDaniel, & Poole, 1994; Daley, 1997; Duchin & Sherwood, 1990; Pulley et al., 2007) and can be used for a variety of purposes such as serving to remind the public of the importance of getting a flu shot. Posters serve as an important teaching tool to help bring about a change of behavior by adding knowledge, reinforcing information, or appealing to attitudes. By using short, simple, and eye-catching imagery, posters ensure that a message can be

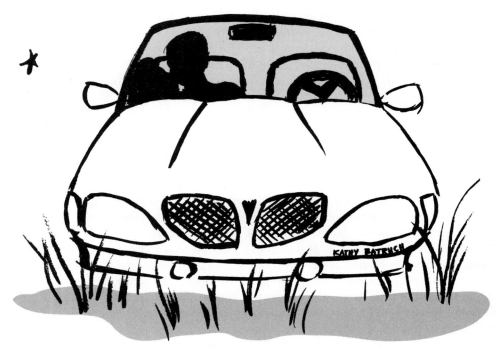

Last night Jennifer had a fatal accident. She just doesn't know it yet.

Figure 12–5 Example of an effective poster for AIDS awareness

Line drawing courtesy of Katherine Batruch-Meadows.

circulated quickly and simultaneously to many potential learners in a variety of health-care and community-based settings (Saldana, 2014). These demonstration materials also can be used with individuals and small groups to transmit or reinforce information with or without the nurse present. In addition, they are relatively inexpensive and easy to produce.

With practice, and with access to today's computer technology, a nurse can become skilled at creating attractive, impressive posters in an efficient and timely manner. Software programs such as Print Shop Deluxe, PaintShop Pro, Adobe Photoshop, and Microsoft Publisher are excellent resources to produce professional-looking visuals. The major disadvantage of posters is that the content in the final product is static and, therefore, may become quickly dated. Also, if the same poster is kept on display for too long, the potential audience may begin to disregard its message.

The key to a poster's effectiveness lies in its planning and design. Duchin and Sherwood (1990) and Bach et al. (1994) provide guidelines that still remain relevant today for developing attractive, simple, yet effective posters that consider variations in learner needs and patient education settings. Bushy (1991) and Duchin and Sherwood (1990) emphasize the application of design elements, such as color, spacing, graphics, lettering, and borders, required to create posters that not only catch the eye but also ensure that the message persists in memory. Also, effective imagery can take the form of graphic designs or photographs, so great artistic skill is not required to create the graphic elements of posters. Simple pictures, such as schematics, outlines, and stick figure drawings, work well and can be created using colored pencils, markers, construction paper, or computer printouts.

The ability of a poster to influence behavior or increase awareness can be greatly enhanced by careful consideration of all of these factors. Because aesthetic appeal is critical in capturing learners' attention, nurses should adhere to the following tips when making and critiquing a poster for use as a teaching tool (Bach et al., 1994; Bushy, 1991; Duchin & Sherwood, 1990; Haggard, 1989):

- Complementary (opposite-spectrum) color combinations are visually appealing.
- One color should make up as much as 70% of the display. No two colors should be used in equal proportions, and a third color should be used only to accent or highlight printed components such as titles and subheadings. Too many colors make the design appear cluttered and complicated.
- Because a picture is worth a thousand words, graphics should be used to break up blocks of print.
- Use simple, high-quality (but not necessarily sophisticated or ornate) drawings or graphics that can be easily understood.
- Balance the written message with white space (or another background color) and graphics to add variety and contrast.
- Use simple, high-quality photographs with colored borders and of different sizes and shapes.
- Deliver the written message in common, straightforward language, avoiding unfamiliar terms, abbreviations, or symbols.
- Adhere to the KISS principle (keep it simple and smart) when using words to decrease length, detail, and crowding. Simplicity and neatness attract attention.
- Be concise; do not repeat information. Include only essential information, but be sure the message is complete.
- Keep the learning objectives in mind to ensure the appropriate focus of information in this display tool.
- Be sure content is current and free of spelling, grammar, and mathematical errors.
- Add textures, if desired, by using a variety of paper and fabrics.
- Make titles catchy and crisp, using 10 or fewer words (no longer than two lines) and keeping lettering large enough to be read from a distance of at least 20 feet.
- Letters should be straight and at least 1 inch in height to be read easily at a distance of 4 to 6 feet. Avoid using all-capital letters except for very short titles and labels. Use capitals for only the first letter of each word in titles with more than two to three words or as the first word of a sentence.
- Use a title or introductory statement that orients readers to the subject.

- Logically sequence the written and graphic components.
- Use letter-quality script or laser print instead of dot matrix print if using computer-generated type.
- Use arrows, circles, or directional lines to merge the parts to achieve correct focus, flow, sequence, and unity.
- Achieve balance in visual weight on each side by positioning information around an imaginary central axis running vertically and horizontally.
- Handouts can be used to supplement, highlight, and reinforce the messages conveyed by the poster.
- If a poster is to be transported, use durable backboards and overlays (Styrofoam, heavy cardboard, lamination, or acrylic sprays).

Table 12–2 summarizes the basic advantages and disadvantages of demonstration materials.

Audiovisual Materials

Technology has changed the traditional approach to teaching. Nowhere is this trend more evident than with the audiovisual media. **Audiovisual materials** support and enrich the education process by stimulating the senses of seeing and hearing, adding variety to the teaching–learning experience, and instilling visual memories, which have been found to be more permanent than auditory memories (Kessels, 2003). Audiovisual elements have been known to increase understanding and retention of information as well as satisfaction with care by combining what people hear with what they see (Gysels & Higginson, 2007; Jeste, Dunn, Folsom, & Zisook, 2008). Technology software and hardware are exceptional aids because many can influence all three domains of learning (cognitive, affective, and psychomotor) by promoting cognitive development, stimulating attitude change, and helping to build psychomotor skills.

The term **multimedia learning** refers to the use of two or more types of learning modes (e.g., audio, visual, or animation) that can be accessed via a computer to engage the learner in the content. **Blended learning**—a more recent term in education—combines e-learning technology with more traditional instructor-led teaching methods, such as a lecture or demonstration. Audiovisual technologies often offer learners more control over content as well as over the sequencing, pacing, and timing of information, which

Table 12–2 Basic Advantages and Disadvantages of Demonstration Materials

Advantages	Disadvantages
Brings the learner closer to reality through active engagement	Static, easily outdated content
Useful for cognitive learning and psychomotor skill development	Can be time consuming to make
Stimulates learning in the affective domain	Potential for overuse
Relatively inexpensive	Not suitable for simultaneous use with large audiences
Opportunity for repetition of the message	Not suitable for visually impaired learners or for learners with poor abstract thinking abilities

allows teaching and learning experiences to be tailored to meet behavioral objectives for each individual. In our increasingly technological age, nurses have to be aware of which audiovisual tools are available, how tools actually and potentially affect the ability to learn, and how they might apply the various tools at their disposal effectively and efficiently. When and to what extent nurses should use such tools to enhance teaching depends on many variables, not the least of which is the nurse's comfort level and expertise in operating these technological devices. Also, it should not be forgotten that some adult learners may have difficulty becoming oriented to the newer modes of teaching and learning and that some patients may have physical or cognitive limitations that require the nurse to avoid certain types of audiovisual tools.

As with any instructional materials, major concerns affecting which tools nurses choose include accuracy and appropriateness of content, resources available for the purchase or rental of software programs and hardware equipment, and the time, money, and expertise needed to either introduce new technologies or self-produce audiovisual materials.

Audiovisual materials can be categorized into five major types of media: projected, audio, video, telecommunications, and computer formats. Computer technology, in particular, is rapidly altering the ways in which nurses share information and interact with patients.

PROJECTED LEARNING RESOURCES

The projected learning resources category of media includes overhead transparencies, PowerPoint slides, SMART Board systems, and other computer outputs that are projected onto a screen. These media types are appropriate for audiences of various sizes. A SMART Board is a large whiteboard that uses touch technology to project messages via a personal computing input system, such as a mouse or keyboard. Although very flexible and one of the newest technology instruments for teaching, they are still costly to purchase and not widely adopted yet for patient education (SMART, 2009).

Microsoft PowerPoint

Microsoft's computer-generated slideshow software program, PowerPoint, has replaced conventional slides and overheads as tools for instruction. PowerPoint slides are easy to design, economical to produce, effective as an instructional tool if used properly, and an impressive medium by which to share information with a large or small audience (deWet, 2006). The software program offers the flexibility to make changes in the slides whenever necessary as well as flexibility during the presentation to repeat slides, add new slides, or skip slides to move ahead to other content.

PowerPoint slides have many advantages. They are an excellent medium for conveying a message because they are an attractive mode for learning at all ages in a manner that facilitates retention and recall. They can enhance an oral presentation by adding visual dimensions to the narration. Presentations can be burned onto a CD or DVD, transferred to a flash drive, or downloaded from a server for presentation through a portable notebook computer. Digital photographs and graphics can easily be scanned and added to PowerPoint slides. Animation also can be included as a feature. Finally, slides can be personalized or tailored to meet specific learner needs.

Careful composition of slides is necessary to avoid clutter. Too much detail makes it difficult for the viewer to identify the major message (Brown, 2001; Polyakova-Norwood, 2009). DuFrene and Lehman (2004) provide a four-step process for assisting nurses to develop and deliver lively PowerPoint presentations designed to avoid the "death by PowerPoint" experience for intended audiences. Nurses should adhere to the following suggestions when preparing a PowerPoint slide presentation:

- Illustrate one idea per slide.
- Keep images simple by using clear pictures, symbols, or diagrams. Put long lists of words or complex figures on handouts that supplement the slides.
- Avoid distorted images by keeping the images' proportion of height to width at 2:3.
- Use large, easily readable, and professional-looking lettering.

Remember—visuals should *enrich* the message, not *become* the message. Overuse of slides may discourage audience participation, potentially sacrificing rich interactive discussions (Brown, 2001; DuFrene & Lehman, 2004). Dickerson (2005) reminds nurses that audiovisual resources are simply tools that they should use to help achieve teaching objectives.

Table 12–3 summarizes the basic advantages and disadvantages of PowerPoint slides.

AUDIO LEARNING RESOURCES

Audio technology, although it has existed for a long time, has not been used to any great extent for patient education purposes until recently. For years, audiotapes and radio have been useful tools to get information for people who are visually impaired or blind or for those with serious motor impairment who could not easily get to a location for an education session. However, with significant advances in audio software and hardware, as well as the adoption of audio technology for more than purely commercial use, CDs, digital sound players (e.g., MP3 players, iPods), radio, and podcasts have become more popular tools for teaching and learning. These resources can be used to deliver many different types of messages, can help learners who benefit from repetition and reinforcement, and are well suited for those individuals who enjoy or prefer auditory learning (Heinich, Molenda, Russell, & Smaldino, 2002). They are also useful media resources for teaching individuals who are illiterate or have low literacy (Santo, Laizner, & Shohet, 2005).

Table 12–3 Basic Advantages and Disadvantages of PowerPoint Slides

Advantages	Disadvantages
Most effectively used with groups	May stifle active learner participation if overused
May be especially beneficial for hearing-impaired, low-literate patients	May encourage learners only to think in bullet points
Good for teaching skills in all domains	Easy to pack too much content into each slide, making the print too difficult to read and presenting more than one concept per slide
Flexible to add, delete, or revise slides easily and quickly	Animations, sounds, and fancy transitions may be distracting
Do not require darkened room for projection	Lack of time for cognitive processing if too many slides included for the scheduled teaching session

Compact Discs and Digital Sound Players

Digital sound files and CDs, which have replaced traditional vinyl records and audio-tapes, are very popular formats today. Use of these media for teaching has been growing because they have major advantages, such as being small in size, portable, inexpensive, simple to operate, easy to prepare or duplicate, and offering superior sound that does not deteriorate over time.

Digital sound files and CDs (software) in conjunction with digital sound players (hardware) are powerful tools to enhance, reinforce, or supplement information previously presented in other formats or to expose learners to information not otherwise easily available or accessible. Such audio media on a variety of health topics, from stress reduction to programs on how to quit smoking, can be prepared specifically to meet the needs of patients by reinforcing facts, giving feedback and directions, or providing support. As early examples of the effective use of audio media, Hagopian (1996) described how audiotapes increased knowledge and self-care behaviors of persons undergoing radiation therapy, and Naperstek (1993) developed a large line of CDs on guided imagery for use by patients dealing with illness, surgery, and broad treatment modalities. Feldman (2004) described the development, implementation, and evaluation of self-directed learning using audiocassettes and pictures to teach basic child care, health, and safety skills to parents with intellectual disabilities. This study indicated that a significant number of these parents were able to improve their parenting skills with these low-cost, low-tech materials.

If digital sound files and CDs are instructor made, the learner will derive much comfort from hearing the nurse's familiar voice and reassuring words. Learners can listen to this information at their leisure and can review it as often as necessary. These media can be used almost anywhere, such as in the home, office, clinic, or hospital setting, and can be played while simultaneously driving a car or fixing a meal, thereby filling what normally would be considered wasted time.

The versatility of CDs and digital sound players for application to education is currently growing at a rapid rate for teaching patients and their family members. As with all technologies, over time the cost of digital sound players is becoming very reasonable, and the software availability of digital sound files and CDs for healthcare education is rapidly increasing.

The disadvantages of using this type of medium are few. The biggest drawback is that they address only one sense—hearing—and, therefore, cannot be used by individuals with hearing impairment. Also, some learners may be easily distracted from the information being presented unless they have visuals to accompany the recorded information. There is also no opportunity for interactive feedback between the listener and the speaker. As with any instructional tool, digital sound files and CDs should be used only as supplements to the various methods of teaching.

Radio and Podcasts

The radio has tremendously affected all of our lives for many years and is one of the oldest forms of audio technology. As early as the 1930s, the effectiveness of radio for health education was reported as influencing listeners' health behaviors (Turner,

Drenckhahn, & Bates, 1935). Because of its commercial nature and appeal to mass audiences, it has typically been used more for pleasure than for education.

In recent years, the medium of radio has been exploited by both public and private radio stations, which have begun airing community service and medical talk shows for public education on health issues (Hussain, 2008). Radio is serving as a medium for patient education campaigns because it can reach large numbers of listeners at great distances at relatively low unit cost, it functions in real time, and it is purely auditory, which stimulates the listeners' imagination and abstract thinking abilities. Also, it is effective in teaching those who are illiterate or low literate (Duby, 1990). These programs are helpful in delivering a message and, because of the convenience and popularity of radio as a communication tool, represent a useful vehicle for teaching and learning.

Podcasts are becoming an increasingly popular form of patient education as well. With this technology, audiences of learners are able to download lectures and informational sessions about various health topics. They can then listen to these broadcasts on their computers or digital audio players.

The disadvantage of radio and podcasts relates to the difficulty of consistently delivering information on major topics to general as well as specific populations. That is, the nurse as teacher has little control over the variety and depth of topics discussed or how regularly learners listen to a program. In addition, the general nature of radio programs and podcasts is not tailored to meet individual needs. Unlike CDs and digital sound files, radio does not allow the opportunity for repetition of information. However, because of its widespread use and versatility, it has the potential for becoming a major source for important and useful healthcare information, especially if airtime is funded by private foundations or sponsored by special groups or agencies dedicated to health teaching.

Table 12–4 summarizes the basic advantages and disadvantages of audio learning resources.

VIDEO LEARNING RESOURCES

Digital video files and DVDs (software), along with camcorders, DVD recorders, television sets, and computer monitors as electronic devices (hardware) with which to view them, have become commonplace in homes. Nurses are using these resources extensively for teaching in a variety of settings. The webinar format, which allows for interaction between speaker and participants even though sessions are virtual, and streaming

Table 12–4 Basic Advantages and Disadvantages of Audio Learning Resources

Advantages	Disadvantages
Widely available	Relies only on sense of hearing
May be especially beneficial for visually impaired, low-literacy patients	Expensive in some forms
May be listened to repeatedly	Lack of opportunity for interaction between instructor and learner
Usually practical, cheap, small in size, and portable	

technology, which plays audio and visual files from the Internet, are cost effective, easy to use, time efficient, and available wherever the Internet is accessible (Beranova & Sykes, 2007; Manny, 2006; Smaldino, Lowther, & Russell, 2012).

In a review of research studies, Jeste et al. (2008) found that multimedia DVDs for educating consumers about illness management and treatment decision increased learners' understanding of medical information and enabled both patients and their caregivers to take a more active role in making healthcare choices. Video files and DVDs are among the major nonprint media tools for enhancing patient and family education because tapes can be simultaneously entertaining and educational (Beranova & Sykes, 2007; Bussey-Smith & Rosen, 2007; Gysels & Higginson, 2007).

Video, although a logical technology to use for patient care, has not yet been used to its fullest extent. Clark and Lester (2000) conducted a research study on video interventions with an older adult population. They found this instructional tool to be as effective in changing behaviors in this group as in teaching and learning of adolescents and younger adults.

Digital video files and DVDs, which incorporate the sound quality of CDs and superior images of video by way of digital technology, have incredible storage qualities (similar to CDs) that allow for long-term use. The market for this technology has increased as the cost of the software and hardware has become more reasonable (Heinich et al., 2002). Originally designed for entertainment purposes only, today these discs are popular with a wide range of audiences for patient and family education. Healthcare facilities often broadcast patient education segments via video files and DVDs over in-house televisions. The convenience and flexibility of these instructional tools allow nurses to use video learning resources for individual patient teaching situations as well as for large-group instruction.

The usefulness of video derives from the combination of color, motion, different angles, and sound that enhances learning through visual as well as auditory senses. For example, Leiner, Handal, and Williams (2004) compared the effectiveness of printed information about polio vaccination from the Centers for Disease Control with the same message converted into a production of animated cartoons using marketing and advertising techniques. The findings showed that the animated cartoon was more effective in delivering the same message than the written instructional materials.

The disadvantage of purchased digital video files and DVDs is that they may be beyond the viewers' level of understanding, inappropriate for learner needs, or too long. This digital technology has become very inexpensive, and the ready portability of recorders allows patient educators to capture situations unavailable elsewhere for reinforcement of learning.

Williams, Wolgin, and Hodge (1998) have outlined detailed steps for creating educational videos. They suggest striving for network-quality production by following these guidelines:

- Write a script for the program. Rehearse thoroughly.
- With a small budget, use a single camera with zoom capacity. A larger budget may allow a professional to be hired to edit the final product.
- Consider hiring a video technician on a per-hour or per-diem basis to yield a quality production in a time-efficient and cost-effective manner. The operator

Table 12–5 **Basic Advantages and Disadvantages of Video Learning Resources**

Advantages	Disadvantages
Widely used educational tool	Viewing formats limited depending on availability of hardware in healthcare settings, especially in patient homes
Inexpensive, for the most part	
Uses visual and auditory senses	Expense of some commercial products
Flexible for use with different audiences	Excessive length or inappropriateness for the audience of some purchased materials
Powerful tool for role modeling, demonstration, teaching psychomotor skills	

of the recorder needs to be knowledgeable about motion picture technology, such as the use of close-ups, dramatization of situations, and angle effects, which are not in the usual skill set of many nurses.

- Always be mindful of the learning objectives to avoid going astray with the informational message.
- Keep the teaching session short. The attention spans of learners vary, but the longer the video, the more risk of losing viewer interest. A video that is 5 to 10 minutes long is ideal.

Table 12-5 summarizes the basic advantages and disadvantages of video learning resources.

TELECOMMUNICATIONS LEARNING RESOURCES

Telecommunications is a means by which information can be transmitted via television, telephone, related modes of audio and video teleconferencing, and closed-circuit, cable, and satellite broadcasting. Telecommunications devices have allowed messages to be sent to many people at the same time in a variety of places at great distances (Austin & Husted, 1998; Tones & Tilford, 2001).

Television

The television—a very common device in American homes—has been used for many years as an entertainment tool. Today, there are more televisions than telephones in private residences. The TV is also well suited for educational purposes and has become a popular teaching–learning tool in homes, schools, businesses, and healthcare settings (MDM Commercial, 2015). TV has been found to be more effective than using only written information and as effective as any other audiovisual tool based on a review of over 30 studies on the use of the TV as a patient education aid. This medium has a definite role to play in increasing knowledge and skills and influencing behavior change (Nielson & Sheppard, 1988). The power to influence cognitive, affective, and psychomotor behavior is well demonstrated by television commercials, whose messages are simple, direct, and repetitive to effectively influence the behavior of intended audiences.

Cable TV is legally obligated to provide public access programming by offering channels for community members and organizations to air their own programs. Health education, if placed on the cable system, can be seen in any home with cable access. The advantage of this national and international option is that distribution of programs is relatively inexpensive (Palmer, n.d.). The disadvantage is that there is no control over who is watching, and this medium cannot serve as an interactive question-and-answer experience unless call-in phone lines are provided.

Closed-circuit TV, in contrast, allows for education programs to be sent to specific locations, such as patient rooms. The learner can request a particular program at any given time, much like a guest in a hotel can choose on demand from a variety of movies day and night (Falvo, 2010). Such telecommunications technology allows programs to be played intermittently or continuously, with program availability clearly advertised. Because the learner controls program viewing, the nurse must follow up to answer questions and determine whether learning has, in fact, occurred.

Satellite broadcasting—a much more sophisticated form of telecommunications— can reach far more distant locations and carry a number of programs at any given time. Because of its expense, not many institutions send health information via this mode, but many receive it. More types of satellite systems are being developed to make this form of communication for educational purposes available on a worldwide basis.

Telephones

It is almost impossible to imagine being without the telephone as a daily tool. Americans have come to depend on their wireless cell phones and land-based phone lines as fundamental means of communication. It is not surprising, therefore, that the telephone can be used effectively for education.

In recognition of this fact, many healthcare associations have begun to provide telephone services with messages about disease treatment and prevention. The American Cancer Society, for example, has established a toll-free number for the public to obtain short taped messages about various types of cancer. Hospitals, too, have set up call-in services about a variety of health-related topics and sources for referral. Telephones for support and education interventions have been used to help patients adjust to breast cancer as well as carry out self-care management of diabetes and other chronic diseases (Chamberlain, Tulman, Coleman, Stewart, & Samarel, 2006; Handley, Shumway, & Schillinger, 2008; Kivela, Elo, Kyngas, & Kaariainen, 2014; Mons et al., 2013). Telephone consultation also is becoming a popular strategy for patient follow-up after hospital and clinic visits (Eisenburg, Hwa, & Wren, 2014; ElHalwagy & Otify, 2009), and telephone support has been used to motivate patients to increase their physical activity levels (B. B. Green et al., 2002).

Such services are relatively inexpensive and can be operated by someone with minimal medical knowledge because the taped message by experts contains the substance of the content. Moreover, this type of service is available in most cases around the clock. The disadvantage is that there is no opportunity for questions to be answered directly.

Telecommunications as an instructional tool is becoming increasingly popular and refined. Many hospitals and healthcare agencies have already established hotline consumer information centers, which are staffed by knowledgeable healthcare personnel so that information can be personalized and appropriate feedback can be given on the spot. The poison control hotline is a good example of the use of this medium.

Table 12–6 summarizes the basic advantages and disadvantages of telecommunications learning resources.

Table 12–6 Basic Advantages and Disadvantages of Telecommunications Learning Resources

Advantages	Disadvantages
Influences cognitive, affective, and psychomotor domains	Complicated to set up interactive capability
Relatively inexpensive hardware and software devices	Expensive to broadcast via satellite
A large number of programs on a variety of topics	Occasional inability of formats to provide for repetition of information
Widely accessible for distribution to many users at a distance	
Appealing to many learners because of convenience and flexibility	Cannot control how many and what type of viewer audiences are reached

COMPUTER LEARNING RESOURCES

In our technological society, the computer has changed lives dramatically and has found widespread application in industry, business, schools, and homes. Only recently, however, has computer-assisted instruction been used for patient education in healthcare settings, such as a medical office or clinic waiting rooms (Wofford, Smith, & Miller, 2005). The computer can store large amounts of information and is designed to display pictures, graphics, and text. The presentation of information can be changed depending on user input. Although computer technology is a relatively recent addition to the educational field, it is becoming very common, especially with the rapid increase of computer literacy among the general public (Rice, Trockel, King, & Remmert, 2004). Computers, as a multimedia approach to teaching and learning, usually stimulate learners and transform learning into "an active, engaging process" that promotes problem solving and the development of critical-thinking skills (Huang, 2005, p. 224).

Computer-assisted instruction (CAI), also called computer-based learning and computer-based training, promotes learning in primarily the cognitive domain (Grunwald & Corsbie-Massay, 2006). Research has revealed that CAI increases both the efficiency of learning and the retention of information (Lewis, 1999). Computers are an efficient instructional tool, computer programs can influence affective and psychomotor skill development, and retention of information potentially can be improved by the interactive exchange between learner and computer, even though the instructor is not actually present (DiGiacinto, 2007). Illustrations (visual information), along with narration (verbal information) via computer, increase learners' recall and comprehension.

Lewis (1999) summarized the findings from a large number of studies on computer-based education and concluded that teaching and learning by computers is an effective strategy for transfer of knowledge and skill development in patients. For example, telemedicine technology has been found to be as effective an educational tool as in-person teaching for diabetes control (Izquierdo et al., 2003). In addition, use of interactive videodisc programs shows promise in improving retention and understanding of information (M. J. Green et al., 2004).

CAI has many advantages. Instruction can be individualized to the learner, lessons can be varied readily, and the learner can control the pace of the learning experience (Heinich et al., 2002). Without time constraints, the learner can move as quickly or as slowly as desired to master content without penalty for mistakes or performance speed.

For instance, many educational computer games are designed to teach a subject at a variety of skill levels. Instructions that present to learners more problems with increasing complexity at a pace of the learners' own choosing can be selected. The ability of computers to internally change the rules or the format of games makes them endlessly challenging and novel to the user.

Another advantage of CAI is that a nurse can easily track the level of understanding of the learner because the computer has the ability to ask questions and analyze responses to perform ongoing learner assessment. Computers can be programmed to provide feedback to the nurse regarding the learner's grasp of concepts, the speed of learning, and those aspects of learning that need reinforcement. The interactive features of this medium also provide for immediate feedback to the learner.

Computers also represent a valuable instructional tool for those persons with aphasia, motor difficulties, visual and hearing impairments, or learning disabilities. Assistive technologies, such as screen readers that convert electronic text to spoken language, are available to individuals with learning or visual disabilities. Hoffman, Hartley, and Boone (2005) address specific problems of access to computer resources for individuals who are disabled. They provide an excellent resource list for nurses and learners who want more information on organizations and websites specializing in assistive technologies. In addition, the Center for Applied Special Technology is a nonprofit educational, research, and development organization whose mission is to expand opportunities for individuals with disabilities through the development of innovative, technology-based educational resources and strategies (http://www.cast.org). Nurses can visit this organization's website for additional information.

The major disadvantage of CAI is the expense of both the hardware and the software, which makes this option not feasible for implementation in some learning situations. In most cases, programs must be purchased because they are too time consuming and too complex for the nurse to develop. Even if a nurse has programming skills, it can take as long as 500 hours to produce 1 hour of instructional material (Boyd et al., 1998). **Table 12–7** provides examples of companies that supply patient education materials.

Another barrier to education via a computer is the lack of computer literacy or comfort level with computers among some learners and even some health professionals (Prensky, 2001). In particular, many older adults are computer shy, are computer illiterate, or lack easy access to computers even if they understand how to use this technology. This situation is beginning to change, though, as computers become more of a household item. Although multimedia resources may be important tools to enhance learning in the older adult, much more research also needs to be conducted on age-related cognitive changes that could have implications for the design and use of multimedia learning environments for this growing population of learners (Pass, VanGerven, & Tabbers, 2014).

In addition, people with reading problems unfortunately may experience difficulty in making sense of the information on the screen. However, a recent study on CAI with patients of varying health literacy levels found that those who had low health literacy also had limited computer experience. Nevertheless, the majority of these patients completed the computer-based educational program on screening for colorectal cancer without assistance and claimed they understood the information better than they would have if asked to read a brochure (Duren-Winfield, Onsomu, Case, Pignone, & Miller, 2015).

Table 12–7 Some Examples of Internet Sites and Companies That Provide Technology-Based Patient Education Materials

Accessible Online Through the Internet (Available to the Public)

General Resources

Health Library from EBSCO Publishing—assists hospitals and other medical facilities to enhance their patient education websites and services (www.epnet.com).

MedlinePlus (www.medlineplus.gov)—a service of the U.S. National Library of Medicine and the National Institutes of Health (NIH) (www.nih.gov)

Mayoclinic.org (www.mayoclinic.org)

WebMD.com (www.webmd.com)

National Cancer Institutes (www.cancer.gov)

Family Doctor—covers information on prevention and wellness and diseases and conditions by name, symptom, and drug information (http://familydoctor.org)

American Diabetes Association—creates written and video information in English (www.diabetes.org/research-and-practice/we-support-your-doctor/patient-education-materials.html) and Spanish (www.diabetes.org/es/)

Centers for Disease Control and Prevention—provides materials in English, Spanish and French on different types of diseases, illnesses, and prevention measures (http://www.cdc.gov/hepatitis/resources/patientedmaterials.htm)

5Minute Consult—over 1000 patient education materials listed in alphabetical order for easy searching in simple language, and in English and Spanish versions (http://5minuteconsult.com)

Videos and Animations

Wired.MD—provides interactive, online videos (www.wired.md)

pCare—videos in multiple languages for targeted patient education populations on 7000 diagnoses, procedures, and medicines that are designed by leading content producers and reviewed by health literacy and medical experts (www.pcareinteractive.com/education.html)

Pritchett & Hull—uses extensive graphics with a lower reading level in many formats and subjects; online ordering available (www.p-h.com)

Hazelden—emphasis on addiction, recovery, sobriety, and similar health issues; Adobe Reader needed. To locate videos, go to www.hazelden.org/OA_HTML/ibeCCtpSctDspRte.jsp?section＝10021 and use Search Bookstore, selecting Videos under All Products

Milner-Fenwick Online—free previews covering most health topics, many available in Spanish and with closed captioning (www.milner-fenwick.com)

MedlinePlus in English and Spanish—interactive tutorials on diseases and conditions, specific tests and diagnostic procedures, surgery and treatment options, and prevention and wellness (e.g., hypertension—slides with audio) (www.medlineplus.gov; www.medlineplus.gov/spanish)

The PatientChannel—GE Health care (www.gehealthcare.com)

(continued)

Accessible Online Through the Internet (Expanded Applications May Be Available Through the Intranet of Individual Organizations)

Print Resources

Krames on Demand—electronic patient education solutions; self-care guides in Spanish and English; publisher of choice for American Heart Association, American Stroke Association, American Lung Association, and National Cancer Institute (www.kramesstore.com)

Hopkins Medicine—self-management patient education materials on many diseases that can be printed off and given to patients (http://hopkinsmedicine.org/gim/core_resources/patient%20Handouts/)

Micromedex (www.micromedex.com)—medications, diseases, procedures, home care

Cengage Learning—source for healthcare information and interactive tools for teaching and learning and improving health literacy (www.adam.com)

ExitCare—interactive videos, educational handouts, and medication management tools to help build meaningful communications with patients and engage patients through education (www.exitcare.com)

HealthWise—print guides, website information, and healthcare organization websites on a wide range of health content, decision aids, and health coaching (www.healthwise.org)

American Academy of Allergy, Asthma, and Immunology—provides low-literacy patient education materials, such as games, puzzles, posters, quizzes, and printed materials in English and Spanish (www.aaaai.org)

Video Resources

Emmi Solutions—outcome-driven patient education communications (www.emmisolutions.com)

Videos—DVD Companies for Purchasing Individual Titles

Context Media—videos specifically designed for TV projection in office waiting rooms (http://www.contextmediahealth.com)

Milner-Fenwick—videos and digital media for health professionals providing patient education on most healthcare topics across the continuum of care—free previews; most in Spanish language and closed captioning (http://www.milner-fenwick.com)

Aquarius Health Care Media—all videos have an inspirational message of hope and healing; award-winning videos and DVDs on disabilities, cancer, caregiving, children, diseases and health, death and dying, end of life, bereavement, and mental health (www.academicvideostore.com)

NIMCO—education products, such as posters, DVDs, displays (www.nimcoinc.com)

Also, learners with physical limitations, such as arthritis, neuromuscular disorders, pain, fatigue, paralysis, or vision impairment, may similarly find computers challenging to use.

Moreover, it should not be forgotten that the computer is a machine, so the learner is necessarily deprived of the personal, compassionate, one-to-one interaction that only a teacher can provide to facilitate learning. Because of the independent nature of the computer learning experience, the CAI format is not recommended for nondirected or poorly motivated learners.

Despite these caveats, the tremendous growth of the Internet has opened new doors for many learners to gain access to libraries and to direct learning experiences, such as online discussions with nurses at great distances. **Table 12–8** summarizes the basic advantages and disadvantages of computer learning resources.

Table 12–8 Basic Advantages and Disadvantages of Computer Learning Resources

Advantages	Disadvantages
Promotes quick feedback, retention of learning	Primarily promotes learning in cognitive domain; but can influence affective and psychomotor skill development
Potential database enormous	
Can be individualized to suit different types of learners or different paces for learning	Expensive software and hardware, therefore less accessible to a wide audience
Time efficient	Too complex and time consuming for most nurses to prepare independently
	Limited use for many elderly, low-literate learners, and those with physical limitations

Evaluating Instructional Materials

Choosing the right tools for patient education calls for judgment on the part of the nurse, who must take into consideration the variables of the learner, the medium, and the task. Decisions as to which instructional materials are or are not appropriate depend on the size and characteristics of the audience, the preset behavioral objectives to be achieved, and the effectiveness and availability of media resources. The values of these three variables in combination with one another result in the selection of different teaching tools by the nurse, who is faced with multiple situations, different learners, and varying circumstances on a daily basis. In particular, the evaluation of tools for teaching involves appraising the content, the instructional design, the technical production, and the packaging of any given instructional materials. **Figure 12–6** provides a patient education materials assessment tool (PEMAT) for selecting and evaluating print and audiovisual instructional materials (Shoemaker, Wolf, & Brach, 2013).

Printed materials, as the most popular tool available for patient education, require the nurse to determine the reading levels prior to distribution to learners. This is an essential factor when selecting brochures, pamphlets, information sheets, and the like to be sure they are suitable for a given audience of learners. **Figure 12–7** illustrates the learning pyramid. It emphasizes an important learning principle: According to numerous research studies, people retain information at a higher rate if they are actively involved in the learning process (National Training Laboratories, n.d.). The effectiveness of teaching and learning is, therefore, greatly enhanced when instructional materials stimulate multiple senses and modes of learning.

In making their final media selections, nurses must ask themselves which material(s) will best support teaching and learning to achieve the behavioral outcomes for their particular audience. They must remember that active learner involvement and using materials and objects that most closely resemble the real thing (realia) are the best choices for enhancing retention of information. Above all else, nurses should remember that instructional materials should be used to support learning only by complementing and supplementing the teaching, not by substituting for it.

Domain: Understandability

Topic: Content

Item 1: The material makes its purpose completely evident (P and A/V).

Item 2: The material does not include information or content that distracts from its purpose (P).

Topic: Word Choice and Style

Item 3: The material uses common, everyday language (P and A/V).

Item 4: Medical terms are used only to familiarize audience with the terms. When used, medical terms are defined (P and A/V).

Item 5: The material uses the active voice (P and A/V).

Topic: Use of Numbers

Item 6: Numbers appearing in the material are clear and easy to understand (P).

Item 7: The material does not expect the user to perform calculations (P).

Topic: Organization

Item 8: The material breaks or chunks information into short sections (P and A/V).

Item 9: The material's sections have informative headers (P and A/V).

Item 10: The material presents information in a logical sequence (P and A/V).

Item 11: The material provides a summary (P and A/V).

Topic: Layout and Design

Item 12: The material uses visual cues (e.g., arrows, boxes, bullets, bold, larger font, highlighting) to draw attention to key points (P and A/V).

Item 13: Text on the screen is easy to read (A/V).

Item 14: The material allows the user to hear the words clearly (e.g., not too fast, not garbled) (A/V).

Topic: Use of Visual Aids

Item 15: The material uses visual aids whenever they could make content more easily understood (e.g., illustration of healthy portion size) (P).

Item 16: The material's visual aids reinforce rather than distract from the content (P).

Item 17: The material's visual aids have clear titles or captions (P).

Item 18: The material uses illustrations and photographs that are clear and uncluttered (P and A/V).

Item 19: The material uses simple tables with short and clear row and column headings (P and A/V).

Domain: Actionability

Item 20: The material clearly identifies at least one action the user can take (P and A/V).

Item 21: The material addresses the user directly when describing actions (P and A/V).

Item 22: The material breaks down any action into manageable, explicit steps (P and A/V).

Item 23: The material provides a tangible tool (e.g., menu planners, checklists) whenever it could help the user take action (P).

Item 24: The material provides simple instructions or examples of how to perform calculations (P).

Item 25: The material explains how to use the charts, graphs, tables, or diagrams to take actions (P and A/V).

Item 26: The material uses visual aids whenever they could make it easier to act on the instructions (P).

P = Patient Education Materials Assessment Tool for Printed Materials (PEMAT-P)

A/V = Patient Education Materials Assessment Tool for Audiovisual Materials (PEMAT-A/V)

Figure 12–6 The Patient Education Materials Assessment Tool (PEMAT) for evaluating instructional materials

Reproduced from Shoemaker, S. J., Wolf, M. S., & Brach, C. (2013). *The Patient Education Materials Assessment Tool (PEMAT) and User's Guide*. Rockville, MD: Agency for Healthcare Research and Quality. Retrieved from http://www.ahrq.gov/prefessionals/prevention-chronic-care/improve/self-mgmt/pemat/index.html

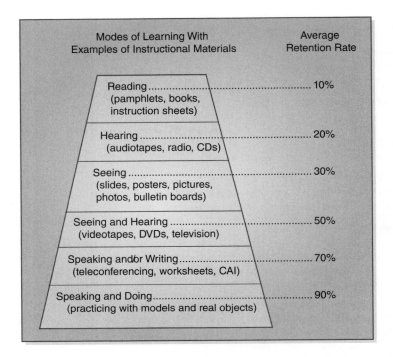

Figure 12–7 Learning pyramid: Information retention based on level of active learner involvement

Modified from NTL Institute for Applied Behavioral Science, 8380 Colesville Road, Suite 560, Silver Spring, MD 20910. 301-565-3200.

Summary

This chapter reviewed the major categories of instructional material, identified how to select tools from a range of possible options based on their advantages and disadvantages, and addressed how to evaluate their effectiveness. Nurses are expected to be able to make choices for teaching methods and materials every day, whether it be to meet the needs of an individual learner or to design an educational program to satisfy a broader, more diverse group of learners. In this chapter, the importance of considering characteristics of the learner, the medium, and the task when choosing instructional materials was emphasized. The importance of using instructional materials only to supplement teachings was also stressed, as was the need to keep the behavioral objectives in focus when selecting these materials as adjuncts to instruction.

Print media include both commercially prepared and instructor-composed materials. The problem of matching literacy and cognitive levels of learners to printed instructional tools is a real concern. The major advantages of printed tools are that they are widely available, patients are able to refer back to these materials for review at any time and at their own pace, and the materials have potential to reinforce information. Disadvantages include the limited opportunity for nurses and patients to give and receive feedback. For some learners, the readability level and complexity of information may be significant barriers to their ability to take full advantage of printed tools. Several guidelines that nurses can use in selecting or developing printed materials appropriate to both the audience and the task were presented.

Demonstration materials include many types of visual, hands-on tools, such as models and real equipment, as well as displays such as posters, bulletin boards, and whiteboards. In particular, these materials stimulate the senses of sight and touch. They are especially useful for cognitive and psychomotor skill development and may even influence attitudes, feelings, and values in the affective domain. Other advantages include bringing the learner closer to reality through active involvement and the opportunity for repetition of information.

The major disadvantage of demonstration materials is the potential for content to become outdated or be overused because they are often costly and time consuming to prepare. Because of workload demands, nurses may be reluctant or unable to revise these materials frequently. In addition, most of these materials are not suitable for simultaneous viewing by large audiences, for learners with visual impairments, or for individuals with poor abstraction abilities.

Audiovisual materials make up the fastest growing category of instructional tools. Their ability to stimulate the senses of sight and hearing enhances their power to actively engage learners and to potentially increase retention of information. Many audiovisual tools can influence all three domains of learning by promoting cognitive development, influencing attitude change, and helping to build psychomotor skills.

The audiovisual materials section of the chapter examined the five major categories of audiovisual media—projected, audio, video, telecommunications, and computer formats. Consideration was given to how appropriate each of these tools is depending on learner characteristics, expense of the software and hardware, and convenience of use. General guidelines for selecting and developing audiovisual materials were presented, and the principal advantages and disadvantages of the five categories were described. Learners with low literacy skills may benefit from most categories of these media except computer formats. Audio materials are most appropriate for learners with visual impairments, while projected video with captions and computer resources most benefit learners with hearing impairments.

Review Questions

1. How do instructional materials differ from teaching methods?
2. What are the general principles to consider when determining the effectiveness of instructional tools?
3. What are the three major variables that must be taken into account when selecting, developing, and evaluating printed, demonstration, and audiovisual tools?
4. What are the three primary components of instructional materials to be kept in mind when evaluating their appropriateness as tools for teaching?
5. Which instructional materials are examples of illusionary representations?
6. Why are numbers as well as oral and written words known to be the most abstract forms of messages?

7. Which factors must be considered when reviewing commercially prepared print materials for use in teaching and learning?
8. What are the guidelines to be followed to make sure instructor-composed printed education materials are clearly written and appropriate?
9. What are some examples of demonstration materials? Of audiovisual materials?
10. What are the major advantages and disadvantages of computer learning resources?
11. Why is it that instructional materials should not be selected before behavioral objectives are determined?

Case Study

Carlos Padia, RN, a longtime staff member on a medical unit of Midland Health Center, has been assigned to care for Mr. Harry Goldberg, a patient who was admitted late last evening for cardiac monitoring and treatment. Carlos is beginning an initial needs assessment to develop with Mr. Goldberg a teaching plan for patient education during his stay in the hospital and for follow-up care upon his discharge to home.

Mr. Goldberg is a 52-year-old man with a strong family history of heart disease. He never completed high school but did manage to finish the 11th grade. He has been a self-employed carpenter all of his working life, is married, and has three children.

Mr. Goldberg was diagnosed a year ago with coronary artery disease and secondary hypertension; however, he had symptoms indicating cardiovascular problems for a couple of years prior to his diagnoses. His fasting cholesterol levels have ranged from 250 to 300 mg/dL, his triglycerides and HDL levels are also significantly above normal, and his blood pressure readings have averaged 180 systolic and 100 diastolic. His doctor describes these findings as numbers Mr. Goldberg absolutely must decrease to more normal limits for the chance to have a longer, healthier life. At the time of initial diagnoses, he was advised to take medication, increase his exercise, and control his diet to lose weight (at least 25 lbs.), but he has made little progress toward these recommended goals.

During his first contact with Mr. Goldberg, Carlos explores many aspects of his patient's situation and understanding of his medical status. When asked about monitoring his blood pressure at home, the patient states, "I have one of those blood pressure gadgets, but I don't use it. What good would it do for me to know the numbers? The doctor already sees that they are high."

The three major variables to help make the appropriate choice of instructional materials are: *characteristics of the learner*, *characteristics of the medium*, and *characteristics of the task*.

1. What are the characteristics of Mr. Goldberg as a learner that must be taken into account when planning for patient education?
2. What behavioral objectives and domain(s) for learning should be discussed with him as the tasks to be accomplished?
3. Which two types of instructional materials would likely benefit this patient?
   a. Discuss the advantages and disadvantages of each.
   b. Identify the three components of each of these instructional materials.

References

Aldridge, M. D. (2009). Using models to teach congenital heart defects. *Dimensions of Critical Care Nursing, 28*(3), 116–122.

Austin, L. S., & Husted, K. (1998). Cost effectiveness of television, radio, and print media for public mental health education. *Psychiatric Services of the American Psychiatric Association, 49*(6). 808–811. Retrieved from http://dx.doi.org/10.1176/ps.49.6.808

Babcock, D. E., & Miller, M. A. (1994). *Client education: Theory and practice.* St. Louis, MO: Mosby–Year Book.

Bach, C. A., McDaniel, R. W., & Poole, M. J. (1994). Posters: Innovative and cost-effective tools for staff development. *Journal of Nursing Staff Development, 10*(2), 71–74.

Beranova, E., & Sykes, C. (2007). A systematic review of computer-based software for educating patients with coronary heart disease. *Patient Education and Counseling, 66*(1), 21–28.

Boyd, M. D., Gleit, C. J., Graham, B. A., & Whitman, N. J. (1998). *Health teaching in nursing practice: A professional model* (3rd ed.). Stamford, CT: Appleton & Lange.

Brown, D. G. (2001, March). Judicious PowerPoint. *Syllabus, 14*(8), 27.

Brownson, K. (1998). Education handouts: Are we wasting our time? *Journal for Nurses in Staff Development, 14*(4), 176–182.

Bushy, A. (1991). A rating scale to evaluate research posters. *Nurse Educator, 16*(1), 11–15.

Bussey-Smith, K. L., & Rossen, R. D. (2007). A systematic review of randomized control trials evaluating the effectiveness of interactive computerized asthma patient education programs, *Annals of Allergy and Asthma Immunology, 98*(6), 507–516.

Campbell, M. K., DeVellis, B., Strecher, V. J., Ammerman, A. S., DeVellis, R. S., & Sandler, R. S. (1994). Improving dietary behavior: The effectiveness of tailored messages in primary care settings. *American Journal of Public Health, 84*, 783–787.

Chamberlain, W. M., Tulman, L., Coleman, E. A., Stewart, C. B., & Samarel, N. (2006). Women's perceptions of the effectiveness of telephone support and education on their adjustment to breast cancer. *Oncology Nursing Forum, 33*(1), 138–144.

Clark, M. C., & Lester, J. (2000). The effect of video-based interventions on self-care. *Western Journal of Nursing Research, 22*(8), 895–911.

Cobussen-Boekhorst, J. G. L., Van Der Weide, M., Feitz, W. F. J., & DeGier, R. P. E. (2000). Using an instructional model to teach clean intermittent catheterization to children. *BJU International, 85*, 551–553.

D'Allessandro, D. M., Kingsley, P., & Johnson-West, J. (2001). The readability of pediatric patient education materials on the World Wide Web. *Journal of the American Medical Association, 155*(7), 807–812.

Daley, E. (1997). Effectiveness of poster for nutrition education in an acquired immunodeficiency syndrome clinic. *Journal of the American Dietetic Association, 97*(9), A28–A30. doi:10.1016/S0002-8223(97)00419-7. Retrieved from http://www.sciencedirect.com/science/article/pii/S0002822397004197

deWet, C. F. (2006). Beyond presentations: Using PowerPoint as an effective instructional tool. *Gifted Child Today, 29*(4), 29–39.

Dickerson, P. S. (2005). Nurturing critical thinkers. *Journal of Continuing Education in Nursing, 36*(3), 68–72.

DiGiacinto, D. (2007). Using multimedia effectively in the teaching–learning process. *Journal of Allied Health, 36*(3), 176–179.

Doak, C. C., Doak, L. G., Friedell, G. H., & Meade, C. D. (1998). Improving comprehension for cancer patients with low literacy skills: Strategies for clinicians. *CA: A Cancer Journal for Clinicians, 48*(3), 151–162.

Doak, C. C., Doak, L. G., & Root, J. H. (1996). *Teaching patients with low literacy.* Philadelphia, PA: J. B. Lippincott.

Duby, A. (1990). The effectiveness of radio as an educational medium. *Educational Media International, 27*(3), 154–157. Retrieved from http://www.freepaperdownload.us/678/article37523.htm

Duchin, S., & Sherwood, G. (1990). Posters as an educational strategy. *Journal of Continuing Education in Nursing, 21*(5), 205–208.

DuFrene, D. D., & Lehman, C. M. (2004). Concepts, content, construction, and contingencies: Getting the horse before the PowerPoint cart. *Business Communication Quarterly, 67*, 84–88.

Duren-Winfield, V., Onsomu, E. O., Case, D. L., Pignone, M., & Miller, D. (2015). Health literacy and computer-assisted instruction: Usability and patient preference. *Journal of Health Communication: International Perspectives, 20*(4), 491–498.

Eisenburg, D., Hwa, K., & Wren, S. M. (2014). Telephone follow-up by a midlevel provider after laparoscopic inquinal hernia repair instead of face-to-face clinic visit. *Journal of the Society of Laparoendoscopic Surgeons, 19*(1). doi:10.4293/JSLS.2014.00205

ElHalwagy, H., & Otify, M. (2009). Long term outcome of a telephone follow up clinic. *The Internet Journal of Healthcare Administration, 7*(1). Retrieved from http://ispub.com/IJHCA/7/1/13392

Estey, A., Musseau, A., & Keehn, L. (1994). Patients' understanding of health information: A multihospital comparison. *Patient Education and Counseling, 24*, 73–78.

Falvo, D. (2010). *Effective patient education: A guide to increased adherence* (4th ed.). Sudbury, MA: Jones & Bartlett.

Feldman, M. A. (2004). Self-directed learning of child-care skills by parents with intellectual disabilities. *Infants and Young Children, 17*(1), 17–31.

Flournoy, E., Turner, G., & Combs, D. (2000). Innovative teaching: Read the writing on the wall. *Dimensions of Critical Care Nursing, 19*(4), 36–37.

Frantz, R. A. (1980). *Selecting media for patient education. Topics in Clinical Nursing.* Rockville, MD: Aspen.

Fraze, J., Griffith, J., Green, D., & McElroy, L. (2010). So many materials, so little time: A checklist to select printed education materials for clinical practice. *Journal of Midwifery & Women's Health, 55*(10), 70–73.

Friedman, A. J., Cosby, R., Boyko, S., Hatton-Bauer, J., & Turnbull, G. (2011). Effective teaching strategies and methods of delivery for patient education: A systematic review and practice guidelines recommendations. *Journal of Cancer Education, 26*, 12–21.

Giguere, A., Legare, F., Grimshaw, J., Turcotte, S., Fiander, M., Grudniewicz, A., . . . Gagnon, M. P. (2012). Printed educational materials: Effects on professional practice and healthcare outcomes. *Cochrane Database Systematic Reviews.* doi:10-1002/14651858.CD004398.pub3. Retrieved from http://ncbi.nlm.nih.gov/pubmed/23076904

Green, B. B., McAfee, T., Hindmarsh, M., Madsen, L., Caplow, M., & Buist, D. (2002). Effectiveness of telephone support in increasing physical activity levels in primary care patients. *American Journal of Preventive Medicine, 22*(3), 177–183. Retrieved from http://www.pubfacts.com/detail/11897462

Green, M. J., Peterson, S. K., Baker, M. W., Harper, G. R., Friedman, L. C., Rubenstein, W. S., & Mauger, D. T. (2004). Effect of a computer-based decision aid on knowledge, perceptions, and intentions about genetic testing for breast cancer susceptibility: A randomized controlled trial. *Journal of the American Medical Association, 492*(4), 442–452.

Grunwald, T., & Corsbie-Massay, C. (2006). Guidelines for cognitively efficient multimedia learning tools: Educational strategies, cognitive load, and interface redesign. *Academic Medicine, 81*(3), 213–223.

Gysels, M., & Higginson, I. J. (2007). Interactive technologies and videotapes for patient education in cancer care: Systematic review and meta-analysis of randomised trials. *Support Cancer Care Journal, 15*(1), 7–20.

Haggard, A. (1989). *Handbook of patient education.* Rockville, MD: Aspen.

Hagopian, G. A. (1996). The effects of informational audiotapes on knowledge and self-care behaviors of patients undergoing radiation therapy. *Oncology Nursing Forum, 23*(4), 697–700.

Handley, M. A., Shumway, M., & Schillinger, D. (2008). Cost-effectiveness of automated telephone self-management support with nurse care management among patients with diabetes. *Annals of Family Medicine*, 6(6), 512–518. doi:10-1370/afm.889. Retrieved from http://www.ncbi.nlm.nih.gov/pubmed/19001303

Heinich, R., Molenda, M., Russell, J. D., & Smaldino, S. E. (2002). *Instructional media and technologies for learning* (7th ed.). Upper Saddle River, NJ: Pearson.

Hoffman, B., Hartley, K., & Boone, R. (2005, January). Reaching accessibility: Guidelines for creating and refining digital learning materials. *Interventions in School and Clinic*, 40(3), 171.

Houts, P. S., Bachrach, B., Witmer, J. T., Tringali, C. A., Bucher, J. A., & Localio, R. A. (1998). Using pictographs to enhance recall of spoken medical instructions. *Patient Education and Counseling*, 35, 83–88.

Houts, P. S., Doak, C. C., Doak, L. G., & Loscalzo, M. J. (2006). The role of pictures in improving health communication: A review of research on attention, comprehension, recall, and adherence. *Patient Education and Counseling*, 61(2), 173–190. Retrieved from http://www.ncbi.nlm.nih.gov/pubmed/16122896

Huang, C. (2005). Designing high-quality interactive multimedia learning modules. *Computerized Medical Imaging and Graphics*, 29, 223–233.

Hussain, F. (2008, July). Interactivity in radio-based distance education: An overview. In F. Hussain (Ed.), *Effectiveness of technological interventions for education and information services in rural South Asia* (pp. 133–143). PhD dissertation, Carnegie Melon University, Pittsburgh, PA. Available at http://books.google.com/books?isbn=0549974334

Ilic, D., & Rowe, N. (2013). What is the evidence that poster presentations are effective in promoting knowledge transfer? A state of the art review. *Health Information and Libraries Journal*, 30, 4–12.

Izquierdo, R. E., Knudson, P. E., Meyer, S., Kearns, J., Ploutz-Snyder, R., & Weinstock, R. S. (2003). A comparison of diabetes education administered through telemedicine versus in-person. *Diabetes Care*, 26(4), 1002–1007.

Jeffries, P. R. (2005). A framework for designing, implementing, and evaluating simulations used as teaching strategies in nursing. *Nursing Education Perspectives*, 26(2), 96–103.

Jeste, D. V., Dunn, L. B., Folsom, D. P., & Zisook, D. (2008). Multimedia educational aids for improving consumer knowledge about illness management and treatment decisions: A review of randomized controlled trials. *Journal of Psychiatric Research*, 42, 1–21.

Johnson, A., & Sanford, J. (2005). Written and verbal information versus verbal information only for patients being discharged from acute hospital settings to home: Systematic review. *Health Education Research*, 20(4), 423–429.

Kessels, R. P. C. (2003). Patients' memory for medical information. *Journal of the Royal Society of Medicine*, 96, 219–222.

Kivela, K., Elo, S., Kyngas, H., & Kaariainen, M. (2014). The effects of health coaching on adult patients with chronic diseases: A systematic review. *Patient Education & Counseling*, 97, 147–157.

Leiner, M., Handal, G., & Williams, D. (2004). Patient communication: A multidisciplinary approach using animated cartoons. *Health Education Research*, 19(5), 591–595.

Lerner, E. B., Jehle, D. V. K., Janicke, D. M., & Moscati, R. M. (2000). Medical communication: Do our patients understand? *American Journal of Emergency Medicine*, 18(7), 764–766.

Lewis, D. (1999). Computer-based approaches to patient education: A review of the literature. *Journal of the American Medical Informatics Association*, 6(4), 272–282.

Lowenstein, A. J., Foord, L., & Romano, J. C. (2009). *Teaching strategies for health education and health promotion: Working with patients, families, and communities*. Sudbury, MA: Jones and Bartlett.

Manny, R. (2006, Winter). Multimedia streaming: A big part of the future for CHC [Community Health Care Services Foundation]. *Focus*, 3(1), 1, 4.

Mayer, G., & Villaire, M. (2009). Enhancing written communications to address health literacy. *The Online Journal of Issues in Nursing*, 14(3). doi:10-3912/OJIN,Vol14,No03Man03

Mayer, R. E. (Ed.). (2014). *The Cambridge handbook of multimedia learning* (2nd ed.) New York, NY: Cambridge University Press.

MDM Commercial. (2015). *Journey patient education solution.* Retrieved from http://www.mdm commercial.com/patient-education

Moneyham, L., Ura, D., Ellwood, S., & Bruno, B. (1996). The poster presentation as an educational tool. *Nurse Educator, 21*(4), 45–47.

Mons, U., Raum, E., Kramer, H. U., Ruter, G., Rothenbacher, D., Rosemann, T., . . . Brenner, H. (2013, October 30). Effectiveness of a supportive telephone counseling intervention in type 2 diabetes patients: Randomized controlled study. *PLOS One, 8*(10): e77954. doi:1371/journal.pone.0077954

Naperstek, B. (1993). Guided imagery: A technique that engages the imagination in the healing process. *Health Journeys* [CD]. United Kingdom: GlaxoSmithKline.

National Training Laboratories. (n.d.). *Learning pyramid.* Alexandria, VA: Institute for Applied Behavioral Science. Retrieved from http://homepages.gold.ac.uk/polovina/learnpyramid/about.htm

Nielsen, E., & Sheppard, M. A. (1988). Television as a patient education tool: A review of its effectiveness. *Patient Education and Counseling, 11*(1), 3–16.

Palmer, E. (n.d.). *Television for learning: Our foremost tool in the 21st century.* Opinion article 7, UNESCO. Retrieved from http://www.unesco.org/education/lwf/doc/portfolio/opinion7.htm

Pass, F., VanGerven, P. W. M., & Tabbers, H. K. (2014). The cognitive aging principle in multimedia learning. In R. E. Mayer (Ed.), *The Cambridge handbook of multimedia learning* (pp. 339–351). New York, NY: Cambridge University Press.

Pinto, B. M. (1993). Training and maintenance of breast self-examination skills. *American Journal of Preventive Medicine, 9*(6), 353–358.

Polyakova-Norwood, V. (2009, February 3). *Waking up from "PowerPoint-induced sleep": Effective use of PowerPoint for teaching.* Retrieved from http://www.sc.edu/cte/polyakova-norwood/doc/handout.pdf

Prensky, M. (2001). Digital natives, digital immigrants. *On the Horizon, 9*(5), 1–6.

Pulley, J. M., Brace, M., Bernard, G. R., & Masys, D. (2007). Evaluation of the effectiveness of posters to provide information to patients about DNA database and their opportunity to opt out. *Cell Tissue Bank, 8*(3), 233–241.

Rankin, S. H., & Stallings, K. D. (2005). *Patient education: Principles and practices* (5th ed.). Philadelphia, PA: Lippincott Williams & Wilkins.

Redman, B. K. (2007). *The practice of patient education: A case study approach* (10th ed.). St. Louis, MO: Mosby.

Rice, J., Trockel, M., King, T., & Remmert, D. (2004). Computerized training in breast self-examination: A test in a community health center. *Cancer Nursing, 27*(2), 162–168.

Saldana, R. A. (2014). Assessing the effectiveness of health education posters in community health centers. *GE National Medical Fellowship,* 1–31. Retrieved from http://www.nmfonline.org/file /2014-pclp-projects-for-resource-library/Saldana-Rafael-Paper.pdf

Santo, A., Laizner, A. M., & Shohet, L. (2005). Exploring the value of audiotapes for health literacy: A systematic review. *Patient Education and Counseling, 58*(3), 235–243.

Shoemaker, S. J., Wolf, M. S., & Brach, C. (2013, October). The Patient Education Materials Assessment Tool (PEMAT) and user's guide: An instrument to assess the understandability and actionability of print and audiovisual patient education materials. *Agency for Healthcare Research and Quality.* Rockville, MD: AHRQ.

Siwe, K., Bertero, C., Pugh, C., & Wijma, B. (2009). Use of clinical simulations for patient education: Targeting an untapped audience. *Studies in Health, Technology, and Informatics, 142,* 325–330. Retrieved from http://www.ncbi.nlm.nih.gov/pubmed/19377178

Skinner, C. S., Strecher, V. J., & Hospers, H. (1994). Physician's recommendations for mammography: Do tailored messages make a difference? *American Journal of Public Health, 84,* 43–49.

Smaldino, S. E., Lowther, D. L., & Russell, J. D. (2012). *Instructional technology and media for learning* (10th ed.). Upper Saddle River, NJ: Pearson.

SMART. (2009). Home page. Retrieved from http://smarttech.com

Tones, K., & Tilford, S. (2001). The mass media and health promotion. In K. Tones & S. Tilford (Eds.), *Health promotion effectiveness, efficiency, and equity* (3rd ed., pp. 342–393). Cheltenham, United Kingdom: Nelson Thornes, Ltd.

Turner, C. E., Drenckhahn, V. V., & Bates, M. W. (1935). Effectiveness of radio in health education. *American Journal of Public Health Nations Health, 25*(5), 589–594. Retrieved from http://www.ncbi.nlm.nih.gov/pmc/articles/PMC1559159/?page=1

Weixler, D. (1994). Correcting metered-dose inhaler misuse. *Nursing, 24*(7), 62–65.

Weston, C., & Cranston, P. A. (1986). Selecting instructional strategies. *Journal of Higher Education, 57*(3), 259–288.

Williams, N. H., Wolgin, C. S., & Hodge, C. S. (1998). Creating an educational videotape. *Journal for Nurses in Staff Development, 14*(6), 261–265.

Wofford, J. L., Smith, E. D., & Miller, D. P. (2005). The multimedia computer for office-based patient education: A systematic review, *Patient Education and Counseling, 59*(2), 148–157.

Technology in Patient Education

Deborah L. Sopczyk

Chapter Highlights

- Health Education in the Information Age
- The Impact of Technology on the Teacher and the Learner
- Strategies for Using Technology in Healthcare Education
  - *The World Wide Web*
  - *Healthcare Consumer Education and the World Wide Web*
  - *Social Media*
- The Internet
  - *E-Mail/Texting*
  - *Electronic Discussion Groups*
  - *Mailing Lists*
  - *Other Forms of Online Discussion*
  - *Online Chats*
- Issues Related to the Use of Technology

Key Terms

asynchronous
blogs
consumer informatics
digital divide
information age
information literacy
Internet
social media
wiki
World Wide Web

Objectives

After completing this chapter, the reader will be able to

1. Describe changes in patient education that have occurred as a result of information age technology.

2. Define the terms *information age, consumer informatics, computer literacy, World Wide Web, Internet, information literacy, social media,* and *digital divide.*

3. Identify ways in which the resources of the Internet and World Wide Web could be incorporated into healthcare education.

4. Describe the role of the nurse in using technology for patient education.

5. Recognize the issues related to the use of technology in teaching patients and their families.

© wanchai/Shutterstock

459

Life, as we know it today, has been greatly influenced by technological advances of the last half century. The birth of the Internet and the World Wide Web, the development of information technology, the wide-scale accessibility of computers, and the development of user-friendly software have all had an impact on every aspect of people's lives. "In the 21st century, technology will continue to advance and become the norm in healthcare rather than the exception" (Daniels & Wedler, 2015, p. 28). Technology is influencing many aspects of professional nursing practice. Some of the most dramatic changes are occurring in the field of patient, staff, and student education, where technology has and will continue to transform the way learners learn and the way teachers teach (Matthews-DeNatale & Lowenstein, 2014).

In these modern times, learners and teachers alike have access to a world of information instantaneously. Computers and the Internet have made it possible to get information from anyone, anywhere, anytime, with just a click of a mouse or a tap of the fingertip. With the development of mobile devices and gadgets such as smartphones, smart watches, and tablets, most people have computer technology at close hand throughout the day. Virtually all children begin learning on computers when they are in nursery school as young as 3 years of age (National Center for Educational Statistics, 2006), and many parents are exposing their kids to technology even before this age. As a result, children's lifelong exposure to digital technology has shaped the way they think and process information (Prensky, 2001).

This chapter explores the challenges and opportunities resulting from the use of technology as they pertain to health and health care. Technology in education has tremendous potential. Through wise use of technology, nurses can increase access, improve educational practices already in place, and create new strategies that transform teaching and learning experiences for healthcare consumers. Because of the complexity of health care today, "patient education through interactive technology becomes a vital instrument in patients' safety and quality of care" (Cassano, 2015, p. 1). Educating patients with the help of sophisticated electronic devices has been found to enhance their engagement in care planning, improve their self-care efforts, reduce the number of hospital readmissions, improve their outcomes, and increase their satisfaction with care (Cassano, 2014; Roney, 2012).

Of course, technology is not a magic solution that can be implemented without careful planning, monitoring, and evaluation. Even though technology has incredible power, users may find that it has given them results that they neither anticipated nor desired. To use these resources effectively, the nurse who adopts technology to enhance learning must not only have a basic understanding of the technology itself but also be able to integrate the technology into a teaching plan that is based on sound educational principles and that addresses issues such as access, cost, support, equipment, process, and outcomes.

This chapter is designed as an introduction to the application of technology in patient education. This chapter is not intended to give detailed instruction on the mechanics of computers and other types of hardware and software; instead, it presents a basic overview of the technology involved and its implications for the teacher and the learner. Hence, this chapter focuses primarily on the Internet, the World Wide Web, and computer-based hardware and software applications that can be used by nurses to enhance teaching and learning with patients and their family members in any healthcare setting as well as by learners who seek education independently and from a distance.

The Internet, the World Wide Web, and computer-based technologies are developing at a rapid pace that is accelerating with each new generation of discoveries and applications. Because of this phenomenon, consumers are often advised that the computers they buy today are not likely to reflect the state-of-the-art technology of tomorrow. The same caution must be given to readers of books on technology. Given the pace of technology and the development cycle of a textbook, it is impossible to capture all that is new and cutting edge in the world of educational technologies in a text such as this one. Rather, this chapter is meant to serve as a starting point from which readers can begin to investigate the wide array of educational technologies and resources available. Ideally, it will stimulate readers to continue to search for new and exciting ways to integrate technology into their teaching and learning activities.

Health Education in the Information Age

The use of technology in education is a reflection of what is happening on a much larger scale in our communities. Hence, it is useful to think of educational technology within the broader context of the environment in which people live and work. This period of history, often referred to as the **information age**, the computer age, or the digital age, is characterized by a change in focus from industry to information. Beginning in the 1970s, improvements in information technology and the decreasing cost of computers suddenly made information more accessible, resulting in a dramatically different world (Finnis, 2003; Wachter, 2013). New and powerful industries have sprung up, and the world has very quickly become a much smaller place as it is now possible to access people and services from around the world in a blink of an eye and at very low cost.

The demand for technology and for information continues to grow. In the 21st century, adults and children have come to depend on smartphones, media players, electronic readers, and other computer-driven devices. If you think about the many ways in which technology has changed the world, it is clear that computers have become more than tools to make life easier—they have become part of the culture of most societies.

Perhaps the most significant effect of computers on our society, in general, and on education, in particular, is related to their capacity to assist in the collection, management, transportation, and transformation of information at high speed. As a result of this newfound ability to handle information, the world has experienced an "information explosion." People living in this information-driven society benefit from the availability of information but also are challenged to keep up with the vast amounts of information that are continually bombarding them from all directions. Information and knowledge have become valuable commodities, and the ability to gather and evaluate information efficiently and effectively has become a 21st-century life skill.

How can the information age impact health education? Consider the following points:

- The infrastructure now exists to link people around the world to one another, to nurses and other healthcare professionals, and to a vast array of Web-based information.
- Internetworldstats.com (2015), an international website that provides comprehensive and current information on Internet usage, reports that the North American continent is home to approximately 357 million people, of whom 310 million are Internet users and 182 million are Facebook subscribers.

Looking specifically at adults living in the United States, only 15% report not using the Internet (Zickuhr, 2013).

- Approximately 70% of American adults have a high-speed broadband connection in their homes (Zickuhr & Smith, 2013)

The use of information age technology has had such a dramatic influence on health education that a unique and rapidly expanding field of study, consumer informatics (also referred to as consumer health informatics), has emerged. The American Medical Informatics Association, one of the principal professional organizations for people in healthcare informatics, has established a working group to advance consumer informatics through collaboration and dialogue. This group defines **consumer informatics** as a field "devoted to informatics from multiple consumer or patient views including patient-focused informatics, health literacy, and consumer education" (American Medical Informatics Association, 2015).

Researchers and other professionals in the field of consumer informatics are striving to find ways to use technology to strengthen the relationship between patient and healthcare provider as well as to teach and empower patients dealing with issues related to health and wellness. Although much attention has been given to computer-based educational systems, consumer informatics is not restricted to computer-based programs. It includes the study of a wide range of social media that can be employed to deliver health-related information (Pho & Gay, 2013).

Sophisticated technology will continue to make health and healthcare information more accessible and more meaningful to both healthcare consumers and health professionals. However, a number of issues remain to be resolved. One significant area of concern is the limited oversight and control over the content that is posted on the Internet and World Wide Web, two of the major vehicles for delivering information to a global audience.

When the World Wide Web was first introduced, users were primarily consumers of content developed by organizations and commercial enterprises. The increased use of blogs, wikis, and social network sites—many of which are devoted to health and health-related topics—testify to this ease of placing content on the Web (Miller & Pole, 2010). The amount of health information created by individuals without healthcare education or expertise has also increased.

Healthcare professionals are concerned that consumers are making serious healthcare decisions based on information on the Web that has not been reviewed for accuracy, currency, or bias. These concerns are valid as increasing numbers of people are using the Web as a source of health information, and studies have shown that the information they find may be inaccurate or misleading (Fleming, Vandermause, & Shaw, 2014; Modave, Shokar, Peñaranda, & Nguyen, 2014; Seymour, German, Sharif, Zhang, & Kalinderian, 2015). According to a Pew study of adults living in the United States (Fox & Duggan, 2013), the findings are as follows:

- 59% of respondents went to the Web seeking health-related information in the past year.
- 35% went to the Web for the purpose of diagnosing a medical condition for themselves or others.

- 26% learned about someone else's experiences with a health problem or health care.
- 16% of respondents went to the Web looking to find others with a similar health problem.

Healthcare education and informatics professionals are working together to develop codes to guide practice and safeguard healthcare consumers who use educational information and services delivered via the World Wide Web and the Internet. The Internet Healthcare Coalition (http://www.ihealthcoalition.org/ehealth-code/), a not-for-profit group, was founded in 1997 for the purpose of identifying and promoting quality educational resources on the Internet. One of this organization's most significant accomplishments was the establishment of the *e-Health Code of Ethics*, displayed in six languages on its website. The purpose of this code is to ensure confident and informed use of the health-related information found on the Web. The *e-Health Code of Ethics* is based on the principles of candor, honesty, quality, informed consent, privacy, professionalism, responsible partnering, and accountability, as described in more detail in **Table 13–1.**

Table 13–1 Guiding Principles of the *e-Health Code of Ethics*

Candor
Disclose who created the site and its purpose to help users make a judgment about the credibility and trustworthiness of the information or services provided.
Honesty
Be truthful in describing products/services to present information in a way that is not likely to mislead the user.
Quality
Take the necessary steps to ensure that the information provided is accurate and well supported and that the services offered are of the highest quality. Present information in a manner that is easy for users to understand and use. Make available background information about the sources of the content so the user can make a decision about the quality of the product and services being offered.
Informed Consent
Inform users if personal information is collected and allow them to choose whether the information can be used or shared.
Privacy
Take steps to ensure that the user's right to privacy is protected.
Professionalism in Online Health Care
Abide by the ethical code of your profession (e.g., nursing, medicine). Provide users with information about who you are, your credentials, what you can do online, and which limitations may apply to the online interaction.
Responsible Partnering
Take steps to ensure that sponsors, partners, and others who work with you are trustworthy.
Accountability
Implement a procedure for collecting, reviewing, and responding to user feedback. Develop and share procedures for self-monitoring compliance with the *e-Health Code of Ethics*.

Modified from the Internet Healthcare Coalition. (2000). *e-Health code of ethics*. e-Health Ethics Initiative, 2000. http://www.ihealthcoalition.org/ethics/ehcode.html

The Impact of Technology on the Teacher and the Learner

Information age technology has had a significant influence on patient education for a number of reasons. Most important, access to information bridges the gap between teacher and learner. When information is widely available, it is no longer necessary for nurses to locate, interpret, and deliver content to patients and their family members. Therefore, they are no longer the ones who hold all of the answers or who are solely responsible for imparting knowledge (Cassano, 2015).

Nurses in the information age are becoming facilitators of learning rather than providers of information. They must structure their approach to teaching to be consistent with the needs of patients by striving to create collaborative atmospheres in their teaching and learning environments. Nurses also must be willing to encourage and support patients in their attempts to seek the knowledge they require. As information becomes more and more accessible, the need for patients to memorize facts becomes less important than the ability to think critically. Hence, patient educators in the information age must help individuals learn how to refine a problem, to find the information they need, and to critically evaluate the information they find.

The information age has been witness to some dramatic changes in the behavior of healthcare consumers, making inevitable the role changes for patients and nurses as described previously. Technology and the increased accessibility to information it offers have empowered and enlightened these consumers, encouraging them to form new partnerships with their healthcare providers (Cassano, 2015; Fox, 2011; Kaplan & Brennan, 2001; Shaw et al., 2006). Even those patients who are reluctant to assume more responsibility for managing their own health care are moving in that direction as changes in the health delivery system have forced them to assume more active roles. As a result, healthcare consumers in the information age are eager to learn about and make use of the many information resources available to them.

Today's consumers often enter the healthcare arena with information in hand. They are prepared to engage in a dialogue with their healthcare providers about their diagnoses and treatments. Surveys of the 113 million consumers who have gone online to find health information show that the information they found caused them to make decisions about treatment of a condition and made them more confident in asking questions of their care provider (Fox, 2011; Fox & Duggan, 2013).

A survey conducted by Fox and Duggan (2013) found that 65% of consumers who go to the Web for health information will follow up with a healthcare provider, while the remaining 35% will use the information to treat themselves at home. Based on this trend, nurses can no longer assume that the patients they see in a hospital or clinic will have only the information that has been provided to them by healthcare providers. Furthermore, nurses cannot assume that patients will unquestioningly accept what is told to them.

Whereas healthcare consumers of the past were often isolated from others with similar diagnoses and were dependent upon healthcare providers for information, today's e-consumers and e-caregivers have the means to easily access networks of other patients and healthcare providers worldwide. Online support groups, blogs, and discussion groups where healthcare consumers can share experiences are readily available. Consumers who are being treated for health problems can readily find detailed information about their diagnoses, treatments, and prognoses from a variety of sources via the computer or other digital devices.

In this dynamic environment, it is not surprising that the teaching needs of today's healthcare consumers and the expectations they hold for those who will be teaching them are changing. The role of the nurse has not been diminished, but it has changed. Nurses must now be prepared not only to use technology in education but also to help patients to access information, evaluate the information they find, and engage in discussions about the information that is available.

Strategies for Using Technology in Healthcare Education

The World Wide Web

In simple terms, the **World Wide Web** is a virtual space for information. It is almost impossible to track its size because there are billions of webpages in existence, with several million new pages being added every month. These webpages cover a wide range of topics and display a variety of formats, including text, audio, graphic, and video.

A user moves around the World Wide Web by way of a Web browser, a special software program that locates and displays webpages. Mozilla Firefox, Apple Safari, and Microsoft Internet Explorer are examples of Web browsers. Search engines and search directories are computer programs that allow the user to search the Web for particular subject areas. Google is an example of a search engine, and Yahoo! is an example of a search directory. The **Internet** is a huge global network of computers established to allow the transfer of information from one computer to another. Unlike the World Wide Web, which was created to *display* information, the Internet was created to *exchange* information. The World Wide Web resides on a small section of the Internet and would not exist without the Internet's computer network.

A report produced by the Pew Foundation revealed that 72% of Americans who use the Internet have accessed the World Wide Web to obtain health-related information (Fox & Duggan, 2013). Healthcare consumers can find websites ranging from those that present videos of surgical procedures to those where they can ask questions as well as receive information. The number of healthcare sites on the World Wide Web is difficult to capture with any accuracy, as new sites are being introduced on a daily basis. Nevertheless, there are clearly thousands of health-related websites available to consumers offering a wide range of information, products, and services.

Also, health-related information on the World Wide Web is becoming increasingly accessible to consumers through the development of mobile technology, which takes the concept of information anytime/anywhere to a new realm. A survey by Fox and Duggan (2012) found that 53% of Americans own a smartphone that provides Web access, with 1 in 3 smartphone owners reporting that they use their phones to find health-related information. Another study found that 25% of Americans own a tablet, another mobile device with easy access to the Web (Rainie, 2012).

Knowledge of the World Wide Web is critical for nurses who work with and educate healthcare consumers. This is true for the following reasons:

- Nurses can expect to see patients enter the healthcare arena having already searched the Web for information. In fact, a Pew study found that many consumers go to the Web to seek information about a problem they are experiencing to help them decide whether it is necessary to see a healthcare provider (Fox & Duggan, 2013). Therefore, familiarity with the type of information found on the Web helps direct the assessment of patients prior to teaching to identify the needs of the learner and to determine whether follow-up is necessary.
- The World Wide Web is a tremendous resource for both consumer and professional education. To use the Web effectively, nurses must possess information literacy skills and be prepared to teach these same skills to patients, including how to access the information on the Web and how to evaluate the information found.
- The World Wide Web provides a powerful mechanism for nurses to offer healthcare education to a worldwide audience. An increasing number of health organizations are creating websites with pages dedicated to presenting healthcare information for consumers.

Healthcare Consumer Education and the World Wide Web

A preteaching assessment of a patient must begin with questions about computer use. Despite the widespread use of computers in our society, not everyone has access to a computer or has interest in using a computer. Adults older than the age of 65, African Americans, individuals who have less than a high school education, and individuals living in a home without children remain less likely to be online than others (Jones & Fox, 2009; Horrigan, 2009).

However, it is important to note that these figures are changing with time. For example, a recent survey of older adults found that although older Americans lag behind younger people in computer use, the percentage of Americans 65 or older who were using a computer had increased to 53%, with 70% of these respondents indicating that they used their computer daily (Zickuhr & Madden, 2012). Therefore, it is important to determine whether a patient has a computer or smartphone in his or her home, has access to the Internet, is knowledgeable about using a computer, and has interest in using a computer to obtain information and resources regarding his or her health care.

If a patient does not have a computer but has interest in using one to access resources on the Web, places where he or she may access a computer should be discussed. Libraries, senior centers, and community centers commonly have computers with Internet access for public use and typically offer instruction and assistance for new users.

Patients who use computers should be asked about their use of the Web. A Pew Foundation study revealed that Web users in the United States found information on the Web that did one of the following:

1. Influenced their decisions about how to treat an illness
2. Led them to ask questions
3. Led them to seek a second medical opinion
4. Affected their decision about whether to seek the assistance of a healthcare provider (Fox, 2006; Fox & Duggan, 2013)

Because the Web can be so influential, it is imperative to determine that the information a patient has found is accurate, complete, and fully understood. Only 15% of Web users report that they always check the source and date of the information found, and many report feeling overwhelmed, confused, or frightened by the complexity and amount of information presented (Fox, 2006; Hartzband & Groopman, 2010).

These findings are not surprising. The World Wide Web contains information designed for both professional and consumer audiences. Healthcare consumers may not have the background necessary to comprehend professional literature and other types of information designed for healthcare professionals. When healthcare consumers do a search on a topic, they will access websites designed for them as well as for health professionals. Consumers should not be discouraged from accessing these sites, but nurses must help patients find information written for them at their level of readability and comprehension. Even websites specifically designed for consumers may be difficult for the general public to understand. For example, in a review of 25 websites on menopause, Charbonneau (2012) found that the average reading level was grade 10, significantly higher than the recommended sixth-grade level.

The Web also contains information that may be biased, inaccurate, or misleading (Hartzband & Groopman, 2010; Lewis, Gundwardena, & Saadawi, 2005). Many of the health-related websites are sponsored by commercial enterprises trying to sell a product. Others contain information posted by nonprofessionals and may be opinion rather than fact based. Because the Web has the potential to change so quickly, it is difficult to regulate. Even webpages sponsored by physicians, nurses, and university medical centers may contain errors or information that is misleading or difficult to decipher.

Patients may find that the Web has provided too much information, information they are not ready to handle, or information they do not fully understand (Hartzband & Groopman, 2010). For example, a patient newly diagnosed with a serious illness may be overwhelmed with the detailed information found on the Web regarding the course of the disease, prognosis, and treatment. For nurses, then, it is important to ask patients if they are using the Web to find health-related information and to explore the types of information they have found.

Patients may or may not initially feel comfortable talking about information they have gathered. They may fear nurses will interpret their research as a lack of trust in the care they receive. Some may be embarrassed to talk about information they do not fully understand. Others may be anxious about how to bring up information that conflicts with what they have been told or how they are being treated.

For these reasons, it is important for nurses to establish early in their relationships with patients that they are interested in talking with them about the information they have gathered from the Web or other resources they have available to them. Patients need to feel that nurses are open to discussing whatever information they find. They need to understand that nurses are their partners in seeking the best information available.

For patients who are being treated for a condition over an extended period of time, it is also important to continue the conversation about their Web searches throughout their treatment. Simply asking "What interesting information have you found on the Web lately?" will keep the dialogue open and provide the nurse with the opportunity to respond to whatever questions or concerns patients may have.

When conducting a patient education session, computer availability during teaching can accomplish several goals. First, it will provide the nurse with the opportunity to review Web-based information with the patient. Not only can the nurse introduce websites that are relevant to the patient's needs, but some of the sites the patient has been using can be reviewed. This will allow the nurse to determine the type and amount of information to which the patient has been exposed, assess the patient's knowledge, and identify areas in which the patient may have need for further teaching. Also, the nurse may find information that needs further discussion. For example, a patient may have visited a website that provides distressing information about side effects of treatment, prognosis, or disease progression. Looking at the site together will enable the nurse and patient to talk about what has been discovered and do additional teaching if needed.

A second important advantage of reviewing websites with a patient is that this activity provides a chance to teach the patient information literacy skills. **Information literacy** is defined as the ability of individuals to demonstrate the following four competencies:

1. The capacity to identify the information needed
2. The skills to access the information needed
3. The knowledge of how to evaluate the information found
4. The skills to apply the information considered valid and useful

In essence, if patients are to make effective use of the vast array of information on the Web, they must be able to identify the questions they need answered, find the information they are looking for, judge whether the information they find is trustworthy, and decide how they will use the information to meet their needs.

Information literacy is *not* synonymous with computer literacy. A patient who is information literate knows how to find the information needed and can evaluate the information found for accuracy, currency, and bias. By comparison, a patient who is computer literate has the technical skills and knowledge required to use contemporary computer hardware and software and can adapt to new technologies that emerge (Williams, 2003).

Although patients and their families may not have the background knowledge to evaluate information to the same extent as a healthcare professional, they can be taught some simple steps to develop their information literacy skills and to help them begin to identify which websites are useful and which are problematic. These steps include the following:

1. *Reduce a problem or topic to a searchable command that can be used with a search engine or search directory.* If patients do not know how to narrow their topics to a few key words, they will be unable to find the information they desire.
2. *Categorize webpages according to their purpose.* A patient should be taught to look for the person or organization responsible for the website and then place the website into a category the reflects its main purpose; for example marketing, sales, advocacy, informational, personal, or instructional.
3. *Identify sources of potential bias that may influence the content or the manner in which the content is presented.* For example, an advocacy website is likely to present information that favors one side of a debate. A marketing or sales site will

have a tendency to include information that is supportive of a particular product or service.

4. *Make a judgment as to the likelihood that the information found on the webpage is accurate and reliable.* For example, patients can be taught to look for the credentials of authors of reports or articles found on the Web. They can also be encouraged to look at more than one site to see if they can find similar claims or suggestions.

5. *Make a decision as to the completeness or comprehensiveness of the information presented.* Because patients may not have the background knowledge needed to quickly recognize when information is missing, they should be encouraged to look at more than one site when researching an area of interest. If nurses know that patients are using the Web to investigate a particular topic, they can help them identify a list of things to look for in articles or webpages addressing the topic.

6. *Determine the currency of the information on a webpage.* Consumers need to know the importance of looking for a creation or modification date or other signs that the information on a website is up to date.

7. *Identify resources to answer questions or verify assumptions made about the content of a webpage.* If questions arise, patients should be encouraged to check out information with their healthcare provider and should know how and when to report information found on the Web that is potentially harmful to others (Lau, Gabarron, Fernandez-Luque, & Amoyones, 2012).

In years past, patients and their families were not encouraged to research health topics or treatment options, but rather to rely on their healthcare providers for all of their health-related information. Providers, including nurses, feared that patients would not understand the information they found or that they would find information they would not be able to handle. Today, nurses have more confidence in the ability of patients to manage their own health care.

More than ever before, nurses are empowering their patients by teaching and encouraging them to take advantage of the resources at their disposal. Computers are being placed in waiting rooms set to appropriate websites. Teaching materials on how to use the Web are being distributed, and websites are being created for patient use. Given concerns about the quality of information available on the Web, some professionals are working together to create trusted websites that provide information and resources for specific patient populations (Fox, Duggan, & Purcell, 2013; Lewis et al., 2005).

There are many reasons why teaching patients where to go on the Web to find information is good practice. Web-based information can be obtained quickly, the cost of Internet access in the home is minimal, and Web access is free in libraries and other community service organizations. Many healthcare consumers would benefit from having their questions answered quickly and inexpensively.

For example, families with young children are likely to have frequent questions related to childhood illnesses, growth and development, and behavior problems, but they may not have the time or money to make a visit to the pediatrician to have such questions answered. Senior citizens may have questions about the health problems encountered with aging but may have difficulty getting to a healthcare provider because of transportation and financial issues. People with chronic illness may gain some sense of control over their lives when they are able to access information on the Web about their conditions. Healthy people may have many questions but few opportunities to talk with a health provider to get answers.

Even when patients do have the opportunity to meet with a health provider, they often leave with unanswered questions. Sometimes they forget to ask, at times they are hesitant to ask, and in today's healthcare delivery system, they may not be given sufficient time to ask the many questions that arise when people are dealing with health issues. The nurse can teach patients who access the Web to use this resource more effectively and can be proactive in encouraging others to give it a try.

A helpful approach to patient education is to compile lists of websites appropriate to the needs of different client populations. **Table 13–2** provides examples of the various types of websites that are available for consumer use. As illustrated in the table, the type of sites range from general sites covering a broad range of topics to sites with a specific focus or theme.

Table 13–2 Sample Websites for Healthcare Consumers

Title	URL	Sponsor/Author	Description
Medline Plus	http://www.nlm.nih.gov/medlineplus	National Library of Medicine	Example of a government site that provides access to extensive information about specific diseases/conditions, links to consumer health information from the National Institutes of Health, dictionaries, lists of hospitals and physicians, health information in Spanish and other languages, and clinical trials. There is no advertising on this site.
Aplastic Anemia and MDS International Foundation, Inc.	http://www.aamds.org	Aplastic Anemia and MDS International Foundation, Inc.	Example of a disease-specific website that provides a range of services, including free educational materials and access to a help line where consumer questions will be researched and answered.
Mayo Clinic	http://www.mayoclinic.org	Mayo Clinic	Example of a comprehensive hospital site that provides information as well as a variety of interactive tools to help healthcare consumers manage a healthy lifestyle, research disease conditions, and make healthcare decisions. Advertising helps support this site.
Cancer Net	http://www.nci.nih.gov	National Cancer Institute	Example of a government site devoted to all aspects of cancer. Provides both professional and consumer-oriented information and resources.
Band-Aides and Blackboards	http://www.lehman.cuny.edu/faculty/jfleitas/bandaides/sitemap.html	Nursing faculty at Lehman College in Bronx, NY	Site provides personal rather than factual information about growing up with health problems from the perspectives of kids, teens, and adults.
NetWellness	http://www.netwellness.org	University of Cincinnati, Ohio State University, and Case Western Reserve University	Nonprofit consumer health website that provides high-quality information created and evaluated by medical and health professional faculty at several universities.

In selecting websites to share with patients, it is important that the nurse review these sources carefully. In recent years, multiple rating scales have been developed to assist in the evaluation of such sites. Most scales include criteria that address the accuracy of the content, design, and visual appeal of the site; disclosure of the authors; sponsors of the site; currency of information; authority of the source; ease of use; and accessibility and availability of the site. Links to multiple sources for tips on how to evaluate websites for accuracy and reliability can be found at www.usa-document.com/lb/evaluating%20 websites.pdf (Ham, 2014).

Table 13–3 summarizes the questions that should be asked in evaluating a health-related website. Resource lists made up of quality sites will not only serve as references for patients but also provide examples of the types of sites they should be accessing.

Finally, nurses can create their own websites to bring their healthcare messages to Web users around the world. Table 13–2 provides two examples of websites that exemplify the types of roles nurses can play to bring health information to various consumers via the World Wide Web. Band-Aides and Blackboards is a creative site designed by a nurse to facilitate understanding of the problems faced by children growing up with

Table 13–3 Criteria for Evaluating Health-Related Websites

Accuracy
• Are supportive data provided?
• Are the supportive data current and from reputable sources?
• Can you find the same information on other websites?
• Is the information provided comprehensive?
• Is more than one point of view presented?

Design
• Is the website easy to navigate?
• Is there evidence that care was taken in creating the site? Do the links work? Are there typographical errors?
• Is the information presented in a manner that is appropriate for the intended audience?
• Do the graphics serve a purpose other than decoration?

Authors/Sponsors
• Are the sponsors/authors of the site clearly identified?
• Do the authors provide their credentials?
• Do the authors/sponsors provide a way to contact them or give feedback?
• Do the authors/sponsors clearly identify the purpose of the site?
• Is there reason for the sponsors/authors to be biased about the topic?

Currency
• Is there a recent creation or modification date identified?
• Is there evidence of currency (e.g., updated bibliography reference to current events)?

Authority
• Are the sponsors/authors credible? (e.g., is it a government agency, educational institution, or healthcare organization site versus a personal page?)
• Are the author's credentials appropriate to the purpose of the site?

health problems. This site is thought provoking rather than factual. The nurse who created it uses the words and drawings of children and parents to bring a real-life perspective to the thoughts, feelings, and experiences of growing up with illness. Band-Aides and Blackboards teaches important messages about not being alone, about ways to solve common problems, and about what really matters to this population.

NetWellness, another site in which nurses play a predominant role, is a very different site than Band-Aides and Blackboards. NetWellness is a noncommercial, electronic consumer health information service that has been in existence since the mid-1990s. Information on the website is created and evaluated in collaboration by more than 500 multidisciplinary professionals from three different universities. Information on this site is checked for accuracy, and each revision made is stamped with its date so that users can easily determine its currency. NetWellness continues to be a wonderful Web resource for healthcare consumers. Individuals can submit health-related questions to the site's panel of experts, with nurses and other health professionals then responding to these queries. The panel of experts also provides information for the section of the site devoted to hot topics.

Development of a website is typically a team effort. In addition to content experts such as nurses who contribute the material to be included on the site, Web designers with technical and layout expertise can provide valuable assistance with practical aspects of the site's development. Many resources are available to healthcare professionals interested in developing websites. For example, the Research Based Web Design and Usability Guidelines website (http://www.usability.gov/pdfs/guidelines.html) is sponsored by the U.S. Department of Health and Human Services. This resource contains guidelines that can be used in designing health-related websites. Not only are the guidelines provided on this site based on research studies and supporting information from the field, but ratings are also assigned to each guideline according to the strength of the evidence available.

A number of issues must be considered before engaging in health education via a website. Websites have the potential to reach millions of users over an extended period of time. The healthcare consumers who use the Web have varying levels of sophistication, and they may or may not know to check the dates on which the website was created and modified. Given this diversity of the audience, it is very important that the information on the site be accurate and updated as often as necessary. Depending on the topics covered, it may be necessary to include a disclaimer about the importance of checking with a healthcare provider.

If the site is interactive and the nurse will be responding to questions submitted by users of the site, liability issues must be carefully considered. Nurses who respond to questions from Web users are providing advice and guidance to people whom they do not see and cannot assess. Nurses need to determine whether their malpractice insurance covers this type of activity. They also need policies and procedures for responding to questions that might be considered urgent (Dizon et al., 2012). Depending on the nature of the site, it may be advisable to include an attorney on the website development and maintenance team to provide advice when needed. It is important to determine if there are relevant legal issues related to practice activities of the nurse on the website.

Although new technology has opened the door to many unique and exciting opportunities, it has also raised many questions about telepractice and licensure. Because technology makes it so easy to provide healthcare services to patients across state lines, the provision of nursing, medical, and other types of technology-facilitated healthcare services to patients at a distance has been thrust into the spotlight. Multistate licensure and other types of legislation have and will continue to be proposed, and new practice guidelines are likely to be enacted.

Finally, the time commitment required to respond to questions from Web users cannot be underestimated. If a website provides an opportunity for consumers to ask questions, responses must be researched and checked for accuracy before they are posted. Healthcare consumers are online 24 hours a day, 7 days a week. Therefore, consumers must be advised how long they will likely wait before responses to their questions are posted. Adequate coverage must be arranged so that questions are answered on a regular basis and service is not interrupted for long periods of time.

Social Media

Social media, also referred to as Web 2.0, "are Internet sites and applications that allow users to create, share, edit and interact with on-line content" (Gagnon & Sabus, 2015, p. 407). Although many different definitions of social media can be found in the literature, in the broadest sense, the term encompasses communities of people who gather online to participate in blogs, wikis, and services such as Facebook, Twitter, YouTube, Instagram, and other similar forums (Boulos & Wheeler, 2007). Because of their quick communication and engaging formats, social media have experienced dramatic growth in their use and popularity in recent years. In 2005, only about 7% of Americans participated in social media. In 2015, that number grew to 65% or two-thirds of adults living in the United States (Perrin, 2015).

The healthcare industry has begun to recognize the potential of social media to educate and empower people, to quickly send messages to a worldwide audience, and to gather information about public perceptions of health issues (Knight, Werstine, Rasmussen-Pennington, Fitzsimmons, & Petrella, 2015; Prasad, 2013; Thackery, Neiger, Smith, & Van Wagenen, 2012). For example, the Mayo Clinic's Center for Social Media was established to "lead the social media revolution in health care by accelerating effective application of social media tools throughout Mayo Clinic and spurring broader and deeper engagement in social media by hospitals, medical professionals and patients" (Mayo Clinic, 2012). Through its Center for Social Media, the Mayo Clinic reports being able to establish a popular medical provider channel on YouTube, offer an active Facebook page, and have more than 400,000 followers on Twitter.

Another example is the Healthcare Hashtag Project, which was created to make Twitter more accessible to individuals interested in healthcare issues. The Healthcare Hashtag project has grown very rapidly. It currently has over 3000 contributors and has registered over 1 billion tweets covering over 15,000 health-related topics (Healthcare Hashtag Project, 2015).

BLOGS

Several of the more common forms of social media are addressed in this section.

First developed in the late 1990s, **blogs** (Web logs) are an increasingly popular mechanism for individuals to share information and experiences related to a given topic.

Although sometimes referred to as Web diaries, blogs are much more than that; for example, they may include images, media objects, and links that allow for public responses (Maag, 2005). Blog entries are typically viewed in reverse chronological order (most recent first) and are easy to follow. Other common blog features include archives, a blogroll (list of recommended blogs), and a reader comment section (Miller & Pole, 2010).

The number of blogs available on the Web has increased dramatically in recent years. A decade ago, the Pew Internet and American Life Project (Lenhart & Fox, 2006) reported that approximately 12 million Americans had created a blog, and another 57 million read blogs on the World Wide Web. Specific to health care, just 5 years later about 35% (over 100 million) of Internet users in the United States reported reading someone else's commentary on a healthcare issue on a blog or similar application, and another 4% actually posted comments or questions on a blog (Fox, 2011).

Many of the blogs found on the Web are health related and often tell the story of the creator's experience with a given disease or treatment (Harvard Health Blog, 2015). For example, a search of the Web will uncover numerous blogs on breast cancer. These blogs cover everything from the stories of cancer survivors and family experiences to information-based blogs describing various breast cancer treatments. Many blog creators provide a picture with a limited or absent biography. A review of 398 blog posts by Buis and Carpenter (2009) also found that commentary on external media—for example, health-related books and newspaper articles—is another common topic in postings.

Given the growing popularity of blogs, it is reasonable to assume that healthcare consumers, particularly young people, might turn to blogs for health-related information and support. The Pew Internet and American Life Project's report on blogging (Lenhart & Fox, 2006) noted that bloggers tend to be men and women younger than the age of 30 who use a pseudonym rather than their own name. Most are heavy Internet users. Other blogs, however, are written by health professionals and by consumers who have a story to tell (Buis & Carpenter, 2009). For this reason, patients who are getting information from blogs must be taught the importance of evaluating the credentials of the author as well as the content of the blog.

Because of the ease of use and the popularity of this form of electronic communication, blogs remain an effective way to provide consumers with health-related information. As with other forms of communication, nurses who use blogs to teach must implement a plan for regular maintenance and updating of the site. Furthermore, given the time commitment required, nurses should regularly evaluate the use, readership, and impact of the blog (Adams, 2011).

WIKIS

Another form of online communication is a **wiki**. In comparison to blogs, wikis are more social in their construction. That is, multiple users come together on a wiki to collaboratively write the content of a collection of webpages. Such a collection is easily expanded, and all users have the ability to add to, edit, and remove content. Wikipedia (www.wikipedia .org) is one of the best-known wikis.

Wikis are **asynchronous**, meaning that they allow users to work together but not necessarily at the same time. Therefore, authors may contribute to the webpages at their individual convenience. Wikis also have the capacity to hold multimedia content such as text, videos, audio, and photographs (Erardi & Hartmann, 2008), making them a potentially exciting and engaging source of information. Participants can also link to other content or to media by way of hyperlinks.

Health-related wikis such as WikiMD (www.wikimd.org) are promising tools for consumer education (Boulos, Maramba, & Wheeler, 2006; Boulos & Wheeler, 2007). Health providers can contribute to or create wikis to disseminate healthcare information and evidence. The resulting communication tool can be either open to the general public or accessible to only a select group of people. In the open version of a wiki, anyone can access the information posted to the webpages.

OTHER FORMS OF SOCIAL MEDIA

Facebook, Twitter, and YouTube are other social media tools that can be employed by nurses for patient education purposes. With these media, users create their own profile pages where information, pictures, and other forms of media such as blogs for comments can be posted. The unlimited storage capacity on the site is a major advantage for users.

Facebook, originally designed in 2004 as a college network at Harvard University, has grown to be an international networking site with more than 500 million members, including a growing number of healthcare professionals. Of all of the social media tools available, Facebook remains the most popular (IBT Reporter, 2014). It is used by approximately 57% of adults living in the United States, and about 73% of adolescents report visiting one or more Facebook sites on a daily basis (Smith, 2015). Facebook also hosts a number of health and professional organizations, illness-based support groups, and nursing and other professional journals (George, 2011). It has been used not only by healthcare consumers to chronicle their experiences with illness and health care but also by health professionals and health organizations to convey health-related information.

Twitter is a social media service that offers free microblogging to its members. Microblogging is defined as the sharing and receiving of tweets—messages that contain 140 or fewer characters—with the members of one's personal network (George, 2011). Twitter can be used by nurses and other health professionals and healthcare organizations in a number of ways. Formal Twitter chats can be arranged to allow for exploration of specific topics or questions, or for more general discussions. Hashtags—that is, keywords preceded by the # symbol that are attached to each message—allow the tweets to be linked together to create a virtual conversation (Mayo Clinic, 2012). Tweets also can be used to provide streamlined messages to patients or other health professionals, keeping them updated on important news or information.

YouTube differs from the Web platforms previously discussed in that it is a video-sharing platform where users upload, view, and share videos of varying lengths. Established in 2005, YouTube's popularity has grown at an astonishing rate. Today, YouTube has more than 1 billion unique users who have shared the more than 300 hours of video that is uploaded to the site every minute (Smith, 2015; YouTube, 2015). Users who search on the YouTube site can find multiple video clips on virtually any illness, surgery, or procedure. Videos available on the site have been designed for both professional and lay audiences.

The advantages of social media platforms for health education are numerous. Local or worldwide communities of learners can be created in a relatively simple and cost-effective manner. Learning experiences on these sites can be media rich and enticing, especially for the younger population. Although some patients may need instruction on how to find, register, and use the site, the sites themselves are easy to use and can be accessed from computers or mobile devices (Morgan, 2015).

Despite the many advantages of using social media to disseminate health-related information, some concerns have been raised about their potential risks (Rosenblum & Bates, 2012). Professional organizations in nursing and other health professions have developed an array of policy and procedure documents to assist health professionals to reduce these risks. For example, the American Nurses Association has published a set of principles for social networking as well as a tool kit to guide the nurse's use of these communication mechanisms (American Nurses Association, 2015).

When using social media, nurses should be aware of the following:

- Many social media sites have been used to market products such as tobacco, to show unhealthy or harmful behaviors such as various forms of abuse, and to convey bullying or biased messages that can result in psychological harm (Lau et al., 2012). Public health officials are concerned about suicide risk, particularly among vulnerable populations who may be subject to bullying behavior on these sites (Luxton, June, & Fairall, 2012).
- As with other forms of electronic communication, it may be wise to obtain legal advice before engaging in online client–professional relationships to avoid unintentionally violating state and federal privacy laws (Dizon et al., 2012).
- Maintaining patient privacy and confidentiality is of utmost importance. Patient information, photographs, and derogatory comments about patients should not be posted (Barry & Hardiker, 2012).
- Professional nurse/patient boundaries should be upheld. "Friending" patients or other activities that may alter the nurse–patient relationship should be avoided (Barry & Hardiker, 2012).
- Remember that everything posted on a social media site is public information and may be widely distributed.

The Internet

As mentioned previously, the World Wide Web is merely a small component of the much larger computer network called the Internet. Although the Internet does not provide the eye-catching webpages and the multimedia found on the World Wide Web, it does offer a wide range of services, many of which can be used to deliver health and healthcare education to patients. The Internet services most likely to be of interest to nurses include those that allow computer-facilitated communication.

While the World Wide Web provides opportunities to send healthcare messages to large groups of people in the form of educational webpages, the Internet can be used to enhance teaching by enabling individuals to communicate with one another and with groups of people via the computer. E-mail, real-time chat, and e-mail discussion or Usenet newsgroups have all been used to communicate with people about health and health care, some in very creative ways.

E-Mail/Texting

In a discussion of health care in the 21st century, the National Institute of Medicine (2001) predicted that both patients and clinicians could benefit from the use of Internet-based communication, which improves the timeliness of sending and receiving messages. Electronic mail (e-mail) is a commonly used Internet technology that has demonstrated great potential for improving care, communication, and health education. Although electronic communication was once thought to be reserved for the younger generation, it is now widely used and accepted across generations and provides a simple and efficient way for nurses to connect with patients (Mattison, 2012).

As early as the turn of the century, studies suggested that many patients had interest in communicating with their healthcare providers via e-mail. One survey found that one third of online health seekers would consider switching healthcare providers if they could communicate with them via e-mail (Kassirer, 2000). Indeed, e-mail is now universally used among all age groups and is a very popular form of communication by Internet users. However, a survey of healthcare consumers revealed that although people in general like to use e-mail, only a small but growing number of patients actually used e-mail to contact their healthcare provider (Baker, Wagner, Singer, & Bundoff, 2003; Graham, 2014).

E-mail offers a quick, inexpensive way to communicate with patients. It has the advantage of being asynchronous—that is, a message can be sent at the convenience of the sender, and the same message can be read when the receiver is online and ready to read it. Messages can be sent and responded to at any time, day or night.

As a form of enhanced communication with patients, e-mail is an approach worthy of further study by nurses. An e-mail message system gives patients who identify questions after leaving a healthcare facility a chance to get answers from a reliable source familiar with their history. Patients who are not sure how to phrase a question or feel rushed when instructions are being given in a clinical setting have a chance to compose their thoughts at home and prepare an e-mail message. Also, from the nurse's perspective, an e-mail message system provides a simple way to check on patients—that is, to see whether they understood the instructions they were given and to respond to new questions that have arisen.

In some ways, an e-mail system is preferable to a voice messaging system. For patients who are anxious about asking questions, e-mail allows them all the time they need to gather their thoughts. In addition, patients do not have to remember the answers they are given by the nurse, as the e-mail message provides a written record of the nurse's response.

In contrast, many voicemail systems are time limited. Patients are sometimes cut off in the middle of a voice message if the message is long or if patients are struggling to make themselves understood. Other patients may hesitate to leave a voice mail in the evening or night hours when they know no one is there to respond. However, by virtue of the way e-mail is designed, patients can feel comfortable sending messages at any time.

Unless a mechanism is in place by which patients can contact the nurse with questions, patients may be at risk for making a mistake with their self-care that may have serious consequences for their health. Simply telling patients to call if they have questions is often inadequate. A call to a busy office or clinic usually results in a call back by the nurse and the patient having to wait by the phone for an answer. Even calling hours can be problematic because they imply that the patient is free to call only at the designated hour.

An e-mail message system is simple to implement. Patient e-mail addresses need to be identified as part of the routine information-gathering process for new patients. Because e-mail addresses are likely to change, they need to be updated, just like telephone numbers, whenever a patient visits the office, clinic, or other setting within the healthcare delivery system.

It is a good idea to have more than one person be responsible for responding to e-mail messages, so that questions and concerns can be addressed even when a staff member is away due to vacation or other time out of the office. One way to accomplish this goal is to have messages sent to a mailbox rather than to an individual. Because more than one person can be given access to an electronic mailbox, continuous coverage can be established. If continuous coverage is not provided, it is important that patients know how long they can expect to wait to receive answers to their questions.

E-mail systems can be set up to serve a variety of purposes. If postteaching follow-up is desired, for example, e-mail offers one way for the nurse to initiate contact after the patient has left the healthcare delivery system. The nurse can get in touch with the patient via e-mail following a teaching session to convey interest in how he or she is doing with a medication regimen, treatment, or other types of instructions given. For example, the e-mail message could stress important points that were made during the teaching session, such as, "Remember to take your pill around the same time every day." Also, an e-mail message could be used to assess the patient's understanding of what was taught. For example, a nurse might ask, "At what time of day have you decided to give your child his medication?"

Informational resources also can be shared via e-mail by embedding links to websites in the e-mail message. In all cases, the nurse should encourage the patient to get in touch if questions remain. Any follow-up system will take time and commitment on the part of the organization. Time and resources must be allocated if the system is to work effectively.

An e-mail system also can be established as a mechanism to answer questions and exchange health-related information with patients who have received services at a particular healthcare organization. An e-mail question box can provide simple access to the nurse or other health professional who can serve as a reliable source of information. For this type of system to work, the e-mail address for the mailbox needs to be widely distributed and easy to remember. For example, a mailbox address such as Questions@RDClinic.org would be easy to remember because it includes the purpose of the mailbox and the name of the organization. The e-mail address can be placed on the bottom of written instructions, teaching materials, appointment cards, and other sources of communication with the patient.

A description of the service and instructions for use should be distributed as well. For example, it may be helpful for patients to know who will be answering their questions, the types of questions that can be submitted, and the typical response time. Also, it is very important that patients understand that an e-mail message system is not intended to replace a visit or phone call when they need to see or talk with a healthcare provider about an immediate problem.

When sending e-mail messages, nurses should remember that electronic communication differs in several ways from face-to-face communication:

- Without cues such as facial expressions, tone of voice, and body posture, e-mail messages can appear cold and unfeeling. While emoticons (symbols like smiley faces used to express emotion) are commonly used by people who send e-mail messages, they may not be appropriate for all professional correspondences. However, a carefully constructed e-mail message can convey the intent of the sender.
- Electronic communication may take longer in that the sender could wait hours or days before the message is received and answered. For this reason, it is very important that an e-mail response to a patient question be clear and provide sufficient detail so that it does not generate more questions that cannot be answered immediately. Furthermore, using e-mail may be inappropriate for communicating urgent issues or messages that need to be read or responded to quickly.
- E-mail messages provide a written record. A printed copy can serve as a handy reference for a patient and eliminates any question about which information was shared. Conversely, e-mail messages can serve as documentation of inaccurate or inappropriate information. When responding to a patient question, it is vital that the patient's record be reviewed and that the response to the question be accurate and carefully thought out. Copies of the e-mail message sent to the patient should be placed in the patient's record.
- Electronic communication can never be assumed to be private. This reminder is especially important in the era of Health Insurance Portability and Accountability Act (HIPAA) regulations. The healthcare provider must take steps to ensure privacy at both the healthcare facility and the patient's computer. It is suggested that patients sign a consent form if health-related information is to be shared via e-mail and that they be given instructions for safe use of the e-mail system (American Medical Association, 2015).

Not all information may be appropriate to share in an e-mail message. For example, it may not be appropriate to send abnormal test results to a patient in electronic form. It is also important that both nurses and patients understand that violations of privacy can occur in many ways. For example, patients who send e-mail messages from work may not be aware of the fact that their messages may be stored on servers and hard drives even after they have been deleted. In some cases, the employer may have legal access to this information (Kassirer, 2000).

E-mail messages can also be easily forwarded. The nurse, therefore, should assume that the patient may choose to share a response with others. Privacy also can be ensured at healthcare facilities by requiring a password-protected screen saver at all workstations (American Medical Association, 2015).

E-mail communication between nurse and patient has tremendous potential to enhance teaching. However, despite the increased use of e-mail among the general population, it is important to remember that not every patient has a computer, computer skills, or access to e-mail. For this reason, a backup system such as voice mail should be made available so that the needs of all clients will be met.

In recent years, texting has become a common form of electronic communication, especially among the younger population. Among adolescents, texting has replaced e-mail as the preferred method of communication (Woolford, Blake & Clark, 2013). Texting, which is also referred to as text messaging, involves the process of sending short messages via cell phone or other handheld devices. Although texting holds promise as a potential vehicle for communicating with young patients, nurses must be very cautious in using this mechanism because text messages are typically not considered to be secure. Text messages are not encrypted, and there is much less certainty that the intended patient is the sole person receiving the message. In addition, text messages are sometimes stored by a wireless carrier (HealthIT.gov, 2015).

Electronic Discussion Groups

In addition to blogs and other social media sites, the Internet also provides opportunities for patients to participate in electronic discussion groups with people who share a common interest. Common interests can focus on a particular healthcare problem such as cancer, a life circumstance such as death of a spouse, or a health interest such as nutrition.

Although different types of electronic discussion groups are available, all share a common feature—the ability to connect people asynchronously from various locations via computer. People like electronic discussion groups because they are easy to use and are available 24 hours a day. Because electronic discussion involves faceless communication with strangers from all over the world, there is a sense of anonymity even when real names are used.

Even though Facebook, blogs, and social media sites that facilitate discussion are growing in popularity, electronic discussion groups remain a viable choice in that mail can be distributed to individual subscribers and messages can be posted in a way that makes them accessible to group participants. Email-based electronic discussion groups can be structured in many different ways. Some are moderated, whereas others have little or no oversight. Some electronic discussion groups have thousands of subscribers, whereas others are very small closed groups created for specific purposes.

For the nurse, electronic discussion groups can serve a number of purposes. Such groups can be used as vehicles for teaching or as learning resources to share with patients and other healthcare professionals. The nurse who chooses to create an electronic discussion group can use it to reach large or small groups of healthcare consumers or healthcare professionals from within the immediate vicinity or worldwide.

Whether the group is large or small, the asynchronous nature of electronic discussion groups makes it possible for people to communicate with one another despite different time zones and work schedules. Also, no matter whether the nurse chooses to create an electronic discussion group or uses one already in existence, this form of online communication provides for a creative way to learn and to teach.

Mailing Lists

Automated mailing lists are one of the most popular means of setting up an electronic discussion group. With an automated mailing list, people communicate with one another by sharing e-mail messages. The principle by which these groups work is simple. Individuals who have subscribed to the mailing list send their e-mail messages to a designated address, where a software program then copies the message and distributes it to all subscribers. Therefore, when a message is sent to the group, everyone gets to see it. There are multiple software programs available to manage electronic mailing lists. A popular e-mail list management software program is LISTSERV. Although LISTSERV refers to a commercial product, automated mailing lists are sometimes incorrectly referred to as "Listservs."

Although mailing lists are owned or managed by an individual, much of the work involved in running the list is automated by the software program that is used. Subscribers are given two e-mail addresses to use when interacting with the mailing list: one to use when posting messages to the entire group and another to use for administrative issues such as requests to stop mail for a period of time. Both functions—distributing messages and handling routine requests—are automated and handled by the software program rather than by a person. Subscribers must use the correct address and precisely worded commands when attempting to interact with the list because the computer program cannot problem solve.

Upon enrolling in the mailing list, subscribers are sent directions and a list of properly worded commands that should be used when communicating with the software program. New subscribers are encouraged to save the instructions and refer to them as needed. Despite these precautions, new users frequently make mistakes. It is not uncommon to read messages from frustrated subscribers who cannot stop their mail because they are either posting to the wrong address or failing to use the correct command.

Automated mailing groups are wonderful tools for the nurse when used as a means for delivering education to patients. Mailing lists are easy to use once a user understands how the system works. Multiple free tutorials are available on the Web to help the novice subscriber.

With multiple automated mailing lists available, it is possible to find an online group that covers one of a variety of possible issues. The quality of the messages is usually very high. Nurses who choose to create a group rather than to participate in an established one can learn to manage a large or small electronic mailing list without too much difficulty. Even so, it is helpful for list managers to have either the support of computer professionals in their institution or the knowledge and skill necessary to handle the routine computer problems that arise from time to time.

Mailing lists can be used effectively as vehicles for education or information exchange with groups desiring such connections over time. Because mailing lists facilitate group rather than individual communication, they work especially well with groups that are interested in collaborative learning or learning from the experiences of others. Most of these automated mailing lists are quite active, and at any given time, several discussion topics can be addressed by the group. Members post questions, ask advice, and comment on current issues. Relationships between active members are established over time, and group members come to count on others in the group for their counsel.

For these same reasons, automated mailing lists have become popular as mechanisms for online support for health consumers (Fox & Fallows, 2003; Shaw et al., 2006). With the increased use of computers by the general population, a greater number of people have turned to their computers to access information and resources that can help them deal with their health issues. As a result, the need for electronic discussion groups devoted to particular health problems has been identified, and online support groups have been established.

For example, the Association of Cancer Online Resources, Inc. (ACOR, 2009), has been a major player in the move to bring online support to healthcare consumers. This nonprofit organization, which is devoted to assisting people with cancer, has established 142 different online support groups since 1996, each devoted to a particular type of cancer or cancer-related problem. Memberships in the various groups range from about 25 people in the smaller groups to almost 2000 individuals in the larger groups.

Other individuals and organizations have established similar online groups covering a wide range of healthcare issues. Sometimes these groups are started by individuals who have an interest in a particular topic; others are started by professional or advocacy groups interested in providing service to a particular group of people. In addition to the many public groups that have open enrollments, private groups can be established to meet the needs of a group of people associated with a specific healthcare provider or organization (Thompson, Parrott, & Nussbaum, 2011).

Online support groups are particularly relevant to the discussion of technology for education. As early as 2001, subscribers of an online support group for parents of children with cancer were surveyed, and it was found that 76% of participants cited information giving and receiving as the main benefit of the online group (Han & Belcher, 2001). A review of the purposes and goals of several online support groups revealed education and information sharing as the reason for starting and maintaining a group.

The emphasis on information sharing in online support groups is not surprising. Many people join online support groups after they or their loved ones have been diagnosed with a serious illness. They come to the support group not only to receive reassurance and encouragement but also to gather as much information as possible so that they can begin to make necessary decisions about treatment. By joining an online support group, they are turning to people who know what they are going through and who can give practical advice based on real-life experience. The desire to share the most current information is commonly what brings group members together, and a discussion of new treatments and other discoveries found in the literature is commonplace (Han & Belcher, 2001; Mou & Coulson, 2013; Thompson et al., 2011).

Nurses may wish to teach their patients about the benefits of online support groups. If an appropriate group is not available, nurses can start an online support group of their own. Online support groups may be especially helpful to people who find it difficult to leave home because of illness or care responsibilities.

Patients who are unfamiliar with online communication should be reassured that there is no pressure for them to contribute to the discussion and that many people benefit just from reading the comments of others. Patients who are insecure about their ability to express themselves in written format may find it helpful to initially compose their messages using a word processor so that they can take the time to think about what they want to say and use the spelling and grammar check function to edit their remarks. Patients who are unsure if an online support group will meet their needs should be encouraged to give one a try. There are no costs involved other than the cost of being online, and users are under no obligation to continue their participation. Subscribers can withdraw from a group at any time.

Online support groups have some disadvantages that should be shared with patients who are thinking about joining one. Most people who have participated in a LISTSERV or other type of mailing list note that the volume of messages received each day can be problematic (Han & Belcher, 2001). Some lists report an average of 50 or more messages per day.

Experienced users learn to sort messages and delete the unnecessary or irrelevant ones quickly. Others find requesting that messages be sent in digest form (in which all messages received in a day are combined and sent in one mailing) helps control the volume of e-mails received. In any case, the daily volume of messages initially can be overwhelming and may present a problem for people with low literacy levels or for people for whom English is a second language.

Patients also should be made aware of the fact that most online groups do not have a professional facilitator. Instead, online groups often are run by an individual who is interested in the health problem being discussed, because he or she either has the condition or has a family member with the healthcare problem. As a consequence, inaccurate information may be shared, and problems with group dynamics may not be addressed.

Although online support groups have been found to be beneficial for most individuals, it should be noted that some people report leaving groups because of the intensity of the discussion or because they felt that some participants were unkind to others. It has been suggested that the anonymity associated with the online format may result in some individuals feeling less inhibited, which results in people posting remarks that may not have been made in a face-to-face environment (Hammond, 2015).

Although this chapter classifies online support groups within the category of automated mailing groups, it should be noted that online support groups take many forms. Many groups use the mailing list or LISTSERV format described here. Others use Facebook as their platform for group information sharing. Still others maintain a website that provides many avenues for communication, including scheduled and unscheduled chats, bulletin boards, mailing lists, and electronic newsletters. Regardless of the format, online support groups provide a mechanism for meeting the teaching and learning needs of many different patient populations.

Other Forms of Online Discussion

Online discussion can take place through many other mechanisms. Although mailing lists and blogs are two of the more common approaches to online discussion, others are worthy of mention. When choosing a method for teaching or exchanging information online, it is important to consider all of the options and select the method that is most appropriate for the content to be delivered and the audience to be targeted.

Online forums, message boards, and bulletin boards are systems that provide a way for people to post messages for others to read and respond to. These systems are found on websites that allow users to post directly to the discussion board rather than indirectly via e-mail. Many people find discussion boards easier to use.

Although most discussion board–type forums require some system of registration, users can often select a user name of their choosing, and e-mail addresses are not displayed. This added privacy is a benefit to many people who are reluctant to share their names and e-mail addresses with strangers. Online forums, message boards, and bulletin boards for health consumers and healthcare professionals can be found on many health-related sites on the World Wide Web.

Online Chats

Chats differ from e-mail and the other electronic communication formats previously discussed in that they provide an opportunity for online conversation to take place in real time. Although chat conversations take the form of text rather than audio, a chat session shares many features with a telephone conference call. In both scenarios, several people from different locations participate in a conversation at the same time. Both also allow people to join or leave the session as needed.

Patients and healthcare professionals have many opportunities to engage in online chats related to health issues. A search of the World Wide Web can uncover a vast array of scheduled chats where a particular topic is being discussed at a given time as well as ongoing chats where people are invited to stop in at any time to ask questions or engage in conversation with persons who happen to be in the chat room. In addition to public chat rooms, many organizations sponsor chats for their own patients as a way to offer ongoing educational programs or information exchange among groups.

When leading or facilitating a chat group, it is important to plan ahead. The discussion in a chat room can move quickly, and it is very easy to get so involved in the process of chatting that the content to be covered gets lost or forgotten. Also, without adequate control systems in place, chats can experience a number of communication problems, such as multiple ongoing conversations, lack of focus, and periods of silence. The following suggestions may help to organize a successful chat session:

- E-mail or post the purpose of the chat session several days in advance. If appropriate, include an agenda, assignments to be completed ahead of time, or other resources that participants will need to prepare for the session.
- Make a list of the discussion points to be covered during the session. The list should be well organized, easy to follow, and placed so that it can be easily seen during the chat. Chat sessions often move so quickly that there is little time for the facilitator to make sense of crumpled or scribbled notes.

- Depending on the topic and the experience of the facilitator, it may be appropriate to limit the number of participants. The larger the group, the more difficult the challenge of running a smooth and productive online chat.
- Sign on to the chat session early and encourage participants to do so as well. You want to be able to handle unexpected problems before the session begins.
- Watch the clock. Time in a busy chat session goes by quickly. If the chat was designed as a question-and-answer period, it may be helpful to ask people to e-mail important questions ahead of time so they are not forgotten.
- Help the group to follow the conversation taking place. It is easy for chat discussions to become disjointed or off topic. When responding to a question, refer to the query and the person asking it—for example, "Karen asked about pain management. I think . . ." If the group is losing focus, bring the participants back to the agenda and the points being discussed.
- Limit the amount of time spent discussing the detailed questions or concerns of one participant. If someone in the group needs individualized attention, suggest that he or she e-mail or call you after the chat has ended.
- If appropriate, ask participants who have not joined into the conversation if they have any questions. Some participants choose not to make comments during a chat, which is acceptable. However, there may be others who were not quick enough to get their comments online and who have questions that need to be asked. A statement such as "Our conversation moved very quickly tonight, so I want to give those who haven't had a chance some time to ask their questions" may slow down the conversation long enough for everyone to have an opportunity to contribute.
- Begin to wrap up the session about 10 minutes before the scheduled end time. Announce that there are 10 minutes left and ask for final questions or comments.

It may also help to prepare participants for the chat experience. Chat sessions can be overwhelming for new users. The following guidelines for chat participation should be shared with patients who will be joining a chat session for the first time:

- *Allow enough time before the chat starts to download software if it is needed.* First-time users are often required to download software, called a chat client, before beginning. This software is typically offered as freeware or shareware on the Internet and is easy to install.
- *Be prepared to choose a user name.* Participants in public chats with strangers are often advised not to use their real names so as to protect their privacy.
- *Keep comments short and to the point.* If a user takes a long time to compose a message, the group may have moved on to an entirely new topic by the time the message gets posted.
- *Be prepared for chat lingo in public chat rooms.* Abbreviations like BTW (by the way) and emoticons—symbols that represent emotions or facial expressions such as ;) for winking—are commonly used.
- *Do not worry about typographical errors and grammar.* Chat programs do not have spell checks, and not everyone is an experienced typist. People who are frequent chat users learn to overlook spelling errors.

Chat works well as an online communication modality for many people. Patients who are homebound or isolated may benefit from having the opportunity to participate in education programs or to receive answers to their questions without leaving home. The ability to access patient education sessions that allow for real-time discussion and dialogue is a definite plus for them.

However, some limitations of chat must be considered. Because chat requires that people be online at the same time, scheduling conflicts and time-zone issues may result in less accessibility than asynchronous forms of electronic discussion. Also, as mentioned earlier, because of the fast pace of most chat discussions, it may be difficult for some patients to keep up with the dialogue. Patients with certain disabilities, patients who are ill, and patients with low literacy levels may find it difficult to participate if the group moves along quickly.

The future for electronic communication is exciting. The technology to add audio and video components to online conferencing is available and is becoming more refined and less expensive every day. Chat and other types of conferencing software also are becoming more sophisticated, allowing for more control and greater ease of use.

Issues Related to the Use of Technology

Despite the power of computer and Internet technology to enhance learning, the use of these technologies in patient education presents some unique challenges. Think for a moment about the many ways in which technology-driven healthcare education differs from more traditional in-person patient education. The characteristics of the learners, the setting, and the access to hardware, software, and technological support are all likely to be different. In addition, issues related to the information technology itself can create challenges, such as the accuracy of online content and the accessibility of electronic resources.

Whereas traditional patient education is likely to take place in a structured setting, electronic healthcare education takes place in a wide range of settings, many of which are unstructured. Patient access to resources (hardware and software) and technological support can vary considerably among healthcare consumers and in healthcare organizations. In addition, consumers taking advantage of patient education programs may represent a wide range of ages, abilities, and limitations. As patient educators, nurses must be aware of the special issues involved in the use of computer and Internet technology for healthcare education and be prepared to make accommodations as needed.

One of the most widely publicized issues related to the use of computers and Internet technology is the **digital divide**, referring to the gap between those individuals who have access to information technology resources and those who do not. According to a Pew Foundation report, one in five Americans (20%) is disconnected; that is, he or she does not use the Internet (Zickuhr & Smith, 2012). Factors influencing the likelihood that someone will have access to information technology resources include age, income, level of education, and ability (Zickuhr, & Smith, 2012). Those at risk for limited access to computers included people older than 65, those with household incomes of less than $30,000, adults who did not complete high school, and people with disabilities. In addition, households without children are less likely to have Internet access. However,

African Americans and English-speaking minority adults are just as likely as whites to own and use a mobile phone, thereby reducing some of the racial and ethnic disparities of years past (Zickuhr & Smith, 2012).

As a result of the digital divide, some healthcare consumers do not have the resources necessary to gain entry to computer-based and Internet-based health education programs. Thus, although technology can increase access to healthcare education for some people, nurses as patient educators must be aware that some segments of the population will be denied access if attempts are not made to promote digital inclusion. The first step in promoting digital inclusion is recognizing those groups who are at risk for limited access.

For instance, more than half of all Americans older than age 65 do not use the Internet (Zickuhr & Smith, 2012). There are many explanations for this statistic. Older adults are more likely to be retired without employer access to a computer, are less likely to have children in the home who typically bring an enthusiasm for and knowledge of computers with them, may have less disposable income with which to purchase computer hardware and software, and did not grow up using this technology (Prensky, 2001).

Nevertheless, it would be a mistake to discount computer-delivered education as a possibility for the older adult population. Research studies have shown that with education and support, older adults enjoy using and learning from computer-based programs, particularly if they are helped to see the benefits that can be gained through computer usage (Evangelista et al., 2006; Nagle & Schmidt, 2012; Nahm, Preece, Resnick, & Mills, 2004). Although many older adults have limited incomes, numerous government and private initiatives are available to provide free or low-cost computer and Internet access for this population. While some older adults have physiologic and neurologic problems that make computer use difficult, many others enjoy good health and functionality.

Health and healthcare education are important to older adults, and computer-based and Internet-based technology holds much promise for this segment of the population. Therefore, it is important that the nurse be prepared to support electronic learning opportunities for older patients. The following interventions may be helpful in encouraging older adults to engage in computer-based learning activities:

- Reinforce principles of ergonomics by making suggestions about equipment and posture that will minimize physical problems related to computer use. Ergonomics is important for everyone but is an especially critical consideration for older adults, who may have visual problems as well as arthritic changes in the neck, hands, and spine. Proper posture, correct positioning of the keyboard and monitor, adjusted screen colors and font size, a supportive chair, and a reminder to get up and walk around three to four times per hour will help older adults to avoid discouraging physical symptoms that may interfere with computer use.
- Identify resources that will provide computer access and support in older adults' home communities. Supply older adults with a comprehensive resource list identifying places where free computer and Internet access is available, places where computer training is provided for them, and contact people who will assist them if they encounter problems with the technology. In addition to public libraries

and community centers, numerous projects nationwide are committed to digital inclusion for all segments of the population, including the older adult population. Many of these projects and resources can be identified on the Web. For example, AARP (the American Association of Retired People) has a wide range of services designed to promote and support computer use by older adults available on its website.

- Motivate older adults to use a computer by helping them to identify how the computer can meet their needs. It is important to talk to older adults about their needs and abilities. Find out how they like to learn, which kinds of things they enjoy doing, and what their healthcare needs are. Matching a computer program or website to the individual's unique circumstances will encourage computer use. For example, an older adult who is caring for a spouse with cancer might appreciate an online support group if he or she enjoys interacting with and learning from the experiences of others. In this way, you will help to generate interest in learning how to use a computer for health education by starting at a place that attracts the older adult's interest.

- Create a supportive and nonthreatening environment to teach older adults about using a computer for health education. Today's older adults did not grow up with computers and may not have confidence in their ability to learn this new skill at this point in their lives. The language of computers may seem foreign to them, so nurses in the role of patient educators should avoid jargon and define new terms. They should pace their teaching according to the older adults' responses. Also, it may be necessary for nurses to proceed slowly at first and provide opportunities for older adults to practice and reinforce their skills. Written computer instructions should be provided before the teaching session ends so that older adults can go home with answers to technology questions that may arise.

Computers can open up a whole new avenue of support and information to older adults who are struggling with their own health problems and those of their partners. Older adults who enjoy good health can find resources to help them maintain their health and to become educated healthcare consumers. It is important that older adults be given the same opportunities to take advantage of the information age resources that are available to younger patients. The nurse can play a key role in promoting digital inclusion among this segment of the population.

People with disabilities make up another special population who may require additional planning before using technologies in health and healthcare education. Not only are people with disabilities less likely to have computer and Internet access than are members of the general population, but they may also have difficulty using hardware and software (Burgstahler, 2012b). The ability to use a computer without adaptive devices requires the fine motor coordination and mobility necessary to use a mouse and keyboard, the strength to sit and hold the head in an upright position, and the ability to comprehend information presented on the computer screen. Furthermore, individuals who use a wheelchair may find that they require special equipment for mobility, as some wheelchairs do not fit under a standard computer table (Burgstahler, 2012b).

Individuals with visual impairments may have difficulty seeing text or graphics on a computer screen or performing tasks on the computer that require hand–eye coordination. When identifying obstacles related to visual impairments, it is important to think broadly and address the wide range of conditions that affect the way we see. Color blindness, which affects approximately 8% of all males and 0.5% of females, can cause significant problems for computer users if the website or software used does not display the correct color combinations, if the contrast between background and foreground is inadequate, and if color rather than text is used to convey directions (Liu, 2012).

Although hearing impairments cause fewer problems for computer users than visual impairments, some accessibility issues nevertheless need to be addressed for users with such challenges (Burgstahler, 2012a). An individual with a hearing problem may not be able to hear the sounds that are often used as prompts when a wrong key is struck or when an e-mail message is delivered. Accessibility for individuals with hearing impairments is becoming a bigger issue now that it is easier to send audio signals across the Web, and audio messages are becoming more commonplace.

Despite the protections offered by the Americans with Disabilities Act (ADA) and other federal legislation, accessibility issues on the Web and constraints with hardware and software still exist. Federal legislation outlined in Section 508 of the Workforce Investment Act requires government agencies and institutions receiving government funding to make their websites accessible to people with disabilities. However, many websites and programs do not fall under this umbrella of protection (Burgstahler, 2012b).

Nurses who use the Internet and the World Wide Web to teach also need to consider website design when creating or selecting websites that might be used by disabled learners. The World Wide Web contains multiple resources that can be used by Web designers or Web users to learn design principles for accessibility. For example, submitting the search command "color blindness" to a search engine will turn up websites that explain color blindness, illustrate how various types of color blindness affect what might be seen on a website, describe good Web design principles for promoting accessibility, and provide tools that can be used to select color combinations that will not create barriers for individuals with color blindness.

Several resources are available to assist Web developers in creating websites that meet the needs of people with disabilities. The Web Accessibility Initiative website (http://www.w3.org/wai) provides guidelines that are recognized by many as the international standard for accessibility. Another website of note is that created by the Center for Applied Special Technology (CAST; http://www.cast.org).

Age, disabilities, and other factors that place an individual on the wrong side of the digital divide are also factors that can isolate and diminish access to patient education resources. Therefore, every effort should be made to help elderly individuals or individuals with disabilities connect to the wealth of resources that are and can be made available through technology. The nurse can play a vital role in providing the support, education, and advocacy needed to reduce the barriers that still exist for these special groups of people.

Summary

This chapter focused on information age technology and its use in healthcare education for consumers. Specifically, this chapter discussed ways in which the World Wide Web and the Internet could be used by nurses to enhance patient education. The impact of technology on teachers and learners was addressed. Special considerations were identified for the use of technology by older adults and other patient groups, such as those with physical and sensory disabilities, low literacy, and limited socioeconomic and educational backgrounds.

Information age technology has the potential to transform health and healthcare education. The powerful tools of computers and other social media devices must be used thoughtfully and carefully, however. Education is about learning, not technology. Technology is merely a vehicle to deliver patient education in a way that promotes learning.

The benefits of technology-based education are numerous, as are the challenges for teachers and learners. Nurses have a responsibility to adopt new tools to promote health in their patients and for their own professional growth and development. The future looks very bright to continue implementing technology approaches for teaching and learning. Nurses can help to shape the future by thinking creatively about how to use technology in patient education and how to participate in research studies about its effectiveness.

Review Questions

1. What is the information age and the difference between the World Wide Web and Internet as sources of information?
2. How has technology influenced health and healthcare education for consumers?
3. What are the guiding ethical principles that have been created to ensure quality of health-related information available to consumers on the World Wide Web?
4. What is the impact of technology on the roles and responsibilities of nurses and patients in the teaching and learning process?
5. Which information age skills are required by nursing professionals and healthcare consumers to take advantage of the tremendous power of the World Wide Web and social media for patient education?
6. What categories of criteria should be considered when evaluating the accuracy, efficiency, effectiveness, and appeal of health-related websites?
7. What types of social media are available to facilitate electronic communication between and among nurses and consumers for the purpose of sharing health and healthcare information?
8. What services on the Internet enhance the delivery of health and healthcare education to consumers?
9. How has the digital divide limited access to technology resources by certain population groups, such as older adults and people with disabilities, and how can this lack of accessibility be addressed?

Case Study

Sarah is a registered nurse working with Steve, a client in a rehabilitation outpatient clinic. Steve experienced a stroke 2 months ago and has recently returned home. He is now physically able to live independently but is still working on his ability to communicate effectively with others. Since his stroke, Steve has experienced difficulty with finding words when speaking with others. As a retired human resources specialist, this communication barrier is frustrating to Steve.

During her initial patient interview with Steve, Sarah learns that he is hesitant to return to many of his former activities with friends and is feeling socially isolated. Steve feels that his only successful social interactions since returning home are e-mail exchanges with family and friends in different parts of the country. Sarah realizes that because e-mails are written, asynchronous forms of communication, Steve has more time to word find when composing his messages than he would in a spoken conversation. She asks Steve if he has Internet access at home. He indicates that he has a high-speed Internet connection and computer in his living room that he uses daily.

Based on this preassessment of Steve's ability and interest in this technology, Sarah asks him if he has found any online support groups for individuals who have experienced strokes. She explains that such groups would be an excellent resource for information about others' experiences with stroke and would serve as a social venue and as another type of written activity to enhance his interaction with others. Sarah suggests that a support group could be educational and socially engaging, and would offer a chance for Steve to continue building his communication skills during his rehabilitation. Steve expresses interest in this idea, and he and Sarah plan to seek out such groups online during his next clinic visit.

1. Given Steve's condition and age, how can technology be used to foster social participation? What is Sarah's role in encouraging his social engagement?
2. Which potential problems might Steve face when trying to use the Web?
3. As a patient educator, which criteria should Sarah use for evaluating health-related websites? Explain how she can apply each criterion to determine which websites are appropriate for Steve.

References

Adams, R. (2011). Building a user blog with evidence: The health information skills academic library blog. *Evidence Based Library and Information Practice, 6*(3), 84–88.

American Medical Association. (2015). *H-478.997 Guidelines for patient-physician electronic mail.* Retrieved from https://www.ama-assn.org/ssl3/ecomm/PolicyFinderForm.pl?site=www.ama-assn.org&uri=/resources/html/PolicyFinder/policyfiles/HnE/H-478.997.HTM

American Medical Informatics Association. (2015). *Consumer health informatics.* Retrieved from http://www.amia.org/applications-informatics/consumer-health-informatics

American Nurses Association. (2015). *ANA's principles for social networking and the nurse.* Retrieved from http://www.nursesbooks.org/Main-Menu/eBooks/Principles/Social-Networking.aspx

Association of Cancer Online Resources, Inc. (ACOR). (2009). http://www.acor.org

Baker, L., Wagner, T., Singer, S., & Bundoff, K. (2003). Use of the Internet and e-mail for healthcare information. *Journal of the American Medical Association, 289*, 2400–2406.

Barry, J., & Hardiker, N. R. (2012). Advancing nursing practice through social media: A global perspective. *The Online Journal of Issues in Nursing, 17*. Retrieved from http://nursingworld.org/MainMenuCategories/ANAMarketplace/ANAPeriodicals/OJIN/TableofContents/Vol-17-2012/No3-Sept-2012/Advancing-Nursing-Through-Social-Media.html

Boulos, M. N., Maramba, I., & Wheeler, S. (2006). Wikis, blogs, and podcasts: A new generation of Web-based tools for virtual collaborative clinical practice and education. *BMC Medical Education, 6*, 41.

Boulos, M. N. K., & Wheeler, S. (2007). The emerging Web 2.0 social software: An enabling suite of sociable technologies in health and health care education. *Health Information & Libraries Journal, 24*, 2–23.

Buis, L. B., & Carpenter, S. (2009). Health and medical blog content and its relationship with blogger credentials and blog host. *Health Communication, 24*, 703–710.

Burgstahler, S. (2012a). *Working together: Computers and people with sensory impairments*. Retrieved from http://www.washington.edu/doit/Brochures/Technology/wtsense.html

Burgstahler, S. (2012b). *Working together: People with disabilities and computer technology*. Retrieved from http://www.washington.edu/doit/working-together-computers-and-people-sensory-impairments

Cassano, C. (2014). The right balance—Technology and patient care. *Online Journal of Nursing Informatics (OJNI), 18* (2). Retrieved from http://www.himss.org/ResourceLibrary/GenResourceDetail.aspx?ItemNumber=33541

Cassano, C. (2015, March 27). *Technology & patient education*. Retrieved from http://www.himss.org/ResourceLibrary/GenResourceDetail.aspx?ItemNumber=33541

Charbonneau, D. H. (2012). Readability of menopause Web sites: A cross sectional study. *Journal of Women & Aging, 24*, 280–291.

Daniels, M., & Wedler, J. A. (2015). Enhancing childbirth education through technology. *International Journal of Childbirth Education, 30*(3), 28–32.

Dizon, D., Graham, D., Thompson, M. A., Johnson, L., Fisch, M., & Miller, R. (2012). Practical guidance: The use of social media in oncology practice. *American Society of Clinical Oncology, 8*(5), 114–124.

Erardi, L. K., & Hartmann, K. (2008). Blogs, wikis, and podcasts: Broadening our connections for communication, collaboration, and continuing education. *OT Practice, 13*, CE1–CE8.

Evangelista, L. S., Stromberg, A., Westlake, C., Galstanyan, A., Anderson, N., & Dracup, K. (2006). Developing a Web-based education and counseling program for heart failure patients. *Progress in Cardiovascular Nursing, 21*, 196–201.

Finnis, J. A. (2003). *Learning in the information age*. Retrieved from http://dev.twinisles.com/research/learninfoage.pdf

Fleming, S. E., Vandermause, R., & Shaw, M. (2014). First time mothers preparing for birthing in an electronic world: Internet and mobile phone technology. *Journal of Reproductive and Infant Psychology. 32*(3), 240–253.

Fox, S. (2006). *Online health search*. Pew Internet & American Life Project. Retrieved from http://www.pewinternet.org/2006/10/29/online-health-search-2006/

Fox, S. (2011). *The social life of health information, 2011*. Pew Internet and American Life Project. Retrieved from http://pewinternet.org/Reports/2011/Social-Life-of-Health-Info.aspx

Fox, S., & Duggan, M. (2012). *Mobile health 2012*. Retrieved from http://www.pewinternet.org/2012/11/08/mobile-health-2012/

Fox, S., & Duggan, M. (2013). *Health online 2013*. Retrieved from http://www.pewinternet.org/2013/01/15/health-online-2013/

Fox, S., Duggan, M., & Purcell, K. (2013, June 20). *Family caregivers are wired for health.* Retrieved from http://www.pewinternet.org

Fox, S., & Fallows, D. (2003). *Internet health resources.* Retrieved from http://www.pewinternet.org

Gagnon, K., & Sabus, C. (2015). Professionalism in a digital age: Opportunities and considerations for using social media in health care. *Physical Therapy, 95*(1), 406–414.

George, D. (2011). Friending Facebook: A minicourse on the use of social media by health professionals. *Journal of Continuing Education in the Health Professions, 31*(13), 215–219.

Graham, C. (2014). Study: How patients want to communicate with their physician. *Technology Advice.* Retrieved from http://technologyadvice.com/medical/blog/study-patient-portal-communication-2014/

Ham, K. (2014, November 10). *Evaluating health websites.* National Network of Libraries of Medicine. Retrieved from http://nnlm.gov/outreach/consumer/evalsite.html

Hammond, H. (2015). Social interest, empathy and online support groups. *The Journal of Individual Psychology, 71*(2), 174–181.

Han, H.-R., & Belcher, A. (2001). Computer-mediated support group use among parents of children with cancer: An exploratory study. *Computers in Nursing, 19*(1), 27–33.

Hartzband, P., & Groopman, J. (2010, March 25). Untangling the Web—Patients, doctors, and the Internet. *New England Journal of Medicine, 362,* 1063–1066. doi:10.1056/NEJMp0911938

Harvard Health blog. (2015). Patient Education Center. Harvard Medical School, Harvard University, Health Media Network, Harvard Health Publications. Retrieved from http://www.patienteducation center.org/health-blog/

Healthcare Hashtag Project. (2015). Retrieved from http://www.symplur.com/healthcare-hashtags/

HealthIT.gov. (2015). *Can you use texting to communicate health information, even if it is to another provider or professional?* Retrieved from https://www.healthit.gov/providers-professionals/faqs/can-you-use-texting-communicate-health-information-even-if-it-another-p

Horrigan, J. (2009). *Access for African Americans.* Pew Internet & American Life Project. Retrieved from http://www.pewinternet.org/Reports/2009/12-Wireless-Internet-Use/6-Access-for-African-Americans/1-Overview.aspx

IBT Reporter. (2014). *A breakdown of Facebook, Instagram and Twitter users.* Retrieved from http://www.ibtimes.com/breakdown-facebook-instagram-twitter-users-infographic-1616600

Internetworldstats.com. (2015). Retrieved from http://www.internetworldstats.com

Jones, S., & Fox, S. (2009). *Generations online in 2009.* Retrieved from http://www.pewinternet.org/2009/01/28/generations-online-in-2009/

Kaplan, B., & Brennan, P. F. (2001). Consumer informatics: Supporting patients as co-producers of quality. *Journal of the American Medical Informatics Association, 8*(4), 309–315.

Kassirer, J. P. (2000). Patients, physicians and the Internet. *Health Affairs, 19*(6), 115–123.

Knight, E., Werstine, R., Rasmussen-Pennington, D., Fitzsimmons, D., & Petrella, R. J. (2015). Physical therapy 2.0: Leveraging social media to engage patients in rehabilitation and health promotion. *Physical Therapy, 95*(3), 389–396.

Lau, A. Y. S., Gabarron, E., Fernandez-Luque, L., & Amoyones, M. (2012). Social media in health: What are the safety concerns for health consumers? *Health Information Management Journal, 41*(2), 31–35.

Lenhart, A., & Fox, S. (2006). *Bloggers: A portrait of the Internet's new storytellers.* Retrieved from http://www.pewinternet.org/files/old-media/Files/Reports/2006/PIP%20Bloggers%20Report%20July%2019%202006.pdf.pdf

Lewis, D., Gundwardena, S., & Saadawi, G. (2005). Caring connection: Developing an Internet resource for family caregivers of children with cancer. *CIN: Computers, Informatics, Nursing, 23,* 265–274.

Liu, J. (2012). *Color blindness.* Retrieved from http://www.usability.gov/articles/newsletter/pubs/022010new.html

Luxton, D., June, J. D., & Fairall, J. M. (2012). Social media and suicide: A public health perspective. *American Journal of Public Health, 102*(S2), 196–200.

Maag, M. (2005). The potential use of blogs in nursing education. *CIN: Computers, Informatics, Nursing, 23,* 16–26.

Matthews-DeNatale, G., & Lowenstein, A. J. (2014). Educational use of technology: E-communication that fosters connection between people and ideas. Chapter 19, pp. 297-310. In Bradshaw & Lowenstein (Eds.). *Innovative Teaching Strategies* (6th ed., pp. 297–310). Burlington, MA: Jones & Bartlett Learning.

Mattison, M. (2012). Social work in the digital age: E-mail as a direct practice methodology. *Social Work, 57*(3), 249–258.

Mayo Clinic. (2012). *Mayo Clinic Center for Social Media.* Retrieved from http://socialmedia .mayoclinic.org/

Miller, E. A., & Pole, A. (2010). Diagnosis blog: Checking up on health blogs in the biosphere. *American Journal of Public Health, 100*(8), 1514–1519.

Modave, F., Shokar, N., Peñaranda, E., & Nguyen, N. (2014). Analysis of the accuracy of weight loss information search engine results in the Internet. *American Journal of Public Health, 104*(10), 1971–1978.

Morgan, K. K. (2015, May). Patient uprising. *American Way,* 67–68, 72–77.

Mou, P., & Coulson, N. (2013). Online support group use and psychological help for individuals living with HIV/AIDS. *Patient Education and Counseling, 93*(3), 426–432.

Nagle, S., & Schmidt, L. (2012). Computer acceptance of older adults. *Work, 41,* 3541–3548.

Nahm, E., Preece, J., Resnick, B., & Mills, M. (2004). Usability of Web sites for older adults. *CIN: Computers, Informatics, Nursing, 22,* 326–334.

National Center for Educational Statistics. (2006). *Computer and Internet use by students in 2003: Statistical analysis report.* NCES 2006-065. Washington, DC: U.S. Department of Education, Institute of Educational Sciences.

National Institute of Medicine. (2001). *Crossing the quality chasm: A new health system for the 21st century.* Washington, DC: National Academy Press.

Perrin, A. (2015). *Social media usage 2005-2015.* Retrieved from http://www.pewinternet.org/2015 /10/08/social-networking-usage-2005-2015/

Pho, K., & Gay, S. (2013). *Establishing, managing, and protecting your online reputation: A social media guide to physicians and medical practices.* Phoenix, MD: Greenbranch Publishing.

Prasad, B. (2013). Social media, healthcare, and social networking. *Journal of Gastrointestinal Endoscopy, 77*(3), 492–495.

Prensky, M. (2001). Digital natives, digital immigrants. *On the Horizon, 9*(5), 1–6.

Rainie, L. (2012). *25% of Americans own tablet computers.* Retrieved from http://www.pewinternet .org/2012/10/04/25-of-american-adults-own-tablet-computers/

Roney, K. (2012, August 31). Interactive patient education reduces readmissions, increases satisfaction: Kaiser Permanente Panorama Hospital case study. *Becker's Health IT & CIO Review.* Retrieved from http://www.beckershospitalreview.com

Rosenblum, R., & Bates, D. W. (2012). Patient-centred healthcare, social media and the Internet: The perfect storm? *British Medical Journal Quality & Safety.* doi: 10.1136/bmjqs-2012-0017441. Retrieved from http://qualitysafety.bmj.com

Seymour, B., German, R., Sharif, A., Zhang, L. H., & Kalinderian, E. (2015). When advocacy obscures accuracy online: Digital pandemics of public health misinformation through an anti-fluoride case study. *American Journal of Public Health, 105*(3), 517–523.

Shaw, B. R., Hawkins, R., Aroroa, N., McTavish, F., Pingree, S., & Gustafson, D. H. (2006). An exploratory study of predictors of participation in a computer support group for women with breast cancer. *CIN: Computer, Informatics, Nursing, 23*, 18–27.

Smith, C. (2015). *By the numbers: 120+ amazing YouTube statistics.* Digital Marketing (DMR). Retrieved from http://expandedramblings.com/index.php/youtube-statistics/

Thackery, R., Neiger, B. L., Smith, A. K., & Van Wagenen, S. (2012). Adoption and use of social media among public health departments. *BMC Public Health, 12*(242), 1–7.

Thompson, T. L., Parrott, R., & Nussbaum, J. F. (2011). *The Routledge handbook of health communication* (2nd ed.). New York, NY: Routledge.

Wachter, B. (2013, February 18). *The transformation of healthcare in the information age.* Retrieved from http://www.kevinmd.com/blog/2013/02/transformation-healthcare-information-age.html

Williams, K. (2003). Literacy and computer literacy: Analyzing the NCRs being fluent with information technology. *Journal of Literacy and Technology, 3*(1). Retrieved from http://citeseerx.ist.psu.edu/viewdoc/download?doi=10.1.1.455.719&rep=rep1&type=pdf

Woolford, S., Blake, N., & Clark, S. (2013).Texting, tweeting and talking: E-communication with adolescents in primary care. *Contemporary Pediatrics, 30*(6), 12–18.

YouTube. (2015). *Statistics.* Retrieved from http://www.youtube.com/yt/press/statistics.html

Zickuhr, K. (2013). *Who's not online and why.* Pew Internet & American Life Project. Retrieved from http://www.pewinternet.org/2013/09/25/whos-not-online-and-why/

Zickuhr, K., & Madden, M. (2012). *Older adults and Internet use.* Retrieved from http://www.pewinternet.org/2012/06/06/older-adults-and-internet-use/

Zickuhr, K., & Smith, A. (2012). *Digital differences.* Pew Internet & American Life Project. Retrieved from http://www.pewinternet.org/~/media//Files/Reports/2012/PIP_Digital_differences_041312.pdf

Zickuhr, K., & Smith, A. (2013). *Home broadband 2013.* Pew Internet & American Life Project. Retrieved from http://www.pewinternet.org/2013/08/26/home-broadband-2013/

Evaluation in Healthcare Education

CHAPTER 1

Priscilla Sandford Worral

Chapter Highlights

- Evaluation, Evidence-Based Practice, and Practice-Based Evidence
- Evaluation Versus Assessment
  - *Determining the Focus of Evaluation*
- Evaluation Models
  - *Process (Formative) Evaluation*
  - *Content Evaluation*
  - *Outcome (Summative) Evaluation*
  - *Impact Evaluation*
  - *Total Program Evaluation*
- Designing the Evaluation
  - *Design Structure*
  - *Evaluation Methods*
  - *Evaluation Instruments*
  - *Barriers to Evaluation*
- Conducting the Evaluation
- Analyzing and Interpreting Data Collected
- Reporting Evaluation Results
  - *Be Audience Focused*
  - *Stick to the Evaluation Purpose*
  - *Use Data as Intended*

Key Terms

assessment
content evaluation
evaluation
evidence-based practice
external evidence
impact evaluation
internal evidence
outcome (summative)
    evaluation
practice-based evidence
process (formative)
    evaluation
total program evaluation

Objectives

After completing this chapter, the reader will be able to

1. Define the term *evaluation*.
2. Discuss the relationships among evaluation, evidence-based practice, and practice-based evidence.

3. Describe the difference between the terms *evaluation* and *assessment*.
4. Identify the purposes of evaluation.
5. Distinguish between five basic types of evaluation: process, content, outcome, impact, and program.
6. Discuss characteristics of various models of evaluation.
7. Recognize the similarities and differences between evaluation and research.
8. List the major barriers to evaluation.
9. Examine methods for conducting an evaluation.
10. Explain the variables that must be considered in selecting appropriate evaluation instruments for the collection of different types of data.
11. Identify guidelines for reporting the results of evaluation.

Evaluation, in general, is defined as a systematic process that judges the worth or value of something—in this case, teaching and learning. Evaluation can provide evidence about what nurses do as patient educators that makes a value-added difference in the care they provide. The importance of evaluating patient education has never been more critical than in today's healthcare environment (London, 2009). Patients must be educated about their health needs and how to manage their own care so that patient outcomes are improved and healthcare costs are decreased (Institute for Healthcare Improvement, 2012; Schaefer, Miller, Goldstein, & Simmons, 2009).

Preparing patients for safe discharge from hospitals or from home care must be efficient so that the time patients are under the supervision of nurses is reduced, and it also must be effective in preventing unplanned readmissions (Stevens, 2015). For example, monitoring the hospital return rates of patients is not a new idea as a way to evaluate effectiveness of patient education efforts. The Institute for Healthcare Improvement (2012) has been sponsoring and conducting studies since 2009 linking hospital admissions and readmissions to patient education programs that are primarily nurse driven (Bates, O'Connor, Dunn, & Hasenau, 2014).

Evaluation is critical to decision making in nursing practice and is a vital component of the education process. Evaluation is the final step in this process. Because the education process is cyclical, evaluation serves as the critical bridge at the end of one cycle that provides evidence to guide direction of the next cycle.

The sections of this chapter follow the steps in conducting an evaluation. These steps are: (1) determining the focus of the evaluation, including evaluation models used; (2) designing the evaluation; (3) conducting the evaluation; (4) determining methods to analyze and interpret the data collected; (5) and reporting a summary of the findings from data collection. Each of these aspects of the evaluation process is important, but all of them are meaningless if the results of evaluation are not used to guide future action in planning and carrying out patient education interventions. In other words, the results of evaluation provide practice-based evidence to either support continuing an educational intervention as it has been designed or support revising that intervention to enhance learning.

Evaluation, Evidence-Based Practice, and Practice-Based Evidence

One definition of **evidence-based practice** (EBP) is "the conscientious use of current best evidence in making decisions about patient care" (Melnyk & Fineout-Overholt, 2011, p. 4). More broadly, EBP may be described as "a lifelong problem-solving approach to clinical practice that integrates . . . the most relevant and best research, . . . one's own clinical expertise, . . . and patient preferences and values" (p. 4). The definition of a related term, known as evidence-based medicine, includes these same three primary components but also adds "patient circumstances" (p. 1) to account for both the patient's clinical state and the clinical setting in which the care has been delivered (Straus, Richardson, Glasziou, & Haynes, 2005).

The strongest evidence upon which to base practice decisions, especially decisions about treatment, comes from what are known as systematic reviews of clinically relevant, well designed and conducted quantitative studies or qualitative studies that provide a more thorough understanding of patient experiences within the setting in which care is provided (Flemming, 2007; Goethals, Dierckx de Casterlé, & Gastmans, 2011; Taylor, Shaw, Dale, & French, 2011). Evidence from such research studies is called **external evidence**, because the findings can be applied (generalized or transferred) to patients who are external to the study but are similar to study patients.

However, as is discussed later in this chapter, the results from carrying out evaluations, unlike the findings that come from research, are not considered external evidence. Instead, evaluation findings are considered to be **internal evidence**. That is because results from evaluations are not intended to be generalized, but rather are conducted to determine the effectiveness of a specific intervention in a specific setting with an identified individual or group.

Although not considered external evidence, results of a systematically conducted evaluation are still important from an EBP perspective. When research is not available, results from a well-conducted evaluation are appropriate in determining the effectiveness of patient education in changing patients' knowledge of, attitudes toward, and skills regarding self-care (Melnyk & Fineout-Overholt, 2011). Perhaps the most common example of internal evidence is what comes from a well-designed and systematically conducted quality improvement project.

Nurses' understanding and use of EBP have evolved and expanded over the past two decades. One aspect of this growth in recent years has been the adoption of the term **practice-based-evidence** (Brownson & Jones, 2009; Girard, 2008; Green, 2008; Horn, Gassaway, Pentz, & James, 2010). Defined as "the systematic collection of data about client progress generated during treatment to enhance the quality and outcomes of care"

(Girard, 2008, p. 15), practice-based evidence is made up of internal evidence that can be used both to identify whether a problem exists and to determine whether an intervention effectively resolved a problem. Put another way, practice-based evidence can be equally useful for assessment and for evaluation.

Conducting an audit of medical records in preparation for a visit from an accrediting agency to learn whether patient teaching has been adequately documented is one example of collecting practice-based evidence that determines the quality of nursing care. If audit results demonstrate that patient education has not been documented, nurses might be given a checklist to help them remember to record their teaching interventions. Evidence for evaluation depends on good documentation. Following introduction of the checklist, a reaudit of records is needed to learn whether documentation has improved. This is an example of collecting practice-based evidence to evaluate the usefulness of a checklist.

The results of evaluations, the outcomes of expert-delivered patient-centered care, and the results of quality improvement projects all represent internal evidence. This information should be gathered by nurses and other healthcare providers on an ongoing basis as an important component of professional practice. Recognizing these findings about current practice as a source of evidence to guide future practice requires that nurses think critically before acting, and carry out ongoing evaluations during and after each nurse–patient interaction.

Evaluation Versus Assessment

Although assessment and evaluation are highly interrelated and the terms are often used interchangeably, they are two different things. The process of **assessment** focuses on initially gathering, summarizing, interpreting, and using data to decide a direction for action. In contrast, the process of **evaluation** involves gathering, summarizing, interpreting, and using data after an activity has been completed to determine the extent to which an action was successful.

Thus, the primary differences between these two terms are in the timing and purpose of each process. For example, education of a patient and significant others begins with an assessment of their learning needs and other learner characteristics, such as hearing loss or visual acuity, that might influence how those needs can best be met. While the education is being conducted, periodic evaluation lets the nurse know whether changes in patient or caregiver behavior is progressing as planned. After education is completed, evaluation identifies whether and to what extent identified needs were met and learning outcomes were achieved.

An important note of caution: Although an evaluation is often considered after education is completed, that is not the time to plan it. Evaluation as an afterthought is, at best, a poor idea and, at worst, a dangerous one. For example, consider patient education for the safe discharge of an older adult who is going to his daughter's home so she can provide his care until he is able to function independently. In this situation, both assessment of learning needs and evaluation of learning outcomes must include the patient, the daughter, and the patient and daughter as a pair. Ideally, assessment and evaluation planning should be activities that occur at the same time. "If only . . ." is an all-too-frequently heard complaint, which can be avoided or minimized by planning ahead.

Determining the Focus of Evaluation

In planning any evaluation, the first and most crucial step is to determine the focus of the evaluation. The importance of a clear, specific, and realistic understanding of the purpose and direction of evaluation cannot be overemphasized. Useful and accurate results of an evaluation depend heavily on how well the evaluation is initially planned. This focus then guides evaluation design, conduct, data analysis, and reporting of results.

Evaluation focus consists of five basic components: (1) audience, (2) purpose, (3) questions, (4) scope, and (5) resources (Ruzicki, 1987). To identify these components, ask the following:

1. For which audience is the evaluation being conducted?
2. For which purpose is the evaluation being conducted?
3. Which questions will be asked in the evaluation?
4. What is the scope of the evaluation?
5. Which resources are available to conduct the evaluation?

AUDIENCE

The audience includes the persons or groups for whom the evaluation is being conducted (Dillon, Barga, & Goodin, 2012; Ruzicki, 1987). The primary audience are those individuals or groups who requested the evaluation or who will use the evaluation results, and the general audience are all those who might benefit from the findings of an evaluation. Thus, the primary audience for an evaluation might include peers, other health professional colleagues, the manager of a unit or ambulatory care area, a supervisor, the chief nursing officer, the staff development director, the executive officer or president of the institution or agency, a group of community leaders, or patients and their family members. For example, staff nurses during their careers may find institutional leaders as the primary audience interested in whether patients taught by a particular nurse or group of nurses are among those with longer lengths of stay or unplanned readmissions within 30 days of discharge. Nurses who have the lead role as direct care providers will have patients and families as their most frequent general audience.

When the results of the evaluation are reported, all members of the audience must receive feedback. In focusing the evaluation, however, the nurse carrying out the evaluation must first consider the primary audience. Giving priority to the individual or group that requested the evaluation makes it easier to focus the evaluation. This is especially true if evaluation results will be used by more than one group representing different interests. This chapter will focus on patients and their families, healthcare colleagues, and the nurse in the role of teacher as the audience most interested in the results of evaluation of an educational activity.

PURPOSE

The purpose answers the question, "Why is the evaluation being conducted?" For example, the purpose might be to decide whether to continue a particular education program or to determine the effectiveness of the teaching. If a particular individual or group has a primary interest in the results of an evaluation, then this interest clarifies the reason for doing it.

An important note of caution: Why an evaluation is being done is not the same as who or what is being evaluated. For example, nursing literature on patient education commonly distinguishes among three types of evaluations: (1) learner (e.g., patient), (2) teacher (e.g., nurse), and (3) educational activity (e.g., self-care at home). This distinction answers the question of *who or what will be evaluated* and is extremely useful in designing and conducting an evaluation. The question of *why undertake an evaluation of a learner*, for example, is answered by the need to know how well the learner performed. If the purpose for evaluating learner performance is to determine whether the patient gained sufficient skill to perform a self-care activity (e.g., foot care), the nurse might design an evaluation that measures content by observing one or more return demonstrations by the patient prior to hospital discharge. If the purpose for evaluating learner performance is to determine whether the patient is able to conduct the same self-care activity at home on a regular basis, the nurse might design an evaluation measuring outcomes by observing both the patient performing the activity in his or her home environment and measuring other related clinical parameters of good foot care (e.g., skin integrity), which would improve and be maintained with regular and ongoing self-care. Content evaluation and outcome evaluation are terms that will be defined and discussed in more detail later in this chapter.

In stating the purpose of an evaluation, an excellent rule of thumb is to keep it singular. In other words, the evaluator should state, "The purpose is . . .," not "The purposes are . . ." Keeping the purpose singular and focused on the audience helps avoid the all-too-frequent tendency to attempt to do too much in one evaluation.

QUESTIONS

Questions should be directly related to the purpose for conducting the evaluation, must be specific, and must yield measurable answers. Examples of such questions include "How satisfied are patients with the cardiac discharge teaching program?" and "Is the patient's daughter able to help her mother transfer correctly from bed to chair prior to discharge to the daughter's home?" Asking the right questions is essential if the evaluation is to fulfill the intended purpose. As discussed later in this chapter, formulating clear, concise, and appropriate questions is both the first step in selecting the evaluation design and the basis for analyzing the data that are collected from evaluation.

SCOPE

Scope considers the extent of what is being examined, such as "How much will be evaluated?" "How many individuals or representative groups will be evaluated?" and "What time period is to be evaluated?" For example, will the evaluation focus on the learning experiences for one patient or for all patients being taught a particular skill? The scope of an evaluation is determined in part by the purpose for conducting the evaluation and in part by available resources. For example, an evaluation to determine whether a patient understands each step in a teaching and learning session on how to self-administer heparin injections is narrow in scope, is focused on a particular point in time, and requires expertise in clinical practice and observation.

RESOURCES

Resources include time, expertise, personnel, materials, equipment, and facilities. A realistic determination of which resources are accessible and available relative to the resources that are required is crucial in focusing any evaluation. Anyone who is conducting an evaluation should remember that time and expertise are required to analyze data collected during the evaluation as well as to prepare the report of the evaluation results.

Evaluation Models

Evaluation can be classified into different types or levels. A number of evaluation models have been developed that define these evaluation types and how different levels of evaluation relate to one another (Abruzzese, 1992; Frye & Hemmer, 2012; Milne, 2007; Noar, 2012; Ogrinc & Batalden, 2009; Rankin & Stallings, 2005; Rouse, 2011). Because not all models define types of evaluation in the same way, the nurse in the role of teacher should choose the model that is most appropriate and most realistic based on the purpose of the evaluation and the resources available.

Abruzzese (1992) constructed the Roberta Straessle Abruzzese (RSA) model for classifying types of educational evaluation into different levels. Although developed in 1978 and originally designed to evaluate staff development education, the RSA model remains useful from a patient education perspective. The RSA model provides a visual of five basic types of evaluation in relation to one another based on the purpose, components of the evaluation focus, related questions, scope, and resources available (**Figure 14–1**).

The five types of evaluation are process, content, outcome, impact, and total program. Abruzzese describes the first four types as levels of evaluation leading from the simple (process evaluation) to the complex (impact evaluation). Total program evaluation encompasses and summarizes all of these four levels.

Process (Formative) Evaluation

The purpose of **process evaluation**, also known as **formative evaluation**, is to make adjustments to an education activity as soon as they are needed, such as making changes in personnel, materials, facilities, teaching methods, learning objectives, or even the educator's own attitude. One or more adjustments may need to be made after a teaching session and before the next is taught, or even in the middle of a single learning experience. Consider, for example, evaluating the process of teaching an adolescent with

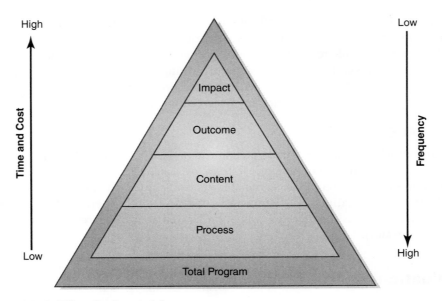

Figure 14–1   RSA evaluation model

newly diagnosed type 1 diabetes and her family how to administer insulin. The nurse might facilitate learning by first injecting himself or herself with normal saline so that the learners can see someone maintain a calm expression during an injection. If the nurse educator had planned to have the parent give the first injection but the child seems less fearful, the nurse might consider revising the teaching plan to let the patient first perform self-injection.

Process evaluation is part of the ongoing education cycle of assessment, planning, and implementation. Process evaluation helps the nurse anticipate and prevent problems before they occur or identify problems as they arise. Milne's (2007) evaluation framework consists of the elements of structure–content–outcomes–procedures–processes– efficiencies (SCOPPE). Noar's (2012) framework for evaluation includes the elements of audience–channel–message–evaluation (ACME). Both of these frameworks focus on the characteristics of the teacher and the learner as well as on examining instructional materials and teaching methods as aspects of process evaluation. Noar (2012) speaks to the importance of using a consistent theoretical framework for designing, conducting, and evaluating education.

Consistent with the purpose of process evaluation, the primary question here is, "How can teaching be improved to facilitate learning?" The nurse's teaching effectiveness, the elements of the education process, and the learner's responses are monitored on an ongoing basis. Abruzzese (1992) describes process evaluation as a "happiness index." While teaching and learning are ongoing, learners are asked their opinions about the teacher(s), learning objectives, content, teaching methods, instructional materials, physical facilities, and overall learning experience. For the nurse as the patient educator, specific questions could include the following:

- Am I giving the patient and/or family members time to ask questions?
- Is the information I am giving orally consistent with information included in instructional materials being provided?
- Are the patient and family members actively participating?
- Is the environment, such as room temperature, privacy, and level of distraction, conducive to learning?
- Should I include more opportunities for return demonstration or teach-back?

The scope of process evaluation generally is limited in breadth and time period to a specific learning experience, such as a teaching session or workshop, yet is sufficiently detailed to include as many aspects of the specific learning experience as possible while they occur. Thus, learner behavior, teacher behavior, learner–teacher interaction, learner response to teaching methods and materials, and characteristics of the environment are all aspects of the learning experience within the scope of process evaluation. Resources usually are less costly and more readily available for process evaluation than for the other types of evaluation, such as impact or total program evaluation. Although process evaluation occurs more frequently—during and throughout every learning experience—than any other type of evaluation, it occurs at the same time that teaching is happening. Therefore, the need for additional time and resources to conduct process evaluation is minimal and limited.

From the perspective of EBP, process evaluation is important in providing patient-centered care based on clinical practice guidelines (CPGs). CPGs also are sometimes referred to as "clinical pathways" or "critical pathways" (Habel, 2005), although they are at different levels of precision or exactness. A well-constructed CPG includes not only the specific intervention, such as teaching a patient how to take his discharge medication, but also how to evaluate the effectiveness of that intervention.

Developing a CPG is intended as a guide in caring for all patients who have similar characteristics and learning needs. If a patient has unique learning needs or responses to teaching, the nurse should use informal process evaluation to vary from the guideline to ensure that the patient is able to learn and is receiving individualized patient-centered care. Because CPGs are written as step-by-step guidelines, the nurse, when delivering patient education, can use them to choose teaching and learning activities specific to the behavioral outcomes to be achieved (Bradshaw, 2014).

EBP is not a cookbook approach to providing health care. Similarly, CPGs are not intended to disregard the individual learner's needs. As attention to practice-based evidence evolves, the importance of using internal evidence gathered from process evaluation is becoming an increasingly critical aspect of every teaching–learning experience.

For instance, Chan, Richardson, and Richardson (2012) describe a process evaluation conducted to examine which factors might support successful delivery of an intervention to improve symptom management for patients receiving palliative radiation therapy for their lung cancer. Although two nurses were using the same procedure to provide the intervention, patients were more satisfied with the nurse who had prior experience in oncology. Patients also were less likely to practice their muscle relaxation protocol if they had not yet experienced the level of pain that the muscle relaxation was intended to alleviate. Based on these findings, Chan and colleagues modified the intervention protocol to have patient education be provided by nurses with prior oncology experience and to allow patients flexibility to decide on the frequency with which they practiced muscle relaxation techniques. As another example, Jurasek, Ray, and Quigley (2010) describe use of a questionnaire to ask adolescents with epilepsy and their caregivers about the benefit of attending a clinic developed to ease the adolescents' transition from pediatric to adult care. As a result of the findings from the questionnaire, the information provided to adolescents now is prioritized according to what they identify as their greatest concerns.

Content Evaluation

The purpose of **content evaluation** is to determine whether patients and their significant others have acquired the knowledge or skills taught during the learning experience. Abruzzese (1992) described content evaluation as taking place immediately after the learning experience to answer the guiding question, *To what degree did the learners learn what they were taught?* or *To what degree did learners achieve pre-set behavioral objectives?* Asking a patient to give a return demonstration at the completion of a teaching session on psychomotor skill development is an example of content evaluation.

The RSA model shows content evaluation as the level in between process and outcome evaluation. In other words, the purpose of content evaluation is to focus on how the teaching–learning process affected immediate, short-term outcomes. A question to be asked is: "Were specified objectives met as a result of teaching?"

The scope of content evaluation is limited to a specific learning experience and to specifically stated objectives for that experience. Content evaluation occurs immediately after completion of teaching but takes into account all teaching–learning activities included in that specific learning experience. Data are obtained from all learners involved in a specific teaching session. For example, if both parents and the adolescent patient with diabetes are taught insulin administration, all three are asked to complete a return demonstration. Also, resources used to teach content can be evaluated as to how well that content was learned. For example, the exact equipment used in teaching a patient how to change a dressing also can be used by the patient to perform a return demonstration.

Content evaluation, like process evaluation, focuses on collecting internal evidence to determine whether objectives for a specific group of learners were met. Gathering data about the learner prior to a teaching session and then collecting data again immediately after the teaching session can be used to compare if any change in learner behavior occurred. Walker (2012) describes development and implementation of Skin Protection for Kids, a primary prevention education project aimed at school-aged children, their parents, and their teachers to decrease unnecessary sun exposure. Content evaluation included pretests conducted prior to providing informational materials and posttests conducted 24 to 48 hours later. Teachers' scores, for example, improved from an average of 56.25% on the pretest to an average of 87.5% on the posttest, indicating that the project helped teachers to improve their short-term knowledge of sun safety.

An important rule of thumb when collecting data: If any individual is asked to spend his or her time to complete a quiz, survey, or any similar activity, then the nurse collecting those data should promise to use them appropriately to improve nursing practice.

Outcome (Summative) Evaluation

The purpose of **outcome evaluation**, also known as **summative evaluation**, is to determine the results of patient teaching efforts by nurses. Outcome evaluation measures the changes that result from teaching and learning. This type of evaluation summarizes what happened as a result of education. Changes in learning can include patients demonstrating a new technique, an increase in knowledge, or a change in attitudes. The behaviors measured are based on the objectives established as a result of an initial needs assessment. Guiding questions in outcome evaluation include the following:

- Was teaching appropriate?
- Did the individual(s) learn?
- Were behavioral objectives met?
- Did the patient who learned a skill before discharge use that skill correctly once home?

Unlike process evaluation that occurs during the teaching–learning experience, outcome evaluation occurs after teaching has been completed or after an educational program has been carried out. Abruzzese (1992) clearly explains the difference in scope between outcome evaluation and content evaluation. She notes that outcome evaluation measures more long-term change that "persists after the learning experience" (p. 243). Thus, the scope of outcome evaluation focuses on a longer time period than does content evaluation. Whereas evaluating the accuracy of a patient's return demonstration of a skill prior to discharge may be appropriate for content evaluation, outcome evaluation should include measuring a patient's competency with a skill in the home setting after discharge. Abruzzese (1992) suggests that outcome data be collected 6 months after the original baseline data to determine whether a change has really taken place.

Resources required for outcome evaluation are more costly and more complex than those needed for process or content evaluation. Compared to the resources required for the first two types of evaluation in the RSA model, outcome evaluation requires greater expertise to develop measurement and data collection strategies, more time to conduct the evaluation, knowledge of baseline data establishment, and ability to collect reliable and valid data for comparison purposes after the learning experience has occurred. Postage to mail surveys, and time and personnel to complete patient/family telephone interviews are specific examples of resources that may be necessary to conduct an outcome evaluation.

From an EBP perspective, outcome evaluation might arguably be considered as "where the rubber meets the road." Once a need for change has been identified, the search for evidence on which to base future changes commonly begins with a structured clinical question that will guide an efficient search of the literature. This question is also known as a PICO question, where the letters *P*, *I*, *C*, and *O* stand for *population* (patient, family member, or other caregiver), *intervention*, *comparison*, and *outcome*, respectively.

For example, nurses caring for an outpatient population of adults with heart failure might discover that many patients are not following their prescribed treatment regimen. Upon questioning these patients, the nurses learn that a majority of the patients do not recognize symptoms resulting from failure to take their medications on a consistent basis. To search the literature efficiently for ways in which they might better educate their patients, the nurses would pose the following PICO question: Does nurse-directed patient education on symptoms and related treatment for heart failure provided to adult outpatients with heart failure result in improved compliance with treatment regimens? In this example, the *P* is the population of adult outpatients with heart failure, the *I* is the nurse-directed patient education intervention on symptoms and related treatment for heart failure, the *C* is the comparison of the education currently being provided (or lack of education, if that is the case), and the *O* is the outcome that, it is hoped, will result in improved compliance with treatment regimens.

The Skin Protection for Kids program (Walker, 2012) included outcome evaluation as well as the content evaluation described earlier in this chapter. Whereas content evaluation of teachers' knowledge was conducted 24 to 48 hours after the educational activity, outcome evaluation took place several months later to measure whether sun-safety practices were implemented by the children who were enrolled in this program.

Prior to making a change in practice, especially if that change will require additional resources or might increase patient risk if unsuccessful, several well-conducted studies providing external evidence directly relevant to a PICO question should be reviewed. Implementation of the Skin Protection for Kids program (Walker, 2012) is an excellent example of a practice change based on extensive external evidence, which included a critique of 39 studies plus peer-reviewed guidelines and systematic reviews that focused on sun-safety measures for children.

Impact Evaluation

The purpose of **impact evaluation** is to obtain information that will help decide whether continuing an educational activity is worth its cost, based on the effect it has on the institution or the community (Adams, 2010). An example of a question appropriate for impact evaluation is "What is the effect of a cardiac discharge teaching program on long-term frequency of rehospitalization among patients who have completed the program?"

The scope of impact evaluation is broader, more complex, and usually more long term than that of process, content, or outcome evaluation. For example, whereas outcome evaluation focuses on whether specific teaching results in achievement of specific outcomes, impact evaluation goes beyond that point to measure the effect or worth of those outcomes. In other words, outcome evaluation focuses on a learning objective, whereas impact evaluation focuses on a goal for learning. Consider, for instance, a class on healthy food choices for patients who have had bariatric surgery. The objective is that patients will choose healthy foods regardless of whether they are in a restaurant or in the grocery store. The goal is for these patients to increase and sustain their weight loss.

Like good science that is rarely inexpensive and never quick, good impact evaluation shares the same characteristics. The resources needed to design and conduct an impact evaluation generally include reliable and valid instruments, trained data collectors, personnel with research and statistical expertise, equipment and materials necessary for data collection and analysis, and access to populations who may be culturally diverse or geographically spread out. Kobb, Lane, and Stallings (2008) describe an impact evaluation of e-learning as a method for building telehealth skills that spanned the entire Veterans Health Administration system and that was initiated 3 years after implementing e-learning. The scope and time frame for this project is commonly found with this type of evaluation. For example, impact evaluation can be global in nature as described by Padian et al. (2011) in their discussion of challenges faced by those persons who have conducted large-scale evaluations of a number of HIV prevention programs.

Because impact evaluation requires many resources, including time, money, and research expertise, this type of evaluation is usually beyond the scope of the individual nurse responsible for patient education. However, the current managed care environment requires justification for every health dollar spent. The value of patient education may be assumed to be beneficial in improving the quality of care, but evidence of the positive impact of education must be demonstrated if it is to be recognized, valued, and funded.

Total Program Evaluation

Within the framework of the RSA model (Abruzzese, 1992), the purpose of **total program evaluation** is to determine the extent to which all activities for an entire department or program over a specified period of time meet or exceed the goals originally established. A guiding question appropriate for a total program evaluation is "How well did patient education activities implemented throughout the year meet annual goals established for the institution's patient education program?"

The scope of program evaluation is broad, generally focusing on overall goals rather than on specific learning objectives. Given its scope, total program evaluation is also complex, usually focusing on the learner *and* the teacher *and* the educational activity, rather than on just one of these three components. Abruzzese (1992) describes the scope of program evaluation as encompassing all aspects of educational activities (e.g., process, content, outcome, impact) with input from all of the participants (e.g., learners, teachers, institutional representatives, and community stakeholders).

It is not surprising, then, that a number of models and related theories have been developed as a way to frame and organize total program evaluation. Kirkpatrick's four-level model, known as the logic model, consists of four components: inputs, activities, outputs, and outcomes (Rouse, 2011). Frye and Hemmer (2012) have authored a guide for choosing a program evaluation model and to help those evaluating educational programs to appreciate and adequately account for how complex program evaluation really is.

Given the complexity of program evaluation, the resources required may include a combination of all resources necessary to conduct process, content, outcome, and impact evaluations. Also, the time period over which data are collected may extend from several months to one or more years. Rouse (2011), for example, used Kirkpatrick's four-level model, which closely matches the Abruzzese model, to demonstrate just how extensive this type of evaluation is. He describes a comprehensive evaluation of the effectiveness of health information management programs. The first level of evaluation addresses the immediate reactions of the attendees to the setting, the instructor, the materials, and the learning activities. What Abruzzese describes as a happiness index, Rouse labels a "smile sheet," commenting that although satisfaction does not necessarily result in learning, dissatisfaction may prevent it. Kirkpatrick's second, third, and fourth levels are learning, behavior, and results, respectively. Rouse describes these levels, in turn, as evaluation of knowledge immediately after education is completed, evaluation of whether actual change has occurred in the workplace, and evaluation of system-wide impact of the program.

L. M. Haggard and Burnett (2006) describe their use of the logic model to evaluate the impact of a Web-based data system that asks the public about their access to data on health information. The authors highlight the ability of the logic model to demonstrate to their stakeholders how resources—dollars and personnel—are directly tied to education activities, which in turn are directly related to learning outcomes.

As stated earlier, the RSA model remains useful as a general framework for categorizing the basic types of evaluation: process, content, outcome, impact, and total program. As this model demonstrates, differences between these types are largely a matter of degree. For example, process evaluation occurs most frequently, whereas total program evaluation occurs least frequently. Content evaluation focuses on immediate effects of teaching, while impact evaluation concentrates on more long-term effects of teaching. Conducting process evaluation requires fewer resources compared with impact and program evaluation, which require extensive resources for their implementation. The RSA model further illustrates one way that process, content, outcome, and impact evaluations can be considered together as components of total program evaluation.

A. Haggard (1989) described three dimensions in evaluating the effectiveness of patient education. Also, Rankin and Stallings (2005) explained four levels of evaluation of patient learning. The three dimensions described by A. Haggard and the four levels identified by Rankin and Stallings are consistent with the basic types of evaluation included in Abruzzese's RSA model, as shown in **Table 14–1**. As depicted in this table, models developed from an education theory base, such as the RSA model, have much in common with models developed from a patient care theory base, such as the other two models put forth by A. Haggard and Rankin and Stallings.

At least one important point about the difference between the RSA and other models needs to be mentioned, however. That difference is depicted in the learner evaluation

Table 14–1 Comparison of Types of Evaluation Across Education Evaluation Models

Abruzzese (1992)	A. Haggard (1989)	Rankin and Stallings (2005)
Process	Patient assimilation of information during teaching	Patient education interventions
Content	Patient information retention after teaching	Patient/family performance following learning
Outcome	Patient use of information in day-to-day life	Patient/family performance at home
Impact	N/A	Overall self-care and health maintenance
Program	N/A	N/A

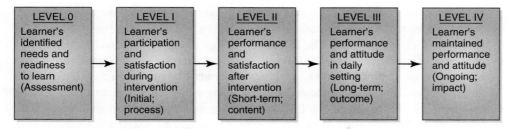

Figure 14–2 Five levels of learner evaluation

Data from Rankin, S. H., & Stallings, K. D. (2005). *Patient education in health and illness* (5th ed.). Philadelphia, PA: Lippincott Williams & Wilkins; Rouse, D. (2011). Employing Kirkpatrick's evaluation framework to determine the effectiveness of health information management courses and programs. *Perspectives in Health Information Management, 8*, 1c–5c.

model shown in **Figure 14–2**. This learner-focused model emphasizes the continuum of learner participation determined from needs assessment to learner performance over time. This model and the RSA model have value in focusing and planning any type of evaluation but are especially important for impact and program evaluations.

Designing the Evaluation

Nurses in the role of patient educators must design an evaluation that is consistent with its purpose, questions, and scope and that must be realistic given the available resources. It must be noted here that evaluation and research are not the same thing, but they are related activities. Traditionally, the primary difference between the two has been with respect to the purpose for conducting the evaluation or the study. The purpose for evaluating education is to measure whether a practice change is effective in a specific setting with a specific group of learners or teachers during a specific period of time. In contrast, the purpose of research is to generate new knowledge that can be used across settings and individuals with similar characteristics (Melnyk & Fineout-Overholt, 2011).

Evaluation designs that measure the success of patient education activities include at least three interrelated components: structure, methods, and instruments. The following describe these design elements.

Design Structure

An important question to be answered in designing an evaluation is "How detailed should the evaluation be?" The obvious answer is that all evaluations should have some level of what is known as rigor, which means they are precise, logical, and exact. In other words, all evaluations should be carefully and thoroughly planned and systematically structured before they are conducted. How rigorous the design structure should be depends on the questions to be answered, how complex the scope of the evaluation is, and how evaluation results will be used. The more the questions address cause and effect, the more complex the scope of the evaluation. Likewise, the more critical and broad-reaching the expected use of results, the more complicated the structure of the evaluation design will be.

The structure of an evaluation design depends on whether one individual is being evaluated or a number of individuals in a group are to be included in the evaluation, as in the case of a childbirth class. The evaluation design also is influenced by the number or frequency of evaluations and the time sequence between an educational intervention and evaluation of that intervention, as in the case of one-to-one instruction of patients.

A process evaluation might be conducted during a single patient education activity where the nurse demonstrates a skill and then observes patient behavior during return demonstration. Process evaluation also is carried out when engaging the patient in a question-and-answer exchange as part of this teaching and learning encounter. Because the purpose of process evaluation is to facilitate better learning while that learning is happening, in this case, education and evaluation occur at the same time.

Also, evaluation may be conducted immediately after an educational intervention has been completed. This structure is probably the most common approach to evaluating teaching and learning, although it is not necessarily the most appropriate. If the purpose for doing an evaluation is to determine whether learners who have just been exposed to a teaching session know specific content that they did not know before participating, then a structure that begins with collecting baseline data is more appropriate. For example, a pretest can be used to collect baseline data, which then can be compared with data collected via a posttest at one or more points in time after learners have completed the educational activity. This approach provides an opportunity for the nurse to measure whether change has really occurred. The ability to measure change in a particular skill or level of knowledge, for example, also requires that the same instruments be used for pretest and posttest data collection at both points in time. Data collection is discussed in more detail later in this chapter.

If the purpose of conducting an evaluation is to determine whether learners know content or can perform a skill as a direct result of an educational intervention, the most appropriate structure would be to include at least two groups: one receiving the new educational intervention and one receiving the usual education or standard care. Both groups are evaluated at the same time, even though only one group is exposed to the new education. For example, suppose a nurse wants to learn whether providing written material as well as in-class education will improve patients' ability to remember healthy eating tips. Patients on nursing Unit A would receive the pamphlet on healthy eating to read prior to attending a class, while patients on nursing Unit B would attend the class without first reading the pamphlet. Patients in both groups would be asked the same questions before the intervention began. If patients on both units had about the same number of correct answers to the questions asked before the intervention, and then the patients on Unit A had more correct answers after the class ended, the nurse would have internal evidence to demonstrate that adding the pamphlet resulted in a positive outcome for patients on Unit A.

This chapter provides only a few examples of evaluation designs that nurses are most likely to find useful in the practice setting. Many more complex and more rigorous evaluation designs exist for those times when the results of an evaluation will be used to make major financial or program decisions. The literature on evaluating the effectiveness of patient education has become an increasingly rich source of examples of how to conduct high-level, complex evaluation.

Evaluation Methods

The choice of design structure provides the basis for determining what methods of evaluation should be used to collect information. All evaluation methods deal in some way with data and data collection. Answers to the following questions can assist in selecting the most appropriate and realistic methods when conducting a particular evaluation in a particular setting and for a specific purpose:

- Which types of data will be collected?
- What data will be collected and from whom?
- How, when, and where will data be collected?
- Who will collect the data?

TYPES OF DATA TO COLLECT

Evaluation of patient education includes collecting data about people, about the educational program or activity, and about the environment in which the educational activity takes place. The types of data that are collected about people can be classified as demographic (e.g., age, gender, health status) as well as cognitive, affective, and/or psychomotor behaviors. The types of data that are collected about educational activities or programs generally include such factors as cost, length of the activity or program, number of educators required, teaching–learning methods used, amount and type of materials required, and so on. The types of data that are collected about the environment in which a program or activity is conducted generally include such environmental characteristics as temperature, lighting, location, layout, space, and noise level.

Given the possibility that an unlimited and overwhelming amount of data could be collected, how do you decide which data should be gathered? The most straightforward answer to this question is that you should collect data that will answer the questions that were asked when deciding the evaluation focus. The likelihood that the evaluator will collect the right amount of the right type of data to answer evaluation questions can be significantly improved by (1) remembering that any data collected must be used and (2) using operational definitions allows everyone who is involved to understand what is being evaluated.

An operational definition must clearly define one or more words or phrases being used and must be written in measurement terms. Patient compliance, for example, can be defined as the patient's regular and consistent adherence to a prescribed treatment regimen. For use in outcome evaluation of a particular educational activity, patient compliance might be operationally defined as the patient's demonstration of unassisted and error-free completion of all steps in the sterile dressing change as observed in the patient's home on three separate occasions at 2-week time intervals. These examples show that an operational definition states exactly which data will be collected.

In addition to data being categorized as describing people, programs, or the environment, data also can be categorized as quantitative or qualitative. Quantitative data are expressed in numbers and generally are stated as statistics, such as the frequency, average (mean), or ratio (proportion) with which something occurs. Numbers can be used to answer questions of how much, how many, how often, and so on, in terms that are commonly understood by the audience for the evaluation. Analysis of data can demonstrate, for example, how much improvement in a learner's knowledge or skill is the result of patient education.

Qualitative data, on the other hand, include feelings, behaviors, and words or phrases that generally are summarized into themes or categories. Such data provide the richness and insight into the responses of individuals about their experiences. Qualitative data can be used to measure such value-laden or conceptual terms as *satisfaction* or *quality*.

WHAT DATA TO COLLECT AND FROM WHOM

What data to collect when measuring patient education are described as outcome factors related to either the effectiveness of a program or patient achievement of behavioral change. Program evaluation indicates the extent of how well a program has functioned, such as measuring the use of healthcare resources that potentially saves money for the institution. Patient outcome measures include medical factors (such as health status, use of healthcare services, or levels of risk), behavioral factors (such as knowledge and skills for self-management), and psychosocial factors (such as beliefs, attitudes, perceived quality of life, well-being, or support systems). What patient outcomes to evaluate and how to evaluate them are described by Lorig and Laurent (2007).

Data can be collected directly from the individuals whose behavior or knowledge is being evaluated, from family caregivers or significant others as representatives of these individuals, from patient records documenting care, or from databases that have already been created to collect information. In the case of process evaluation, for example, data should be collected from all learners and all nurses while they are participating in a specific educational activity. Content and outcome evaluations should include data from all learners at the completion of one or more educational activities.

Because impact and total program evaluations have a broader scope than do process, content, and outcome evaluations, collecting data from all individuals who participated in an educational program over an extended period of time may be impossible. This difficulty occurs because data collectors may not be able to locate every participant, or they may lack sufficient resources to gather data from such a large number of people. When all participants cannot be counted or located, data may be collected from a sample (subset) of participants who are considered to represent the entire group.

HOW, WHEN, AND WHERE TO COLLECT DATA

Methods for how data can be collected include the following (Euromed Info, n.d.):

- Observation
- Interview
- Questionnaire or written examination
- Record review

Which method is selected depends, first, on the type of data being collected and, second, on the available resources. When possible, data collected using more than one method can provide the nurse with more information about the education being evaluated than could be accomplished using a single method. A nurse in the role of teacher might use both observation and teach-back, for example, to determine whether a patient is able to correctly perform a dressing change plus explain why each step of the dressing change is important (Visiting Nurse Associations of America, 2012).

The timing of data collection, or when data collection takes place, has already been addressed both in discussion of different types of evaluation and in descriptions of evaluation design structures. Process evaluation, for example, generally occurs during or just after a patient education activity. Content evaluation takes place immediately after completion of the patient education session. Outcome evaluation occurs some-time after completion of patient education activities, for example, when a patient has been discharged from the hospital to the setting where he or she is expected to use new knowledge or perform a new skill. Impact evaluation generally is conducted from weeks to years after the educational program because its purpose is to determine which change has occurred within the community or institution as a whole as a result of an educational intervention.

The timing of data collection for program evaluation is less obvious than for other types of evaluation. As discussed earlier, Abruzzese (1992) describes data collection for program evaluation as occurring over a prolonged period. This is because program evaluation is itself the culmination of process, content, outcome, and impact evaluations already conducted.

Where an evaluation is conducted can have a major effect on evaluation results. Those conducting an evaluation must be careful not to make the decision about where to collect data on the basis of convenience for the data collector. For example, an appropriate setting for conducting a content evaluation may be at the bedside or in the ambulatory services area where patients have just completed instruction or training. As another example, outcome evaluation to determine whether discharge teaching in the hospital enabled the patient to provide self-care at home requires that data collection, or observation of the patient's performance, be conducted in the home. What if available resources are insufficient to allow for home visits by the evaluator? To answer this question, keep in mind that the focus of the evaluation is on performance by the patient—not performance by the evaluator. Training a family member, a visiting nurse, or even the patient to observe and record his or her performance at home is preferable to bringing the patient to a place of convenience for the evaluator.

WHO COLLECTS DATA

The nurse who is conducting patient education activities or teaching sessions is the one who most commonly collects evaluation data. That is because the nurse in the role of teacher is already present and interacting with learners. Combining the role of evaluator with that of teacher is an appropriate method for conducting a process evaluation because instruction and evaluation are aspects of the teaching–learning process. Inviting another nurse or a patient representative to observe an individual or group teaching session can provide additional data from the perspective of someone who does not have to divide his or her attention between delivering education and evaluating it. This second, and perhaps less biased, input can strengthen the accuracy and usefulness of the evaluation results.

The individuals who are chosen to carry out data collection become an extension of the evaluation instrument. If the data that are collected are to be reliable, unbiased, and accurate, the data collectors must likewise be unbiased and sufficiently expert at the task. Use of unbiased expert data collectors is especially important for collecting observation and interview data because these data in part depend on the subjective interpretation by the data collector.

Also, data collectors can influence the information that is obtained in other ways. For example, if parents-to-be are asked to complete a survey on their satisfaction with the childbirth classes they attended and the nurse instructor is the one who collects the surveys, certain problems are likely to occur. Might some of these learners be hesitant to provide negative scores on particular items, even though they hold one or more negative opinions about their teaching and learning experiences?

With the emphasis on continuous quality improvement in healthcare organizations, nurses and other professionals are expected to become more knowledgeable about what data are needed and how to use measurement techniques to collect evidence of their daily satisfaction in their work setting (Joint Commission on Accreditation of Healthcare Organizations, 2006). One benefit of this change in practice is that nurses as patient educators have within the organization people with the expertise, the motivation, and the available instruments to carry out data collection activities.

Evaluation Instruments

In the selection, revision, or development of evaluation instruments, nurses must consider some key points. Whenever possible, an evaluation of patient education should be conducted using existing instruments. This is because instrument development not only requires considerable amounts of expertise, time, and money, but also requires testing to be sure the instrument, whether it is in the form of a questionnaire or a type of equipment, is reliable and valid before it is used for measuring data. This testing can take several months to several years to determine the usefulness of the tool (Osborne, Elsworth, & Whitfield, 2007).

Multiple questionnaires, scales, and other types of instruments exist to measure patient and healthcare provider characteristics, such as traits, perceptions, beliefs, attitudes, activity levels, conflicts, communication skills, and relationships. Many measurement tools are already available and have been tested for how well and how consistently they perform in collecting data related to patient education. Redman (2003) describes many of these useful evaluation instruments. Monsivais and Reynolds (2003) describe how to evaluate patient education materials using an instrument to measure effectiveness for patient teaching and learning. Also, a patient education materials assessment tool (PEMAT) is an instrument recently developed to evaluate whether patients are able to understand and take action on information available in print and audiovisual formats that are used so frequently for patient education (Shoemaker, Wolf, & Brach, 2013).

One helpful step in instrument selection for evaluation of patient education is to review materials used to provide that education. Did the educator use a step-by-step checklist to teach the patient how to flush a urinary catheter? That same checklist might be used to observe whether the patient remembers each step during return demonstration. A checklist for the purpose of both teaching and evaluation almost guarantees that the nurse is measuring the performance being evaluated exactly as that performance was operationally defined prior to instruction and evaluation.

An appropriate instrument also must be documented for its reliability and validity and used only with individuals who are as closely matched as possible with the people on whom the instrument was tested. For example, when evaluating the ability of older adult patients to complete activities of daily living, an instrument developed to evaluate the ability of young orthopedic patients to complete routine activities should not be used on this population of older adults. Also, similarities in reading level, visual acuity, and cognitive abilities should exist if the instrument being evaluated is a questionnaire or scale that participants will complete themselves. Also, existing instruments being considered for use in conducting an evaluation must be affordable, must be feasible for use in the location planned for conducting data collection, and should require minimal training on the part of data collectors.

Barriers to Evaluation

If evaluation is so important to healthcare education, why is evaluation often an afterthought or even overlooked entirely? The reasons given for not conducting evaluations are many and varied but rarely, if ever, are impossible to overcome. Barriers to evaluation must first be identified and understood; then, the nurse educator must design and conduct the evaluation in a way that minimizes or eliminates as many identified barriers as possible.

Barriers to conducting an evaluation can be classified into three broad categories:

1. Lack of clarity
2. Lack of ability
3. Fear of punishment or loss of self-esteem

LACK OF CLARITY

If the focus for evaluation is unclear, unstated, or not well defined, then undertaking an evaluation is difficult if the purpose of an evaluation or what will be done with evaluation results is unknown. A clearly stated purpose must explain why the evaluation is being conducted and what decision(s) will be made based on evaluation results. For example, if the purpose for teaching a patient about his medications is so that he can be independent in self-care at home, then the nurse must evaluate both the knowledge and physical ability of the patient to take his medicines correctly prior to discharge. Using teach-back can inform the nurse whether the patient understands what the medications are for, how frequently and in what dosage they should be taken, and what might be side effects that should prompt the patient to immediately contact his primary care provider. Filling the prescriptions in advance before discharge can allow the nurse to observe whether the patient is able to read the labels, open the containers, and take the medications as directed (Visiting Nurse Associations of America, 2012).

LACK OF ABILITY

Inability to conduct patient education evaluations most often results from lack of knowledge, confidence, interest, or resources needed to carry out this process. For instance, a survey tool recently was developed to evaluate the perceptions of pediatric nurses in carrying out their role as patient educators, but the self-designed instrument required outside experts to determine if the survey content was valid (Lahl, Modic, & Siedlecki, 2013). In another study, interviews with nurses revealed that they needed much more professional education on how to teach children and their families, including the use of multi-method evaluation techniques (Kelo, Martikainen, & Eriksson, 2013). Lack of knowledge about evaluation techniques can be resolved by enlisting the assistance of individuals who have expertise and are willing to collaborate or provide consultation services. Remember that patient care is a team activity. If a patient, for example, needs to learn how to use crutches correctly before being discharged, the nurse can appropriately request a physical therapist who is expert in evaluating the patient's ability to safely do so.

In addition, because timely discharge of patients is essential in controlling healthcare costs, time also is among the scarcest of resources available to nurses in preparing patients for discharge. Collaborating with other healthcare professionals is essential in providing the highest possible quality of care. The help of a physical therapist to evaluate the patient's readiness to ambulate on his own is most appropriate but time to do so is among the scarcest resources available to nurses and other healthcare professionals.

FEAR OF PUNISHMENT OR LOSS OF SELF-ESTEEM

Evaluation might be perceived as a judgment of someone's value or personal worth. Evaluation of patient education includes determining how well the patient has learned as well as how well the nurse has taught. Both the learner and the teacher may fear that anything less than a perfect performance will result in criticism, punishment, or evidence that their mistakes will result in their being labeled as incompetent (Lahl et al., 2013). These fears form one of the greatest barriers to conducting an evaluation.

Unfortunately, these fears also may not easily be overcome, especially for individuals who have had negative experiences with teaching and learning in the past. Consider, for example, traditional quality assurance monitoring, where results are used to correct deficiencies often through punitive measures, such as losing the opportunity for promotion or losing respect from colleagues. As another example, many times a patient educator has interpreted learner dissatisfaction with a teaching style as learner dislike for the nurse as a person. In addition, it is unfortunate yet not unusual for parents of pediatric patients to say, "If you don't do it right, the doctor won't let you go home . . . and we will be very disappointed in you." And everyone probably has experienced test anxiety as a learner at some point in life.

The first step in overcoming this barrier is to realize that the potential for its existence may be close to 100%. Individuals whose performance or knowledge is being evaluated are not likely to state outright that evaluation represents a threat to them. Rather, they are far more likely to demonstrate self-protective behaviors or attitudes that can range from failing to participate in a teaching session or attend a class that has a posttest, to providing socially desirable answers on a questionnaire, or to responding with anxiety or anger to evaluation questions. It is even possible that an individual may intentionally choose to fail an evaluation as a method for controlling the uncertainty of success.

The second step in overcoming the barrier of fear or threat in being evaluated is to remember that "the person is more important than the performance or the product" (Narrow, 1979, p. 185). If the purpose of an evaluation is to facilitate better learning, as in process evaluation, then the focus is on the process. For example, in teaching a patient how to perform urinary self-catheterization using the same clean technique as she will use at home, the nurse carefully and thoroughly explains each step of the process, observing the patient's responses (e.g., level of attention or nonverbal reactions) during the explanation. When the patient tries to demonstrate the steps, however, she is unable to begin. Why? One answer may be that the use of an auditory teaching style does not match the patient's visual learning style. Another possibility might be that too many distractions are present in the immediate environment, making concentration on learning all but impossible. And yet another reason may be psychosocial, such as embarrassment about carrying out this procedure. The nurse must attend to these teaching and learning factors for patient education to be successful.

A third step in overcoming fear of being evaluated on the outcomes of patient education is to point out achievements, if they exist, or to continue to encourage effort if success in learning has not been achieved. For example, the nurse should praise the efforts of the learner honestly, focusing on the task at hand.

Also, communication of information about why an evaluation is being done is very important to those who are the subjects of an evaluation as much as for those who will conduct the evaluation. If learners or patient educators know and understand the focus of an evaluation, they may be less fearful than if such information is left to their imaginations.

Finally, failure to provide reassurance to patients that their privacy will be protected and their health information will be held in confidence may contribute to their unwillingness to be evaluated. For example, any evaluative data about an individual that can be identified with that specific person should be collected only with the individual's informed consent. The ethical and legal importance of informed consent as a protection of human rights must be a central concern and responsibility of anyone involved in collecting data for evaluation purposes.

Conducting the Evaluation

How smoothly an evaluation is carried out depends primarily on how thoroughly that evaluation was planned and how carefully the instruments for data collection were selected or developed. However, these two factors alone do not always guarantee success. To minimize the effects of unexpected events that occur when carrying out an evaluation, the following three methods are likely to add to successful achievement of the process:

1. Do a pilot test first, especially of the instrument(s) selected.
2. Include extra time to complete all of the evaluation steps.
3. Keep a sense of humor throughout the experience.

A pilot test or trial run of the evaluation allows the nurse to try out the data collection methods, instruments, and plan for data analysis with a few individuals who are the same as or very similar to those who will be included in the actual evaluation. If one or more newly developed instruments will be used to collect data, they must be tested first to be sure they are reliable, valid, and relatively reasonable to use. Also, if a full evaluation will be expensive or time consuming to conduct or is one on which major decisions will be based, a pilot test should be carried out prior to implementation. Process evaluation generally is not pilot tested unless a new instrument will be used for data collection, but pilot testing should be considered prior to conducting outcome, impact, or program evaluations.

Ream, Richardson, and Evison (2005) describe a pilot test conducted to evaluate the feasibility of a multidisciplinary education and support group program for patients with cancer treatment–related fatigue. Results provided important information about how to involve team members from different disciplines to best meet patients' needs from a patient-centered perspective. Because only six patients were included in the pilot test, findings were not intended to show a significant effect of the education; rather, they were intended to indicate whether a more expanded program might be beneficial.

Including extra time while conducting an evaluation means leaving room for unexpected delays. Almost always, more time is needed than anticipated for evaluation planning, data collection, analysis of evaluation results, and reporting the results that will be meaningful and useful by the primary audience.

Because delays not only likely will occur but also are likely to crop up at inconvenient times during evaluation, keeping a sense of humor is very important. An evaluator with a sense of humor is more likely to maintain a realistic perspective on the evaluation process as well as when reporting results that include negative findings.

Analyzing and Interpreting Data Collected

The purposes for conducting data analysis are twofold: (1) to organize data so that they can provide meaningful information and (2) to provide answers to evaluation questions. The terms *data* and *information* are not the same. Data, as a mass of numbers or a mass of comments, does not become information until it has been organized into understandable tables, graphs, or categories relevant to the purpose for conducting the evaluation.

Basic decisions about how data will be analyzed are dictated by the nature of the data and by the questions used to focus the evaluation. As described earlier, data can be either quantitative or qualitative. Qualitative data, such as verbal comments obtained during interviews and written comments obtained from open-ended questionnaires, are summarized, or themed, into categories of similar comments. Each category or theme is qualitatively described by directly quoting one or more comments that are typical of that category.

The first step in analyzing quantitative data consists of organizing and summarizing the data using statistics, such as frequencies and percentages that describe the sample or population. A description of learners in a sample and from a larger population, for example, might include such information as presented **Table 14–2.**

Table 14–2 Participants in a Breast-Feeding Teaching Session Compared to All Women Eligible for the Teaching Session During the Same Time Frame

Demographic Characteristics	Teaching Session Participants (n=50)	All Eligible Women (n=98)
	Group Averages	Group Averages
Age	27.5 years	25.5 years
Length of time employed	3.5 years	7.5 years
Years of post-high school education	2.0 years	2.0 years

The next step in analyzing quantitative data is to select the statistical procedures appropriate for the type of data collected to answer the questions asked during the planning phase of evaluation. Nurses are encouraged to enlist the assistance of someone with experience to make sense of the data collected.

Reporting Evaluation Results

Results of an evaluation must be reported if the evaluation is to be of any use. Such a statement seems obvious, but many times an evaluation is carried out, yet its results are never made public. Many times people participate in an evaluation but never receive feedback or see the final report. How many times have nurses conducted an evaluation without sharing their findings? Almost all health professionals, if they are honest, would have to answer that they have been guilty of this on more than one occasion.

Reasons for not reporting evaluation results are many and varied. The following are four major reasons why evaluation data never make the trip from the spreadsheet to the customer:

1. Ignorance of who should receive the results
2. Belief that the results are not important or will not be used
3. Lack of ability to translate findings into language useful in producing a final report
4. Fear that results will be misused

Listed below are a few guidelines that can significantly increase the likelihood that results of the evaluation will be reported to the appropriate individuals or groups, in a timely manner, and in usable form:

- Be audience focused.
- Stick to the evaluation purpose.
- Use data as intended.

Be Audience Focused

The purpose for conducting an evaluation is to provide information for decision making by the primary audience. The report of evaluation results must, therefore, be consistent with that purpose. One rule of thumb: Always begin an evaluation report with a summary of the evaluation process and findings that is no longer than one page. No matter who the audience members are, their time is important to them, and they want something quick to read.

A second rule of thumb is to present evaluation results in a format and language that the audience can understand and use. This statement means that in the body of the report, important information should be written using nontechnical terms. For example, graphs and charts generally are easier to understand than are tables of numbers. If a secondary audience of clinical experts will also receive the report of evaluation results, it should include an appendix containing the more detailed or clinically specific information.

A third rule of thumb is that the evaluator should make every effort to present results in person as well as in writing. A direct presentation, which should include specific recommendations or suggestions for how evaluation results might be used, provides an opportunity for the evaluator to answer questions and to assess whether the report meets the needs of the audience. Giving specific recommendations may increase the likelihood that the results of evaluation actually will be used.

Stick to the Evaluation Purpose

Evaluators should keep the main body of an evaluation report focused on information that fulfills the purpose for conducting the evaluation. The main aspects of how the evaluation was conducted and answers to the questions asked also should be provided.

Use Data as Intended

Evaluators should maintain consistency with actual data when reporting and interpreting findings. A question not asked cannot be answered, and data not collected cannot be interpreted. For instance, if evaluators did not measure or observe a family member give the patient an injection, they should not draw conclusions about the adequacy of the family member's skill in performing that activity. Similarly, if the only measures of patient performance were those conducted in the hospital, the evaluators must not interpret successful inpatient performance as successful performance by the patient at home or at work. These examples might seem obvious, but conceptual leaps from the data collected to the conclusions drawn from those data are an all-too-common occurrence.

A discussion of any limitations of the evaluation is an important part of the evaluation report. For example, if several patients were unable to complete a questionnaire because they could not understand it or because they were too fatigued, the report should say so. Knowing that evaluation results do not include data from patients below a certain educational level or physical status can help the audience realize that they cannot make decisions about those patients based on the evaluation. Discussion of limitations also provides useful information for what not to do the next time a similar evaluation is conducted.

Summary

Conducting evaluations of patient education involves gathering, summarizing, interpreting, and using data to determine the extent to which an educational activity is efficient, effective, and useful for those who participate in that activity as learners or teachers. Five types of evaluation were discussed in this chapter: (1) process, (2) content, (3) outcome, (4) impact, and (5) program evaluations. Each of these types focuses on a specific purpose, scope, and questions to be asked of an educational activity or program to meet the needs of those who can benefit from its results. Each type of evaluation also requires some level of available resources for the evaluation to be conducted.

The number and variety of evaluation models, designs, methods, and instruments are growing in importance as evaluation becomes widely accepted and expected in today's healthcare environment. A number of guidelines, rules of thumb, suggestions, and examples were included in this chapter to help nurses as patient educators go about selecting the most appropriate model, design, methods, and instruments for a particular type of evaluation.

Since the introduction of the concept of EBP, the importance of evaluation to gather internal evidence has gained momentum. That momentum continues to grow as the public demand for a balance between healthcare costs and healthcare quality increases. Perhaps the most important point to remember is this: Each aspect of the evaluation process is important, but all of these considerations are meaningless if the results of evaluation are not used to guide future action in planning, carrying out, and improving patient education interventions.

Review Questions

1. How is the term *evaluation* defined?
2. How does the process of evaluation differ from the process of assessment?
3. How is evidence-based practice (EBP) related to evaluation?
4. How does internal evidence differ from external evidence?
5. What is the first and most important step in planning any evaluation?
6. What are the five basic components included in determining the focus of an evaluation?
7. How does formative evaluation differ from summative evaluation, and what is another name for each of these two types of evaluation?
8. What are the five basic types (levels) of evaluation, in order from simple to complex, as identified in Abruzzese's RSA evaluation model?
9. What is the purpose of each type (level) of evaluation as described by Abruzzese in her RSA evaluation model?
10. Which data collection methods can be used in conducting an evaluation of patient education?
11. What are the three major barriers to conducting an evaluation?
12. What are three guidelines to follow in reporting the results of an evaluation?

Case Study

Sharon has been employed as a registered nurse for the past 6 years in an adult on-cology unit of a large medical center. Having recently completed her bachelor's degree in nursing, she is eager to put her education into practice to benefit the patients she cares for. Sharon meets with her nurse manager to learn about the priority issues on which she should focus. She learns that the primary concern on the unit is the need to better prepare cancer patients to cope with their physical as well as their psychosocial challenges after they are discharged to home. Her manager comments, "Some of our patients either aren't being taught what they need to know, they don't believe what they're hearing, or they don't understand what they're hearing. As a result, I'm being told by ambulatory service nurses that our discharged patients aren't taking their medications properly, aren't following suggested changes in diet or exercise, or aren't taking advantage of resources to help them adjust to changes in their appearance or lifestyle."

Sharon next meets with Eric, a certified nurse educator at the hospital. He reminds her that a teaching plan must be in place for all patients and at least one other family member prior to discharge. Nurses must be sure that the patient and his or her personal caregiver(s) understand how to manage self-care at home.

1. Which type(s) of evaluation would be most relevant to the nurse manager's concerns?
2. Putting yourself into Sharon's place, describe in detail how you would conduct an evaluation of teaching and learning with the patients and family members.
3. If evaluation of patient education is so crucial to the delivery of quality care, what are some of the reasons why it is often an afterthought or is even over-looked by staff nurses?

References

Abruzzese, R. S. (1992). Evaluation in nursing staff development. In R. S. Abruzzese (Ed.), *Nursing staff development: Strategies for success* (pp. 235–248). St. Louis, MO: Mosby–Year Book.

Adams, R. J. (2010). Improving health outcomes with better patient understanding and education. *Dovepress, 2010*(3), 61–72. Retrieved from http://www.ncbi.nlm.nih.gov/pubmed/22312219

Bates, O. L., O'Connor, N., Dunn, D., & Hasenau, S. M. (2014). Applying STAAR interventions in incremental bundles: Improving post-CABG surgical patient care. *Worldviews on Evidence-Based Nursing, 11*(2), 89–97.

Bradshaw, M. J. (2014). The clinical pathway: A tool to evaluate clinical learning. In M. J. Bradshaw & A. J. Lowenstein (Eds.), *Innovative teaching strategies in nursing and related health professions* (6th ed., pp. 507–516). Burlington, MA: Jones & Bartlett Learning.

Brownson, R. C., & Jones, E. (2009). Bridging the gap: Translating research into policy and practice. *Preventive Medicine, 49*, 313–315.

Chan, C. W. H., Richardson, A., & Richardson, J. (2012). Evaluating a complex intervention: A process evaluation of a psycho-education program for lung cancer patients receiving palliative radiotherapy. *Contemporary Nurse, 40*(2), 234–244.

Dillon, K. A., Barga, K. N., & Goodin, H. J. (2012). Use of the logic model framework to develop and implement a preceptor recognition program. *Journal for Nurses in Staff Development, 28*(1), 36–40.

Euromed Info. (n.d.). *Evaluating teaching and learning.* Retrieved from http://www.euromedinfo.eu/evaluating-teaching-and-learning.html/

Flemming, K. (2007). Synthesis of qualitative research and evidence-based nursing. *British Journal of Nursing, 16*(10), 616–620.

Frye, A. W., & Hemmer, P. A. (2012). Program evaluation models and related theories: AMEE Guide No. 67. *Medical Teacher, 34*, e288–e299.

Girard, N. J. (2008). Practice-based evidence. *AORN Journal, 87*(1), 15–16.

Goethals, S., Dierckx de Casterlé, B., & Gastmans, C. (2011). Nurses' decision-making in cases of physical restraint: A synthesis of qualitative evidence. *Journal of Advanced Nursing, 68*(6), 1198–1210.

Green, L. W. (2008). Making research relevant: If it is an evidence-based practice, where's the practice-based evidence? *Family Practice, 20*, i20–i24.

Habel, M. (2005). How to be an effective teacher. Getting your message across: Patient Teaching, Part 4. In *Patient Education Update* (Chapter 2, pp. 1–5). Retrieved from http://www.patienteducationupdate.com/2006-09-01/article3.asp

Haggard, A. (1989). Evaluating patient education. In A. Haggard (Ed.), *Handbook of patient education* (pp. 159–186). Rockville, MD: Aspen.

Haggard, L. M., & Burnett, S. J. (2006). Measuring the impact of a web-based data query system: The logic model as a tool in the evaluation process. *Journal of Public Health Management & Practice, 12*(2), 189–195.

Horn, S. D., Gassaway, J., Pentz, L., & James, R. (2010). Practice-based evidence for clinical practice improvement: An alternative study design for evidence-based medicine. *Studies in Health Technology and Informatics, 151*, 446–460.

Institute for Healthcare Improvement. (2012). *Self-management support for people with chronic conditions.* Retrieved from http:///www.ihi.org/knowledge/pages/changes/selfmanagement.aspx

Joint Commission on Accreditation of Healthcare Organizations. (2006). *Accreditation manual for hospitals.* Oakbrook Terrace, IL: Author.

Jurasek, L., Ray, L., & Quigley, D. (2010). Development and implementation of an adolescent epilepsy transition clinic. *Journal of Neuroscience Nursing, 42*(4), 181–189.

Kelo, M., Martikainen, M., & Eriksson, E. (2013). Patient education of children and their families: Nurses' experiences. *Pediatric Nursing, 39*(2), 71–79.

Kobb, R. F., Lane, R. J., & Stallings, D. (2008). E-learning and telehealth: Measuring your success. *Telemedicine Journal & E-Health, 14*(6), 576–579.

Lahl, M., Modic, M. B., & Siedlecki, S. (2013, July/August). Perceived knowledge and self-confidence of pediatric nurses as patient educators. *Clinical Nurse Specialist,* 188–193. doi:10.1097/NUR.0b013e3182955703

London, F. (2009). *No time to teach: The essence of patient and family education for healthcare providers* (2nd ed.). Atlanta, GA: Pritchett & Hull Associates, Inc.

Lorig, K., & Laurent, D. (2007, April). *Primer for evaluating outcomes: Chronic disease self-management program.* Stanford Patient Education Research Center, Stanford University, 1–7. Retrieved from http://patienteducation.stanford.edu

Melnyk, B. M., & Fineout-Overholt, E. (2011). *Evidence-based practice in nursing and healthcare: A guide to best practice* (2nd ed.). Philadelphia, PA: Lippincott Williams & Wilkins.

Milne, D. (2007). Evaluation of staff development: The essential "SCOPPE." *Journal of Mental Health, 16*(3), 389–400.

Monsivais, D., & Reynolds, A. (2003). Developing and evaluating patient education materials. *The Journal of Continuing Education in Nursing, 34*(4), 172–176.

Narrow, B. (1979). *Patient teaching in nursing practice: A patient and family-centered approach.* New York, NY: Wiley.

Noar, S. M. (2012). An audience–channel–message–evaluation (ACME) framework for health communication campaigns. *Health Promotion Practice, 13*(4), 481–488.

Ogrinc, G., & Batalden, P. (2009). Realist evaluation as a framework for the assessment of teaching about the improvement of care. *Journal of Nursing Education, 48*(12), 661–667.

Osborne, R. H., Elsworth, G. R., & Whitfield, K. (2007). The Health Education Impact Questionnaire (heiQ): An outcomes and evaluation measure for patient education and self-management interventions for people with chronic conditions. *Patient Education and Counseling, 66,* 192–201.

Padian, N. S., McCoy, S. I., Manian, S., Wilson, D., Schwartlander, B., & Bertozzi, S. M. (2011). Evaluation of large-scale combination HIV prevention programs: Essential issues. *Journal of Acquired Immune Deficiency Syndromes, 58*(2), e23–e28.

Rankin, S. H., & Stallings, K. D. (2005). *Patient education in health and illness* (5th ed.). Philadelphia, PA: Lippincott Williams & Wilkins.

Ream, E., Richardson, A., & Evison, M. (2005). A feasibility study to evaluate a group intervention for people with cancer experiencing fatigue following treatment. *Clinical Effectiveness in Nursing, 9,* 178–187.

Redman, B. K. (2003). *Measurement tools in patient education* (2nd ed.). New York, NY: Springer.

Rouse, D. (2011). Employing Kirkpatrick's evaluation framework to determine the effectiveness of health information management courses and programs. *Perspectives in Health Information Management, 8,* 1c–5c.

Ruzicki, D. A. (1987). Evaluating patient education: A vital part of the process. In C. E. Smith (Ed.), *Patient education: Nurses in partnership with other health professionals* (pp. 233–248). Orlando, FL: Grune & Stratton.

Schaefer, J., Miller, D., Goldstein, M. G., & Simmons, L. (2009). *Partnering in self-management support: A toolkit for clinicians.* Robert Wood Johnson Foundation, 1–26, Cambridge, MA: Institute for Healthcare Improvement. Retrieved from http://www.ihi.org

Shoemaker, S. J., Wolf, M. S., & Brach, C. (2013). *The patient education materials assessment tool (PEMAT) and user's guide.* Agency for Healthcare Research and Quality. Rockville, MD. Retrieved from http://www.ahrq.gov/professionals/prevention-chronic-care/improve/self-mgmt/pemat/index.html/

Straus, S. E., Richardson, W. S., Glasziou, P., & Haynes, R. B. (2005). *Evidence-based medicine: How to practice and teach EBM* (3rd ed.). New York, NY: Elsevier.

Stevens, S. (2015). Preventing 30-day readmissions. *Nursing Clinics of North America, 50*(1), 123–137.

Taylor, C. A., Shaw, R. L., Dale, J., & French, D. P. (2011). Enhancing delivery of health behavior change interventions in primary care: A meta-synthesis of views and experiences of primary care nurses. *Patient Education and Counseling, 85,* 315–322.

Visiting Nurse Associations of America. (2012, September). *Patient education—Evaluation of learning.* Section: 18.02, 559. Retrieved from http://vnaa.org

Walker, D. K. (2012). Skin Protection for (SPF) Kids program. *Journal of Pediatric Nursing, 27,* 233–242.

Glossary

abstract conceptualization A term used by Kolb to describe a dimension of perceiving information; known as the *thinking mode.*

accommodator One of the four learning style types according to Kolb's theory, combining the learning modes of concrete experience and active experimentation.

acculturation The willingness of an individual to adapt to the customs, values, beliefs, and behaviors of another culture.

active experimentation A term used by Kolb to describe a dimension of processing information; known as the *doing mode.*

adaptive computing The professional services and the technology (both hardware and software) that make computing technology accessible for persons with disabilities.

adherence Commitment or attachment to a prescribed, predetermined regimen.

affective domain One of three domains in the taxonomy of behavioral objectives; deals with attitudes, values, and beliefs.

ageism Prejudice against the older adult that perpetuates the negative stereotyping of aging as a period of decline.

aids The resources or vehicles used to help communicate information, which include both print and nonprint (audiovisual) media, to enhance teaching and learning by stimulating the various senses such as vision and hearing. These are intended to supplement, not replace, teaching methods. Synonymous terms are *instructional materials/tools.*

analogue A type of model that uses analogy to explain something by comparing it to something else. The model performs like the real object, although its actual appearance may differ. A dialysis machine and the extracorporeal circulation pump to explain how the kidneys and the heart and lung work, respectively, are examples.

andragogy The art and science of helping adults learn; a term coined by Malcolm Knowles to describe his theory of adult learning.

anomic aphasia Individuals with this disorder understand what is being said to them and are able to speak in full sentences, but they have difficulty finding the right noun or verb to convey their thoughts. They speak in a roundabout way to fill in the gaps as they struggle to recall the right word or name.

Asperger syndrome A developmental disability that falls at the high end of the autism spectrum and is caused by a brain dysfunction that is typically genetic in origin, which is diagnosed in 2 out of 10,000 children in the United States.

assess To gather, summarize, and interpret pertinent data about the learner to make a decision or plan.

assessment The process of systematically collecting data to determine the relative magnitude, importance, or value of needs, problems, and strengths of the learner to decide a direction for action.

assessment phase The first part of the educational cycle, which provides the foundation for the rest of the educational process.

assimilation The willingness of a person immigrating to a new culture to gradually adopt and incorporate the characteristics of the prevailing culture.

assimilator One of the four learning style types, according to Kolb's theory, combining the learning modes of abstract conceptualization and reflective observation.

asynchronous Of or relating to a message that can be sent via the computer at the convenience of the sender, with the message then being read when the receiver is online and ready to read it; messages that can be sent and responded to any time, day or night.

attention deficit/hyperactivity disorder (ADHD) A condition of children with prominent cognitive difficulties as demonstrated by inattention and impulsivity that are signs of developmentally inappropriate behavior.

audio resources Instructional tools that stimulate the learners' sense of hearing as a mechanism for teaching. Audiotapes and recorders are examples.

audiovisual materials (tools) Nonprint instructional media that can influence all three domains of learning and stimulate the senses of hearing and/or

sight to help convey the message to the learner. This category includes five major types: projected, audio, video, telecommunications, and computer formats.

auditory processing disorder A broad term used to describe a condition that results in the inability of the central nervous system to efficiently process or interpret sound impulses.

augmentative and alternative communication Devices, such as computers, that allow people who are unable to speak or whose speech is difficult to understand to be able to communicate with others. These devices have added a whole new dimension and quality to their lives.

augmented feedback An opinion or conveyance of a message through oral or body language by the teacher to the learner about how well he or she performed a psychomotor skill; often referred to as extrinsic feedback.

autonomy The right to self-determination.

barriers to teaching Those factors that impede the nurse's ability to deliver educational services.

behavioral (learning) objectives Intended outcomes of the education process that are action oriented rather than content oriented and learner centered rather than teacher centered.

behaviorist learning One of the five major learning theories. According to theorists, the focus for learning is mainly on what is directly observable, and learning is viewed as the product of the stimulus conditions (S) and the responses (R) that follow. It is sometimes termed the *S–R model of learning.*

beneficence The principle of doing good.

blended learning A more recently used term in education that combines electronic instruction (e-learning) technology with the more traditional teaching methods, such as lecture or demonstration.

blogs One of the newer forms of online communication, also known as Web logs or Web diaries; an increasingly popular mechanism for individuals to share information and/or experiences about a given topic that includes images, media objects, and links allowing for public responses.

bodily-kinesthetic intelligence A term used by Gardner to describe children who learn by processing knowledge through bodily sensations.

causal thinking The ability of school-aged children to understand cause and effect through logic, concrete thinking, and inductive and deductive reasoning.

causality That which causes something to happen.

characteristics of the learner One of the three major variables that refers to the individual's perceptual abilities, reading ability, self-direction, and learning style, which must be considered when making appropriate choices of instructional materials.

characteristics of the medium One of the three major variables that refers to the form through which information will be communicated, which must be considered when making appropriate choices of instructional materials.

characteristics of the task One of the three major variables defined by the behavioral objectives in the cognitive, affective, and psychomotor domains of learning, which must be considered when making appropriate choices of instructional materials.

chronic illness A disease or disability that is permanent and can never be completely cured. It constitutes the number one medical malady of people in the United States and affects the physical, psychosocial, economic, and spiritual aspects of an individual's life.

cloze test A standardized test to measure comprehension of written materials (particularly recommended for health education literature) based on systematically deleting every fifth word from a portion of a text and having the reader fill in the blanks.

code of ethics Nine provisions for professional values and moral obligations in relation to the nurse–patient relationship, developed and adopted by the American Nurses Association in 1950. These provisions have been revised and updated several times, most recently in 2015.

cognitive ability The extent to which information can be processed. It is indicative of the level at which the learner is capable of learning; of major importance when designing instruction.

cognitive development The process of acquiring more complex and adaptive ways of thinking as an individual grows from infancy to adulthood according to Piaget's four stages of cognitive maturation: sensorimotor, preoperational, concrete operations, and formal operations.

cognitive development perspective Focuses on the qualitative changes in perceiving, thinking, and reasoning as individuals grow and mature based on how external events are conceptualized, organized, and represented within each person's mental framework or schema.

cognitive domain One of three domains in the taxonomy of behavioral objectives; deals with aspects of behavior focusing on the way in which someone thinks in acquiring facts, concepts, principles, etc.

cognitive learning One of the five major learning theories. Theoretically, in order to learn, individuals change as a result of the way they perceive, process, interpret, and organize information based on what is already known; the reorganization of information leads to new insights and understanding.

commercially prepared materials Predesigned, cost-effective printed educational materials that are widely available on a wide range of topics for purchase by educators as supplements to teaching–learning, such as brochures, pamphlets, books, and posters.

compliance Submission or yielding to predetermined goals through regimens prescribed or established by others.

comprehension The degree to which individuals understand what they have read or heard; the ability to grasp the meaning of a verbal or nonverbal message.

computer-assisted instruction (CAI) An individualized method of self-study using technology to deliver an educational activity, which allows learners to proceed at their own pace with immediate and continuous feedback on their progress as they respond to a software program. Primarily used to achieve cognitive domain skills.

computer literacy The ability to use the necessary computer hardware and software to meet the needs for information.

concrete experience A term used by Kolb to describe a dimension of perceiving; known as the *feeling mode*.

concrete operations period As defined by Piaget, this is the third stage in the cognitive development of children when the school-aged child (ages 6 to 12 years) is capable of logical thought processes and the ability to reason but is still incapable of abstract thinking.

confidentiality A binding social contract or covenant; a professional obligation to respect privileged information between the health professional and the client.

conservation The concept that a certain quantity of something will stay at that quantity even if it is manipulated, such as by moving or placing it into containers of various sizes.

consumer informatics A discipline that analyzes learners' needs for information, studies and implements methods of making information accessible to them, and models and integrates their preferences into medical information systems.

content The actual information that is communicated to the learner through various teaching methods and tools.

content evaluation A systematic assessment taking place immediately after the learning experience to determine the degree to which learners have acquired the knowledge or skills taught during a teaching/learning session.

converger One of the four learning style types according to Kolb's theory, combining the learning modes of abstract conceptualization and active experimentation.

corpus callosum The connector between the two hemispheres of the brain.

cosmopolitan orientation Persons with a worldly perspective on life who are receptive to new ideas and opportunities to learn new ways of doing things; a component of experiential readiness.

cost benefit Money well spent. Expenditures for services (e.g., education) ensure return of satisfied clients and stability of the economic base of a healthcare facility.

cost recovery Occurs when revenues generated are equal to or greater than expenditures.

cost savings Monies realized through decreased use of expensive services, shortened length of stay, or fewer complications resulting from preventive services or patient education.

crystallized intelligence The intellectual ability developed over a lifetime; includes such elements as vocabulary, general information, understanding of social interactions, arithmetic reasoning, and capacity to evaluate experiences, which tends to increase over time as a person ages.

cueing Using prompts and reminders to get a learner to perform routine tasks by focusing on an appropriate combination of time and situation.

cultural assessment An organized, systematic appraisal of beliefs, values, and practices of an individual or group to determine client needs as a basis for planning nursing care interventions.

cultural awareness The process of becoming sensitive to the interactions with other cultural groups by examining one's biases and prejudices toward others of another culture or ethnic background.

cultural competence The ability to demonstrate knowledge and understanding of another person's culture and accept and respect cultural differences by adapting interventions to be congruent with that specific culture when delivering care.

cultural diversity A term used to describe the variety of cultures that exist within a society.

cultural encounter The process of exposing oneself in nursing practice to cross-cultural interactions with clients of diverse cultural backgrounds.

cultural knowledge The process of acquiring an educational foundation about various cultural worldviews.

cultural literacy The ability of knowing how to communicate with someone from another culture without having to explain undertones, voice intonations, and message contexts during a conversation.

cultural phenomena Six factors (communication patterns, personal space, social organization, time perspective, environmental control, and biological variations) that need to be taken into account when assessing a client's cultural response to health care.

cultural relativism The belief that the behaviors and practices of individuals or a group of people should be judged only from the context of their cultural system.

cultural skill The process of learning how to conduct an accurate cultural assessment.

culture A complex concept that is an integral part of each person's life and includes knowledge, beliefs, values, morals, customs, traditions, and habits acquired by the members of a society.

defense mechanism A psychodynamic concept that may be employed to protect the self when an individual's ego is threatened; short-term use is a way of coming to grips with reality, but long-term reliance allows individuals to avoid reality and may act as a barrier to learning and the transfer of learning.

delivery system The physical form of instructional materials, including durable equipment used to present these materials, such as film and projectors, audiotapes and tape players, and computer programs and computers.

demonstration A traditional teaching method by which the learner is shown by the nurse how to perform a particular psychomotor skill.

demonstration materials Tools that stimulate the senses by combining sight with touch, smell, and sometimes even taste with the advantage of helping to teach cognitive and psychomotor skill development. Major forms of media in this category include many types of nonprint media, such as models, real equipment, diagrams, charts, posters, displays, photographs, and drawings.

desirable needs Learning necessities of the patient that are not life dependent but related to well-being and can be met by the overall ability of nursing staff to provide quality care.

determinants of learning Consist of learning needs, readiness to learn, and learning styles.

developmental disability A disorder that manifests itself during the developmental period when a child demonstrates below average general intellectual functioning with simultaneous deficits in adaptive behaviors. Sometimes referred to as mental retardation or developmental delay.

developmental stages Milestones marking changes in the physical, cognitive, and psychosocial growth of an individual over time from infancy to old age.

digital divide The gap between those individuals who have access to and use information technology resources and those who do not or cannot access these resources.

direct costs Tangible, predictable financial outlays associated with expenditures for personnel, equipment, etc.

disability Inability to perform some key life functions; often used interchangeably with the term *functional limitation*.

discharge planning An interdisciplinary process, highly dependent on patient educational interventions for effectiveness, by which members of the healthcare team (often led by nurses) plan and coordinate services for the purpose of providing continuity of care to patients and their families between various care settings.

displays Type of demonstration materials, frequently regarded as static, which may be permanently installed or portable. Included in this category are chalkboards, flip charts, and posters.

distance learning A flexible telecommunications method of instruction using video or computer technology to transmit live, online, or taped messages directly between the instructor and the learner, who are separated from one another by time and/or location.

distributed practice Learning information over successive periods of time, which is much more effective for remembering facts and forging memories than massed practice or cramming, which does not allow for long-term recall of information.

diverger One of the four learning style types according to Kolb's theory, combining the learning modes of concrete experience and reflective observation.

domains of learning Cognitive, psychomotor, and affective are the three areas in which change in behavior due to acquisition of knowledge occurs.

Dunn and Dunn learning style Identification of how individuals prefer to function, learn, concentrate, and perform in learning activities based on five basic stimuli.

duty Responsibility; professional expectation.

dysarthria Difficulty with voluntary muscle control of speech due to damage to the central or peripheral nervous system that controls muscles essential to speaking and swallowing. Types of this disorder include flaccid, spastic, ataxic, hypokinetic, and mixed. Persons with degenerative neurologic diseases often suffer with this disorder.

dyscalculia A severe learning disability that impairs those parts of the brain involved in mathematical processing; an inability to understand sets of numbers; inability to comprehend the relationship between a numerical symbol and the objects it represents.

dyslexia A neurodevelopmental learning disorder that is characterized by slow and inaccurate word recognition; affects approximately 10–15% of the U.S. population.

e-health literacy Refers to how well an individual can read, interpret, and comprehend health information from electronic sources and apply the knowledge gained to maintain an optimal level of wellness.

e-mail An Internet-based activity that is a quick, inexpensive, and popular way to communicate asynchronously via the computer.

education An umbrella term used to describe the process, including the components of teaching and instruction, of producing observable or measurable behavioral changes (in knowledge, attitudes, and/or skills) in the learner through planned educational activities.

education process A systematic, sequential, planned course of action that parallels the nursing process and consists of two interdependent operations, teaching and learning, which form a continuous cycle to include assessment of the learner, establishment of a teaching plan, implementation of teaching methods and tools, and evaluation of the learner, teacher, and education program.

emoticons Symbols commonly used to represent emotions, such as :) (smiley face) or ;) (winking), by people who are sending e-mail messages.

emotional readiness A state of psychological willingness to learn, which is dependent on such factors as anxiety level, support system, motivation, risk-taking behavior, frame of mind, and psychosocial developmental stage.

ethical dilemma A type of moral conflict in which two or more principles apply but support conflicting courses of action.

ethical rights and duties A term that refers to the norms or standards of behavior of healthcare professionals.

ethics Guiding principles of human behavior.

ethnic group A population of people, also referred to as a subculture, that has different experiences from those of the dominant culture.

ethnocentrism A concept in which the belief is held that one's own culture is superior and all other cultures are less sophisticated.

evaluation A systematic and continuous process by which the significance of something is judged; the process of collecting and using information to determine what has been accomplished and how well it has been accomplished to guide decision making.

evidence-based practice (EBP)
The conscientious use of current best evidence in making decisions about patient care; a problem-solving approach to clinical practice using the most relevant and best research.

experiential readiness A state of willingness to learn based on such factors as an individual's past experiences with learning, cultural background, previous coping mechanisms, and locus of control.

expressive aphasia An absence or impairment of the ability to communicate through speech or writing due to a dysfunction in the Broca's area of the brain, which is the center of the cortex that controls motor abilities.

external evidence Findings from research studies that can be generalized or transferred beyond a particular study setting or sample of patients to other patients in other healthcare settings.

external locus of control An individual's motivation to learn comes from outside oneself, attributing success or failure of an action to luck, the nature of the task, or the efforts of someone else.

extraversion-introversion (EI) Describes behavior that reflects an orientation to either the outside world of people or to the inner world of concepts and ideas; one of four dichotomous preference dimensions in the Myers-Briggs typology.

extrinsic feedback Also known as augmented or enhanced feedback, this information is provided to the learner from an outside source, such as the teacher or significant other; often used in relation to a psychomotor skill performance.

feedback Can either be intrinsic (inherent or internal), which comes from sensory and perceptual information within the individual, or extrinsic (augmented or enhanced), which is information provided to the learner from an outside source, such as the teacher or significant other.

fixed costs Predictable and controllable expenses that remain stable over time.

Flesch-Kincaid formula An objective, statistical measurement tool for readability of written materials between fifth grade and college level, based on a count of the two basic language elements of average sentence length and average word length (measured as syllables per 100 words) of selected samples.

fluid intelligence The intellectual capacity to perceive relationships, to reason, and to perform abstract thinking, which declines over time as degenerative changes occur with aging.

Fog formula An index appropriate for use in determining readability of materials from fourth grade to college level based on average sentence length and the percentage of multisyllabic words in a 100-word passage.

formal operations period As defined by Piaget, this is the fourth and final stage of cognitive development in which the adolescent (ages 12 to 18 years) and the adult learner are capable of abstract thought, internalization of ideas, complex logical reasoning, and understanding causality.

formative evaluation A systematic and continuous assessment of success of the teaching process made during the implementation of materials, methods, and activities to control, ensure, or improve the quality of performance in delivery of an educational program. Also referred to as *process evaluation*.

Fry formula A measurement tool for testing the readability of materials (especially books, pamphlets, and brochures) at the level of first grade through college by using a graph to plot the number of syllables of words and the number of sentences in three 100-word samples.

functional illiteracy The lack of fundamental education skills needed by adults to read, write, and comprehend information below the fifth-grade level of difficulty to function effectively in today's society; the inability to read well enough to understand and interpret written information for use as intended.

functional magnetic resonance imaging (FMRI) A type of advanced technology that has revolutionized the field of neuroscience by making colorful images of the brain on computer monitors to determine the possible areas of nerve activity involved in the processes of thinking, emotions, and recall.

gaming A nontraditional instructional method requiring the learner to participate in a competitive activity (which may or may not reflect reality) with preset rules.

Gardner's seven types of intelligence A theory that describes the styles of learning in children.

gender bias A preconceived notion about the abilities of women and men that interferes with or prevents individuals from pursuing their own interests and achieving their potentials.

gender gap The behavioral and biological differences between males and females.

gender-related cognitive abilities A comparison between the sexes as to how males and females act, react, and perform in situations affecting every sphere of life as a result of genetic and environmental influences on behavior.

gender-related personality behaviors The observed differences between the sexes in personality and affective behaviors that are thought to be largely determined by culture, but to some extent are a result of interaction between environment and heredity.

gerogogy The art and science of teaching the elderly.

gestalt perspective The oldest of psychological theories, which emphasizes the importance of perception from a cognitive perspective, reflecting the maxim that "the whole is greater than the sum of its parts."

global aphasia The most severe form of aphasia that produces deficits in both the ability to speak and the ability to understand language as well as difficulty with reading and writing as a result of extensive damage to the left side of the brain.

goal A desirable outcome to be achieved by the learner at the end of the teaching–learning process; they are global and more future oriented and long-term in nature than the specific, short-term objectives that lead step by step to the final achievement.

group discussion A commonly employed, traditional method of instruction whereby 3–20 learners (ideally) gather together to exchange information, feelings, and opinions with each other and the teacher; the activity is learner centered and subject centered.

habilitation Includes all the activities and interactions that enable individuals with a disability to develop new abilities to achieve their maximum potential.

hardware Part of the delivery system for many types of media (e.g., computers, projectors, tape players).

health belief model A framework or paradigm used to explain or predict health behavior composed of the interaction among individual perceptions, modifying factors, and likelihood of action.

health education A participatory educational approach, often used interchangeably with the term *patient education* or *client education*, aimed at preventing disease, promoting positive health, and incorporating the physical, mental, and social aspects of learning needs.

health literacy Refers to how well an individual can read, interpret, and comprehend health information for maintaining an optimal level of wellness.

health promotion model A framework that describes the interaction of healthful activity factors, including cognitive perceptual factors, modifying factors, and likelihood of participation in such behaviors.

healthcare-related setting One of three classifications of instructional locations or situations, in which healthcare-type services are offered as a complementary function of a quasihealth agency. Examples: American Heart Association, American Cancer Society, Muscular Dystrophy Association, and Leukemia Society of America.

healthcare setting One of three classifications of instructional locations or situations, in which the delivery of health care is the primary or sole function of an institution, organization, or agency. Examples: hospitals, visiting nurse associations, public health departments, outpatient clinics, physician offices, health maintenance organizations, extended-care facilities, and nurse-managed centers.

healthcare team An interdisciplinary group of professionals and nonprofessionals who work together to provide services to the patient and family members in an attempt to maximize optimal health and well-being of the client to whom their activities are directed.

hearing impairment A general term used to categorize an auditory sensory deficit that includes either complete loss or a reduction in sensitivity to sounds by persons who are fully or partially deaf.

hidden costs Expenses that cannot be predicted or accounted for until after the fact.

hierarchy of needs Theory of human motivation based on integrated wholeness of the individual and levels of satisfaction of basic human requirements organized by potency.

humanistic learning One of the five major learning theories, which views learning as being facilitated by curiosity, needs, a positive self-concept, and open situations where freedom of choice and individuality are promoted and respected.

ideology Thoughts, attitudes, and beliefs that reflect the social needs and desires of an individual or ethnocultural group.

illiteracy The total inability of adults to read, write, or comprehend information.

illiterate The total inability to read, write and comprehend or the inability to read, write, understand, and interpret information at or below the fourth-grade level.

illusionary representations A category of instructional materials that lack realism, such as dimensionality, but offer visual and/or auditory stimuli. Examples are photographs, drawings, and audiotapes, which depend on imagination to fill in the gaps and provide the learner experiences that simulate reality.

imaginary audience A belief or obsession by adolescents that everyone is focusing on them and their activities, which has considerable influence over teenagers' behavior.

impact evaluation The process of assessing outcomes or effects of an educational activity that extend beyond the activity itself to address organizational and/or societal effects.

indirect costs Expenses that may be fixed but are not necessarily directly related to an educational activity (e.g., heating, electricity, housekeeping).

informal teaching Unplanned or spontaneous sessions in which teaching–learning takes place.

information age The present period of time, in which sweeping advances in computer and data technology have transformed the economic, social, and cultural life of society.

information literacy The ability to access, evaluate, organize, and use data from a variety of sources.

information processing perspective Emphasizes the process of memory functioning in the way facts are encountered, organized, stored, and retrieved.

input disability A general category of learning incapacity, such as dyslexia and short- and long-term memory disorders, that refers to problems of receiving and recording information in the brain, which includes visual, auditory, perceptual, and integrative processing.

instruction As one component of the educational process, it is a deliberate, intentional act of communicating information to the learner in response to identified learning needs with the objective of producing learning to achieve desired behavioral outcomes. See *teaching*.

instructional materials/tools The resources or vehicles used to help communicate information, which include both print and nonprint media, to aid teaching-learning by stimulating the various senses such as vision and hearing. These are intended to supplement, not replace, actual teaching. Synonymous terms are *educational aids* and *audiovisual materials*.

instructional setting A situation or area in which health teaching takes place as classified on the basis of what relationship health education has to the primary function of an organization, agency, or institution in which the teaching occurs.

instructional strategy See *teaching strategy*.

intellectual disability A developmental condition that originates before the age of 18 and results in impaired reasoning, learning, problem solving, and adaptive behavior that affects approximately 6.5 million people in the United States; a score of less than 75 on an IQ test is one of the major indicators.

internal evidence Findings that are not generated from research but are appropriate for use when, for example, they are derived from a systematically conducted evaluation.

internal locus of control Individuals are motivated from within to learn, attributing success or failure to their own ability or effort.

Internet A huge global computer network, of which the World Wide Web is a component, established to allow transfer (exchange) of information from one computer to another; it provides a diverse range of services used to deliver information to large numbers of people and to enable people to communicate with one another, such as via e-mail, real-time chat, electronic discussion groups, or Usenet newsgroups.

interpersonal intelligence A term used by Gardner to describe children who learn best in groups.

intrapersonal intelligence A term used by Gardner to describe children who learn well with independent, self-paced instruction.

intrinsic feedback A response that is generated within the self, giving learners a sense of or a feel for how they have performed; often used in relation to a psychomotor skill performance.

judgment-perception (JP) Descriptions of behavior that reflects the way a person comes to a conclusion about something or becomes aware of something; one of four dichotomous preference dimensions in the Myers-Briggs typology.

justice The equal distribution of benefits and burdens.

knowledge deficit A gap in what a learner needs or wants to know; this category of nursing diagnosis can include learning needs in the cognitive, affective, and psychomotor domains.

knowledge readiness A state of willingness to learn dependent on such factors as the learner's present knowledge base, the level of learning capability, and the preferred style of learning.

Kolb's cycle of learning An experiential learning model that includes four modes of learning reflecting the dimensions of perception and processing.

law A clearly stated pronouncement of a binding custom, enforceable by a controlling body.

layout The arrangement of printed and/or graphic information on a flat surface. Effective use of white space, graphics, and wording will depend heavily on this arrangement.

learner characteristics One of the three major variables that refers to the individual's perceptual abilities, reading ability, self-direction, and learning style, which must be considered when making appropriate choices of instructional materials.

learning A conscious or unconscious, relatively permanent change in behavior as a result of a lifelong, dynamic process by which individuals acquire new knowledge, skills, and/or attitudes that can be measured and can occur at any time or in any place due to exposure to environmental stimuli.

learning contract A mutually agreed-on specific plan of action between the patient and the nurse that clearly defines the specific behavioral objectives and predetermined goal to be achieved by the patient as a result of teaching by the nurse.

learning curve Also sometimes referred to as the experience curve, it is a record of an individual's improvement in psychomotor skill development made by measuring his or her ability at different stages during a specified time period, which includes six stages: negligible progress, increasing gains, decreasing gains, plateau, renewed gains, and approach to limit.

learning disability (LD) A generic term that refers to a heterogeneous group of disorders manifested by significant difficulties with learning. Inattention and impulsivity are signs of this group of disorders that indicate developmentally inappropriate behavior.

learning needs Gaps in knowledge that exist between a desired level of performance and the actual level of performance; what the learner is required to know.

learning styles The manner by which (how) individuals perceive and then process information. Some of these characteristics are biological in origin, whereas others are sociologically developed as a result of environmental influences.

learning theory A coherent framework and set of integrated constructs and principles that describe, explain, or predict how people learn.

lecture The oldest, most commonly used, and most traditional instructional method by which the teacher verbally transmits information in a highly structured format directly to a group of learners.

legal rights and duties Rules governing behavior or conduct of healthcare professionals that are enforceable under threat of punishment or penalty, such as a fine, imprisonment, or both.

legally blind Condition in which a person's vision is 20/200 or less in the better eye with correction, or if visual field limits in both eyes are within 20 degrees diameter.

linguistic intelligence A term used by Gardner to describe children who have highly developed auditory skills and think in words.

listening test A standardized test to measure comprehension using a selected passage from instructional material written at approximately the fifth-grade level that is read aloud at a normal rate to determine what a person understands and remembers about what he or she heard.

LISTSERV An automated mailing list software program that copies messages and distributes them to all subscribers.

literacy The ability of adults to read, understand, and interpret information written at the eighth-grade level or above. An umbrella term used to describe socially required and expected reading and writing abilities; the relative ability of persons to use printed and written material commonly encountered in daily life.

literate The ability to write and to read, understand, and interpret information written at the eighth-grade level or above.

locus of control (LOC) The location of the regulation of behaviors as either self-directed or directed by others. Persons with the internal or external type differ particularly in the degree of responsibility taken for their own actions. See also *internal locus of control* and *external locus of control.*

logical-mathematical intelligence A term used by Gardner to describe children who are strong in exploring patterns, categories, and relationships of objects.

low literacy The ability of adults to read, write, and comprehend information between the fifth- and the eighth-grade level of difficulty (also referred to as marginally literate or marginally illiterate).

malpractice Failure to exercise an accepted degree of professional skill or learning by one rendering professional services that result in injury, loss, or damage to the recipient of those services.

mandatory needs Requisites to be learned for survival or situations where the learner's life or safety is threatened.

marginally illiterate A term to describe a person with low literacy skills; also known as *marginally literate*.

marginally literate A term to describe a person with low literacy skills; also known as *marginally illiterate*.

massed practice Learning information all at once, which is much less effective for remembering facts than learning information over successive periods of time; similar to cramming.

media characteristics One of the three major variables that refers to the form through which information will be communicated, which must be considered when making appropriate choices of instructional materials.

media/medium The form in which information or ideas are conveyed to learners.

mental practice Imagining or visualizing a skill without body movement that can have positive effects on the performance of the skill. Motor skill acquisition is enhanced when mental practice is used together with physical practice.

models Three-dimensional instructional tools that allow the learner to immediately apply knowledge and psychomotor skills by observing, examining, manipulating, handling, assembling, and disassembling objects while the teacher provides feedback. Types include replicas, analogues, and symbols, which all enhance instruction by means that range from concrete to abstract.

moral rights and duties Refers to an internal value system that is expressed externally in ethical behaviors of healthcare professionals; often used interchangeably with the terms *morality* and *morals*.

moral values An internal belief system or what one believes to be right.

morals Synonymous with *ethics*; a personal value system.

motivation A psychological force that moves a person to take action in the direction of meeting a need or goal, evidenced by willingness or readiness to act.

motivational axioms Premises on which an understanding of motivation is based, such as a state of optimum anxiety, learner readiness, realistic goal setting, learner satisfaction/success, and uncertainty-reducing or uncertainty-maintaining dialogue.

motivational incentives Factors that influence motivation in the direction of the desired goal.

motivational interviewing (MI) A method of staging readiness to change for the purpose of promoting desired health behaviors, which is an individualized, flexible, client-centered approach that is supportive, empathetic, and goal directed.

motor learning A set of processes associated with practice or experience leading to relatively permanent changes in the capability for movement.

motor performance Acquisition of a motor skill but not necessarily retention of that skill.

multimedia learning The use of two or more types of learning modes (e.g., audio, visual, and/or animation) that can be accessed via a computer to engage the learner in the content being taught.

musical intelligence A term used by Gardner to describe children who are talented in playing musical instruments, singing, dancing, and keeping rhythm and who often learn best with music playing in the background.

Myers-Briggs typology A self-report inventory that uses forced-choice questions and word pairs to measure four dichotomous dimensions of behavior.

needs assessment The process of determining through data collection what a person, group, organization, or community must learn or wants to learn to provide appropriate education programs to meet the requirements of the learners.

negligence Conduct that falls below professional legal standards and puts a person at risk for harm. Doing or nondoing of an act, pursuant to a duty, that a reasonable person in the same circumstances would or would not do; the acting or the nonacting is the proximate cause of injury to another person or property.

nonadherence Occurs when the patient intentionally or unintentionally does not follow treatment recommendations that are mutually agreed upon. Five sets of factors (socioeconomically related, patient related, condition related, therapy related, and healthcare team or system related) contribute to someone not following a prescribed regimen of care.

noncompliance Nonsubmission or resistance of the individual to follow a prescribed, predetermined regimen.

nonhealthcare setting One of three classifications of instructional places or situations in which health care is an incidental or supportive function of an organization, such as a business, industry, or school system.

nonmalfeasance The notion of doing no harm.

nonprint instructional materials Include the full range of audiovisual teaching–learning items, such as audiotapes and CDs, videotapes and DVDs, pictures, models, and displays.

numeracy The ability to read and interpret numbers.

nurse–client negotiations model A model developed for the purpose of cultural assessment and planning for care of culturally diverse people that recognizes the popular, professional, and folk arenas (sectors) as concepts to bridge the gap between the scientific perspectives of the nurse and the cultural perspectives of the patient.

nurse practice acts Legal provisions of each state defining nursing and the standards of nursing practice, usually including patient teaching as a professional responsibility to protect the public from incompetent practitioners.

nursing process A model for nursing practice using the problem-solving approach, which includes the phases of assessment, nursing diagnosis, planning, implementation, and evaluation of patient care that parallel education phases.

OARS A mneumonic to describe specific strategies in motivational interviewing (**o**pen-ended questions, **a**ffirmation of the positives, **r**eflective listening, and **s**ummaries of the interactions) that can be used by the nurse to build motivation in patients for behavior change throughout the entire care process.

objectives (behavioral) Statements defining specific health activities, quantitatively measurable and descriptive of the intended results (rather than the process) of instruction, to be competently achieved by the learner in a finite period of time. When well-stated, they reflect the characteristic components of performance, condition, and criteria.

obstacles to learning Those factors that negatively affect the ability of the learner to attend to and process information.

one-to-one instruction A common, traditional instructional method for exchange of information whereby the teacher delivers individual verbal instruction of learning activities in a format designed specifically to meet the needs of a particular learner.

operant conditioning Focuses on the behavior of an organism as a result of a positive or negative reinforcer (stimulus or event) applied after a response that strengthens the probability that the response will be performed again; nonreinforcement and punishment decrease the likelihood that a response will continue to be performed.

oral literacy How well someone understands information given to him or her verbally. A deficit in this type of literacy has been referred to as iloralcy.

outcome The result of actions that may be intended or unintended; synonymous with *stated goals*.

outcome evaluation Systematic assessment of the degree to which individuals have learned or objectives have been met as a result of education intervention. See *summative evaluation*.

output disability A general category of learning disability that refers to orally responding and performing physical tasks, which include language and motor disorders.

pacing The speed at which information is presented to a learner.

parochial orientation Persons who tend to be more conservative in thinking, are less willing to accept change, and place trust in traditional authority figures; a component of experiential readiness.

patient education A process of assisting consumers of health care to learn how to incorporate health-related behaviors (knowledge, skills, and/or attitudes) into everyday life with the purpose of achieving the goal of optimal health.

pedagogy The art and science of helping children to learn.

PEMs The most common type of teaching tools; these include handouts, leaflets, books, pamphlets, brochures, and instruction sheets, which may be purchased or instructor developed. See *printed education materials*.

people-first language The practice of putting the person first before the disability in writing and speaking so as to describe what a person has, not what a person is (e.g., a person with diabetes, not a diabetic person).

personal fable A belief by adolescents that they are invincible and invulnerable to outside forces.

physical maturation Change in an individual's bodily characteristics as a result of normal body growth and development during the aging process.

physical readiness A state of willingness to learn that is dependent on such factors as measures of physical ability, complexity of task, health status, and gender.

pooled ignorance Lack of knowledge or information about issues or problems prior to a group discussion session, whereby clients cannot adequately learn from one another if they do not possess a basic, accurate understanding of a subject to draw on for purposes of discourse.

positron emission tomography (PET) A type of technology that has revolutionized the field of neuroscience by making images of the brain to detect which areas of the brain are possibly used for thinking, feeling, and remembering.

possible needs Nice to know information that is not essential at a given point in time or in situations in which learning is not directly related to daily activities.

posters A hybrid type of demonstration instructional material that combines print and often visual illustrations (diagrams, graphs, charts, photographs, and/or drawings) to help convey a message.

poverty cycle A process whereby parents who are of low income and educational level produce children of low income and educational attainment, who grow up and repeat the process with their own children; a situation in which generation after generation are born into poverty by many factors, such as poor health care, limited resources, family stress, and low-paying jobs.

practice Repeated performance so as to become proficient in a skill is the most important factor in retaining motor skills. The amount, type, and variability all affect how well a skill is acquired and retained.

practice acts Documents that define a profession, describe that profession's scope of practice, and provide guidelines for state professional boards to grant entry into a profession via licensure and to take disciplinary actions against a professional when necessary.

practice-based evidence Data derived from practice rather than from research, such as the results of a systematically conducted evaluation, patients' responses to care delivered on the basis of clinical expertise, or a systematically conducted quality improvement project.

precausal thinking Unawareness by preschoolers of causation by invisible and mechanical forces.

preoperational period As defined by Piaget, this is the second key milestone in the cognitive development of children when children of the preschool age group (3 to 6 years) are acquiring language skills and gaining experience but thinking is precausal, animistic, egocentric, and intuitive, with only a vague understanding of relationships and multiple classifications of objects.

presentation The form in which the message (content) is put forth, occurring along a continuum from real objects to symbols.

primary characteristics of culture Factors that influence an individual's identification with an ethnic group and that cause the individual to share a group's worldview, such as nationality, race, color, gender, age, and religious affiliation.

printed education materials (PEMs) The most common type of instructional tools; these include handouts, leaflets, books, pamphlets, brochures, and instruction sheets, which may be purchased or teacher developed.

process evaluation A systematic and continuous assessment of success of the teaching process made during the implementation of materials, methods, and activities to control, ensure, or improve the quality of performance in delivery of patient education. See *formative evaluation*.

Prochaska's change model A model developed by Prochaska that informs the phenomenon of health behaviors of the learner, particularly applied to addictive and problem behaviors, and includes the six distinct stages of change: precontemplation, contemplation, preparation, action, maintenance, and termination. See *stages of change model*.

program evaluation A systematic assessment to determine the extent to which all activities for an entire department or program over a specified time period have accomplished the goals originally established.

projection resources Audiovisual instructional formats that depend primarily on the learners' sense of sight as the means through which messages are received. These resources require equipment to display images, usually in a darkened room, and include movies, slides, overhead transparencies, and others.

psychodynamic learning One of the five major learning theories. Largely a theory of motivation stressing emotions rather than cognition and responses; this perspective emphasizes the importance of conscious and unconscious forces derived from earlier childhood experiences and conflicts that guide and change behavior.

psychomotor domain One of three domains in the taxonomy of behavioral objectives, which is concerned with the physical activities of the body, such as coordination, reaction time, and muscular control, related to the acquisition of a skill or task.

psychosocial development The process of adjustment as an individual grows from infancy to adulthood according to Erickson's eight stages of the maturation of humans: trust versus mistrust; autonomy versus shame and doubt; initiative versus guilt; industry versus inferiority; identity versus role confusion; intimacy versus isolation; generativity versus self-absorption and stagnation; and ego integrity versus despair.

Purnell model of transcultural health care A framework for cultural competence to understand and respond to the complex phenomena of culture and ethnicity.

reachable moment The time when a nurse truly connects with the patient by directly meeting the individual on mutual terms; it allows for the mutual exchange of concerns and options without the nurse being inhibited by prejudice or bias and sets the stage for the teachable moment.

readability The level of difficulty at which printed teaching tools are written. A measure of those elements in a given text of printed material that influence with what degree of success a group of readers will be able to understand the information; the ease, or, conversely, the difficulty, with which a person can understand or comprehend the style of writing of a selected printed passage.

readiness to learn The time when the learner is receptive to learning and is willing and able to participate in the learning process; preparedness or willingness to learn.

reading Also known as *word recognition*, it is the process of transforming letters into words and being able to pronounce them correctly.

READS A mneumonic to help the nurse remember the five general principles of motivational interviewing (**r**oll with resistance, **e**xpress empathy, **a**void argumentation, **d**evelop discrepancy. and **s**upport self-efficacy.

realia The most concrete form of stimuli that can be used to deliver information. Example: a person or a model being used to demonstrate a procedure such as breast self-examination.

REALM (rapid estimate of adult literacy in medicine) A reading skills test to measure a patient's ability to read medical and health-related vocabulary.

receptive aphasia An absence or impairment of the ability to comprehend what is read or heard due to a dysfunction in the Wernicke's area of the brain, which controls sensory abilities. Although hearing is unimpaired, the person is unable to understand the significance of the spoken word and is unable to communicate verbally.

reflective observation A term used by Kolb to describe a dimension of processing; known as the *watching mode.*

rehabilitation The relearning of previous skills, which often requires an adjustment to altered functional abilities and altered lifestyle.

religiosity An individual's adherence to beliefs and ritualistic practices associated with religious institutions.

repetition A technique that strengthens learning by aiding in retention of information of new or difficult material through reinforcement of important points.

replica A facsimile constructed to scale that resembles the features or substance of the original object. It may be examined or manipulated by the learner to get an idea of how something works. Example: resuscitation dolls.

respondent conditioning Emphasizes the importance of stimulus conditions and the associations formed in the learning process, whereby, without thought or awareness, learning takes place when a newly conditioned stimulus (CS) becomes associated with a conditioned response (CR); also termed *classical* or *Pavlovian conditioning.*

return demonstration A traditional instructional method by which the learner attempts to perform a psychomotor skill, with cues or prompting as needed from the teacher.

revenue generation Income earned that is over and above costs of the programs offered.

role modeling The use of self as a role model, often overlooked as an instructional method, whereby the learner acquires new behaviors and social roles by identification with the role model.

role play A method of teaching by which learners participate in an unrehearsed dramatization, acting out an assigned part of a character as they think the character would act in reality.

RSA model Named after the developer, Roberta Straessle Abruzzese, this model classifies educational evaluation into 5 levels (process, content, outcome, impact, and total program) from simple to complex and provides a visual of these five basic types of evaluation in relation to one another with respect to purpose, questions asked, scope, and resources available.

SAM (suitability assessment of materials) An evaluation instrument designed to measure the appropriateness of print materials, illustrations, and video- and audiotaped instructions for a given patient population.

scaffolding The incremental approach to sequencing distinct steps of a procedure that provides the learner with a clear and exact image of each stage of skill development.

secondary characteristics of culture Factors that influence an individual's identification with an ethnic group and that cause the individual to share a group's worldview, such as SES (socioeconomic status), physical characteristics (e.g., clothing, length of hair, manners of expression), educational status, occupational status, and place of residence.

selective attention The process of recognizing and choosing appropriate and inappropriate stimuli.

self-composed instructional materials Printed instructional materials created by individual instructors for the purposes of supplementing teaching.

self-efficacy theory A framework that describes the belief that one is capable of accomplishing a specific behavior.

self-instruction A method of instruction used by a teacher to provide or design teaching materials and activities that guide the learner in independently achieving the objectives of learning.

sensing-intuition (SN) Describes how individuals perceive the world, either directly through the five senses or indirectly by way of the unconscious; one of four dichotomous preference dimensions in the Myers-Briggs typology.

sensorimotor period As defined by Piaget, this is the first key milestone in the cognitive development of children in the age group of infancy to toddlerhood when learning is enhanced through movement and manipulation of objects in the environment via visual, auditory, tactile, olfactory, taste, and motor stimulation.

sensory disabilities A category of common physical disabilities or deficits that includes, in particular, hearing and visual impairments.

settings for teaching Places of practice where nurses teach health education; settings are classified into three categories (healthcare setting, healthcare-related setting, and non-healthcare setting) according to the relationship that health education has to the primary purpose of the organization or agency where nurses may be employed.

silent epidemic The literacy problem in the United States; also known as the *silent barrier* or *silent disability*.

simulation A nontraditional method of instruction whereby an artificial or hypothetical experience that engages the learner in an activity reflecting real-life conditions is created but without the risk-taking consequences of an actual situation.

simulation laboratory A type of learning environment that contains realistic equipment in a lifelike setting but that allows the learner to practice manipulating and using this equipment as a prelude to performing a task in a real-life situation. Frequently used to teach the development of psychomotor skills.

skill inoculation The opportunity for repeated practice of a behavioral task to learn that task.

SMOG formula A relatively easy-to-use, popular, valid test of readability based on 100% comprehension of printed material from grade 4 to college level.

social cognition An aspect of cognitive theory that highlights the influence of social factors on perception, thought, motivation, and behaviors.

social learning One of five major learning theories, this theory is seen as a mixture of behaviorist, cognitive, and psychodynamic influences; much of learning is a process that occurs by observation and watching other people's behavior to see what happens to them. Role modeling is a central concept of this theory, with cognitive or psychodynamic aspects of internal processing and motivation sometimes considered in the learning process.

social media Online communication tools, such as blogs, wikis, Twitter, and Facebook.

socioeconomic status (SES) Variation in health, health behavior, or learning abilities among individuals of different social and income levels.

software Computer programs and other instructional materials such as videotapes and overhead transparencies.

spatial intelligence A term used by Gardner to describe children who learn by images and pictures.

spirituality A belief in a higher power or a sacred power that exists in all things.

spontaneous recovery A response, which appears to be extinguished, that reappears at any time (even years later), especially when stimulus conditions are similar to those in the initial learning experience.

stages of change model A model developed by Prochaska that informs the phenomenon of health behaviors of the learner, particularly applied to addictive and problem behaviors, and includes the six distinct stages of change: precontemplation, contemplation, preparation, action, maintenance, and termination.

stages of motor learning A classic model of sequential learning that includes three phases, the cognitive, the associative, and the autonomous stages, which provide a framework for nurses to use as they organize learning strategies when teaching patients to acquire motor skills; similar to the concept of the learning curve for psychomotor skill development.

stereotyping An oversimplified conception, opinion, or belief about some aspect of an individual or group.

subculture An ethnocultural group of people who have experiences different from those of the dominant culture.

subobjectives A specific statement of a short-term behavior that is written to reflect an aspect of the main objective leading to the achievement of the primary objective.

suitability assessment of materials An evaluation instrument designed to measure the appropriateness of print materials, illustrations, and video- and audiotaped instructions for a given patient population. See *SAM*.

summative evaluation Systematic assessment of the degree to which individuals have learned or objectives have been met as a result of education intervention; also referred to as *outcome evaluation*.

support system Resources and significant others, such as family and friends, on whom the patient relies or is dependent for information or assistance in managing activities of daily living and who may serve as a positive or negative influence on teaching efforts.

syllogistic reasoning The ability of school-aged children to consider two premises and draw a logical conclusion from them.

symbol A type of model that conveys a message to the learner through the use of abstract constructs, such as words, pictures, or numbers, that stand for the real thing. Cartoons and printed materials are examples of this form of a message.

symbolic representations Numbers and words, symbols written and spoken to convey ideas or denote objects, which are the most common form of communication and yet are the most abstract types of messages.

systematic desensitization A technique based on respondent conditioning that is used by psychologists to reduce fear or anxiety by unlearning or extinguishing it through teaching relaxation techniques or introducing a fear-producing stimulus at a nonthreatening level.

tailored instruction Personalizing the message so that the content, structure, and image fit an individual patient's learning needs by using such techniques as highlighting in a pamphlet the most important information while verbally reviewing it with the patient, writing the patient's name on the cover of a pamphlet that you are giving to her, or using checklists that help a patient or family member learn specific care tasks in a step-by-step fashion.

tailoring Coordinating a patient's treatment regimens into his or her daily schedules by allowing new tasks to be associated with old behaviors.

task characteristics One of the three major variables defined by the behavioral objectives in the cognitive, affective, and psychomotor domains of learning, which must be considered when making appropriate choices of instructional materials.

taxonomic hierarchy A form of classifying cognitive, affective, and psychomotor domains of behaviors into rank order according to their degree or level of complexity. See *taxonomy*.

taxonomy A form of hierarchical classification of cognitive, affective, and psychomotor domains of behaviors according to their degree or level of complexity.

teach back approach A way of assessing how well and how much patients and/or their family members understood the information given to them; asking patients to explain in their own words what they have been taught to determine if there are any gaps in their interpretation and remembering of information given to them; repeating back to the nurse or other healthcare provider the essential points that have been taught is a way to be sure that the content has been learned; also known as tell back or show me.

teachable moment As defined by Havighurst, that point in time when the learner is most receptive to an instructional situation; it can occur at any hour that a patient, family member, staff member, or nursing student has a question or needs information.

teaching As one component of the educational process, it is a deliberate, intentional act of communicating information to the learner in response to identified learning needs with the objective of producing learning to achieve desired behavioral outcomes.

teaching method A traditional or nontraditional technique or approach used by the teacher to bring the learner into contact with the content to be learned; a way or a process to communicate and share information with the learner.

teaching plan Overall blueprint or outline for instruction clearly defining the relationship between the essential components of behavioral objectives, instructional content, teaching methods, resources, time frame for teaching, and methods of evaluation that fit together in a logical pattern of flow to achieve a predetermined goal.

teaching role An expected and legally mandated standard of practice by the nurse that supports, encourages, and assists the learner to acquire behaviors (knowledge, skills, and attitudes) and put them into meaningful parts and wholes to reach an optimum potential of functioning.

teaching strategy An overall plan of action for instruction that anticipates barriers to teaching, resources needed, and obstacles to learning to achieve specific behavioral objectives.

Technological Devices for the Deaf (TDD) Important resources for patient education when teaching people who are deaf or hearing impaired that include such tools as television decoders for closed caption programs and caption films, which are considered reasonable accommodations to enhance communication.

telecommunications resources Tools for instruction used to help convey information via electrical energy from one place to another such as telephones, televisions, and computers.

theory of planned behavior (TPB) A new learning theory model developed by Ajzen that added a third element, the concept of perceived behavioral control, to his original theory of reasoned action.

theory of reasoned action (TRA) A framework that is concerned with prediction and understanding of human behavior within a social context.

therapeutic alliance model An interpersonal provider–patient model that addresses the continuum of compliance, adherence, and collaboration in healing relationships.

thinking-feeling (TF) An approach used by individuals to arrive at judgments through impersonal, logical, subjective, or empathetic processes; one of four dichotomous preference dimensions in the Myers-Briggs typology.

TOFHLA (test of functional health literacy in adults) A relatively new instrument for measuring patients' literacy levels by using actual hospital materials, such as prescription labels, appointment slips, and informed consent documents, to determine their reading and numeracy skills.

tools The resources or vehicles used to help communicate information, which include both print and nonprint media, to aid teaching and learning by stimulating the various senses such as vision and hearing. These are intended to supplement, not replace, actual teaching. Synonymous terms are *audiovisual materials, aids, and instructional materials.*

total program evaluation Within the framework of the RSA model, the purpose is to determine the extent to which all activities for an entire department or program over a specified period of time meet or exceed the goals originally established.

transcultural nursing A formal area of study and practice comparing and analyzing different cultures and subcultures with respect to cultural care, health practices, and illness beliefs with the goal of using these insights to provide culture-specific and culture-universal care to diverse groups of people.

transfer of learning The effects of learning one skill on the subsequent performance of another related skill.

Usenet A global discussion system made up of a cooperative network of computers that distribute and archive messages posted to topic-specific electronic discussion groups called newsgroups.

variable costs Not predictable, volume-related expenses.

veracity Truth telling; honesty.

vicarious reinforcement A concept from social learning theory that involves determining whether role models are perceived as rewarded or punished for their behavior.

visual impairment A reduction or complete loss of vision due to infection, accident, poisoning, or congenital degeneration of the eye(s).

wiki A relatively new form of online communication. Unlike blogs, wikis are more social in their construction in that multiple users come together to collaboratively write the content of a collection of Web pages that users have the ability to add to, edit, and remove. Wikipedia is one of the best known wikis.

World Wide Web A computer network of information servers around the world that are connected to the Internet; it is a technology-based educational resource that was created as a virtual space for the display of information.

worldview The way individuals or groups of people look at the universe to form values and beliefs about their lives and the world around them.

WRAT (wide range achievement test) technique A word recognition screening test used to assess a person's ability to recognize and pronounce a list of words out of context as a criterion for measuring comprehension of written materials. The level I test is designed for children ages 5 to 12 years; level II is intended to test persons over 12 years of age.

Index

Note: Page numbers followed by *f* and *t* indicate material in figures and tables respectively